Lippincott
Illustrated Reviews:
Pharmacology
Sixth Edition

Lippincott
Illustrated Reviews:
Pharmacology
Sixth Edition

Karen Whalen, Pharm.D., BCPS

Department of Pharmacotherapy and Translational Research

University of Florida

College of Pharmacy

Gainesville, Florida

Collaborating Editors

Richard Finkel, Pharm.D.

Department of Pharmaceutical Sciences

Nova Southeastern University

College of Pharmacy

Fort Lauderdale, Florida

Thomas A. Panavelil, Ph.D., MBA

Department of Pharmacology

Nova Southeastern University

College of Medical Sciences

Fort Lauderdale, Florida

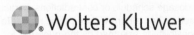

Philadelphia • Baltimore • New York • London
Buenos Aires • Hong Kong • Sydney • Tokyo

Acquisitions Editor: Tari Broderick
Product Development Editor: Stephanie Roulias
Production Project Manager: Marian A. Bellus
Design Coordinator: Holly McLaughlin
Illustration Coordinator: Jennifer Clements
Manufacturing Coordinator: Margie Orzech
Marketing Manager: Joy Fisher-Williams
Prepress Vendor: SPi Global

Sixth edition

Library of Congress Cataloging-in-Publication Data
Pharmacology (Whalen)
  Pharmacology / [edited by] Karen Whalen ; collaborating editors, Richard Finkel, Thomas A. Panavelil. – Sixth edition.
      p. ; cm. – (Lippincott illustrated reviews)
  Includes index.
  Preceded by Pharmacology / Michelle A. Clark ... [et al.]. 5th ed. c2012.
  ISBN 978-1-4511-9177-6
 I. Whalen, Karen, editor. II. Finkel, Richard (Richard S.), editor. III. Panavelil, Thomas A., editor. IV. Title. V. Series: Lippincott illustrated reviews.
  [DNLM: 1. Pharmacology–Examination Questions. 2. Pharmacology–Outlines. QV 18.2]
  RM301.14
  615.1076–dc23
                                                                              2014021450

This work is provided "as is," and the publisher disclaims any and all warranties, express or implied, including any warranties as to accuracy, comprehensiveness, or currency of the content of this work.

This work is no substitute for individual patient assessment based upon healthcare professionals' examination of each patient and consideration of, among other things, age, weight, gender, current or prior medical conditions, medication history, laboratory data and other factors unique to the patient. The publisher does not provide medical advice or guidance and this work is merely a reference tool. Healthcare professionals, and not the publisher, are solely responsible for the use of this work including all medical judgments and for any resulting diagnosis and treatments.

Given continuous, rapid advances in medical science and health information, independent professional verification of medical diagnoses, indications, appropriate pharmaceutical selections and dosages, and treatment options should be made and healthcare professionals should consult a variety of sources. When prescribing medication, healthcare professionals are advised to consult the product information sheet (the manufacturer's package insert) accompanying each drug to verify, among other things, conditions of use, warnings and side effects and identify any changes in dosage schedule or contradictions, particularly if the medication to be administered is new, infrequently used or has a narrow therapeutic range. To the maximum extent permitted under applicable law, no responsibility is assumed by the publisher for any injury and/or damage to persons or property, as a matter of products liability, negligence law or otherwise, or from any reference to or use by any person of this work.

Shawn Anderson, Pharm.D., BCACP
Department of Pharmacy
North Florida/South Georgia VA Medical Center
Gainesville, Florida

Angela K. Birnbaum, Ph.D.
Department of Experimental and Clinical
Pharmacology
University of Minnesota
College of Pharmacy
Minneapolis, Minnesota

Nicholas Carris, Pharm.D., BCPS
Department of Pharmacotherapy and Translational
Research
University of Florida
Colleges of Pharmacy and Medicine
Gainesville, Florida

Lisa Clayville Martin, Pharm.D.
Department of Pharmacotherapy and Translational
Research
University of Florida
College of Pharmacy
Orlando, Florida

Patrick Cogan, Pharm.D.
Department of Pharmacotherapy and Translational
Research
University of Florida
College of Pharmacy
Gainesville, Florida

Jeannine M. Conway, Pharm.D., BCPS
Department of Experimental and Clinical
Pharmacology
University of Minnesota
College of Pharmacy
Minneapolis, Minnesota

Eric Dietrich, Pharm.D., BCPS
Department of Pharmacotherapy and Translational
Research
University of Florida
Colleges of Pharmacy and Medicine
Gainesville, Florida

Eric Egelund, Pharm.D., Ph.D.
Department of Pharmacotherapy and Translational
Research
University of Florida
College of Pharmacy
Gainesville, Florida

Richard Finkel, Pharm.D.
Department of Pharmaceutical Sciences
Nova Southeastern University
College of Pharmacy
Fort Lauderdale, Florida

Timothy P. Gauthier, Pharm.D., BCPS (AQ-ID)
Department of Pharmacy Practice
Nova Southeastern University
College of Pharmacy
Fort Lauderdale, Florida

Andrew Hendrickson, Pharm.D.
Department of Pharmacy
North Florida/South Georgia VA Medical Center
Gainesville, Florida

Jamie Kisgen, Pharm.D., BCPS
Department of Pharmacy
Sarasota Memorial Health Care System
Sarasota, Florida

Kourtney LaPlant, Pharm.D., BCOP
Department of Pharmacy
North Florida/South Georgia VA Medical Center
Gainesville, Florida

Paige Louzon, Pharm.D., BCOP
Department of Pharmacy
North Florida/South Georgia VA Medical Center
Gainesville, Florida

Kyle Melin, Pharm.D., BCPS
Department of Pharmacy Practice
University of Puerto Rico
School of Pharmacy
San Juan, Puerto Rico

Robin Moorman Li, Pharm.D., BCACP
Department of Pharmacotherapy and Translational
Research
University of Florida
College of Pharmacy
Jacksonville, Florida

Carol Motycka, Pharm.D., BCACP
Department of Pharmacotherapy and Translational
Research
University of Florida
College of Pharmacy
Jacksonville, Florida

Kristyn Mulqueen, Pharm.D., BCPS
Department of Pharmacy
North Florida/South Georgia VA Medical Center
Gainesville, Florida

Thomas A. Panavelil, Ph.D., MBA
Department of Pharmacology
Nova Southeastern University
College of Medical Sciences
Fort Lauderdale, Florida

Charles A. Peloquin, Pharm.D.
Department of Pharmacotherapy and
Translational Research
University of Florida
College of Pharmacy
Gainesville, Florida

Joanna Peris, Ph.D.
Department of Pharmacodynamics
University of Florida
College of Pharmacy
Gainesville, Florida

Jason Powell, Pharm.D.
Department of Pharmacotherapy and Translational
Research
University of Florida
College of Pharmacy
Gainesville, Florida

Rajan Radhakrishnan, B.S. Pharm., M.S., Ph.D.
Roseman University of Health Sciences
College of Pharmacy
South Jordan, Utah

Jose A. Rey, Pharm.D., BCPP
Department of Pharmaceutical Sciences
Nova Southeastern University
College of Pharmacy
Fort Lauderdale, Florida

Karen Sando, Pharm.D., BCACP
Department of Pharmacotherapy and Translational
Research
University of Florida
College of Pharmacy
Gainesville, Florida

Elizabeth Sherman, Pharm.D.
Department of Pharmacy Practice
Nova Southeastern University
College of Pharmacy
Fort Lauderdale, Florida

Dawn Sollee, Pharm.D., DABAT
Florida/USVI Poison Information Center
UF Health – Jacksonville
Jacksonville, Florida

Joseph Spillane, Pharm.D., DABAT
Department of Pharmacy
UF Health – Jacksonville
Jacksonville, Florida

Sony Tuteja, Pharm.D., BCPS
Department of Medicine
Perelman School of Medicine at the
University of Pennsylvania
Philadelphia, Pennsylvania

Nathan R. Unger, Pharm.D.
Department of Pharmacy Practice
Nova Southeastern University
College of Pharmacy
Palm Beach Gardens, Florida

Katherine Vogel Anderson, Pharm.D., BCACP
Department of Pharmacotherapy and Translational
Research
University of Florida
Colleges of Pharmacy and Medicine
Gainesville, Florida

Karen Whalen, Pharm.D., BCPS
Department of Pharmacotherapy and Translational
Research
University of Florida
College of Pharmacy
Gainesville, Florida

Thomas B. Whalen, M.D.
Diplomate, American Board of Anesthesiology
Ambulatory Anesthesia Consultants, PLLC
Gainesville, Florida

Venkata Yellepeddi, B.S. Pharm, Ph.D.
Roseman University of Health Sciences
College of Pharmacy
South Jordan, Utah

Reviewer

Ashley Castleberry, Pharm.D., M.A.Ed.
University of Arkansas for Medical Sciences
College of Pharmacy
Little Rock, Arkansas

Illustration and Graphic Design

Michael Cooper
Cooper Graphic
www.cooper247.com

Claire Hess
hess2 Design
Louisville, Kentucky

Contents

Pharmacokinetics

1

Venkata Yellepeddi

I. OVERVIEW

Pharmacokinetics refers to what the body does to a drug, whereas pharmacodynamics (see Chapter 2) describes what the drug does to the body. Four pharmacokinetic properties determine the onset, intensity, and the duration of drug action (Figure 1.1):

- **Absorption:** First, absorption from the site of administration permits entry of the drug (either directly or indirectly) into plasma.
- **Distribution:** Second, the drug may then reversibly leave the bloodstream and distribute into the interstitial and intracellular fluids.
- **Metabolism:** Third, the drug may be biotransformed by metabolism by the liver or other tissues.
- **Elimination:** Finally, the drug and its metabolites are eliminated from the body in urine, bile, or feces.

Using knowledge of pharmacokinetic parameters, clinicians can design optimal drug regimens, including the route of administration, the dose, the frequency, and the duration of treatment.

II. ROUTES OF DRUG ADMINISTRATION

The route of administration is determined by the properties of the drug (for example, water or lipid solubility, ionization) and by the therapeutic objectives (for example, the desirability of a rapid onset, the need for long-term treatment, or restriction of delivery to a local site). Major routes of drug administration include enteral, parenteral, and topical, among others (Figure 1.2).

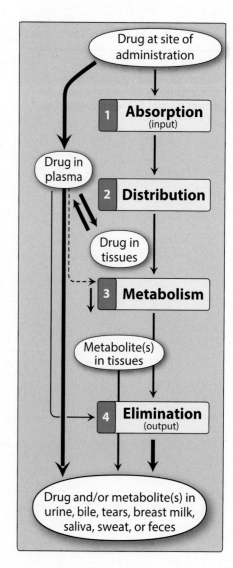

Figure 1.1
Schematic representation of drug absorption, distribution, metabolism, and elimination.

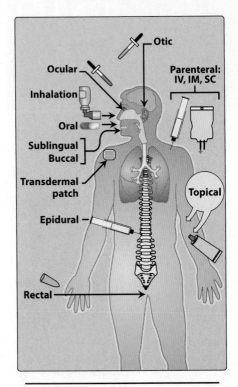

Figure 1.2
Commonly used routes of drug administration. IV = intravenous; IM = intramuscular; SC = subcutaneous.

A. Enteral

Enteral administration (administering a drug by mouth) is the safest and most common, convenient, and economical method of drug administration. The drug may be swallowed, allowing oral delivery, or it may be placed under the tongue (sublingual), or between the gums and cheek (buccal), facilitating direct absorption into the bloodstream.

1. **Oral:** Oral administration provides many advantages. Oral drugs are easily self-administered, and toxicities and/or overdose of oral drugs may be overcome with antidotes, such as activated charcoal. However, the pathways involved in oral drug absorption are the most complicated, and the low gastric pH inactivates some drugs. A wide range of oral preparations is available including enteric-coated and extended-release preparations.

   a. **Enteric-coated preparations:** An enteric coating is a chemical envelope that protects the drug from stomach acid, delivering it instead to the less acidic intestine, where the coating dissolves and releases the drug. Enteric coating is useful for certain drugs (for example, *omeprazole*) that are acid unstable. Drugs that are irritating to the stomach, such as *aspirin*, can be formulated with an enteric coating that only dissolves in the small intestine, thereby protecting the stomach.

   b. **Extended-release preparations:** Extended-release (abbreviated ER or XR) medications have special coatings or ingredients that control the drug release, thereby allowing for slower absorption and a prolonged duration of action. ER formulations can be dosed less frequently and may improve patient compliance. Additionally, ER formulations may maintain concentrations within the therapeutic range over a longer period of time, as opposed to immediate-release dosage forms, which may result in larger peaks and troughs in plasma concentration. ER formulations are advantageous for drugs with short half-lives. For example, the half-life of oral *morphine* is 2 to 4 hours, and it must be administered six times daily to provide continuous pain relief. However, only two doses are needed when extended-release tablets are used. Unfortunately, many ER formulations have been developed solely for a marketing advantage over immediate-release products, rather than a documented clinical advantage.

2. **Sublingual/buccal:** Placement under the tongue allows a drug to diffuse into the capillary network and enter the systemic circulation directly. Sublingual administration has several advantages, including ease of administration, rapid absorption, bypass of the harsh gastrointestinal (GI) environment, and avoidance of first-pass metabolism (see discussion of first-pass metabolism below). The buccal route (between the cheek and gum) is similar to the sublingual route.

B. Parenteral

The parenteral route introduces drugs directly into the systemic circulation. Parenteral administration is used for drugs that are poorly absorbed from the GI tract (for example, *heparin*) or unstable in the GI tract (for example, *insulin*). Parenteral administration is also used if a patient is unable to take oral medications (unconscious patients) and in circumstances that require a rapid onset of action. In addition, parenteral routes have the highest bioavailability and are not subject to first-pass metabolism or the harsh GI environment. Parenteral administration provides the most control over the actual dose of drug delivered to the body. However, these routes of administration are irreversible and may cause pain, fear, local tissue damage, and infections. The three major parenteral routes are intravascular (intravenous or intra-arterial), intramuscular, and subcutaneous (Figure 1.3).

1. **Intravenous (IV):** IV injection is the most common parenteral route. It is useful for drugs that are not absorbed orally, such as the neuromuscular blocker *rocuronium*. IV delivery permits a rapid effect and a maximum degree of control over the amount of drug delivered. When injected as a bolus, the full amount of drug is delivered to the systemic circulation almost immediately. If administered as an IV infusion, the drug is infused over a longer period of time, resulting in lower peak plasma concentrations and an increased duration of circulating drug levels. IV administration is advantageous for drugs that cause irritation when administered via other routes, because the substance is rapidly diluted by the blood. Unlike drugs given orally, those that are injected cannot be recalled by strategies such as binding to activated charcoal. IV injection may inadvertently introduce infections through contamination at the site of injection. It may also precipitate blood constituents, induce hemolysis, or cause other adverse reactions if the medication is delivered too rapidly and high concentrations are reached too quickly. Therefore, patients must be carefully monitored for drug reactions, and the rate of infusion must be carefully controlled.

2. **Intramuscular (IM):** Drugs administered IM can be in aqueous solutions, which are absorbed rapidly, or in specialized depot preparations, which are absorbed slowly. Depot preparations often consist of a suspension of the drug in a nonaqueous vehicle such as polyethylene glycol. As the vehicle diffuses out of the muscle, the drug precipitates at the site of injection. The drug then dissolves slowly, providing a sustained dose over an extended period of time. Examples of sustained-release drugs are *haloperidol* (see Chapter 11) and depot *medroxyprogesterone* (see Chapter 26).

3. **Subcutaneous (SC):** Like IM injection, SC injection provides absorption via simple diffusion and is slower than the IV route. SC injection minimizes the risks of hemolysis or thrombosis associated with IV injection and may provide constant, slow, and sustained effects. This route should not be used with drugs that cause tissue irritation, because severe pain and necrosis may occur. Drugs commonly administered via the subcutaneous route include *insulin* and *heparin*.

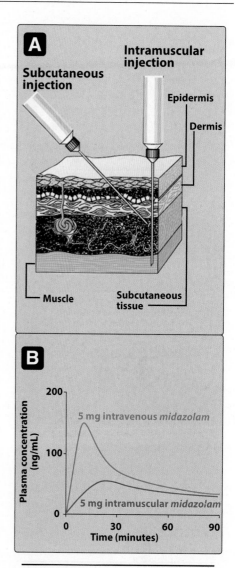

Figure 1.3
A. Schematic representation of subcutaneous and intramuscular injection. **B.** Plasma concentrations of *midazolam* after intravenous and intramuscular injection.

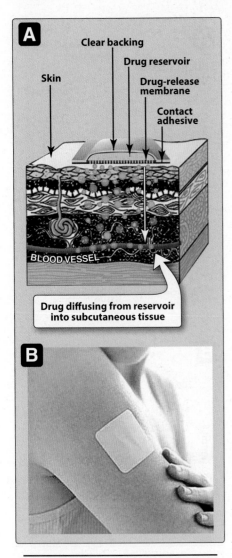

Figure 1.4
A. Schematic representation of a transdermal patch. **B.** Transdermal nicotine patch applied to the arm.

C. Other

1. **Oral inhalation:** Inhalation routes, both oral and nasal (see discussion of nasal inhalation), provide rapid delivery of a drug across the large surface area of the mucous membranes of the respiratory tract and pulmonary epithelium. Drug effects are almost as rapid as those with IV bolus. Drugs that are gases (for example, some anesthetics) and those that can be dispersed in an aerosol are administered via inhalation. This route is effective and convenient for patients with respiratory disorders (such as asthma or chronic obstructive pulmonary disease), because the drug is delivered directly to the site of action, thereby minimizing systemic side effects. Examples of drugs administered via inhalation include bronchodilators, such as *albuterol,* and corticosteroids, such as *fluticasone.*

2. **Nasal inhalation:** This route involves administration of drugs directly into the nose. Examples of agents include nasal decongestants, such as *oxymetazoline,* and corticosteroids, such as *mometasone furoate. Desmopressin* is administered intranasally in the treatment of diabetes insipidus.

3. **Intrathecal/intraventricular:** The blood–brain barrier typically delays or prevents the absorption of drugs into the central nervous system (CNS). When local, rapid effects are needed, it is necessary to introduce drugs directly into the cerebrospinal fluid. For example, intrathecal *amphotericin B* is used in treating cryptococcal meningitis (see Chapter 42).

4. **Topical:** Topical application is used when a local effect of the drug is desired. For example, *clotrimazole* is a cream applied directly to the skin for the treatment of fungal infections.

5. **Transdermal:** This route of administration achieves systemic effects by application of drugs to the skin, usually via a transdermal patch (Figure 1.4). The rate of absorption can vary markedly, depending on the physical characteristics of the skin at the site of application, as well as the lipid solubility of the drug. This route is most often used for the sustained delivery of drugs, such as the antianginal drug *nitroglycerin,* the antiemetic *scopolamine,* and *nicotine* transdermal patches, which are used to facilitate smoking cessation.

6. **Rectal:** Because 50% of the drainage of the rectal region bypasses the portal circulation, the biotransformation of drugs by the liver is minimized with rectal administration. The rectal route has the additional advantage of preventing destruction of the drug in the GI environment. This route is also useful if the drug induces vomiting when given orally, if the patient is already vomiting, or if the patient is unconscious. [Note: The rectal route is commonly used to administer antiemetic agents.] Rectal absorption is often erratic and incomplete, and many drugs irritate the rectal mucosa. Figure 1.5 summarizes the characteristics of the common routes of administration.

ROUTE OF ADMINISTRATION	ABSORPTION PATTERN	ADVANTAGES	DISADVANTAGES
Oral	• Variable; affected by many factors	• Safest and most common, convenient, and economical route of administration	• Limited absorption of some drugs • Food may affect absorption • Patient compliance is necessary • Drugs may be metabolized before systemic absorption
Intravenous	• Absorption not required	• Can have immediate effects • Ideal if dosed in large volumes • Suitable for irritating substances and complex mixtures • Valuable in emergency situations • Dosage titration permissible • Ideal for high molecular weight proteins and peptide drugs	• Unsuitable for oily substances • Bolus injection may result in adverse effects • Most substances must be slowly injected • Strict aseptic techniques needed
Subcutaneous	• Depends on drug diluents: Aqueous solution: prompt Depot preparations: slow and sustained	• Suitable for slow-release drugs • Ideal for some poorly soluble suspensions	• Pain or necrosis if drug is irritating • Unsuitable for drugs administered in large volumes
Intramuscular	• Depends on drug diluents: Aqueous solution: prompt Depot preparations: slow and sustained	• Suitable if drug volume is moderate • Suitable for oily vehicles and certain irritating substances • Preferable to intravenous if patient must self-administer	• Affects certain lab tests (creatine kinase) • Can be painful • Can cause intramuscular hemorrhage (precluded during anticoagulation therapy)
Transdermal (patch)	• Slow and sustained	• Bypasses the first-pass effect • Convenient and painless • Ideal for drugs that are lipophilic and have poor oral bioavailability • Ideal for drugs that are quickly eliminated from the body	• Some patients are allergic to patches, which can cause irritation • Drug must be highly lipophilic • May cause delayed delivery of drug to pharmacological site of action • Limited to drugs that can be taken in small daily doses
Rectal	• Erratic and variable	• Partially bypasses first-pass effect • Bypasses destruction by stomach acid • Ideal if drug causes vomiting • Ideal in patients who are vomiting, or comatose	• Drugs may irritate the rectal mucosa • Not a well-accepted route
Inhalation	• Systemic absorption may occur; this is not always desirable	• Absorption is rapid; can have immediate effects • Ideal for gases • Effective for patients with respiratory problems • Dose can be titrated • Localized effect to target lungs: lower doses used compared to that with oral or parenteral administration • Fewer systemic side effects	• Most addictive route (drug can enter the brain quickly) • Patient may have difficulty regulating dose • Some patients may have difficulty using inhalers
Sublingual	• Depends on the drug: Few drugs (for example, *nitroglycerin*) have rapid, direct systemic absorption Most drugs erratically or incompletely absorbed	• Bypasses first-pass effect • Bypasses destruction by stomach acid • Drug stability maintained because the pH of saliva relatively neutral • May cause immediate pharmacological effects	• Limited to certain types of drugs • Limited to drugs that can be taken in small doses • May lose part of the drug dose if swallowed

Figure 1.5

The absorption pattern, advantages, and disadvantages of the most common routes of administration.

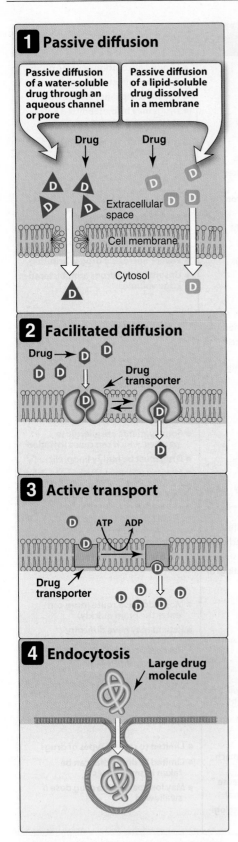

Figure 1.6
Schematic representation of drugs crossing a cell membrane. ATP = adenosine triphosphate; ADP = adenosine diphosphate.

III. ABSORPTION OF DRUGS

Absorption is the transfer of a drug from the site of administration to the bloodstream. The rate and extent of absorption depend on the environment where the drug is absorbed, chemical characteristics of the drug, and the route of administration (which influences bioavailability). Routes of administration other than intravenous may result in partial absorption and lower bioavailability.

A. Mechanisms of absorption of drugs from the GI tract

Depending on their chemical properties, drugs may be absorbed from the GI tract by passive diffusion, facilitated diffusion, active transport, or endocytosis (Figure 1.6).

1. **Passive diffusion:** The driving force for passive absorption of a drug is the concentration gradient across a membrane separating two body compartments. In other words, the drug moves from a region of high concentration to one of lower concentration. Passive diffusion does not involve a carrier, is not saturable, and shows a low structural specificity. The vast majority of drugs are absorbed by this mechanism. Water-soluble drugs penetrate the cell membrane through aqueous channels or pores, whereas lipid-soluble drugs readily move across most biologic membranes due to their solubility in the membrane lipid bilayers.

2. **Facilitated diffusion:** Other agents can enter the cell through specialized transmembrane carrier proteins that facilitate the passage of large molecules. These carrier proteins undergo conformational changes, allowing the passage of drugs or endogenous molecules into the interior of cells and moving them from an area of high concentration to an area of low concentration. This process is known as facilitated diffusion. It does not require energy, can be saturated, and may be inhibited by compounds that compete for the carrier.

3. **Active transport:** This mode of drug entry also involves specific carrier proteins that span the membrane. A few drugs that closely resemble the structure of naturally occurring metabolites are actively transported across cell membranes using specific carrier proteins. Energy-dependent active transport is driven by the hydrolysis of adenosine triphosphate. It is capable of moving drugs against a concentration gradient, from a region of low drug concentration to one of higher drug concentration. The process is saturable. Active transport systems are selective and may be competitively inhibited by other cotransported substances.

4. **Endocytosis and exocytosis:** This type of absorption is used to transport drugs of exceptionally large size across the cell membrane. Endocytosis involves engulfment of a drug by the cell membrane and transport into the cell by pinching off the drug-filled vesicle. Exocytosis is the reverse of endocytosis. Many cells use exocytosis to secrete substances out of the cell through a similar process of vesicle formation. Vitamin B$_{12}$ is transported across the gut wall by endocytosis, whereas certain neurotransmitters (for example, norepinephrine) are stored in intracellular vesicles in the nerve terminal and released by exocytosis.

B. Factors influencing absorption

1. **Effect of pH on drug absorption:** Most drugs are either weak acids or weak bases. Acidic drugs (HA) release a proton (H⁺), causing a charged anion (A⁻) to form:

$$HA \leftrightarrows H^+ + A^-$$

Weak bases (BH⁺) can also release an H⁺. However, the protonated form of basic drugs is usually charged, and loss of a proton produces the uncharged base (B):

$$BH^+ \leftrightarrows B + H^+$$

A drug passes through membranes more readily if it is uncharged (Figure 1.7). Thus, for a weak acid, the uncharged, protonated HA can permeate through membranes, and A⁻ cannot. For a weak base, the uncharged form B penetrates through the cell membrane, but the protonated form BH⁺ does not. Therefore, the effective concentration of the permeable form of each drug at its absorption site is determined by the relative concentrations of the charged and uncharged forms. The ratio between the two forms is, in turn, determined by the pH at the site of absorption and by the strength of the weak acid or base, which is represented by the ionization constant, pK_a (Figure 1.8). [Note: The pK_a is a measure of the strength of the interaction of a compound with a proton. The lower the pK_a of a drug, the more acidic it is. Conversely, the higher the pK_a, the more basic is the drug.] Distribution equilibrium is achieved when the permeable form of a drug achieves an equal concentration in all body water spaces.

2. **Blood flow to the absorption site:** The intestines receive much more blood flow than the stomach, so absorption from the intestine is favored over the stomach. [Note: Shock severely reduces blood flow to cutaneous tissues, thereby minimizing absorption from SC administration.]

3. **Total surface area available for absorption:** With a surface rich in brush borders containing microvilli, the intestine has a surface area about 1000-fold that of the stomach, making absorption of the drug across the intestine more efficient.

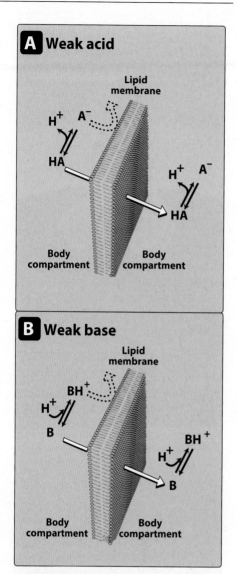

A Weak acid

B Weak base

Figure 1.7
A. Diffusion of the nonionized form of a weak acid through a lipid membrane. **B.** Diffusion of the nonionized form of a weak base through a lipid membrane.

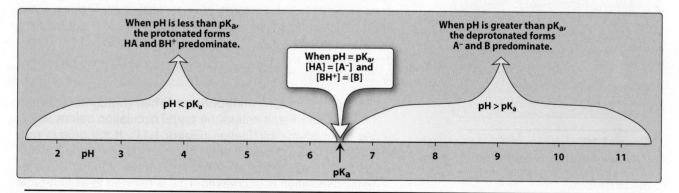

When pH is less than pK_a, the protonated forms HA and BH⁺ predominate.

When pH = pK_a, [HA] = [A⁻] and [BH⁺] = [B]

When pH is greater than pK_a, the deprotonated forms A⁻ and B predominate.

pH < pK_a

pH > pK_a

Figure 1.8
The distribution of a drug between its ionized and nonionized forms depends on the ambient pH and pK_a of the drug. For illustrative purposes, the drug has been assigned a pK_a of 6.5.

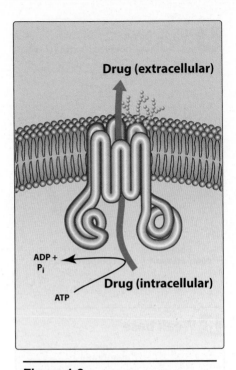

Figure 1.9
The six membrane-spanning loops of the P-glycoprotein form a central channel for the ATP-dependent pumping of drugs from the cell.

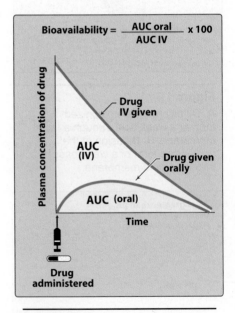

Figure 1.10
Determination of the bioavailability of a drug. AUC = area under curve; IV = intravenous

4. **Contact time at the absorption surface:** If a drug moves through the GI tract very quickly, as can happen with severe diarrhea, it is not well absorbed. Conversely, anything that delays the transport of the drug from the stomach to the intestine delays the rate of absorption of the drug. [Note: The presence of food in the stomach both dilutes the drug and slows gastric emptying. Therefore, a drug taken with a meal is generally absorbed more slowly.]

5. **Expression of P-glycoprotein:** P-glycoprotein is a transmembrane transporter protein responsible for transporting various molecules, including drugs, across cell membranes (Figure 1.9). It is expressed in tissues throughout the body, including the liver, kidneys, placenta, intestines, and brain capillaries, and is involved in transportation of drugs from tissues to blood. That is, it "pumps" drugs out of the cells. Thus, in areas of high expression, P-glycoprotein reduces drug absorption. In addition to transporting many drugs out of cells, it is also associated with multidrug resistance.

C. **Bioavailability**

Bioavailability is the rate and extent to which an administered drug reaches the systemic circulation. For example, if 100 mg of a drug is administered orally and 70 mg is absorbed unchanged, the bioavailability is 0.7 or 70%. Determining bioavailability is important for calculating drug dosages for nonintravenous routes of administration.

1. **Determination of bioavailability:** Bioavailability is determined by comparing plasma levels of a drug after a particular route of administration (for example, oral administration) with levels achieved by IV administration. After IV administration, 100% of the drug rapidly enters the circulation. When the drug is given orally, only part of the administered dose appears in the plasma. By plotting plasma concentrations of the drug versus time, the area under the curve (AUC) can be measured. The total AUC reflects the extent of absorption of the drug. Bioavailability of a drug given orally is the ratio of the AUC following oral administration to the AUC following IV administration (assuming IV and oral doses are equivalent; Figure 1.10).

2. **Factors that influence bioavailability:** In contrast to IV administration, which confers 100% bioavailability, orally administered drugs often undergo first-pass metabolism. This biotransformation, in addition to the chemical and physical characteristics of the drug, determines the rate and extent to which the agent reaches the systemic circulation.

   a. **First-pass hepatic metabolism:** When a drug is absorbed from the GI tract, it enters the portal circulation before entering the systemic circulation (Figure 1.11). If the drug is rapidly metabolized in the liver or gut wall during this initial passage, the amount of unchanged drug entering the systemic circulation is decreased. This is referred to as first-pass metabolism. [Note: First-pass metabolism by the intestine or liver limits the efficacy of many oral medications. For example, more than 90% of *nitroglycerin* is cleared during first-pass metabolism. Hence, it is primarily administered via the sublingual or transdermal route.] Drugs with high first-pass metabolism should be given in doses sufficient to ensure that enough active drug reaches the desired site of action.

b. **Solubility of the drug:** Very hydrophilic drugs are poorly absorbed because of their inability to cross lipid-rich cell membranes. Paradoxically, drugs that are extremely lipophilic are also poorly absorbed, because they are totally insoluble in aqueous body fluids and, therefore, cannot gain access to the surface of cells. For a drug to be readily absorbed, it must be largely lipophilic, yet have some solubility in aqueous solutions. This is one reason why many drugs are either weak acids or weak bases.

c. **Chemical instability:** Some drugs, such as *penicillin G,* are unstable in the pH of the gastric contents. Others, such as *insulin,* are destroyed in the GI tract by degradative enzymes.

d. **Nature of the drug formulation:** Drug absorption may be altered by factors unrelated to the chemistry of the drug. For example, particle size, salt form, crystal polymorphism, enteric coatings, and the presence of excipients (such as binders and dispersing agents) can influence the ease of dissolution and, therefore, alter the rate of absorption.

D. Bioequivalence

Two drug formulations are bioequivalent if they show comparable bioavailability and similar times to achieve peak blood concentrations.

E. Therapeutic equivalence

Two drug formulations are therapeutically equivalent if they are pharmaceutically equivalent (that is, they have the same dosage form, contain the same active ingredient, and use the same route of administration) with similar clinical and safety profiles. [Note: Clinical effectiveness often depends on both the maximum serum drug concentration and the time required (after administration) to reach peak concentration. Therefore, two drugs that are bioequivalent may not be therapeutically equivalent.]

IV. DRUG DISTRIBUTION

Drug distribution is the process by which a drug reversibly leaves the bloodstream and enters the interstitium (extracellular fluid) and the tissues. For drugs administered IV, absorption is not a factor, and the initial phase (from immediately after administration through the rapid fall in concentration) represents the distribution phase, during which the drug

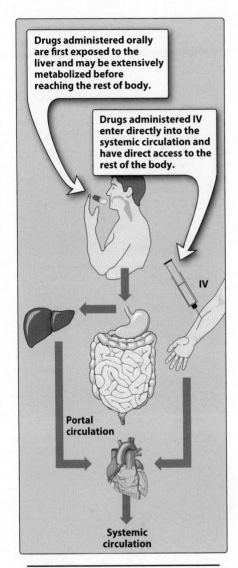

Drugs administered orally are first exposed to the liver and may be extensively metabolized before reaching the rest of body.

Drugs administered IV enter directly into the systemic circulation and have direct access to the rest of the body.

IV

Portal circulation

Systemic circulation

Figure 1.11
First-pass metabolism can occur with orally administered drugs. IV = intravenous.

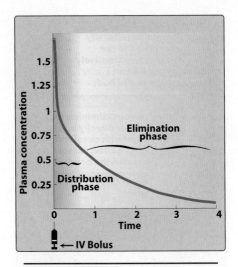

Figure 1.12
Drug concentrations in serum after a single injection of drug. Assume that the drug distributes and is subsequently eliminated.

rapidly leaves the circulation and enters the tissues (Figure 1.12). The distribution of a drug from the plasma to the interstitium depends on cardiac output and local blood flow, capillary permeability, the tissue volume, the degree of binding of the drug to plasma and tissue proteins, and the relative lipophilicity of the drug.

A. Blood flow

The rate of blood flow to the tissue capillaries varies widely. For instance, blood flow to the "vessel-rich organs" (brain, liver, and kidney) is greater than that to the skeletal muscles. Adipose tissue, skin, and viscera have still lower rates of blood flow. Variation in blood flow partly explains the short duration of hypnosis produced by an IV bolus of *propofol* (see Chapter 13). High blood flow, together with high lipophilicity of *propofol,* permits rapid distribution into the CNS and produces anesthesia. A subsequent slower distribution to skeletal muscle and adipose tissue lowers the plasma concentration so that the drug diffuses out of the CNS, down the concentration gradient, and consciousness is regained.

B. Capillary permeability

Capillary permeability is determined by capillary structure and by the chemical nature of the drug. Capillary structure varies in terms of the fraction of the basement membrane exposed by slit junctions between endothelial cells. In the liver and spleen, a significant portion of the basement membrane is exposed due to large, discontinuous capillaries through which large plasma proteins can pass (Figure 1.13A). In the brain, the capillary structure is continuous, and there are no slit junctions (Figure 1.13B). To enter the brain, drugs must pass through the endothelial cells of the CNS capillaries or be actively transported. For example, a specific transporter carries *levodopa* into the brain. By contrast, lipid-soluble drugs readily penetrate the CNS because they dissolve in the endothelial cell membrane. Ionized or polar drugs generally fail to enter the CNS because they cannot pass through the endothelial cells that have no slit junctions (Figure 1.13C). These closely juxtaposed cells form tight junctions that constitute the blood–brain barrier.

C. Binding of drugs to plasma proteins and tissues

1. **Binding to plasma proteins:** Reversible binding to plasma proteins sequesters drugs in a nondiffusible form and slows their transfer out of the vascular compartment. Albumin is the major drug-binding protein and may act as a drug reservoir (as the concentration of free drug decreases due to elimination, the bound drug dissociates from the protein). This maintains the free-drug concentration as a constant fraction of the total drug in the plasma.

2. **Binding to tissue proteins:** Many drugs accumulate in tissues, leading to higher concentrations in tissues than in the extracellular fluid and blood. Drugs may accumulate as a result of binding

to lipids, proteins, or nucleic acids. Drugs may also be actively transported into tissues. Tissue reservoirs may serve as a major source of the drug and prolong its actions or cause local drug toxicity. (For example, acrolein, the metabolite of *cyclophosphamide*, can cause hemorrhagic cystitis because it accumulates in the bladder.)

D. Lipophilicity

The chemical nature of a drug strongly influences its ability to cross cell membranes. Lipophilic drugs readily move across most biologic membranes. These drugs dissolve in the lipid membranes and penetrate the entire cell surface. The major factor influencing the distribution of lipophilic drugs is blood flow to the area. In contrast, hydrophilic drugs do not readily penetrate cell membranes and must pass through slit junctions.

E. Volume of distribution

The apparent volume of distribution, V_d, is defined as the fluid volume that is required to contain the entire drug in the body at the same concentration measured in the plasma. It is calculated by dividing the dose that ultimately gets into the systemic circulation by the plasma concentration at time zero (C_0).

$$V_d = \frac{\text{Amount of drug in the body}}{C_0}$$

Although V_d has no physiologic or physical basis, it can be useful to compare the distribution of a drug with the volumes of the water compartments in the body.

1. **Distribution into the water compartments in the body:** Once a drug enters the body, it has the potential to distribute into any one of the three functionally distinct compartments of body water or to become sequestered in a cellular site.

   a. **Plasma compartment:** If a drug has a high molecular weight or is extensively protein bound, it is too large to pass through the slit junctions of the capillaries and, thus, is effectively trapped within the plasma (vascular) compartment. As a result, it has a low V_d that approximates the plasma volume or about 4 L in a 70-kg individual. *Heparin* (see Chapter 22) shows this type of distribution.

   b. **Extracellular fluid:** If a drug has a low molecular weight but is hydrophilic, it can pass through the endothelial slit junctions of the capillaries into the interstitial fluid. However, hydrophilic drugs cannot move across the lipid membranes of cells to enter the intracellular fluid. Therefore, these drugs distribute into a volume that is the sum of the plasma volume and the interstitial fluid, which together constitute the extracellular fluid (about 20% of body weight or 14 L in a 70-kg individual). Aminoglycoside antibiotics (see Chapter 39) show this type of distribution.

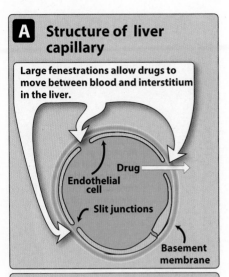

A Structure of liver capillary

Large fenestrations allow drugs to move between blood and interstitium in the liver.

Endothelial cell

Drug

Slit junctions

Basement membrane

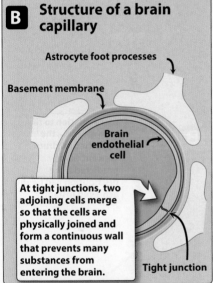

B Structure of a brain capillary

Astrocyte foot processes

Basement membrane

Brain endothelial cell

At tight junctions, two adjoining cells merge so that the cells are physically joined and form a continuous wall that prevents many substances from entering the brain.

Tight junction

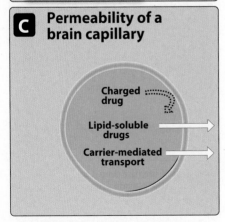

C Permeability of a brain capillary

Charged drug

Lipid-soluble drugs

Carrier-mediated transport

Figure 1.13
Cross section of liver and brain capillaries.

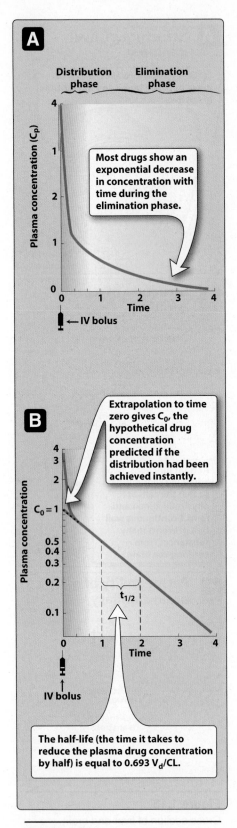

Figure 1.14

Drug concentrations in plasma after a single injection of drug at time = 0. **A.** Concentration data are plotted on a linear scale. **B.** Concentration data are plotted on a log scale.

c. **Total body water:** If a drug has a low molecular weight and is lipophilic, it can move into the interstitium through the slit junctions and also pass through the cell membranes into the intracellular fluid. These drugs distribute into a volume of about 60% of body weight or about 42 L in a 70-kg individual. *Ethanol* exhibits this apparent V_d.

2. **Apparent volume of distribution:** A drug rarely associates exclusively with only one of the water compartments of the body. Instead, the vast majority of drugs distribute into several compartments, often avidly binding cellular components, such as lipids (abundant in adipocytes and cell membranes), proteins (abundant in plasma and cells), and nucleic acids (abundant in cell nuclei). Therefore, the volume into which drugs distribute is called the apparent volume of distribution (V_d). V_d is a useful pharmacokinetic parameter for calculating the loading dose of a drug.

3. **Determination of V_d:** The fact that drug clearance is usually a first-order process allows calculation of V_d. First order means that a constant fraction of the drug is eliminated per unit of time. This process can be most easily analyzed by plotting the log of the plasma drug concentration (C_p) versus time (Figure 1.14). The concentration of drug in the plasma can be extrapolated back to time zero (the time of IV bolus) on the Y axis to determine C_0, which is the concentration of drug that would have been achieved if the distribution phase had occurred instantly. This allows calculation of V_d as

$$V_d = \frac{Dose}{C_0}$$

For example, if 10 mg of drug is injected into a patient and the plasma concentration is extrapolated back to time zero, and C_0 = 1 mg/L (from the graph in Figure 1.14B), then V_d = 10 mg/1 mg/L = 10 L.

4. **Effect of V_d on drug half-life:** V_d has an important influence on the half-life of a drug, because drug elimination depends on the amount of drug delivered to the liver or kidney (or other organs where metabolism occurs) per unit of time. Delivery of drug to the organs of elimination depends not only on blood flow but also on the fraction of the drug in the plasma. If a drug has a large V_d, most of the drug is in the extraplasmic space and is unavailable to the excretory organs. Therefore, any factor that increases V_d can increase the half-life and extend the duration of action of the drug. [Note: An exceptionally large V_d indicates considerable sequestration of the drug in some tissues or compartments.]

V. DRUG CLEARANCE THROUGH METABOLISM

Once a drug enters the body, the process of elimination begins. The three major routes of elimination are hepatic metabolism, biliary elimination, and urinary elimination. Together, these elimination processes decrease the plasma concentration exponentially. That is, a constant fraction of the drug present is eliminated in a given unit of time (Figure 1.14A). Most drugs are eliminated according to first-order kinetics, although some, such as *aspirin* in high doses, are eliminated according to zero-order or nonlinear kinetics. Metabolism leads to production of products with increased polarity, which allows the drug to be eliminated. Clearance (CL) estimates the amount of drug cleared from the body per unit of time. Total CL is a composite estimate reflecting all mechanisms of drug elimination and is calculated as follows:

$$CL = 0.693 \times V_d / t_{1/2}$$

where $t_{1/2}$ is the elimination half-life, V_d is the apparent volume of distribution, and 0.693 is the natural log constant. Drug half-life is often used as a measure of drug CL, because, for many drugs, V_d is a constant.

A. Kinetics of metabolism

1. **First-order kinetics:** The metabolic transformation of drugs is catalyzed by enzymes, and most of the reactions obey Michaelis-Menten kinetics.

$$v = \text{Rate of drug metabolism} = \frac{V_{max}[C]}{K_m + [C]}$$

In most clinical situations, the concentration of the drug, [C], is much less than the Michaelis constant, K_m, and the Michaelis-Menten equation reduces to

$$v = \text{Rate of drug metabolism} = \frac{V_{max}[C]}{K_m}$$

That is, the rate of drug metabolism and elimination is directly proportional to the concentration of free drug, and first-order kinetics is observed (Figure 1.15). This means that a constant fraction of drug is metabolized per unit of time (that is, with each half-life, the concentration decreases by 50%). First-order kinetics is also referred to as linear kinetics.

2. **Zero-order kinetics:** With a few drugs, such as *aspirin, ethanol, and phenytoin,* the doses are very large. Therefore, [C] is much greater than K_m, and the velocity equation becomes

$$v = \text{Rate of drug metabolism} = \frac{V_{max}[C]}{[C]} = V_{max}$$

The enzyme is saturated by a high free drug concentration, and the rate of metabolism remains constant over time. This is called zero-order kinetics (also called nonlinear kinetics). A constant amount of drug is metabolized per unit of time. The rate of elimination is constant and does not depend on the drug concentration.

B. Reactions of drug metabolism

The kidney cannot efficiently eliminate lipophilic drugs that readily cross cell membranes and are reabsorbed in the distal convoluted tubules. Therefore, lipid-soluble agents are first metabolized into more

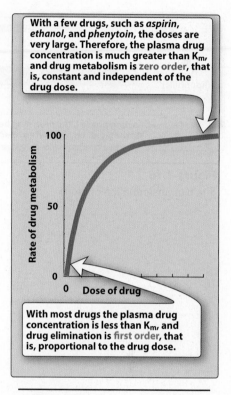

With a few drugs, such as *aspirin, ethanol,* and *phenytoin,* the doses are very large. Therefore, the plasma drug concentration is much greater than K_m, and drug metabolism is zero order, that is, constant and independent of the drug dose.

With most drugs the plasma drug concentration is less than K_m, and drug elimination is first order, that is, proportional to the drug dose.

Figure 1.15
Effect of drug dose on the rate of metabolism.

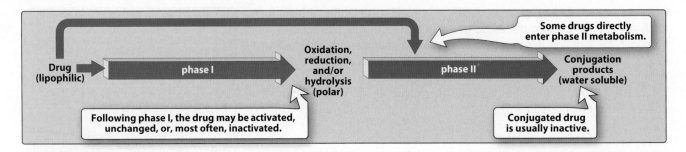

Figure 1.16
The biotransformation of drugs.

polar (hydrophilic) substances in the liver via two general sets of reactions, called phase I and phase II (Figure 1.16).

1. **Phase I:** Phase I reactions convert lipophilic drugs into more polar molecules by introducing or unmasking a polar functional group, such as –OH or –NH$_2$. Phase I reactions usually involve reduction, oxidation, or hydrolysis. Phase I metabolism may increase, decrease, or have no effect on pharmacologic activity.

   a. **Phase I reactions utilizing the P450 system:** The phase I reactions most frequently involved in drug metabolism are catalyzed by the cytochrome P450 system (also called microsomal mixed-function oxidases). The P450 system is important for the metabolism of many endogenous compounds (such as steroids, lipids) and for the biotransformation of exogenous substances (xenobiotics). Cytochrome P450, designated as CYP, is a superfamily of heme-containing isozymes that are located in most cells, but primarily in the liver and GI tract.

      [1] **Nomenclature:** The family name is indicated by the Arabic number that follows CYP, and the capital letter designates the subfamily, for example, CYP3A (Figure 1.17). A second number indicates the specific isozyme, as in CYP3A4.

      [2] **Specificity:** Because there are many different genes that encode multiple enzymes, there are many different P450 isoforms. These enzymes have the capacity to modify a large number of structurally diverse substrates. In addition, an individual drug may be a substrate for more than one isozyme. Four isozymes are responsible for the vast majority of P450-catalyzed reactions. They are CYP3A4/5, CYP2D6, CYP2C8/9, and CYP1A2 (Figure 1.17). Considerable amounts of CYP3A4 are found in intestinal mucosa, accounting for first-pass metabolism of drugs such as *chlorpromazine* and *clonazepam*.

      [3] **Genetic variability:** P450 enzymes exhibit considerable genetic variability among individuals and racial groups. Variations in P450 activity may alter drug efficacy and the risk of adverse events. CYP2D6, in particular, has been shown to exhibit genetic polymorphism. CYP2D6 mutations result in very low capacities to metabolize substrates. Some individuals, for example, obtain no benefit from the opioid

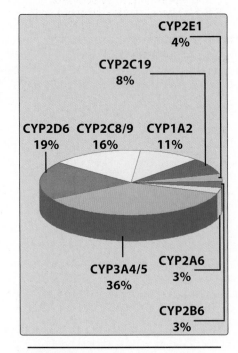

Figure 1.17
Relative contribution of cytochrome P450 (CYP) isoforms to drug biotransformation.

analgesic *codeine,* because they lack the CYP2D6 enzyme that activates the drug. Similar polymorphisms have been characterized for the CYP2C subfamily of isozymes. For instance, *clopidogrel* carries a warning that patients who are poor CYP2C19 metabolizers have a higher incidence of cardiovascular events (for example, stroke or myocardial infarction) when taking this drug. *Clopidogrel* is a prodrug, and CYP2C19 activity is required to convert it to the active metabolite. Although CYP3A4 exhibits a greater than 10-fold variability between individuals, no polymorphisms have been identified so far for this P450 isozyme.

[4] Inducers: The CYP450-dependent enzymes are an important target for pharmacokinetic drug interactions. One such interaction is the induction of selected CYP isozymes. Xenobiotics (chemicals not normally produced or expected to be present in the body, for example, drugs or environmental pollutants) may induce the activity of these enzymes. Certain drugs (for example, *phenobarbital, rifampin,* and *carbamazepine*) are capable of increasing the synthesis of one or more CYP isozymes. This results in increased biotransformation of drugs and can lead to significant decreases in plasma concentrations of drugs metabolized by these CYP isozymes, with concurrent loss of pharmacologic effect. For example, *rifampin,* an antituberculosis drug (see Chapter 41), significantly decreases the plasma concentrations of human immunodeficiency virus (HIV) protease inhibitors, thereby diminishing their ability to suppress HIV replication. *St. John's wort* is a widely used herbal product and is a potent CYP3A4 inducer. Many drug interactions have been reported with concomitant use of *St. John's wort.* Figure 1.18 lists some of the more important inducers for representative CYP isozymes. Consequences of increased drug metabolism include 1) decreased plasma drug concentrations, 2) decreased drug activity if the metabolite is inactive, 3) increased drug activity if the metabolite is active, and 4) decreased therapeutic drug effect.

[5] Inhibitors: Inhibition of CYP isozyme activity is an important source of drug interactions that lead to serious adverse events. The most common form of inhibition is through competition for the same isozyme. Some drugs, however, are capable of inhibiting reactions for which they are not substrates (for example, *ketoconazole*), leading to drug interactions. Numerous drugs have been shown to inhibit one or more of the CYP-dependent biotransformation pathways of *warfarin.* For example, *omeprazole* is a potent inhibitor of three of the CYP isozymes responsible for *warfarin* metabolism. If the two drugs are taken together, plasma concentrations of *warfarin* increase, which leads to greater anticoagulant effect and increased risk of bleeding. [Note: The more important CYP inhibitors are *erythromycin, ketoconazole,* and *ritonavir,* because they each inhibit several CYP isozymes.] Natural substances may also inhibit drug metabolism. For instance, grapefruit juice inhibits CYP3A4

Isozyme: CYP2C9/10	
COMMON SUBSTRATES	**INDUCERS**
Warfarin *Phenytoin* *Ibuprofen* *Tolbutamide*	*Phenobarbital* *Rifampin*

Isozyme: CYP2D6	
COMMON SUBSTRATES	**INDUCERS**
Desipramine *Imipramine* *Haloperidol* *Propranolol*	None*

Isozyme: CYP3A4/5	
COMMON SUBSTRATES	**INDUCERS**
Carbamazepine *Cyclosporine* *Erythromycin* *Nifedipine* *Verapamil*	*Carbamazepine* *Dexamethasone* *Phenobarbital* *Phenytoin* *Rifampin*

Figure 1.18
Some representative cytochrome P450 isozymes. CYP = cytochrome P. *Unlike most other CYP450 enzymes, CYP2D6 is not very susceptible to enzyme induction.

and leads to higher levels and/or greater potential for toxic effects with drugs, such as *nifedipine, clarithromycin,* and *simvastatin,* that are metabolized by this system.

b. **Phase I reactions not involving the P450 system:** These include amine oxidation (for example, oxidation of catecholamines or histamine), alcohol dehydrogenation (for example, ethanol oxidation), esterases (for example, metabolism of *aspirin* in the liver), and hydrolysis (for example, of *procaine*).

2. **Phase II:** This phase consists of conjugation reactions. If the metabolite from phase I metabolism is sufficiently polar, it can be excreted by the kidneys. However, many phase I metabolites are still too lipophilic to be excreted. A subsequent conjugation reaction with an endogenous substrate, such as glucuronic acid, sulfuric acid, acetic acid, or an amino acid, results in polar, usually more water-soluble compounds that are often therapeutically inactive. A notable exception is *morphine-6-glucuronide*, which is more potent than *morphine*. Glucuronidation is the most common and the most important conjugation reaction. [Note: Drugs already possessing an $-OH$, $-NH_2$, or $-COOH$ group may enter phase II directly and become conjugated without prior phase I metabolism.] The highly polar drug conjugates are then excreted by the kidney or in bile.

VI. DRUG CLEARANCE BY THE KIDNEY

Drugs must be sufficiently polar to be eliminated from the body. Removal of drugs from the body occurs via a number of routes, the most important being elimination through the kidney into the urine. Patients with renal dysfunction may be unable to excrete drugs and are at risk for drug accumulation and adverse effects.

A. Renal elimination of a drug

Elimination of drugs via the kidneys into urine involves the processes of glomerular filtration, active tubular secretion, and passive tubular reabsorption.

1. **Glomerular filtration:** Drugs enter the kidney through renal arteries, which divide to form a glomerular capillary plexus. Free drug (not bound to albumin) flows through the capillary slits into the Bowman space as part of the glomerular filtrate (Figure 1.19). The glomerular filtration rate (GFR) is normally about 125 mL/min but may diminish significantly in renal disease. Lipid solubility and pH do not influence the passage of drugs into the glomerular filtrate. However, variations in GFR and protein binding of drugs do affect this process.

2. **Proximal tubular secretion:** Drugs that were not transferred into the glomerular filtrate leave the glomeruli through efferent arterioles, which divide to form a capillary plexus surrounding the nephric lumen in the proximal tubule. Secretion primarily occurs in the proximal tubules by two energy-requiring active transport systems: one for anions (for example, deprotonated forms of weak acids) and one for cations (for example, protonated forms of weak bases). Each of these

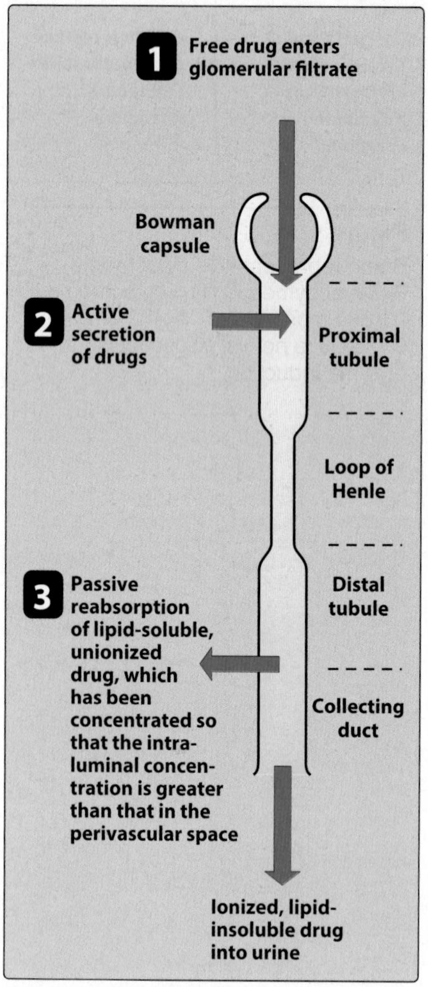

1 Free drug enters glomerular filtrate

Bowman capsule

2 Active secretion of drugs

Proximal tubule

Loop of Henle

3 Passive reabsorption of lipid-soluble, unionized drug, which has been concentrated so that the intra-luminal concentration is greater than that in the perivascular space

Distal tubule

Collecting duct

Ionized, lipid-insoluble drug into urine

Figure 1.19
Drug elimination by the kidney.

transport systems shows low specificity and can transport many compounds. Thus, competition between drugs for these carriers can occur within each transport system. [Note: Premature infants and neonates have an incompletely developed tubular secretory mechanism and, thus, may retain certain drugs in the glomerular filtrate.]

3. **Distal tubular reabsorption:** As a drug moves toward the distal convoluted tubule, its concentration increases and exceeds that of the perivascular space. The drug, if uncharged, may diffuse out of the nephric lumen, back into the systemic circulation. Manipulating the urine pH to increase the fraction of ionized drug in the lumen may be done to minimize the amount of back diffusion and increase the clearance of an undesirable drug. As a general rule, weak acids can be eliminated by alkalinization of the urine, whereas elimination of weak bases may be increased by acidification of the urine. This process is called "ion trapping." For example, a patient presenting with *phenobarbital* (weak acid) overdose can be given *bicarbonate,* which alkalinizes the urine and keeps the drug ionized, thereby decreasing its reabsorption.

4. **Role of drug metabolism:** Most drugs are lipid soluble and, without chemical modification, would diffuse out of the tubular lumen when the drug concentration in the filtrate becomes greater than that in the perivascular space. To minimize this reabsorption, drugs are modified primarily in the liver into more polar substances via phase I and phase II reactions (described above). The polar or ionized conjugates are unable to back diffuse out of the kidney lumen (Figure 1.20).

VII. CLEARANCE BY OTHER ROUTES

Drug clearance may also occur via the intestines, bile, lungs, and breast milk, among others. Drugs that are not absorbed after oral administration or drugs that are secreted directly into the intestines or into bile are eliminated in the feces. The lungs are primarily involved in the elimination of anesthetic gases (for example, *isoflurane*). Elimination of drugs in breast milk may expose the breast-feeding infant to medications and/or metabolites being taken by the mother and is a potential source of undesirable side effects to the infant. Excretion of most drugs into sweat, saliva, tears, hair, and skin occurs only to a small extent. Total body clearance and drug half-life are important measures of drug clearance that are used to optimize drug therapy and minimize toxicity.

A. Total body clearance

The total body (systemic) clearance, CL_{total}, is the sum of all clearances from the drug-metabolizing and drug-eliminating organs. The kidney is often the major organ of elimination. The liver also contributes to drug clearance through metabolism and/or excretion into the bile. Total clearance is calculated using the following equation:

$$CL_{total} = CL_{hepatic} + CL_{renal} + CL_{pulmonary} + CL_{other}$$

where $CL_{hepatic} + CL_{renal}$ are typically the most important.

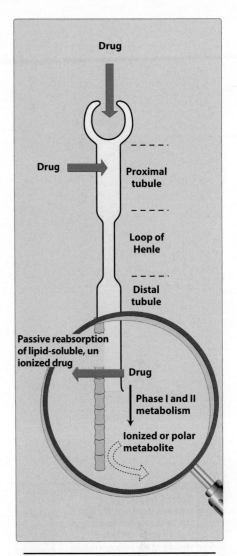

Figure 1.20
Effect of drug metabolism on reabsorption in the distal tubule.

B. Clinical situations resulting in changes in drug half-life

When a patient has an abnormality that alters the half-life of a drug, adjustment in dosage is required. Patients who may have an increase in drug half-life include those with 1) diminished renal or hepatic blood flow, for example, in cardiogenic shock, heart failure, or hemorrhage; 2) decreased ability to extract drug from plasma, for example, in renal disease; and 3) decreased metabolism, for example, when a concomitant drug inhibits metabolism or in hepatic insufficiency, as with cirrhosis. These patients may require a decrease in dosage or less frequent dosing intervals. In contrast, the half-life of a drug may be decreased by increased hepatic blood flow, decreased protein binding, or increased metabolism. This may necessitate higher doses or more frequent dosing intervals.

VIII. DESIGN AND OPTIMIZATION OF DOSAGE REGIMEN

To initiate drug therapy, the clinician must select the appropriate route of administration, dosage, and dosing interval. Selection of a regimen depends on various patient and drug factors, including how rapidly therapeutic levels of a drug must be achieved. The regimen is then further refined, or optimized, to maximize benefit and minimize adverse effects.

A. Continuous infusion regimens

Therapy may consist of a single dose of a drug, for example, a sleep-inducing agent, such as *zolpidem.* More commonly, drugs are continually administered, either as an IV infusion or in oral fixed-dose/fixed-time interval regimens (for example, "one tablet every 4 hours"). Continuous or repeated administration results in accumulation of the drug until a steady state occurs. Steady-state concentration is reached when the rate of drug elimination is equal to the rate of drug administration, such that the plasma and tissue levels remain relatively constant.

1. **Plasma concentration of a drug following IV infusion:** With continuous IV infusion, the rate of drug entry into the body is constant. Most drugs exhibit first-order elimination, that is, a constant fraction of the drug is cleared per unit of time. Therefore, the rate of drug elimination increases proportionately as the plasma concentration increases. Following initiation of a continuous IV infusion, the plasma concentration of a drug rises until a steady state (rate of drug elimination equals rate of drug administration) is reached, at which point the plasma concentration of the drug remains constant.

   a. **Influence of the rate of infusion on steady-state concentration:** The steady-state plasma concentration (C_{ss}) is directly proportional to the infusion rate. For example, if the infusion rate is doubled, the C_{ss} is doubled (Figure 1.21). Furthermore, the C_{ss} is inversely proportional to the clearance of the drug. Thus, any factor that decreases clearance, such as liver or kidney disease, increases the C_{ss} of an infused drug (assuming V_d remains constant). Factors that increase clearance, such as increased metabolism, decrease the C_{ss}.

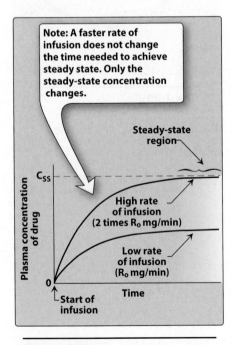

Figure 1.21
Effect of infusion rate on the steady-state concentration of drug in the plasma. R_o = rate of drug infusion; C_{ss} = steady-state concentration.

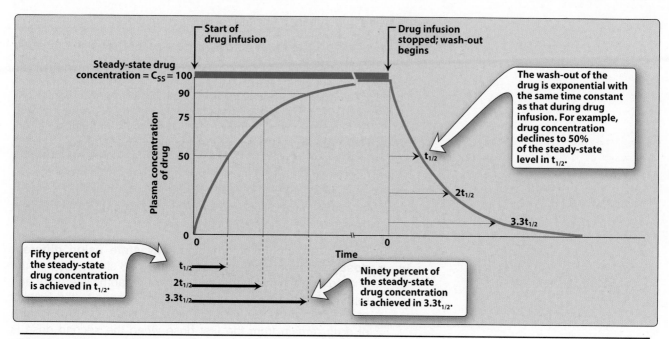

Figure 1.22
Rate of attainment of steady-state concentration of a drug in the plasma after intravenous infusion.

b. Time required to reach the steady-state drug concentration: The concentration of a drug rises from zero at the start of the infusion to its ultimate steady-state level, C_{ss} (Figure 1.21). The rate constant for attainment of steady state is the rate constant for total body elimination of the drug. Thus, 50% of C_{ss} of a drug is observed after the time elapsed, since the infusion, t, is equal to $t_{1/2}$, where $t_{1/2}$ (or half-life) is the time required for the drug concentration to change by 50%. After another half-life, the drug concentration approaches 75% of C_{ss} (Figure 1.22). The drug concentration is 87.5% of C_{ss} at 3 half-lives and 90% at 3.3 half-lives. Thus, a drug reaches steady state in about four to five half-lives.

The sole determinant of the rate that a drug achieves steady state is the half-life ($t_{1/2}$) of the drug, and this rate is influenced only by factors that affect the half-life. The rate of approach to steady state is not affected by the rate of drug infusion. When the infusion is stopped, the plasma concentration of a drug declines (washes out) to zero with the same time course observed in approaching the steady state (Figure 1.22).

B. Fixed-dose/fixed-time regimens

Administration of a drug by fixed doses rather than by continuous infusion is often more convenient. However, fixed doses of IV or oral medications given at fixed intervals result in time-dependent fluctuations in the circulating level of drug, which contrasts with the smooth ascent of drug concentration observed with continuous infusion.

1. Multiple IV injections: When a drug is given repeatedly at regular intervals, the plasma concentration increases until a steady state is reached (Figure 1.23). Because most drugs are given at inter-

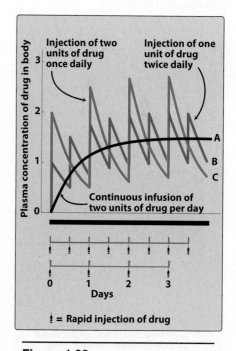

Figure 1.23
Predicted plasma concentrations of a drug given by infusion **(A)**, twice-daily injection **(B)**, or once-daily injection **(C)**. Model assumes rapid mixing in a single body compartment and a half-life of 12 hours.

vals shorter than five half-lives and are eliminated exponentially with time, some drug from the first dose remains in the body when the second dose is administered, some from the second dose remains when the third dose is given, and so forth. Therefore, the drug accumulates until, within the dosing interval, the rate of drug elimination equals the rate of drug administration and a steady state is achieved.

a. **Effect of dosing frequency:** With repeated administration at regular intervals, the plasma concentration of a drug oscillates about a mean. Using smaller doses at shorter intervals reduces the amplitude of fluctuations in drug concentration. However, the C_{ss} is affected by neither the dosing frequency (assuming the same total daily dose is administered) nor the rate at which the steady state is approached.

b. **Example of achievement of steady state using different dosage regimens:** Curve B of Figure 1.23 shows the amount of drug in the body when 1 unit of a drug is administered IV and repeated at a dosing interval that corresponds to the half-life of the drug. At the end of the first dosing interval, 0.50 units of drug remain from the first dose when the second dose is administered. At the end of the second dosing interval, 0.75 units are present when the third dose is given. The minimal amount of drug remaining during the dosing interval progressively approaches a value of 1.00 unit, whereas the maximal value immediately following drug administration progressively approaches 2.00 units. Therefore, at the steady state, 1.00 unit of drug is lost during the dosing interval, which is exactly matched by the rate of administration. That is, the "rate in" equals the "rate out." As in the case for IV infusion, 90% of the steady-state value is achieved in 3.3 half-lives.

2. **Multiple oral administrations:** Most drugs that are administered on an outpatient basis are oral medications taken at a specific dose one, two, or three times daily. In contrast to IV injection, orally administered drugs may be absorbed slowly, and the plasma concentration of the drug is influenced by both the rate of absorption and the rate of elimination (Figure 1.24).

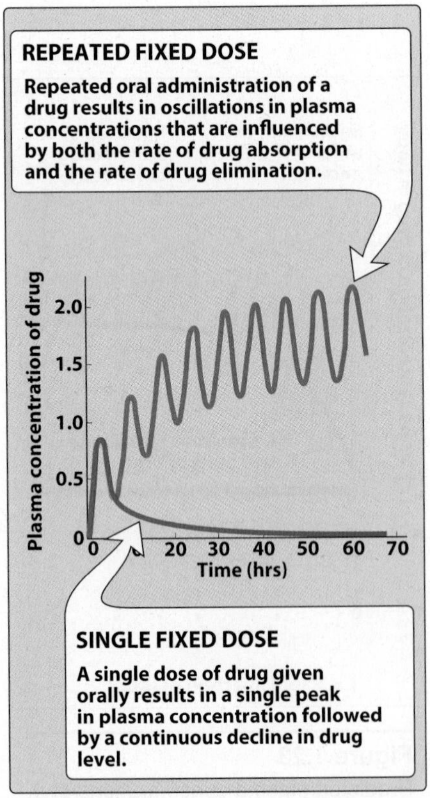

C. Optimization of dose

The goal of drug therapy is to achieve and maintain concentrations within a therapeutic response window while minimizing toxicity and/or side effects. With careful titration, most drugs can achieve this goal. If the therapeutic window (see Chapter 2) of the drug is small (for example, *digoxin, warfarin,* and *cyclosporine*), extra caution should be taken in selecting a dosage regimen, and monitoring of drug levels may help ensure attainment of the therapeutic range. Drug regimens are administered as a maintenance dose and may require a loading dose if rapid effects are warranted. For drugs with a defined therapeutic range, drug concentrations are subsequently measured, and the dosage and frequency are then adjusted to obtain the desired levels.

1. **Maintenance dose:** Drugs are generally administered to maintain a C_{ss} within the therapeutic window. It takes four to five half-lives for a drug to achieve C_{ss}. To achieve a given concentra-

REPEATED FIXED DOSE

Repeated oral administration of a drug results in oscillations in plasma concentrations that are influenced by both the rate of drug absorption and the rate of drug elimination.

SINGLE FIXED DOSE

A single dose of drug given orally results in a single peak in plasma concentration followed by a continuous decline in drug level.

Figure 1.24
Predicted plasma concentrations of a drug given by repeated oral administrations.

tion, the rate of administration and the rate of elimination of the drug are important. The dosing rate can be determined by knowing the target concentration in plasma (Cp), clearance (CL) of the drug from the systemic circulation, and the fraction (F) absorbed (bioavailability):

$$\text{Dosing rate} = \frac{(\text{Target } C_{plasma})(CL)}{F}$$

2. **Loading dose:** Sometimes rapid obtainment of desired plasma levels is needed (for example, in serious infections or arrhythmias). Therefore, a "loading dose" of drug is administered to achieve the desired plasma level rapidly, followed by a maintenance dose to maintain the steady state (Figure 1.25). In general, the loading dose can be calculated as

Loading dose = $(V_d) \times$ (desired steady-state plasma concentration)/F

For IV infusion, the bioavailability is 100%, and the equation becomes

Loading dose = $(V_d) \times$ (desired steady-state plasma concentration)

Loading doses can be given as a single dose or a series of doses. Disadvantages of loading doses include increased risk of drug toxicity and a longer time for the plasma concentration to fall if excess levels occur. A loading dose is most useful for drugs that have a relatively long half-life. Without an initial loading dose, these drugs would take a long time to reach a therapeutic value that corresponds to the steady-state level.

3. **Dose adjustment:** The amount of a drug administered for a given condition is estimated based on an "average patient." This approach overlooks interpatient variability in pharmacokinetic parameters such as clearance and V_d, which are quite significant in some cases. Knowledge of pharmacokinetic principles is useful in adjusting dosages to optimize therapy for a given patient. Monitoring drug therapy and correlating it with clinical benefits provides another tool to individualize therapy.

When determining a dosage adjustment, V_d can be used to calculate the amount of drug needed to achieve a desired plasma concentration. For example, assume a heart failure patient is not well controlled due to inadequate plasma levels of *digoxin*. Suppose the concentration of *digoxin* in the plasma is C_1 and the desired target concentration is C_2, a higher concentration. The following calculation can be used to determine how much additional *digoxin* should be administered to bring the level from C_1 to C_2.

$(V_d)(C_1)$ = Amount of drug initially in the body

$(V_d)(C_2)$ = Amount of drug in the body needed to achieve the desired plasma concentration

The difference between the two values is the additional dosage needed, which equals $V_d (C_2 - C_1)$.

Figure 1.26 shows the time course of drug concentration when treatment is started or dosing is changed.

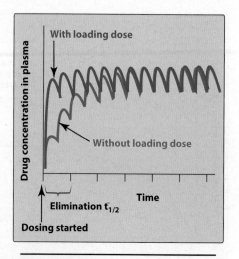

Figure 1.25
Accumulation of drug administered orally without a loading dose and with a single oral loading dose administered at t = 0.

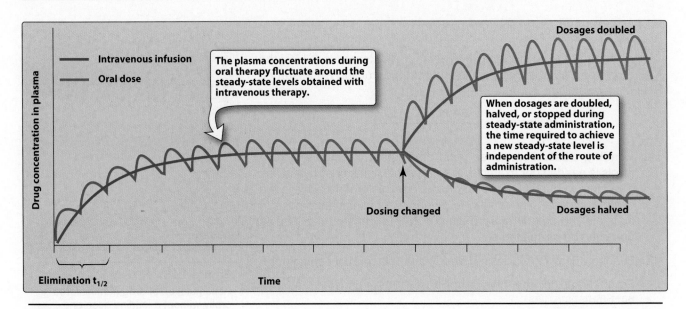

Figure 1.26
Accumulation of drug following sustained administration and following changes in dosing. Oral dosing was at intervals of 50% of $t_{1/2}$.

Study Questions

Choose the ONE best answer.

1.1 An 18-year-old female patient is brought to the emergency department due to drug overdose. Which of the following routes of administration is the most desirable for administering the antidote for the drug overdose?

    A. Intramuscular.
    B. Subcutaneous.
    C. Transdermal.
    D. Oral.
    E. Intravenous.

> Correct answer = E. The intravenous route of administration is the most desirable because it results in achievement of therapeutic plasma levels of the antidote rapidly.

1.2 Chlorothiazide is a weakly acidic drug with a pK_a of 6.5. If administered orally, at which of the following sites of absorption will the drug be able to readily pass through the membrane?

    A. Mouth (pH approximately 7.0).
    B. Stomach (pH of 2.5).
    C. Duodenum (pH approximately 6.1).
    D. Jejunum (pH approximately 8.0).
    E. Ileum (pH approximately 7.0).

> Correct answer = B. Because chlorothiazide is a weakly acidic drug (pKa = 6.5), it will be predominantly in non-ionized form in the stomach (pH of 2.5). For weak acids, the nonionized form will permeate through cell membrane readily.

1.3 Which of the following types of drugs will have maximum oral bioavailability?

A. Drugs with high first-pass metabolism.

B. Highly hydrophilic drugs.

C. Largely hydrophobic, yet soluble in aqueous solutions.

D. Chemically unstable drugs.

E. Drugs that are P-glycoprotein substrates.

Correct answer = C. Highly hydrophilic drugs have poor oral bioavailability, because they are poorly absorbed due to their inability to cross the lipid-rich cell membranes. Highly lipophilic (hydrophobic) drugs also have poor oral bioavailability, because they are poorly absorbed due their insolubility in aqueous stomach fluids and therefore cannot gain access to the surface of cells. Therefore, drugs that are largely hydrophobic, yet have aqueous solubility have greater oral bioavailability because they are readily absorbed.

1.4 Which of the following is *true* about the blood–brain barrier?

A. Endothelial cells of the blood–brain barrier have slit junctions.

B. Ionized or polar drugs can cross the blood–brain barrier easily.

C. Drugs cannot cross the blood–brain barrier through specific transporters.

D. Lipid-soluble drugs readily cross the blood–brain barrier.

E. The capillary structure of the blood–brain barrier is similar to that of the liver and spleen.

Correct answer = D. Lipid-soluble drugs readily cross the blood–brain barrier because they can dissolve easily in the membrane of endothelial cells. Ionized or polar drugs generally fail to cross the blood–brain barrier because they are unable to pass through the endothelial cells, which do not have slit junctions.

1.5 A 40-year-old male patient (70 kg) was recently diagnosed with infection involving methicillin-resistant *S. aureus*. He received 2000 mg of vancomycin as an IV loading dose. The peak plasma concentration of vancomycin was reported to be 28.5 mg/L. The apparent volume of distribution is:

A. 1 L/kg.

B. 10 L/kg.

C. 7 L/kg.

D. 70 L/kg.

E. 14 L/kg.

Correct answer = A. V_d = dose/C = 2000 mg/28.5 mg/L = 70.1 L. Because the patient is 70 kg, the apparent volume of distribution in L/kg will be approximately 1 L/kg (70.1 L/70 kg).

1.6 A 65-year-old female patient (60 kg) with a history of ischemic stroke was prescribed clopidogrel for stroke prevention. She was hospitalized again after 6 months due to recurrent ischemic stroke. Which of the following is a likely reason she did not respond to clopidogrel therapy? She is a:

A. Poor CYP2D6 metabolizer.

B. Fast CYP1A2 metabolizer.

C. Poor CYP2E1 metabolizer.

D. Fast CYP3A4 metabolizer.

E. Poor CYP2C19 metabolizer.

Correct answer = E. Clopidogrel is a prodrug, and it is activated by CYP2C19, which is a cytochrome P450 (CYP450) enzyme. Thus, patients who are poor CYP2C19 metabolizers have a higher incidence of cardiovascular events (for example, stroke or myocardial infarction) when taking clopidogrel.

1.7 Which of the following phase II metabolic reactions makes phase I metabolites readily excretable in urine?

A. Oxidation.

B. Reduction.

C. Glucuronidation.

D. Hydrolysis.

E. Alcohol dehydrogenation.

Correct answer = C. Many phase I metabolites are too lipophilic to be retained in the kidney tubules. A subsequent phase II conjugation reaction with an endogenous substrate, such as glucuronic acid, results in more water-soluble conjugates that excrete readily in urine.

1.8 Alkalization of urine by giving bicarbonate is used to treat patients presenting with phenobarbital (weak acid) overdose. Which of the following best describes the rationale for alkalization of urine in this setting?

A. To reduce tubular reabsorption of phenobarbital.
B. To decrease ionization of phenobarbital.
C. To increase glomerular filtration of phenobarbital.
D. To decrease proximal tubular secretion.
E. To increase tubular reabsorption of phenobarbital.

> Correct answer = A. As a general rule, weak acid drugs such as phenobarbital can be eliminated faster by alkalization of the urine. Bicarbonate alkalizes urine and keeps phenobarbital ionized, thus decreasing its reabsorption.

1.9 A drug with a half-life of 10 hours is administered by continuous intravenous infusion. Which of the following best approximates the time for the drug to reach steady state?

A. 10 hours.
B. 20 hours.
C. 33 hours.
D. 40 hours.
E. 60 hours.

> Correct answer = D. A drug will reach steady state in about four to five half-lives. Thus, for this drug with a half-life of 10 hours, the approximate time to reach steady state will be 40 hours.

1.10 A 55-year-old male patient (70 kg) is going to be treated with an experimental drug, Drug X, for an irregular heart rhythm. If the V_d is 1 L/kg and the desired steady-state plasma concentration is 2.5 mg/L, which of the following is the most appropriate intravenous loading dose for Drug X?

A. 175 mg.
B. 70 mg.
C. 28 mg.
D. 10 mg.
E. 1 mg.

> Correct answer = A. For IV infusion, Loading dose = (V_d) × (desired steady-state plasma concentration). The V_d in this case corrected to the patient's weight is 70 L. Thus, Loading dose = 70 L × 2.5 mg/L = 175 mg.

Drug–Receptor Interactions and Pharmacodynamics

2

Joanna Peris

I. OVERVIEW

Pharmacodynamics describes the actions of a drug on the body and the influence of drug concentrations on the magnitude of the response. Most drugs exert their effects, both beneficial and harmful, by interacting with receptors (that is, specialized target macromolecules) present on the cell surface or within the cell. The drug–receptor complex initiates alterations in biochemical and/or molecular activity of a cell by a process called signal transduction (Figure 2.1).

II. SIGNAL TRANSDUCTION

Drugs act as signals, and their receptors act as signal detectors. Receptors transduce their recognition of a bound agonist by initiating a series of reactions that ultimately result in a specific intracellular response. [Note: The term "agonist" refers to a naturally occurring small molecule or a drug that binds to a site on a receptor protein and activates it.] "Second messenger" or effector molecules are part of the cascade of events that translates agonist binding into a cellular response.

A. The drug–receptor complex

Cells have many different types of receptors, each of which is specific for a particular agonist and produces a unique response. Cardiac cell membranes, for example, contain β receptors that bind and respond to epinephrine or norepinephrine, as well as muscarinic receptors specific for acetylcholine. These different receptor populations dynamically interact to control the heart's vital functions.

The magnitude of the response is proportional to the number of drug–receptor complexes. This concept is closely related to the formation of complexes between enzyme and substrate or antigen and antibody. These interactions have many common features, perhaps the most noteworthy being specificity of the receptor for a given agonist. Most receptors are named for the type of agonist that interacts best with it. For example, the receptor for histamine is called a histamine receptor. Although much

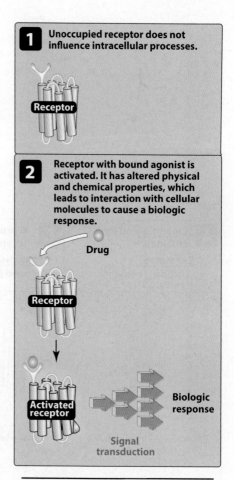

1 Unoccupied receptor does not influence intracellular processes.

Receptor

2 Receptor with bound agonist is activated. It has altered physical and chemical properties, which leads to interaction with cellular molecules to cause a biologic response.

Drug

Receptor

Activated receptor

Biologic response

Signal transduction

Figure 2.1
The recognition of a drug by a receptor triggers a biologic response.

25

of this chapter centers on the interaction of drugs with specific receptors, it is important to know that not all drugs exert their effects by interacting with a receptor. Antacids, for instance, chemically neutralize excess gastric acid, thereby reducing the symptoms of "heartburn."

B. Receptor states

Receptors exist in at least two states, inactive (R) and active (R*), that are in reversible equilibrium with one another, usually favoring the inactive state. Binding of agonists causes the equilibrium to shift from R to R* to produce a biologic effect. Antagonists occupy the receptor but do not increase the fraction of R* and may stabilize the receptor in the inactive state. Some drugs (partial agonists) cause similar shifts in equilibrium from R to R*, but the fraction of R* is less than that caused by an agonist (but still more than that caused by an antagonist). The magnitude of biological effect is directly related to the fraction of R*. Agonists, antagonists, and partial agonists are examples of ligands, or molecules that bind to the activation site on the receptor.

C. Major receptor families

Pharmacology defines a receptor as any biologic molecule to which a drug binds and produces a measurable response. Thus, enzymes, nucleic acids, and structural proteins can act as receptors for drugs or endogenous agonists. However, the richest sources of therapeutically relevant pharmacologic receptors are proteins that transduce extracellular signals into intracellular responses. These receptors may be divided into four families: 1) ligand-gated ion channels, 2) G protein–coupled receptors, 3) enzyme-linked receptors, and 4) intracellular receptors (Figure 2.2). The type of receptor a ligand interacts with

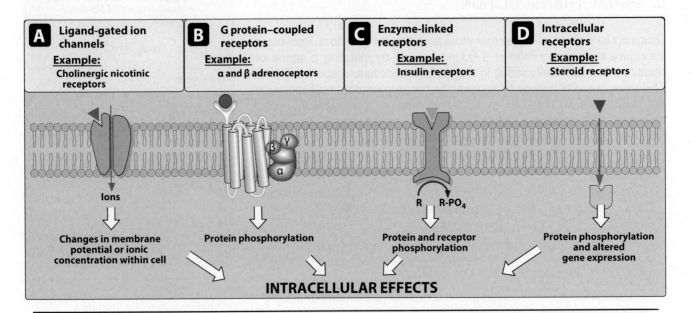

Figure 2.2

Transmembrane signaling mechanisms. **A.** Ligand binds to the extracellular domain of a ligand-gated channel. **B.** Ligand binds to a domain of a transmembrane receptor, which is coupled to a G protein. **C.** Ligand binds to the extracellular domain of a receptor that activates a kinase enzyme. **D.** Lipid-soluble ligand diffuses across the membrane to interact with its intracellular receptor. R = inactive protein.

depends on the chemical nature of the ligand. Hydrophilic ligands interact with receptors that are found on the cell surface (Figures 2.2A, B, C). In contrast, hydrophobic ligands enter cells through the lipid bilayers of the cell membrane to interact with receptors found inside cells (Figure 2.2D).

1. **Transmembrane ligand-gated ion channels:** The extracellular portion of ligand-gated ion channels usually contains the ligand-binding site. This site regulates the shape of the pore through which ions can flow across cell membranes (Figure 2.2A). The channel is usually closed until the receptor is activated by an agonist, which opens the channel briefly for a few milliseconds. Depending on the ion conducted through these channels, these receptors mediate diverse functions, including neurotransmission, and cardiac or muscle contraction. For example, stimulation of the nicotinic receptor by acetylcholine results in sodium influx and potassium outflux, generating an action potential in a neuron or contraction in skeletal muscle. On the other hand, agonist stimulation of the γ-aminobutyric acid (GABA) receptor increases chloride influx and hyperpolarization of neurons. Voltage-gated ion channels may also possess ligand-binding sites that can regulate channel function. For example, local anesthetics bind to the voltage-gated sodium channel, inhibiting sodium influx and decreasing neuronal conduction.

2. **Transmembrane G protein–coupled receptors:** The extracellular domain of this receptor contains the ligand-binding area, and the intracellular domain interacts (when activated) with a G protein or effector molecule. There are many kinds of G proteins (for example, G_s, G_i, and G_q), but they all are composed of three protein subunits. The α subunit binds guanosine triphosphate (GTP), and the β and γ subunits anchor the G protein in the cell membrane (Figure 2.3). Binding of an agonist to the receptor increases GTP binding to the α subunit, causing dissociation of the α-GTP complex from the βγ complex. These two complexes can then interact with other cellular effectors, usually an enzyme, a protein, or an ion channel, that are responsible for further actions within the cell. These responses usually last several seconds to minutes. Sometimes, the activated effectors produce second messengers that further activate other effectors in the cell, causing a signal cascade effect.

A common effector, activated by G_s and inhibited by G_i, is adenylyl cyclase, which produces the second messenger cyclic adenosine monophosphate (cAMP). G_q activates phospholipase C, generating two other second messengers: inositol 1,4,5-trisphosphate (IP_3) and diacylglycerol (DAG). DAG and cAMP activate different protein kinases within the cell, leading to a myriad of physiological effects. IP_3 regulates intracellular free calcium concentrations, as well as some protein kinases.

3. **Enzyme-linked receptors:** This family of receptors consists of a protein that may form dimers or multisubunit complexes. When activated, these receptors undergo conformational changes resulting in increased cytosolic enzyme activity, depending on

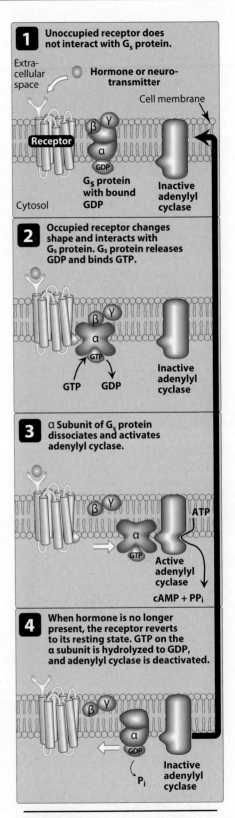

Figure 2.3
The recognition of chemical signals by G protein–coupled membrane receptors affects the activity of adenylyl cyclase. PP_i = inorganic pyrophosphate.

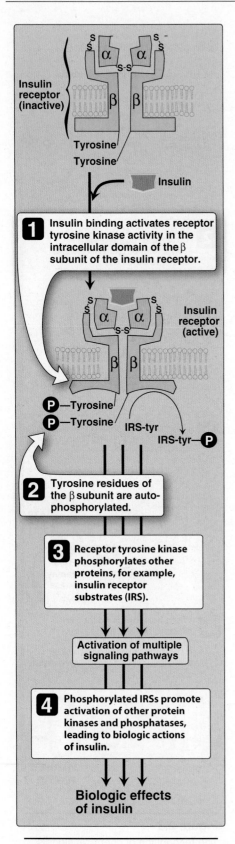

Figure 2.4
Insulin receptor.

their structure and function (Figure 2.4). This response lasts on the order of minutes to hours. The most common enzyme-linked receptors (epidermal growth factor, platelet-derived growth factor, atrial natriuretic peptide, insulin, and others) possess tyrosine kinase activity as part of their structure. The activated receptor phosphorylates tyrosine residues on itself and then other specific proteins (Figure 2.4). Phosphorylation can substantially modify the structure of the target protein, thereby acting as a molecular switch. For example, when the peptide hormone insulin binds to two of its receptor subunits, their intrinsic tyrosine kinase activity causes autophosphorylation of the receptor itself. In turn, the phosphorylated receptor phosphorylates other peptides or proteins that subsequently activate other important cellular signals. This cascade of activations results in a multiplication of the initial signal, much like that with G protein–coupled receptors.

4. **Intracellular receptors:** The fourth family of receptors differs considerably from the other three in that the receptor is entirely intracellular, and, therefore, the ligand must diffuse into the cell to interact with the receptor (Figure 2.5). In order to move across the target cell membrane, the ligand must have sufficient lipid solubility. The primary targets of these ligand–receptor complexes are transcription factors in the cell nucleus. Binding of the ligand with its receptor generally activates the receptor via dissociation from a variety of binding proteins. The activated ligand–receptor complex then translocates to the nucleus, where it often dimerizes before binding to transcription factors that regulate gene expression. The activation or inactivation of these factors causes the transcription of DNA into RNA and translation of RNA into an array of proteins. The time course of activation and response of these receptors is on the order of hours to days. For example, steroid hormones exert their action on target cells via intracellular receptors. Other targets of intracellular ligands are structural proteins, enzymes, RNA, and ribosomes. For example, tubulin is the target of antineoplastic agents such as *paclitaxel* (see Chapter 46), the enzyme dihydrofolate reductase is the target of antimicrobials such as *trimethoprim* (see Chapter 40), and the 50S subunit of the bacterial ribosome is the target of macrolide antibiotics such as *erythromycin* (see Chapter 39).

D. Some characteristics of signal transduction

Signal transduction has two important features: 1) the ability to amplify small signals and 2) mechanisms to protect the cell from excessive stimulation.

1. **Signal amplification:** A characteristic of G protein–linked and enzyme-linked receptors is their ability to amplify signal intensity and duration. For example, a single agonist–receptor complex can interact with many G proteins, thereby multiplying the original signal manyfold. Additionally, activated G proteins persist for a longer duration than does the original agonist–receptor

complex. The binding of *albuterol,* for example, may only exist for a few milliseconds, but the subsequent activated G proteins may last for hundreds of milliseconds. Further prolongation and amplification of the initial signal are mediated by the interaction between G proteins and their respective intracellular targets. Because of this amplification, only a fraction of the total receptors for a specific ligand may need to be occupied to elicit a maximal response. Systems that exhibit this behavior are said to have spare receptors. Spare receptors are exhibited by insulin receptors, where it is estimated that 99% of receptors are "spare." This constitutes an immense functional reserve that ensures that adequate amounts of glucose enter the cell. On the other hand, in the human heart, only about 5% to 10% of the total β-adrenoceptors are spare. An important implication of this observation is that little functional reserve exists in the failing heart, because most receptors must be occupied to obtain maximum contractility.

2. **Desensitization and down-regulation of receptors:** Repeated or continuous administration of an agonist (or an antagonist) may lead to changes in the responsiveness of the receptor. To prevent potential damage to the cell (for example, high concentrations of calcium, initiating cell death), several mechanisms have evolved to protect a cell from excessive stimulation. When a receptor is exposed to repeated administration of an agonist, the receptor becomes desensitized (Figure 2.6) resulting in a diminished effect. This phenomenon, called tachyphylaxis, is due to either phosphorylation or a similar chemical event that renders receptors on the cell surface unresponsive to the ligand. In addition, receptors may be down-regulated such that they are internalized and sequestered within the cell, unavailable for further agonist interaction. These receptors may be recycled to the cell surface, restoring sensitivity, or, alternatively, may be further processed and degraded, decreasing the total number of receptors available. Some receptors, particularly ion channels, require a finite time following stimulation before they can be activated again. During this recovery phase, unresponsive receptors are said to be "refractory." Similarly, repeated exposure of a receptor to an antagonist may result in up-regulation of receptors, in which receptor reserves are inserted into the membrane, increasing the total number of receptors available. Up-regulation of receptors can make the cells more sensitive to agonists and/or more resistant to the effect of the antagonist.

III. DOSE–RESPONSE RELATIONSHIPS

Agonist drugs mimic the action of the original endogenous ligand for the receptor (for example, *isoproterenol* mimics norepinephrine on β₁ receptors of the heart). The magnitude of the drug effect depends on the drug concentration at the receptor site, which, in turn, is determined by both the dose of drug administered and by the drug's pharmacokinetic profile, such as rate of absorption, distribution, metabolism, and elimination.

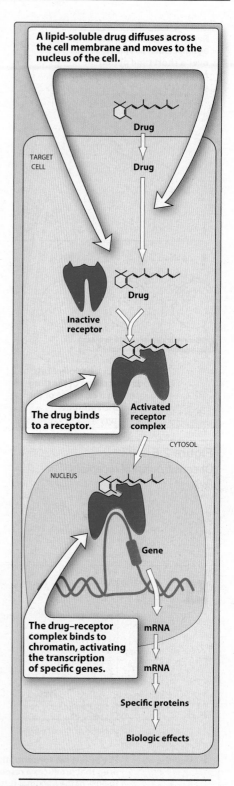

A lipid-soluble drug diffuses across the cell membrane and moves to the nucleus of the cell.

Drug

TARGET CELL

Drug

Drug

Inactive receptor

The drug binds to a receptor.

Activated receptor complex

CYTOSOL

NUCLEUS

Gene

The drug–receptor complex binds to chromatin, activating the transcription of specific genes.

mRNA

mRNA

Specific proteins

Biologic effects

Figure 2.5
Mechanism of intracellular receptors. mRNA = messenger RNA.

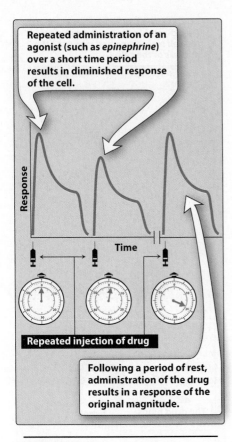

Figure 2.6
Desensitization of receptors.

A. Graded dose–response relations

As the concentration of a drug increases, its pharmacologic effect also gradually increases until all the receptors are occupied (the maximum effect). Plotting the magnitude of response against increasing doses of a drug produces a graded dose–response curve that has the general shape depicted in Figure 2.7A. The curve can be described as a rectangular hyperbola, which is a familiar curve in biology because it can be applied to diverse biological events, such as enzymatic activity, and responses to pharmacologic agents. Two important properties of drugs, potency and efficacy, can be determined by graded dose–response curves.

1. **Potency:** Potency is a measure of the amount of drug necessary to produce an effect of a given magnitude. The concentration of drug producing 50% of the maximum effect (EC_{50}) is usually used to determine potency. In Figure 2.7, the EC_{50} for Drugs A and B indicate that Drug A is more potent than Drug B, because a lesser amount of Drug A is needed when compared to Drug B to obtain 50-percent effect. Therapeutic preparations of drugs reflect their potency. For example, *candesartan* and *irbesartan* are angiotensin receptor blockers that are used to treat hypertension. The therapeutic dose range for *candesartan* is 4 to 32 mg, as compared to 75 to 300 mg for *irbesartan.* Therefore, *candesartan* is more potent than is *irbesartan* (it has a lower EC_{50} value, similar to Drug A in Figure 2.7). Since the range of drug concentrations (from 1% to 99% of the maximal response) usually spans several orders of magnitude, semilogarithmic plots are used so that the complete range of doses can be graphed. As shown in Figure 2.7B, the curves become sigmoidal in shape, which simplifies the interpretation of the dose–response curve.

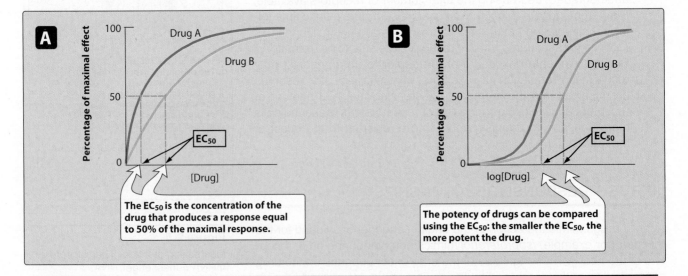

Figure 2.7
The effect of dose on the magnitude of pharmacologic response. **Panel A** is a linear graph. **Panel B** is a semilogarithmic plot of the same data. EC_{50} = drug dose causing 50% of maximal response.

2. Efficacy: Efficacy is the magnitude of response a drug causes when it interacts with a receptor. Efficacy is dependent on the number of drug–receptor complexes formed and the intrinsic activity of the drug (its ability to activate the receptor and cause a cellular response). Maximal efficacy of a drug (E_{max}) assumes that all receptors are occupied by the drug, and no increase in response is observed if a higher concentration of drug is obtained. Therefore, the maximal response differs between full and partial agonists, even when 100% of the receptors are occupied by the drug. Similarly, even though an antagonist occupies 100% of the receptor sites, no receptor activation results and E_{max} is zero. Efficacy is a more clinically useful characteristic than is drug potency, since a drug with greater efficacy is more therapeutically beneficial than is one that is more potent. Figure 2.8 shows the response to drugs of differing potency and efficacy.

B. Effect of drug concentration on receptor binding

The quantitative relationship between drug concentration and receptor occupancy applies the law of mass action to the kinetics of the binding of drug and receptor molecules:

$$\text{Drug} + \text{Receptor} \rightleftarrows \text{Drug–receptor complex} \rightarrow \text{Biologic effect}$$

By making the assumption that the binding of one drug molecule does not alter the binding of subsequent molecules and applying the law of mass action, we can mathematically express the relationship between the percentage (or fraction) of bound receptors and the drug concentration:

$$\frac{[DR]}{[R_t]} = \frac{[D]}{K_d + [D]} \qquad (1)$$

where [D] = the concentration of free drug, [DR] = the concentration of bound drug, [R_t] = the total concentration of receptors and is equal to the sum of the concentrations of unbound (free) receptors and bound receptors, and K_d = the equilibrium dissociation constant for the drug from the receptor. The value of K_d can be used to determine the affinity of a drug for its receptor. Affinity describes the strength of the interaction (binding) between a ligand and its receptor. The higher the K_d value, the weaker the interaction and the lower the affinity, and vice versa. Equation (1) defines a curve that has the shape of a rectangular hyperbola (Figure 2.9A). As the concentration of free drug increases, the ratio of the concentrations of bound receptors to total receptors approaches unity. The binding of the drug to its receptor initiates events that ultimately lead to a measurable biologic response. Thus, it is not surprising that the curves shown in Figure 2.9 and those representing the relationship between dose and effect (Figure 2.7) are similar.

C. Relationship of drug binding to pharmacologic effect

The mathematical model that describes drug concentration and receptor binding can be applied to dose (drug concentration) and response (or effect), providing the following assumptions are met: 1) The magnitude of the response is proportional to the amount of receptors bound or occupied, 2) the E_{max} occurs when all receptors are bound, and 3) binding of the drug to the receptor exhibits no cooperativity. In this case,

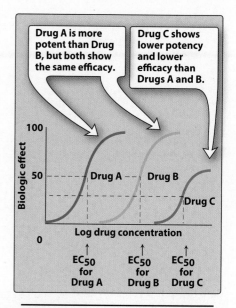

Figure 2.8
Typical dose–response curve for drugs showing differences in potency and efficacy. EC_{50} = drug dose that shows 50% of maximal response.

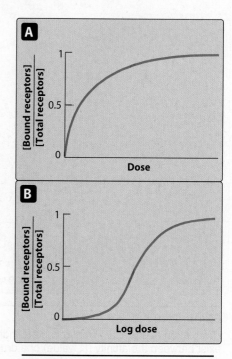

Figure 2.9
The effect of dose on the magnitude of drug binding.

$$\frac{[E]}{[E_{max}]} = \frac{[D]}{K_d + [D]} \tag{2}$$

where [E] = the effect of the drug at concentration [D] and [E_{max}] = the maximal effect of the drug.

Thus, it follows that if a specific population of receptors is vital for mediating a physiological effect, the affinity of an agonist for binding to those receptors should be related to the potency of that drug for causing that physiological effect. It should be remembered that many drugs and most neurotransmitters can bind to more than one type of receptor, thereby causing both desired therapeutic effects and undesired side effects. In order to establish a relationship between drug occupation of a particular receptor subtype and the corresponding biological response, correlation curves of receptor affinity and drug potency are often constructed (Figure 2.10).

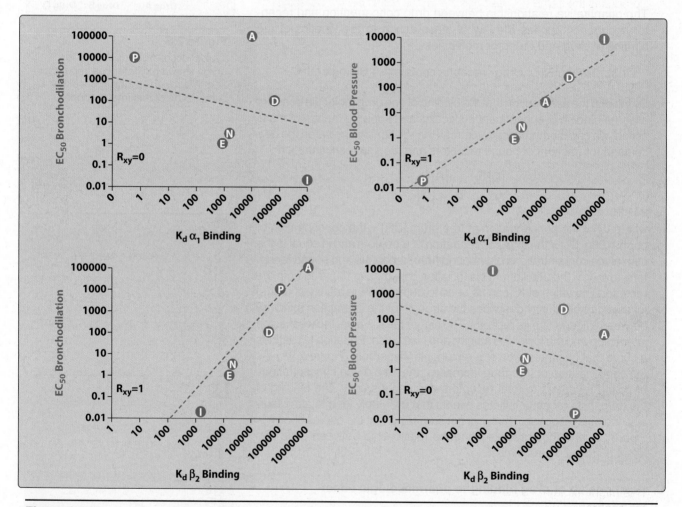

Figure 2.10

Correlation of drug affinity for receptor binding and potency for causing a physiological effect. A positive correlation should exist between the affinity (K_d value) of a drug for binding to a specific receptor subtype and the potency (EC_{50} value) of that drug to cause physiological responses mediated by that receptor population. For example, many drugs have affinity for both α_1 and β_2 adrenergic receptors. The circled letters in the figure represent agonists with varying affinities for α_1 and β_2 receptors. However, from the data provided, it becomes clear that α_1 receptors only mediate changes in blood pressure, while β_2 receptors only mediate changes in bronchodilation.

IV. INTRINSIC ACTIVITY

As mentioned above, an agonist binds to a receptor and produces a biologic response based on the concentration of the agonist and the fraction of activated receptors. The intrinsic activity of a drug determines its ability to fully or partially activate the receptors. Drugs may be categorized according to their intrinsic activity and resulting E_{max} values.

A. Full agonists

If a drug binds to a receptor and produces a maximal biologic response that mimics the response to the endogenous ligand, it is a full agonist (Figure 2.11). Full agonists bind to a receptor, stabilizing the receptor in its active state and are said to have an intrinsic activity of one. All full agonists for a receptor population should produce the same E_{max}. For example, *phenylephrine* is a full agonist at α_1-adrenoceptors, because it produces the same E_{max} as does the endogenous ligand, norepinephrine. Upon binding to α_1-adrenoceptors on vascular smooth muscle, *phenylephrine* stabilizes the receptor in its active state. This leads to the mobilization of intracellular Ca^{2+}, causing interaction of actin and myosin filaments and shortening of the muscle cells. The diameter of the arteriole decreases, causing an increase in resistance to blood flow through the vessel and an increase in blood pressure. As this brief description illustrates, an agonist may have many measurable effects, including actions on intracellular molecules, cells, tissues, and intact organisms. All of these actions are attributable to interaction of the drug with the receptor. For full agonists, the dose–response curves for receptor binding and each of the biological responses should be comparable.

B. Partial agonists

Partial agonists have intrinsic activities greater than zero but less than one (Figure 2.11). Even if all the receptors are occupied, partial agonists cannot produce the same E_{max} as a full agonist. However, a partial agonist may have an affinity that is greater than, less than, or equivalent to that of a full agonist. When a receptor is exposed to both a partial agonist and a full agonist, the partial agonist may act as an antagonist of the full agonist. Consider what would happen to the E_{max} of a receptor saturated with an agonist in the presence of increasing concentrations of a partial agonist (Figure 2.12). As the number of receptors occupied by the partial agonist increases, the E_{max} would decrease until it reached the E_{max} of the partial agonist. This potential of partial agonists to act as both an agonist and antagonist may be therapeutically utilized. For example, *aripiprazole,* an atypical antipsychotic, is a partial agonist at selected dopamine receptors. Dopaminergic pathways that are overactive tend to be inhibited by *aripiprazole*, whereas pathways that are underactive are stimulated. This might explain the ability of *aripiprazole* to improve symptoms of schizophrenia, with a small risk of causing extrapyramidal adverse effects (see Chapter 11).

C. Inverse agonists

Typically, unbound receptors are inactive and require interaction with an agonist to assume an active conformation. However, some

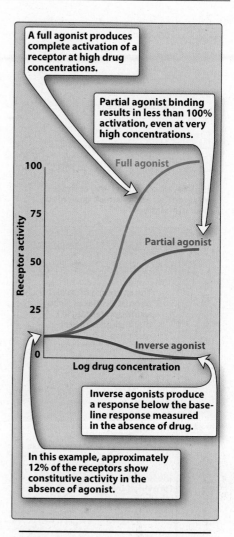

Figure 2.11
Effects of full agonists, partial agonists, and inverse agonists on receptor activity.

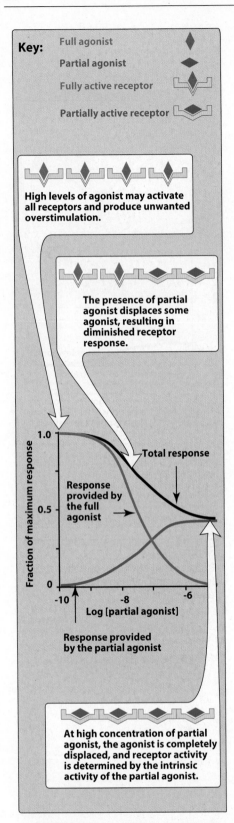

Key:

Full agonist

Partial agonist

Fully active receptor

Partially active receptor

High levels of agonist may activate all receptors and produce unwanted overstimulation.

The presence of partial agonist displaces some agonist, resulting in diminished receptor response.

Total response

Response provided by the full agonist

Response provided by the partial agonist

At high concentration of partial agonist, the agonist is completely displaced, and receptor activity is determined by the intrinsic activity of the partial agonist.

Figure 2.12
Effects of partial agonists.

receptors show a spontaneous conversion from R to R* in the absence of an agonist. Inverse agonists, unlike full agonists, stabilize the inactive R form and cause R* to convert to R. This decreases the number of activated receptors to below that observed in the absence of drug (Figure 2.11). Thus, inverse agonists have an intrinsic activity less than zero, reverse the activity of receptors, and exert the opposite pharmacological effect of agonists.

D. Antagonists

Antagonists bind to a receptor with high affinity but possess zero intrinsic activity. An antagonist has no effect in the absence of an agonist but can decrease the effect of an agonist when present. Antagonism may occur either by blocking the drug's ability to bind to the receptor or by blocking its ability to activate the receptor.

1. **Competitive antagonists:** If both the antagonist and the agonist bind to the same site on the receptor in a reversible manner, they are said to be "competitive." The competitive antagonist prevents an agonist from binding to its receptor and maintains the receptor in its inactive state. For example, the antihypertensive drug *terazosin* competes with the endogenous ligand norepinephrine at α_1-adrenoceptors, thus decreasing vascular smooth muscle tone and reducing blood pressure. However, this inhibition can be overcome by increasing the concentration of agonist relative to antagonist. Thus, competitive antagonists characteristically shift the agonist dose–response curve to the right (increased EC_{50}) without affecting E_{max} (Figure 2.13).

2. **Irreversible antagonists:** Irreversible antagonists bind covalently to the active site of the receptor, thereby reducing the number of receptors available to the agonist. An irreversible antagonist causes a downward shift of the E_{max}, with no shift of EC_{50} values (unless spare receptors are present). In contrast to competitive antagonists, the effect of irreversible antagonists cannot be overcome by adding more agonist (Figure 2.13). Thus, irreversible antagonists and allosteric antagonists (see below) are both considered noncompetitive antagonists. A fundamental difference between competitive and noncompetitive antagonists is that competitive agonists reduce agonist potency (increase EC_{50}) and noncompetitive antagonists reduce agonist efficacy (decrease E_{max}).

3. **Allosteric antagonists:** An allosteric antagonist also causes a downward shift of the E_{max}, with no change in the EC_{50} value of an agonist. This type of antagonist binds to a site ("allosteric site") other than the agonist-binding site and prevents the receptor from being activated by the agonist. An example of an allosteric agonist is picrotoxin, which binds to the inside of the GABA-controlled chloride channel. When picrotoxin is bound inside the channel, no chloride can pass through the channel, even when the receptor is fully activated by GABA.

4. **Functional antagonism:** An antagonist may act at a completely separate receptor, initiating effects that are functionally opposite those of the agonist. A classic example is the functional antagonism by epinephrine to histamine-induced bronchoconstriction. Histamine binds to H_1 histamine receptors on bronchial smooth muscle, causing

bronchoconstriction of the bronchial tree. Epinephrine is an agonist at β_2-adrenoceptors on bronchial smooth muscle, which causes the muscles to relax. This functional antagonism is also known as "physiologic antagonism."

V. QUANTAL DOSE–RESPONSE RELATIONSHIPS

Another important dose–response relationship is that between the dose of the drug and the proportion of a population that responds to it. These responses are known as quantal responses, because, for any individual, the effect either occurs or it does not. Graded responses can be transformed to quantal responses by designating a predetermined level of the graded response as the point at which a response occurs or not. For example, a quantal dose–response relationship can be determined in a population for the antihypertensive drug *atenolol*. A positive response is defined as a fall of at least 5 mm Hg in diastolic blood pressure. Quantal dose–response curves are useful for determining doses to which most of the population responds. They have similar shapes as log dose–response curves, and the ED_{50} is the drug dose that causes a therapeutic response in half of the population.

A. Therapeutic index

The therapeutic index (TI) of a drug is the ratio of the dose that produces toxicity in half the population (TD_{50}) to the dose that produces a clinically desired or effective response (ED_{50}) in half the population:

$$TI = TD_{50} / ED_{50}$$

The TI is a measure of a drug's safety, because a larger value indicates a wide margin between doses that are effective and doses that are toxic.

B. Clinical usefulness of the therapeutic index

The TI of a drug is determined using drug trials and accumulated clinical experience. These usually reveal a range of effective doses and a different (sometimes overlapping) range of toxic doses. Although high TI values are required for most drugs, some drugs with low therapeutic indices are routinely used to treat serious diseases. In these cases, the risk of experiencing side effects is not as great as the risk of leaving the disease untreated. Figure 2.14 shows the responses to *warfarin*, an oral anticoagulant with a low therapeutic index, and *penicillin*, an antimicrobial drug with a large therapeutic index.

1. **Warfarin (example of a drug with a small therapeutic index):** As the dose of *warfarin* is increased, a greater fraction of the patients respond (for this drug, the desired response is a two- to threefold increase in the international normalized ratio [INR]) until, eventually, all patients respond (Figure 2.14A). However, at higher doses of *warfarin*, anticoagulation resulting in hemorrhage occurs in a small percent of patients. Agents with a low TI (that is, drugs for which dose is critically important) are those drugs for which bioavailability critically alters the therapeutic effects (see Chapter 1).

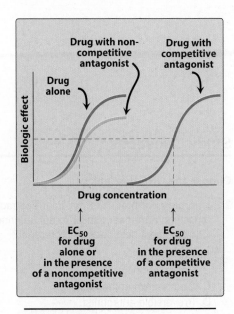

Figure 2.13
Effects of drug antagonists. EC_{50} = drug dose that shows 50% of maximal response.

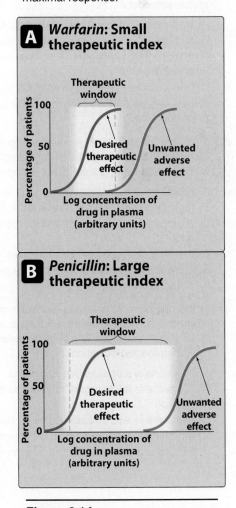

Figure 2.14
Cumulative percentage of patients responding to plasma levels of *warfarin* and *penicillin*.

2. **Penicillin (example of a drug with a large therapeutic index):** For drugs such as *penicillin* (Figure 2.14B), it is safe and common to give doses in excess of that which is minimally required to achieve a desired response without the risk of adverse side effects. In this case, bioavailability does not critically alter the therapeutic or clinical effects.

Study Questions

Choose the ONE best answer.

2.1 Isoproterenol produces maximal contraction of cardiac muscle in a manner similar to epinephrine. Which of the following best describes isoproterenol?

A. Full agonist.

B. Partial agonist.

C. Competitive antagonist.

D. Irreversible antagonist.

E. Inverse agonist.

> Correct answer = A. A full agonist has an E_{max} similar to the endogenous ligand. A partial agonist would only produce a partial effect. An antagonist would block the effects of an endogenous agonist. An inverse agonist would reverse the constitutive activity of receptors and exert the opposite pharmacological effect.

2.2 If 10 mg of naproxen produces the same analgesic response as 100 mg of ibuprofen, which of the following statements is correct?

A. Naproxen is more efficacious than is ibuprofen.

B. Naproxen is more potent than ibuprofen.

C. Naproxen is a full agonist, and ibuprofen is a partial agonist.

D. Naproxen is a competitive antagonist.

E. Naproxen is a better drug to take for pain relief than is ibuprofen.

> Correct answer = B. Without information about the maximal effect of these drugs, no conclusions can be made about efficacy or intrinsic activity. E is false because the maximal response obtained is often more important than the amount of drug needed to achieve it.

2.3 If 10 mg of morphine produces a greater analgesic response than can be achieved by ibuprofen at any dose, which of the following statements is correct?

A. Morphine is less efficacious than is ibuprofen.

B. Morphine is less potent than is ibuprofen.

C. Morphine is a full agonist, and ibuprofen is a partial agonist.

D. Ibuprofen is a competitive antagonist.

E. Morphine is a better drug to take for pain relief than is ibuprofen.

> Correct answer = E. Based on the information presented here, since morphine is more efficacious than is ibuprofen, it is going to provide more pain relief. As long as the situation warrants the necessity of such efficacious pain relief and without any information about differences in side effects caused by the two drugs, morphine is the better choice. Choice C would only be true if both drugs bound to the same receptor population, and that is not the case. The other choices are incorrect statements.

2.4 In the presence of naloxone, a higher concentration of morphine is required to elicit full pain relief. Naloxone by itself has no effect. Which of the following is correct regarding these medications?

A. Naloxone is a competitive antagonist.

B. Morphine is a full agonist, and naloxone is a partial agonist.

C. Morphine is less efficacious than is naloxone.

D. Morphine is less potent than is naloxone.

E. Naloxone is a noncompetitive antagonist.

> Correct answer = A. Since naloxone has no effect by itself, B and C are incorrect. Since it decreases the effect of an agonist but this inhibition can be overcome by giving a higher dose of morphine, naloxone must be a competitive antagonist. No information is given about potency of either drug.

2.5 In the presence of pentazocine, a higher concentration of morphine is required to elicit full pain relief. Pentazocine by itself has a smaller analgesic effect than does morphine, even at the highest dose. Which of the following is correct regarding these medications?

A. Pentazocine is a competitive antagonist.
B. Morphine is a full agonist, and pentazocine is a partial agonist.
C. Morphine is less efficacious than is pentazocine.
D. Morphine is less potent than is pentazocine.
E. Pentazocine is a noncompetitive antagonist.

Correct answer = B. Pentazocine has a lower E_{max} value than does morphine but still has some efficacy. Thus, pentazocine is a partial agonist. Even though pentazocine blocks some of the actions of morphine, since it has some efficacy, it cannot be an antagonist. No information is given about the potency of either drug.

2.6 In the presence of picrotoxin, diazepam is less efficacious at causing sedation, regardless of the dose. Picrotoxin by itself has no sedative effect even at the highest dose. Which of the following is correct?

A. Picrotoxin is a competitive antagonist.
B. Diazepam is a full agonist, and picrotoxin is a partial agonist.
C. Diazepam is less efficacious than is picrotoxin.
D. Diazepam is less potent than is picrotoxin.
E. Picrotoxin is a noncompetitive antagonist.

Correct answer = E. Picrotoxin has no efficacy alone, so B and C are false. Since it decreases the maximal effect of diazepam, it is a noncompetitive antagonist. No information is given about potency of either drug.

2.7 Which of the following statements most accurately describes a system having spare receptors?

A. The number of spare receptors determines the maximum effect.
B. Spare receptors are sequestered in the cytosol.
C. A single drug–receptor interaction results in many cellular response elements being activated.
D. Spare receptors are active even in the absence of an agonist.
E. Agonist affinity for spare receptors is less than their affinity for "non-spare" receptors.

Correct answer = C. One explanation for the existence of spare receptors is that any one agonist–receptor binding event can lead to the activation of many more cellular response elements. Thus, only a small fraction of the total receptors need to be bound to elicit a maximum cellular response. The other choices do not accurately describe spare receptor systems.

2.8 Which of the following would up-regulate postsynaptic β_1 adrenergic receptors?

A. Daily use of amphetamine that causes norepinephrine to be released.
B. A disease that causes an increase in the activity of norepinephrine neurons.
C. Daily use of isoproterenol, a β_1 receptor agonist.
D. Daily use of formoterol, a β_2 receptor agonist.
E. Daily use of propranolol, a β_1 receptor antagonist.

Correct answer = E. Up-regulation of receptors occurs when receptor activation is lower than normal, such as when the receptor is continuously exposed to an antagonist for that receptor. Down-regulation of receptor number occurs when receptor activation is greater than normal because of continuous exposure to an agonist.

The Autonomic Nervous System

3

Rajan Radhakrishnan

I. OVERVIEW

The autonomic nervous system (ANS), along with the endocrine system, coordinates the regulation and integration of bodily functions. The endocrine system sends signals to target tissues by varying the levels of blood-borne hormones. In contrast, the nervous system exerts its influence by the rapid transmission of electrical impulses over nerve fibers that terminate at effector cells, which specifically respond to the release of neuromediator substances. Drugs that produce their primary therapeutic effect by mimicking or altering the functions of the ANS are called autonomic drugs and are discussed in the following four chapters. These autonomic agents act either by stimulating portions of the ANS or by blocking the action of the autonomic nerves. This chapter outlines the fundamental physiology of the ANS and describes the role of neurotransmitters in the communication between extracellular events and chemical changes within the cell.

II. INTRODUCTION TO THE NERVOUS SYSTEM

The nervous system is divided into two anatomical divisions: the central nervous system (CNS), which is composed of the brain and spinal cord, and the peripheral nervous system, which includes neurons located outside the brain and spinal cord—that is, any nerves that enter or leave the CNS (Figure 3.1). The peripheral nervous system is subdivided into the efferent and afferent divisions. The efferent neurons carry signals away from the brain and spinal cord to the peripheral tissues, and the afferent neurons bring information from the periphery to the CNS. Afferent neurons provide sensory input to modulate the function of the efferent division through reflex arcs or neural pathways that mediate a reflex action.

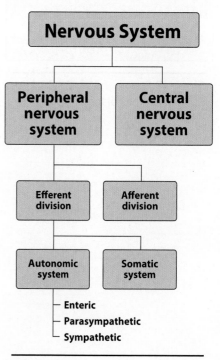

Figure 3.1
Organization of the nervous system.

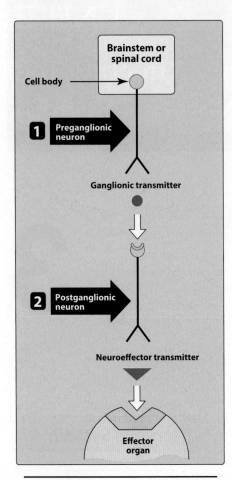

Figure 3.2
Efferent neurons of the autonomic
nervous system.

A. Functional divisions within the nervous system

The efferent portion of the peripheral nervous system is further
divided into two major functional subdivisions: the somatic and the
ANS (Figure 3.1). The somatic efferent neurons are involved in the
voluntary control of functions such as contraction of the skeletal
muscles essential for locomotion. The ANS, conversely, regulates the
everyday requirements of vital bodily functions without the conscious
participation of the mind. Because of the involuntary nature of the
ANS as well as its functions, it is also known as the visceral, vegeta-
tive, or involuntary nervous system. It is composed of efferent neurons that innervate smooth muscle of the viscera, cardiac muscle,
vasculature, and the exocrine glands, thereby controlling digestion,
cardiac output, blood flow, and glandular secretions.

B. Anatomy of the ANS

1. **Efferent neurons:** The ANS carries nerve impulses from the CNS
   to the effector organs by way of two types of efferent neurons: the
   preganglionic neurons and the postganglionic neurons (Figure 3.2).
   The cell body of the first nerve cell, the preganglionic neuron,
   is located within the CNS. The preganglionic neurons emerge
   from the brainstem or spinal cord and make a synaptic connection in ganglia (an aggregation of nerve cell bodies located in the
   peripheral nervous system). The ganglia function as relay stations
   between the preganglionic neuron and the second nerve cell, the
   postganglionic neuron. The cell body of the postganglionic neuron
   originates in the ganglion. It is generally nonmyelinated and terminates on effector organs, such as smooth muscles of the viscera,
   cardiac muscle, and the exocrine glands.

2. **Afferent neurons:** The afferent neurons (fibers) of the ANS are
   important in the reflex regulation of this system (for example, by
   sensing pressure in the carotid sinus and aortic arch) and in signaling the CNS to influence the efferent branch of the system to
   respond.

3. **Sympathetic neurons:** The efferent ANS is divided into the
   sympathetic and the parasympathetic nervous systems, as well
   as the enteric nervous system (Figure 3.1). Anatomically, the
   sympathetic and the parasympathetic neurons originate in the
   CNS and emerge from two different spinal cord regions. The preganglionic neurons of the sympathetic system come from the
   thoracic and lumbar regions (T1 to L2) of the spinal cord, and
   they synapse in two cord-like chains of ganglia that run close to
   and in parallel on each side of the spinal cord. The preganglionic neurons are short in comparison to the postganglionic ones.
   Axons of the postganglionic neuron extend from these ganglia to
   the tissues that they innervate and regulate (see Chapter 6). In
   most cases, the preganglionic nerve endings of the sympathetic
   nervous system are highly branched, enabling one preganglionic neuron to interact with many postganglionic neurons. This
   arrangement enables this division to activate numerous effector
   organs at the same time. [Note: The adrenal medulla, like the
   sympathetic ganglia, receives preganglionic fibers from the sympathetic system. The adrenal medulla, in response to stimulation

by the ganglionic neurotransmitter acetylcholine, secretes epinephrine (adrenaline), and lesser amounts of norepinephrine, directly into the blood.]

4. **Parasympathetic neurons:** The parasympathetic preganglionic fibers arise from cranial nerves III (oculomotor), VII (facial), IX (glossopharyngeal), and X (vagus), as well as from the sacral region (S2 to S4) of the spinal cord and synapse in ganglia near or on the effector organs. [Note: The vagus nerve accounts for 90% of preganglionic parasympathetic fibers in the body. Postganglionic neurons from this nerve innervate most of the organs in the thoracic and abdominal cavity.] Thus, in contrast to the sympathetic system, the preganglionic fibers are long, and the postganglionic ones are short, with the ganglia close to or within the organ innervated. In most instances, there is a one-to-one connection between the preganglionic and postganglionic neurons, enabling discrete response of this system.

5. **Enteric neurons:** The enteric nervous system is the third division of the ANS. It is a collection of nerve fibers that innervate the gastrointestinal (GI) tract, pancreas, and gallbladder, and it constitutes the "brain of the gut." This system functions independently of the CNS and controls the motility, exocrine and endocrine secretions, and microcirculation of the GI tract. It is modulated by both the sympathetic and parasympathetic nervous systems.

C. Functions of the sympathetic nervous system

Although continually active to some degree (for example, in maintaining the tone of vascular beds), the sympathetic division has the property of adjusting in response to stressful situations, such as trauma, fear, hypoglycemia, cold, and exercise (Figure 3.3).

1. **Effects of stimulation of the sympathetic division:** The effect of sympathetic output is to increase heart rate and blood pressure, to mobilize energy stores of the body, and to increase blood flow to skeletal muscles and the heart while diverting flow from the skin and internal organs. Sympathetic stimulation results in dilation of the pupils and the bronchioles (Figure 3.3). It also affects GI motility and the function of the bladder and sexual organs.

2. **Fight-or-flight response:** The changes experienced by the body during emergencies are referred to as the "fight or flight" response (Figure 3.4). These reactions are triggered both by direct sympathetic activation of the effector organs and by stimulation of the adrenal medulla to release epinephrine and lesser amounts of norepinephrine. Hormones released by the adrenal medulla directly enter the bloodstream and promote responses in effector organs that contain adrenergic receptors (see Chapter 6). The sympathetic nervous system tends to function as a unit and often discharges as a complete system, for example, during severe exercise or in reactions to fear (Figure 3.4). This system, with its diffuse distribution of postganglionic fibers, is involved in a wide array of physiologic activities. Although it is not essential for survival, it is nevertheless an important system that prepares the body to handle uncertain situations and unexpected stimuli.

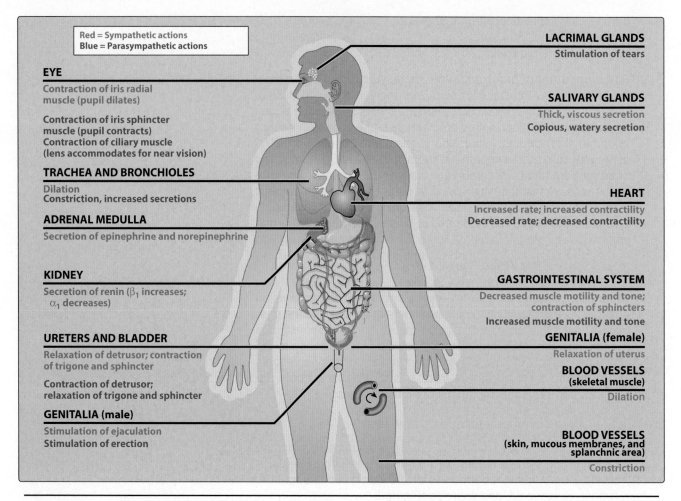

Figure 3.3
Actions of sympathetic and parasympathetic nervous systems on effector organs.

D. Functions of the parasympathetic nervous system

The parasympathetic division is involved with maintaining homeostasis within the body. It is required for life, since it maintains essential bodily functions, such as digestion and elimination of wastes. The parasympathetic division usually acts to oppose or balance the actions of the sympathetic division and generally predominates the sympathetic system in "rest-and-digest" situations. Unlike the sympathetic system, the parasympathetic system never discharges as a complete system. If it did, it would produce massive, undesirable, and unpleasant symptoms, such as involuntary urination and defecation. Instead, parasympathetic fibers innervating specific organs such as the gut, heart, or eye are activated separately, and the system functions to affect these organs individually.

E. Role of the CNS in the control of autonomic functions

Although the ANS is a motor system, it does require sensory input from peripheral structures to provide information on the current state of the body. This feedback is provided by streams of afferent impulses, originating in the viscera and other autonomically innervated structures that travel to integrating centers in the CNS, such as the hypothalamus, medulla oblongata, and spinal cord. These centers respond to the stimuli by sending out efferent reflex impulses via the ANS.

1. **Reflex arcs:** Most of the afferent impulses are involuntarily translated into reflex responses. For example, a fall in blood pressure causes pressure-sensitive neurons (baroreceptors in the heart, vena cava, aortic arch, and carotid sinuses) to send fewer impulses to cardiovascular centers in the brain. This prompts a reflex response of increased sympathetic output to the heart and vasculature and decreased parasympathetic output to the heart, which results in a compensatory rise in blood pressure and tachycardia (Figure 3.5). [Note: In each case, the reflex arcs of the ANS comprise a sensory (or afferent) arm and a motor (or efferent or effector) arm.]

2. **Emotions and the ANS:** Stimuli that evoke strong feelings, such as rage, fear, and pleasure, can modify the activities of the ANS.

F. Innervation by the ANS

1. **Dual innervation:** Most organs in the body are innervated by both divisions of the ANS. Thus, vagal parasympathetic innervation slows the heart rate, and sympathetic innervation increases the heart rate. Despite this dual innervation, one system usually predominates in controlling the activity of a given organ. For example, in the heart, the vagus nerve is the predominant factor for controlling rate. This type of antagonism is considered to be dynamic and is fine tuned continually to control homeostatic organ functions.

2. **Organs receiving only sympathetic innervation:** Although most tissues receive dual innervation, some effector organs, such as the adrenal medulla, kidney, pilomotor muscles, and sweat glands, receive innervation only from the sympathetic system.

G. Somatic nervous system

The efferent somatic nervous system differs from the ANS in that a single myelinated motor neuron, originating in the CNS, travels directly to skeletal muscle without the mediation of ganglia. As noted earlier, the somatic nervous system is under voluntary control, whereas the ANS is involuntary. Responses in the somatic division are generally faster than those in the ANS.

H. Summary of differences between sympathetic, parasympathetic, and motor nerves

Major differences in the anatomical arrangement of neurons lead to variations of the functions in each division (Figure 3.6). The sympathetic nervous system is widely distributed, innervating practically all effector systems in the body. In contrast, the distribution of the parasympathetic division is more limited. The sympathetic preganglionic fibers have a much broader influence than the parasympathetic fibers and synapse with a larger number of postganglionic fibers. This type of organization permits a diffuse discharge of the sympathetic nervous system. The parasympathetic division is more circumscribed,

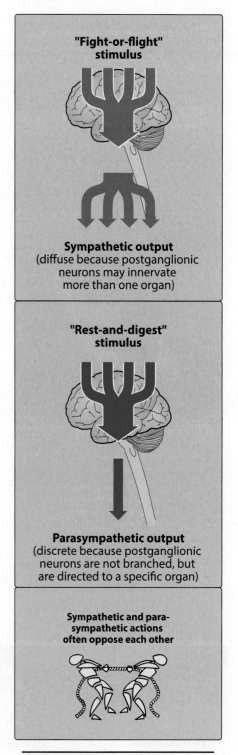

Figure 3.4
Sympathetic and parasympathetic actions are elicited by different stimuli.

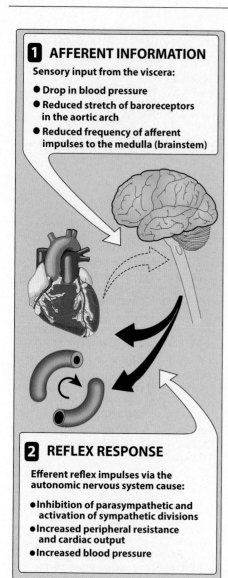

AFFERENT INFORMATION

Sensory input from the viscera:

- Drop in blood pressure
- Reduced stretch of baroreceptors in the aortic arch
- Reduced frequency of afferent impulses to the medulla (brainstem)

2 REFLEX RESPONSE

Efferent reflex impulses via the autonomic nervous system cause:

- Inhibition of parasympathetic and activation of sympathetic divisions
- Increased peripheral resistance and cardiac output
- Increased blood pressure

Figure 3.5
Baroreceptor reflex arc responds to a decrease in blood pressure.

with mostly one-to-one interactions, and the ganglia are also close to, or within, organs they innervate. This limits the amount of branching that can be done by this division. [A notable exception to this arrangement is found in the myenteric plexus, where one preganglionic neuron has been shown to interact with 8000 or more postganglionic fibers.] The anatomical arrangement of the parasympathetic system results in the distinct functions of this division. The somatic nervous system innervates skeletal muscles. One somatic motor neuron axon is highly branched, and each branch innervates a single muscle fiber. Thus, one somatic motor neuron may innervate 100 muscle fibers. This arrangement leads to the formation of a motor unit. The lack of ganglia and the myelination of the motor nerves enable a fast response by the somatic nervous system.

III. CHEMICAL SIGNALING BETWEEN CELLS

Neurotransmission in the ANS is an example of the more general process of chemical signaling between cells. In addition to neurotransmission, other types of chemical signaling include the secretion of hormones and the release of local mediators (Figure 3.7).

A. Hormones

Specialized endocrine cells secrete hormones into the bloodstream, where they travel throughout the body, exerting effects on broadly distributed target cells (see Chapters 24 through 27.)

B. Local mediators

Most cells in the body secrete chemicals that act locally on cells in the immediate environment. Because these chemical signals are rapidly destroyed or removed, they do not enter the blood and are not distributed throughout the body. Histamine (see Chapter 30) and the prostaglandins are examples of local mediators.

C. Neurotransmitters

Communication between nerve cells, and between nerve cells and effector organs, occurs through the release of specific chemical

	SYMPATHETIC	PARASYMPATHETIC
Sites of origin	Thoracic and lumbar region of the spinal cord (thoracolumbar)	Brain and sacral area of the spinal cord (craniosacral)
Length of fibers	Short preganglionic Long postganglionic	Long preganglionic Short postganglionic
Location of ganglia	Close to the spinal cord	Within or near effector organs
Preganglionic fiber branching	Extensive	Minimal
Distribution	Wide	Limited
Type of response	Diffuse	Discrete

Figure 3.6
Characteristics of the sympathetic and parasympathetic nervous systems.

signals (neurotransmitters) from the nerve terminals. This release is triggered by the arrival of the action potential at the nerve ending, leading to depolarization. An increase in intracellular Ca^{2+} initiates fusion of the synaptic vesicles with the presynaptic membrane and release of their contents. The neurotransmitters rapidly diffuse across the synaptic cleft, or space (synapse), between neurons and combine with specific receptors on the postsynaptic (target) cell.

1. **Membrane receptors:** All neurotransmitters, and most hormones and local mediators, are too hydrophilic to penetrate the lipid bilayers of target cell plasma membranes. Instead, their signal is mediated by binding to specific receptors on the cell surface of target organs. [Note: A receptor is defined as a recognition site for a substance. It has a binding specificity and is coupled to processes that eventually evoke a response. Most receptors are proteins (see Chapter 2).]

2. **Types of neurotransmitters:** Although over 50 signal molecules in the nervous system have been identified, norepinephrine (and the closely related epinephrine), acetylcholine, dopamine, serotonin, histamine, glutamate, and γ-aminobutyric acid are most commonly involved in the actions of therapeutically useful drugs. Each of these chemical signals binds to a specific family of receptors. Acetylcholine and norepinephrine are the primary chemical signals in the ANS, whereas a wide variety of neurotransmitters function in the CNS.

    a. **Acetylcholine:** The autonomic nerve fibers can be divided into two groups based on the type of neurotransmitter released. If transmission is mediated by acetylcholine, the neuron is termed cholinergic (Figure 3.8 and Chapters 4 and 5). Acetylcholine mediates the transmission of nerve impulses across autonomic ganglia in both the sympathetic and parasympathetic nervous systems. It is the neurotransmitter at the adrenal medulla. Transmission from the autonomic postganglionic nerves to the effector organs in the parasympathetic system, and a few sympathetic system organs, also involves the release of acetylcholine. In the somatic nervous system, transmission at the neuromuscular junction (the junction of nerve fibers and voluntary muscles) is also cholinergic (Figure 3.8).

    b. **Norepinephrine and epinephrine:** When norepinephrine and epinephrine are the neurotransmitters, the fiber is termed adrenergic (Figure 3.8 and Chapters 6 and 7). In the sympathetic system, norepinephrine mediates the transmission of nerve impulses from autonomic postganglionic nerves to effector organs. [Note: A few sympathetic fibers, such as those involved in sweating, are cholinergic, and, for simplicity, they are not shown in Figure 3.8.]

IV. SIGNAL TRANSDUCTION IN THE EFFECTOR CELL

The binding of chemical signals to receptors activates enzymatic processes within the cell membrane that ultimately results in a cellular response, such as the phosphorylation of intracellular proteins or

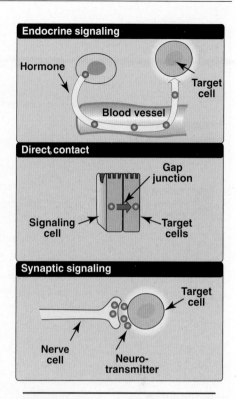

Figure 3.7
Some commonly used mechanisms for transmission of regulatory signals between cells.

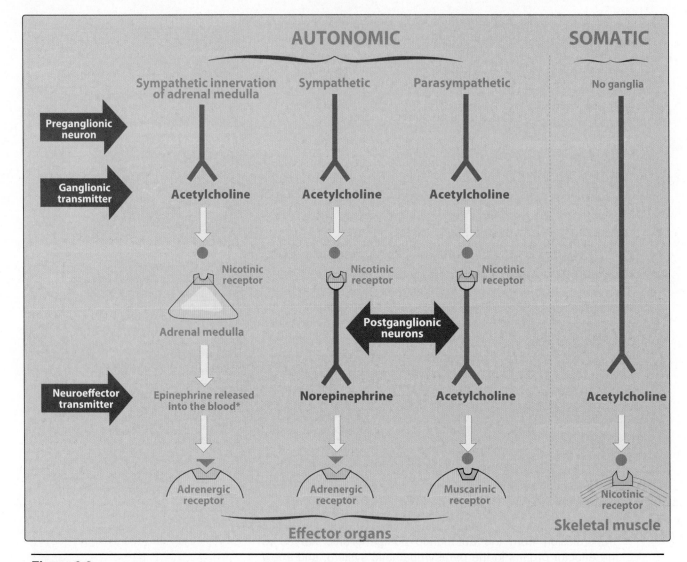

Figure 3.8
Summary of the neurotransmitters released, types of receptors, and types of neurons within the autonomic and somatic nervous systems. Cholinergic neurons are shown in red and adrenergic neurons in blue. [Note: This schematic diagram does not show that the parasympathetic ganglia are close to or on the surface of the effector organs and that the postganglionic fibers are usually shorter than the preganglionic fibers. By contrast, the ganglia of the sympathetic nervous system are close to the spinal cord. The postganglionic fibers are long, allowing extensive branching to innervate more than one organ system. This allows the sympathetic nervous system to discharge as a unit.] *Epinephrine 80% and norepinephrine 20% released from adrenal medulla.

changes in the conductivity of ion channels. A neurotransmitter can be thought of as a signal and a receptor as a signal detector and transducer. Second messenger molecules produced in response to a neurotransmitter binding to a receptor translate the extracellular signal into a response that may be further propagated or amplified within the cell. Each component serves as a link in the communication between extracellular events and chemical changes within the cell (see Chapter 2).

A. Membrane receptors affecting ion permeability (ionotropic receptors)

Neurotransmitter receptors are membrane proteins that provide a binding site that recognizes and responds to neurotransmitter molecules.

Some receptors, such as the postsynaptic nicotinic receptors in the skeletal muscle cells, are directly linked to membrane ion channels. Therefore, binding of the neurotransmitter occurs rapidly (within fractions of a millisecond) and directly affects ion permeability (Figure 3.9A). These types of receptors are known as ionotropic receptors.

B. Membrane receptors coupled to second messengers (metabotropic receptors)

Many receptors are not directly coupled to ion channels. Rather, the receptor signals its recognition of a bound neurotransmitter by initiating a series of reactions that ultimately result in a specific intracellular response. Second messenger molecules, so named because they intervene between the original message (the neurotransmitter or hormone) and the ultimate effect on the cell, are part of the cascade of events that translate neurotransmitter binding into a cellular response, usually through the intervention of a G protein. The two most widely recognized second messengers are the adenylyl cyclase system and the calcium/phosphatidylinositol system (Figure 3.9B, C). The receptors coupled to the second messenger system are known as metabotropic receptors. Muscarinic and adrenergic receptors are examples of metabotropic receptors.

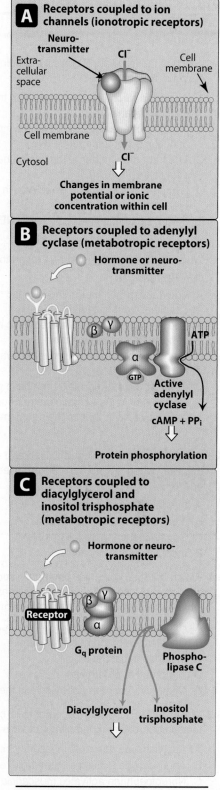

Figure 3.9
Three mechanisms whereby binding of a neurotransmitter leads to a cellular effect.

Study Questions

Choose the ONE best answer.

3.1 Which of the following is correct regarding the autonomic nervous system (ANS)?

 A. Afferent neurons carry signals from the CNS to the effector organs.

 B. The neurotransmitter at the parasympathetic ganglion is norepinephrine (NE).

 C. The neurotransmitter at the sympathetic ganglion is acetylcholine (ACh).

 D. Sympathetic neurons release ACh in the effector organs.

 E. Parasympathetic neurons release NE in the effector organs.

> Correct answer = C. The neurotransmitter at the sympathetic and parasympathetic ganglia is acetylcholine. Sympathetic neurons release NE and parasympathetic neurons release ACh in the effector cells. Afferent neurons carry signals from the periphery to the CNS.

3.2 Which of the following is correct regarding somatic motor neurons?

 A. The neurotransmitter at the somatic motor neuron ganglion is acetylcholine.

 B. The neurotransmitter at the somatic motor neuron ganglion is norepinephrine.

 C. Somatic motor neurons innervate smooth muscles.

 D. Somatic motor neurons do not have ganglia.

 E. Responses in the somatic motor neurons are generally slower than in the autonomic nervous system.

> Correct answer = D. Somatic motor neurons innervate skeletal muscles (not smooth muscle) and have no ganglia. Answers A and B are incorrect, since there are no ganglia. Also, the responses in the somatic motor nervous system are faster compared to the responses in the autonomic nervous system due to the lack of ganglia in the former.

3.3 Which of the following physiological changes could happen when a person is attacked by a grizzly bear?

 A. Increase in heart rate.

 B. Increase in lacrimation (tears).

 C. Constriction of the pupil (miosis).

 D. Increase in gastric motility.

> Correct answer = A. When a person is in the "fight-or-flight" mode, as in the case of a bear attack, the sympathetic system will be activated. Activation of the sympathetic system causes an increase in heart rate and blood pressure and a decrease (not increase) in gastric motility. It also causes dilation (not constriction) of the pupil and inhibition of lacrimation.

3.4 Which of the following changes could theoretically happen in a person when the parasympathetic system is inhibited using a pharmacological agent?

 A. Reduction in heart rate.

 B. Constriction of the pupil (miosis).

 C. Increase in gastric motility.

 D. Dry mouth (xerostomia).

 E. Contraction of detrusor muscle in the bladder.

> Correct answer = D. Activation of the parasympathetic system causes a reduction in heart rate, constriction of the pupil, an increase in gastric motility and salivation, and contraction of the bladder muscle. Therefore, inhibition of the parasympathetic system causes an increase in heart rate, dilation of the pupil, a decrease in gastric motility, dry mouth, and relaxation of detrusor muscles.

3.5 Which of the following statements is correct regarding the sympathetic and parasympathetic systems?

 A. Acetylcholine activates muscarinic receptors.

 B. Acetylcholine activates adrenergic receptors.

 C. Norepinephrine activates muscarinic receptors.

 D. Activation of the sympathetic system causes a drop in blood pressure.

> Correct answer = A. Acetylcholine is the neurotransmitter in the cholinergic system, and it activates both muscarinic and nicotinic cholinergic receptors, not adrenergic receptors. Norepinephrine activates adrenergic receptors, not muscarinic receptors. Activation of the sympathetic system causes an increase in blood pressure (not a drop in blood pressure) due to vasoconstriction and stimulation of the heart.

3.6 Which of the following statements concerning the parasympathetic nervous system is correct?

A. The parasympathetic system uses norepinephrine as a neurotransmitter.

B. The parasympathetic system often discharges as a single, functional system.

C. The parasympathetic division is involved in accommodation of near vision, movement of food, and urination.

D. The postganglionic fibers of the parasympathetic division are long compared to those of the sympathetic nervous system.

E. The parasympathetic system controls the secretion of the adrenal medulla.

Correct answer = C. The parasympathetic nervous system maintains essential bodily functions, such as vision, movement of food, and urination. It uses acetylcholine, not norepinephrine, as a neurotransmitter, and it discharges as discrete fibers that are activated separately. The postganglionic fibers of the parasympathetic system are short compared to those of the sympathetic division. The adrenal medulla is under the control of the sympathetic system.

3.7 Which of the following is correct regarding neurotransmitters and neurotransmission?

A. Neurotransmitters are released from the presynaptic nerve terminals.

B. Neurotransmitter release is triggered by the arrival of action potentials in the postsynaptic cell.

C. Intracellular calcium levels drop in the neuron before the neurotransmitter is released.

D. Serotonin and dopamine are the primary neurotransmitters in the ANS.

Correct answer = A. Neurotransmitters are released from presynaptic neurons, triggered by the arrival of an action potential in the presynaptic neuron (not in the postsynaptic cell). When an action potential arrives in the presynaptic neuron, calcium enters the presynaptic neuron and the calcium levels increase in the neuron before the neurotransmitter is released. The main neurotransmitters in the ANS are norepinephrine and acetylcholine.

3.8 An elderly man was brought to the emergency room after he ingested a large quantity of carvedilol tablets, a drug that blocks α_1, β_1, and β_2 adrenergic receptors, which mainly mediate the cardiovascular effects of epinephrine and norepinephrine in the body. Which of the following symptoms would you expect in this patient?

A. Increased heart rate (tachycardia).

B. Reduced heart rate (bradycardia).

C. Dilation of the pupil (mydriasis).

D. Increased blood pressure.

Correct answer = B. Activation of α_1 receptors causes mydriasis, vasoconstriction, and an increase in blood pressure. Activation of β_1 receptors increases heart rate, contractility of the heart, and blood pressure. Activation of β_2 receptors causes dilation of bronchioles and relaxation of skeletal muscle vessels. Thus, inhibition of these receptors will cause vasorelaxation (α_1 blockade), reduction in heart rate (β_1 blockade), reduction in contractility of the heart (β_1 blockade), reduction in blood pressure, bronchoconstriction (β_2 blockade), and constriction of blood vessels supplying skeletal muscles (β_2 blockade).

3.9 All of the following statements regarding central control of autonomic functions are correct *except*:

A. Baroreceptors are pressure sensors located at various cardiovascular sites.

B. The parasympathetic system is activated by the CNS in response to a sudden drop in blood pressure.

C. The parasympathetic system is activated by the CNS in response to a sudden increase in blood pressure.

D. The sympathetic system is activated by the CNS in response to a sudden drop in blood pressure.

Correct answer = B. When there is a sudden drop in blood pressure, the baroreceptors send signals to the brain, and the brain activates the sympathetic system (not the parasympathetic system) to restore blood pressure to normal values.

3.10 Which of the following is correct regarding membrane receptors and signal transduction?

A. ANS neurotransmitters bind to membrane receptors on the effector cells, which leads to intracellular events.

B. Cholinergic muscarinic receptors are examples of ionotropic receptors.

C. Cholinergic nicotinic receptors are examples of metabotropic receptors.

D. Metabotropic receptors activate ion channels directly.

Correct answer = A. Neurotransmitters generally bind to the membrane receptors on the postsynaptic effector cells and cause cellular effects. Acetylcholine (ACh) binds to cholinergic muscarinic receptors in the effector cells and activates the second messenger pathway in the effector cells, which in turn causes cellular events. These types of receptors that are coupled to second messenger systems are known as metabotropic receptors. Thus, metabotropic receptors do not directly activate ion channels. ACh also binds to cholinergic nicotinic receptors and activates ion channels on the effector cells directly. These types of receptors that activate ion channels directly are known as ionotropic receptors.

Cholinergic Agonists

4

Rajan Radhakrishnan

I. OVERVIEW

Drugs affecting the autonomic nervous system (ANS) are divided into two groups according to the type of neuron involved in their mechanism of action. The cholinergic drugs, which are described in this and the following chapter, act on receptors that are activated by acetylcholine (ACh), whereas the adrenergic drugs (Chapters 6 and 7) act on receptors stimulated by norepinephrine or epinephrine. Cholinergic and adrenergic drugs act by either stimulating or blocking receptors of the ANS. Figure 4.1 summarizes the cholinergic agonists discussed in this chapter.

II. THE CHOLINERGIC NEURON

The preganglionic fibers terminating in the adrenal medulla, the autonomic ganglia (both parasympathetic and sympathetic), and the postganglionic fibers of the parasympathetic division use ACh as a neurotransmitter (Figure 4.2). The postganglionic sympathetic division of sweat glands also uses acetylcholine. In addition, cholinergic neurons innervate the muscles of the somatic system and also play an important role in the central nervous system (CNS).

A. Neurotransmission at cholinergic neurons

Neurotransmission in cholinergic neurons involves six sequential steps: 1) synthesis, 2) storage, 3) release, 4) binding of ACh to a receptor, 5) degradation of the neurotransmitter in the synaptic cleft (that is, the space between the nerve endings and adjacent receptors located on nerves or effector organs), and 6) recycling of choline and acetate (Figure 4.3).

1. **Synthesis of acetylcholine:** Choline is transported from the extracellular fluid into the cytoplasm of the cholinergic neuron by an energy-dependent carrier system that cotransports sodium and can be inhibited by the drug *hemicholinium*. [Note: Choline has a quaternary nitrogen and carries a permanent positive charge and, thus, cannot diffuse through the membrane.] The uptake of choline is the rate-limiting step in ACh synthesis. Choline acetyltransferase catalyzes the reaction of choline with acetyl coenzyme A (CoA) to form ACh (an ester) in the cytosol.

DIRECT ACTING
Acetylcholine MIOCHOL-E
Bethanechol URECHOLINE
Carbachol MIOSTAT, ISOPTO CARBACHOL
Cevimeline EVOXAC
Nicotine NICORETTE
Pilocarpine SALAGEN, ISOPTO CARPINE

INDIRECT ACTING (reversible)
Ambenonium MYTELASE
Donepezil ARICEPT
Edrophonium ENLON
Galantamine RAZADYNE
Neostigmine PROSTIGMIN
Physostigmine ANTILIRIUM
Pyridostigmine MESTINON
Rivastigmine EXELON

INDIRECT ACTING (irreversible)
Echothiophate PHOSPHOLINE IODIDE

REACTIVATION OF ACETYLCHOLINESTERASE
Pralidoxime PROTOPAM

Figure 4.1
Summary of cholinergic agonists.

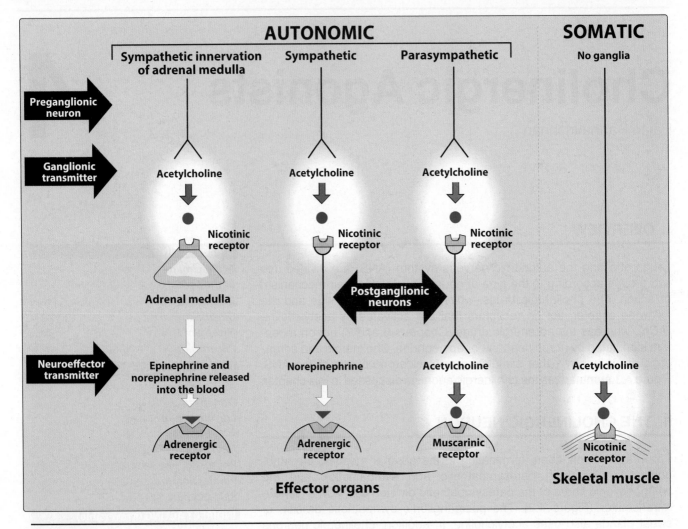

Figure 4.2
Sites of actions of cholinergic agonists in the autonomic and somatic nervous systems.

2. **Storage of acetylcholine in vesicles:** ACh is packaged and stored into presynaptic vesicles by an active transport process coupled to the efflux of protons. The mature vesicle contains not only ACh but also adenosine triphosphate and proteoglycan. Cotransmission from autonomic neurons is the rule rather than the exception. This means that most synaptic vesicles contain the primary neurotransmitter (here, ACh) as well as a cotransmitter that increases or decreases the effect of the primary neurotransmitter.

3. **Release of acetylcholine:** When an action potential propagated by voltage-sensitive sodium channels arrives at a nerve ending, voltage-sensitive calcium channels on the presynaptic membrane open, causing an increase in the concentration of intracellular calcium. Elevated calcium levels promote the fusion of synaptic vesicles with the cell membrane and the release of their contents into the synaptic space. This release can be blocked by botulinum toxin. In contrast, the toxin in black widow spider venom causes all the ACh stored in synaptic vesicles to empty into the synaptic gap.

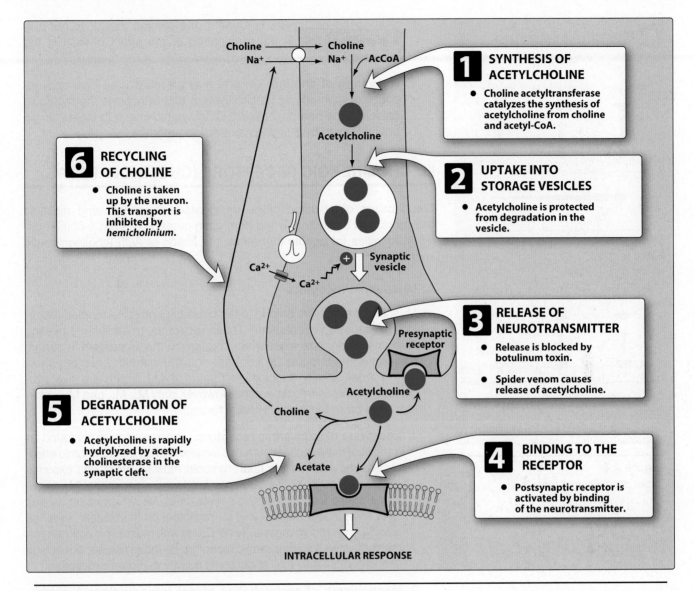

Figure 4.3
Synthesis and release of acetylcholine from the cholinergic neuron. AcCoA = acetyl coenzyme A.

4. **Binding to the receptor:** ACh released from the synaptic vesicles diffuses across the synaptic space and binds to postsynaptic receptors on the target cell, to presynaptic receptors on the membrane of the neuron that released the ACh, or to other targeted presynaptic receptors. The postsynaptic cholinergic receptors on the surface of the effector organs are divided into two classes: muscarinic and nicotinic (Figure 4.2). Binding to a receptor leads to a biologic response within the cell, such as the initiation of a nerve impulse in a postganglionic fiber or activation of specific enzymes in effector cells, as mediated by second messenger molecules.

5. **Degradation of acetylcholine:** The signal at the postjunctional effector site is rapidly terminated, because acetylcholinesterase (AChE) cleaves ACh to choline and acetate in the synaptic cleft (Figure 4.3). [Note: Butyrylcholinesterase, sometimes called

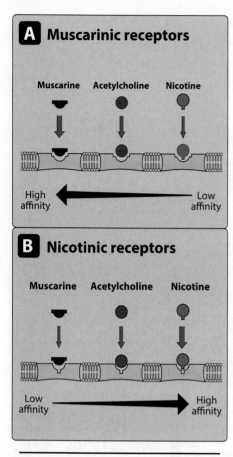

A **Muscarinic receptors**

Muscarine   Acetylcholine   Nicotine

High affinity ← Low affinity

B **Nicotinic receptors**

Muscarine   Acetylcholine   Nicotine

Low affinity → High affinity

Figure 4.4
Types of cholinergic receptors.

pseudocholinesterase, is found in the plasma, but does not play a significant role in the termination of the effect of ACh in the synapse.]

6. **Recycling of choline:** Choline may be recaptured by a sodium-coupled, high-affinity uptake system that transports the molecule back into the neuron. There, it is acetylated into ACh that is stored until released by a subsequent action potential.

III. CHOLINERGIC RECEPTORS (CHOLINOCEPTORS)

Two families of cholinoceptors, designated muscarinic and nicotinic receptors, can be distinguished from each other on the basis of their different affinities for agents that mimic the action of ACh (cholinomimetic agents).

A. Muscarinic receptors

Muscarinic receptors belong to the class of G protein–coupled receptors (metabotropic receptors). These receptors, in addition to binding ACh, also recognize muscarine, an alkaloid that is present in certain poisonous mushrooms. In contrast, the muscarinic receptors show only a weak affinity for nicotine (Figure 4.4A). There are five subclasses of muscarinic receptors. However, only M_1, M_2, and M_3 receptors have been functionally characterized.

1. **Locations of muscarinic receptors:** These receptors are found on ganglia of the peripheral nervous system and on the autonomic effector organs, such as the heart, smooth muscle, brain, and exocrine glands. Although all five subtypes are found on neurons, M_1 receptors are also found on gastric parietal cells, M_2 receptors on cardiac cells and smooth muscle, and M_3 receptors on the bladder, exocrine glands, and smooth muscle. [Note: Drugs with muscarinic actions preferentially stimulate muscarinic receptors on these tissues, but at high concentration, they may show some activity at nicotinic receptors.]

2. **Mechanisms of acetylcholine signal transduction:** A number of different molecular mechanisms transmit the signal generated by ACh occupation of the receptor. For example, when M_1 or M_3 receptors are activated, the receptor undergoes a conformational change and interacts with a G protein, designated G_q, that in turn activates phospholipase C. This ultimately leads to the production of the second messengers inositol-1,4,5-trisphosphate (IP_3) and diacylglycerol (DAG). IP_3 causes an increase in intracellular Ca^{2+}. Calcium can then interact to stimulate or inhibit enzymes or to cause hyperpolarization, secretion, or contraction. Diacylglycerol activates protein kinase C, an enzyme that phosphorylates numerous proteins within the cell. In contrast, activation of the M_2 subtype on the cardiac muscle stimulates a G protein, designated G_i, that inhibits adenylyl cyclase and increases K^+ conductance. The heart responds with a decrease in rate and force of contraction.

3. **Muscarinic agonists:** *Pilocarpine* is an example of a nonselective muscarinic agonist used in clinical practice to treat xerostomia and glaucoma. Attempts are currently underway to develop muscarinic

agonists and antagonists that are directed against specific receptor subtypes. M_1 receptor agonists are being investigated for the treatment of Alzheimer's disease and M_3 receptor antagonists for the treatment of chronic obstructive pulmonary disease. [Note: At present, no clinically important agents interact solely with the M_4 and M_5 receptors.]

B. Nicotinic receptors

These receptors, in addition to binding ACh, also recognize nicotine but show only a weak affinity for muscarine (Figure 4.4B). The nicotinic receptor is composed of five subunits, and it functions as a ligand-gated ion channel. Binding of two ACh molecules elicits a conformational change that allows the entry of sodium ions, resulting in the depolarization of the effector cell. Nicotine at low concentration stimulates the receptor, whereas nicotine at high concentration blocks the receptor. Nicotinic receptors are located in the CNS, the adrenal medulla, autonomic ganglia, and the neuromuscular junction (NMJ) in skeletal muscles. Those at the NMJ are sometimes designated N_M, and the others, N_N. The nicotinic receptors of autonomic ganglia differ from those of the NMJ. For example, ganglionic receptors are selectively blocked by *mecamylamine*, whereas NMJ receptors are specifically blocked by *atracurium*.

IV. DIRECT-ACTING CHOLINERGIC AGONISTS

Cholinergic agonists mimic the effects of ACh by binding directly to cholinoceptors (muscarinic or nicotinic). These agents may be broadly classified into two groups: 1) endogenous choline esters, which include ACh and synthetic esters of choline, such as *carbachol* and *bethanechol*, and 2) naturally occurring alkaloids, such as *nicotine* and *pilocarpine* (Figure 4.5). All of the direct-acting cholinergic drugs have a longer duration of action than ACh. The more therapeutically useful drugs (*pilocarpine* and *bethanechol*) preferentially bind to muscarinic receptors and are sometimes referred to as muscarinic agents. [Note: Muscarinic receptors are located primarily, but not exclusively, at the neuroeffector junction of the parasympathetic nervous system.] However, as a group, the direct-acting agonists show little specificity in their actions, which limits their clinical usefulness.

A. Acetylcholine

Acetylcholine [ah-see-teel-KOE-leen] is a quaternary ammonium compound that cannot penetrate membranes. Although it is the neurotransmitter of parasympathetic and somatic nerves as well as autonomic ganglia, it lacks therapeutic importance because of its multiplicity of actions (leading to diffuse effects) and its rapid inactivation by the cholinesterases. ACh has both muscarinic and nicotinic activity. Its actions include the following:

1. **Decrease in heart rate and cardiac output:** The actions of ACh on the heart mimic the effects of vagal stimulation. For example, if injected intravenously, ACh produces a brief decrease in cardiac rate (negative chronotropy) and stroke volume as a result

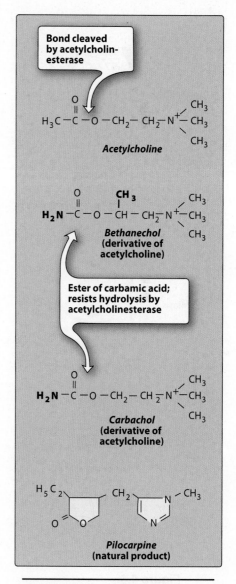

Figure 4.5
Comparison of the structures of some cholinergic agonists.

of a reduction in the rate of firing at the sinoatrial (SA) node. [Note: Normal vagal activity regulates the heart by the release of ACh at the SA node.]

2. **Decrease in blood pressure:** Injection of ACh causes vasodilation and lowering of blood pressure by an indirect mechanism of action. ACh activates M_3 receptors found on endothelial cells lining the smooth muscles of blood vessels. This results in the production of nitric oxide from arginine. Nitric oxide then diffuses to vascular smooth muscle cells to stimulate protein kinase G production, leading to hyperpolarization and smooth muscle relaxation via phosphodiesterase-3 inhibition. In the absence of administered cholinergic agents, the vascular cholinergic receptors have no known function, because ACh is never released into the blood in significant quantities. *Atropine* blocks these muscarinic receptors and prevents ACh from producing vasodilation.

3. **Other actions:** In the gastrointestinal (GI) tract, acetylcholine increases salivary secretion and stimulates intestinal secretions and motility. It also enhances bronchiolar secretions. In the genitourinary tract, ACh increases the tone of the detrusor muscle, causing urination. In the eye, ACh is involved in stimulation of ciliary muscle contraction for near vision and in the constriction of the pupillae sphincter muscle, causing miosis (marked constriction of the pupil). ACh (1% solution) is instilled into the anterior chamber of the eye to produce miosis during ophthalmic surgery.

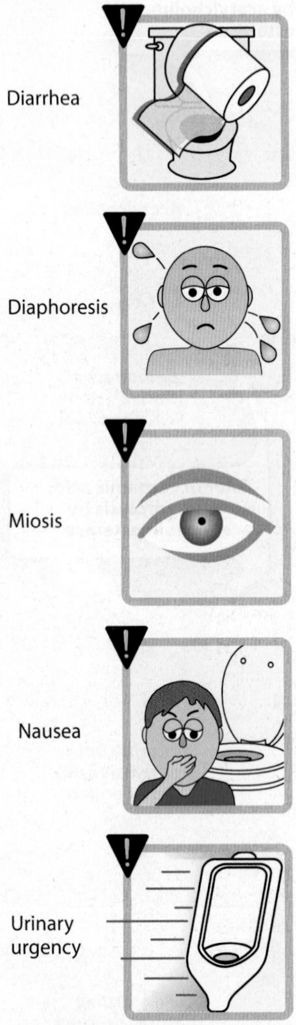

B. Bethanechol

Bethanechol [be-THAN-e-kole] is an unsubstituted carbamoyl ester, structurally related to ACh (Figure 4.5). It is not hydrolyzed by AChE due to the esterification of carbamic acid, although it is inactivated through hydrolysis by other esterases. It lacks nicotinic actions (due to the addition of the methyl group) but does have strong muscarinic activity. Its major actions are on the smooth musculature of the bladder and GI tract. It has about a 1-hour duration of action.

1. **Actions:** *Bethanechol* directly stimulates muscarinic receptors, causing increased intestinal motility and tone. It also stimulates the detrusor muscle of the bladder, whereas the trigone and sphincter muscles are relaxed. These effects produce urination.

2. **Therapeutic applications:** In urologic treatment, *bethanechol* is used to stimulate the atonic bladder, particularly in postpartum or postoperative, nonobstructive urinary retention. *Bethanechol* may also be used to treat neurogenic atony as well as megacolon.

3. **Adverse effects:** *Bethanechol* causes the effects of generalized cholinergic stimulation (Figure 4.6). These include sweating, salivation, flushing, decreased blood pressure, nausea, abdominal pain, diarrhea, and bronchospasm. *Atropine sulfate* may be administered to overcome severe cardiovascular or bronchoconstrictor responses to this agent.

Diarrhea

Diaphoresis

Miosis

Nausea

Urinary urgency

Figure 4.6
Some adverse effects observed with cholinergic agonists.

C. Carbachol (carbamylcholine)

Carbachol [KAR-ba-kole] has both muscarinic and nicotinic actions. Like *bethanechol*, *carbachol* is an ester of carbamic acid (Figure 4.5) and a poor substrate for AChE. It is biotransformed by other esterases, but at a much slower rate.

1. **Actions:** *Carbachol* has profound effects on both the cardiovascular and GI systems because of its ganglion-stimulating activity, and it may first stimulate and then depress these systems. It can cause release of epinephrine from the adrenal medulla by its nicotinic action. Locally instilled into the eye, it mimics the effects of ACh, causing miosis and a spasm of accommodation in which the ciliary muscle of the eye remains in a constant state of contraction.

2. **Therapeutic uses:** Because of its high potency, receptor nonselectivity, and relatively long duration of action, *carbachol* is rarely used therapeutically except in the eye as a miotic agent to treat glaucoma by causing pupillary contraction and a decrease in intraocular pressure.

3. **Adverse effects:** At doses used ophthalmologically, little or no side effects occur due to lack of systemic penetration (quaternary amine).

D. Pilocarpine

The alkaloid *pilocarpine* [pye-loe-KAR-peen] is a tertiary amine and is stable to hydrolysis by AChE (Figure 4.5). Compared with ACh and its derivatives, it is far less potent but is uncharged and can penetrate the CNS at therapeutic doses. *Pilocarpine* exhibits muscarinic activity and is used primarily in ophthalmology.

1. **Actions:** Applied topically to the eye, *pilocarpine* produces rapid miosis and contraction of the ciliary muscle. When the eye undergoes this miosis, it experiences a spasm of accommodation. The vision becomes fixed at some particular distance, making it impossible to focus (Figure 4.7). [Note the opposing effects of *atropine*, a muscarinic blocker, on the eye.] *Pilocarpine* is one of the most potent stimulators of secretions such as sweat, tears, and saliva, but its use for producing these effects has been limited due to its lack of selectivity. The drug is beneficial in promoting salivation in patients with xerostomia resulting from irradiation of the head and neck. Sjögren syndrome, which is characterized by dry mouth and lack of tears, is treated with oral *pilocarpine* tablets and *cevimeline,* a cholinergic drug that also has the drawback of being nonspecific.

2. **Therapeutic use in glaucoma:** *Pilocarpine* is used to treat glaucoma and is the drug of choice for emergency lowering of intraocular pressure of both open-angle and angle-closure glaucoma. *Pilocarpine* is extremely effective in opening the trabecular meshwork around the Schlemm canal, causing an immediate drop in intraocular pressure as a result of the increased drainage of aqueous humor. This action occurs within a few minutes, lasts 4 to 8 hours, and can be repeated. [Note: Topical carbonic anhydrase inhibitors, such as *dorzolamide* and β-adrenergic blockers such as *timolol*, are effective in treating glaucoma but are not used for

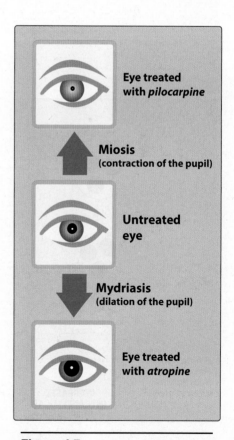

Figure 4.7
Actions of *pilocarpine* and *atropine* on the iris and ciliary muscle of the eye.

emergency lowering of intraocular pressure.] The miotic action of *pilocarpine* is also useful in reversing mydriasis due to *atropine*.

3. **Adverse effects:** *Pilocarpine* can cause blurred vision, night blindness, and brow ache. Poisoning with this agent is characterized by exaggeration of various parasympathetic effects, including profuse sweating (diaphoresis) and salivation. The effects are similar to those produced by consumption of mushrooms of the genus *Inocybe*. Parenteral *atropine*, at doses that can cross the blood–brain barrier, is administered to counteract the toxicity of *pilocarpine*.

V. INDIRECT-ACTING CHOLINERGIC AGONISTS: ANTICHOLINESTERASE AGENTS (REVERSIBLE)

AChE is an enzyme that specifically cleaves ACh to acetate and choline and, thus, terminates its actions. It is located both pre- and postsynaptically in the nerve terminal where it is membrane bound. Inhibitors of AChE (anticholinesterase agents or cholinesterase inhibitors) indirectly provide a cholinergic action by preventing the degradation of ACh. This results in an accumulation of ACh in the synaptic space (Figure 4.8). Therefore, these drugs can provoke a response at all cholinoceptors in the body, including both muscarinic and nicotinic receptors of the ANS, as well as at the NMJ and in the brain. The reversible AChE inhibitors can be broadly classified as short-acting or intermediate-acting agents.

A. Edrophonium

Edrophonium [ed-row-FOE-nee-um] is the prototype short-acting AChE inhibitor. *Edrophonium* binds reversibly to the active center of AChE, preventing hydrolysis of ACh. It is rapidly absorbed and has a short duration of action of 10 to 20 minutes due to rapid renal elimination. *Edrophonium* is a quaternary amine, and its actions are limited to the periphery. It is used in the diagnosis of myasthenia gravis, an autoimmune disease caused by antibodies to the nicotinic receptor at the NMJ. This causes their degradation, making fewer receptors available for interaction with ACh. Intravenous injection of *edrophonium* leads to a rapid increase in muscle strength. Care must be taken, because excess drug may provoke a cholinergic crisis (*atropine* is the antidote). *Edrophonium* may also be used to assess cholinesterase inhibitor therapy, for differentiating cholinergic and myasthenic crises, and for reversing the effects of nondepolarizing neuromuscular blockers after surgery. Due to the availability of other agents, *edrophonium* use has become limited.

B. Physostigmine

Physostigmine [fi-zoe-STIG-meen] is a nitrogenous carbamic acid ester found naturally in plants and is a tertiary amine. It is a substrate for AChE, and it forms a relatively stable carbamoylated intermediate with the enzyme, which then becomes reversibly inactivated. The result is potentiation of cholinergic activity throughout the body.

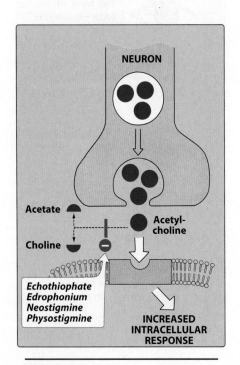

Figure 4.8
Mechanisms of action of indirect cholinergic agonists.

1. **Actions:** *Physostigmine* has a wide range of effects as a result of its action and stimulates not only the muscarinic and nicotinic sites of the ANS but also the nicotinic receptors of the NMJ. Its duration of action is about 30 minutes to 2 hours, and it is considered an intermediate-acting agent. *Physostigmine* can enter and stimulate the cholinergic sites in the CNS.

2. **Therapeutic uses:** The drug increases intestinal and bladder motility, which serves as its therapeutic action in atony of either organ (Figure 4.9). *Physostigmine* is also used in the treatment of overdoses of drugs with anticholinergic actions, such as *atropine.*

3. **Adverse effects:** The effects of *physostigmine* on the CNS may lead to convulsions when high doses are used. Bradycardia and a fall in cardiac output may also occur. Inhibition of AChE at the skeletal NMJ causes the accumulation of ACh and, ultimately, results in paralysis of skeletal muscle. However, these effects are rarely seen with therapeutic doses.

C. Neostigmine

Neostigmine [nee-oh-STIG-meen] is a synthetic compound that is also a carbamic acid ester, and it reversibly inhibits AChE in a manner similar to that of *physostigmine.*

1. **Actions:** Unlike *physostigmine, neostigmine* has a quaternary nitrogen. Therefore, it is more polar, is absorbed poorly from the GI tract, and does not enter the CNS. Its effect on skeletal muscle is greater than that of *physostigmine*, and it can stimulate contractility before it paralyzes. *Neostigmine* has an intermediate duration of action, usually 30 minutes to 2 hours.

2. **Therapeutic uses:** It is used to stimulate the bladder and GI tract and also as an antidote for competitive neuromuscular-blocking agents. *Neostigmine* is also used to manage symptoms of myasthenia gravis.

3. **Adverse effects:** Adverse effects of *neostigmine* include those of generalized cholinergic stimulation, such as salivation, flushing, decreased blood pressure, nausea, abdominal pain, diarrhea, and bronchospasm. *Neostigmine* does not cause CNS side effects and is not used to overcome toxicity of central-acting antimuscarinic agents such as *atropine. Neostigmine* is contraindicated when intestinal or urinary bladder obstruction is present.

D. Pyridostigmine and ambenonium

Pyridostigmine [peer-id-oh-STIG-meen] and *ambenonium* [am-be-NOE-nee-um] are other cholinesterase inhibitors that are used in the chronic management of myasthenia gravis. Their durations of action are intermediate (3 to 6 hours and 4 to 8 hours, respectively) but longer than that of *neostigmine.* Adverse effects of these agents are similar to those of *neostigmine.*

E. Tacrine, donepezil, rivastigmine, and galantamine

Patients with Alzheimer's disease have a deficiency of cholinergic neurons in the CNS. This observation led to the development of

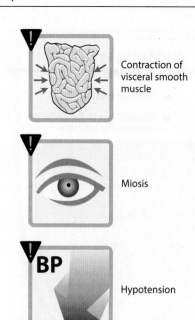

Contraction of visceral smooth muscle

Miosis

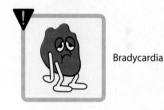

Hypotension

Bradycardia

Figure 4.9
Some actions of *physostigmine.*

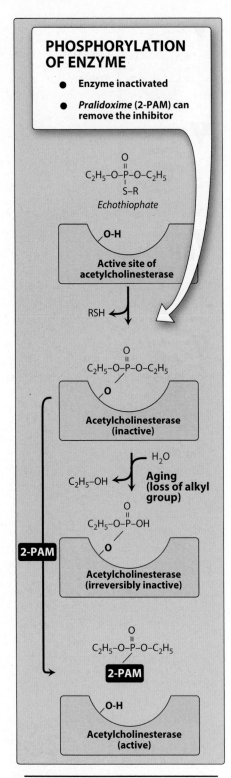

PHOSPHORYLATION OF ENZYME

- **Enzyme inactivated**
- *Pralidoxime* (**2-PAM**) can remove the inhibitor

$$C_2H_5-O-\overset{\overset{\textstyle O}{\|}}{P}-O-C_2H_5$$
$$|$$
$$S-R$$
Echothiophate

O-H

Active site of acetylcholinesterase

RSH

$$C_2H_5-O-\overset{\overset{\textstyle O}{\|}}{P}-O-C_2H_5$$
$$|$$
$$O$$

Acetylcholinesterase (inactive)

H₂O

Aging (loss of alkyl group)

C_2H_5-OH

$$C_2H_5-O-\overset{\overset{\textstyle O}{\|}}{P}-OH$$
$$|$$
$$O$$

2-PAM

Acetylcholinesterase (irreversibly inactive)

$$C_2H_5-O-\overset{\overset{\textstyle O}{\|}}{P}-O-C_2H_5$$

2-PAM

O-H

Acetylcholinesterase (active)

Figure 4.10
Covalent modification of acetylcholinesterase by *echothiophate*. Also shown is the reactivation of the enzyme with *pralidoxime*. R = $(CH_3)_3N^+-CH_2-CH_2-$; RSH = $(CH_3)_3N^+-CH_2-CH_2-S-H$.

anticholinesterases as possible remedies for the loss of cognitive function. *Tacrine* [TAK-reen] was the first to become available, but it has been replaced by others because of its hepatotoxicity. Despite the ability of *donepezil* [doe-NEP-e-zil], *rivastigmine* [ri-va-STIG-meen], and *galantamine* [ga-LAN-ta-meen] to delay the progression of Alzheimer's disease, none can stop its progression. GI distress is their primary adverse effect (see Chapter 8).

VI. INDIRECT-ACTING CHOLINERGIC AGONISTS: ANTICHOLINESTERASE AGENTS (IRREVERSIBLE)

A number of synthetic organophosphate compounds have the capacity to bind covalently to AChE. The result is a long-lasting increase in ACh at all sites where it is released. Many of these drugs are extremely toxic and were developed by the military as nerve agents. Related compounds, such as *parathion* and *malathion*, are used as insecticides.

A. Echothiophate

1. **Mechanism of action:** *Echothiophate* [ek-oe-THI-oh-fate] is an organophosphate that covalently binds via its phosphate group at the active site of AChE (Figure 4.10). Once this occurs, the enzyme is permanently inactivated, and restoration of AChE activity requires the synthesis of new enzyme molecules. Following covalent modification of AChE, the phosphorylated enzyme slowly releases one of its ethyl groups. The loss of an alkyl group, which is called aging, makes it impossible for chemical reactivators, such as *pralidoxime*, to break the bond between the remaining drug and the enzyme.

2. **Actions:** Actions include generalized cholinergic stimulation, paralysis of motor function (causing breathing difficulties), and convulsions. *Echothiophate* produces intense miosis and, thus, has found therapeutic use. Intraocular pressure falls from the facilitation of outflow of aqueous humor. *Atropine* in high dosages can reverse many of the peripheral and some of the central muscarinic effects of *echothiophate*.

3. **Therapeutic uses:** A topical ophthalmic solution of the drug is available for the treatment of open-angle glaucoma. However, *echothiophate* is rarely used due to its side effect profile, which includes the risk of causing cataracts. Figure 4.11 summarizes the actions of some of the cholinergic agonists.

VII. TOXICOLOGY OF ANTICHOLINESTERASE AGENTS

Irreversible AChE inhibitors (mostly organophosphate compounds) are commonly used as agricultural insecticides in the United States, which has led to numerous cases of accidental poisoning with these agents. In addition, they are frequently used for suicidal and homicidal purposes. Organophosphate nerve gases such as sarin are used as agents of warfare and chemical terrorism. Toxicity with these agents is manifested as nicotinic and muscarinic signs and symptoms (cholinergic crisis). Depending on the agent, the effects can be peripheral or can affect the whole body.

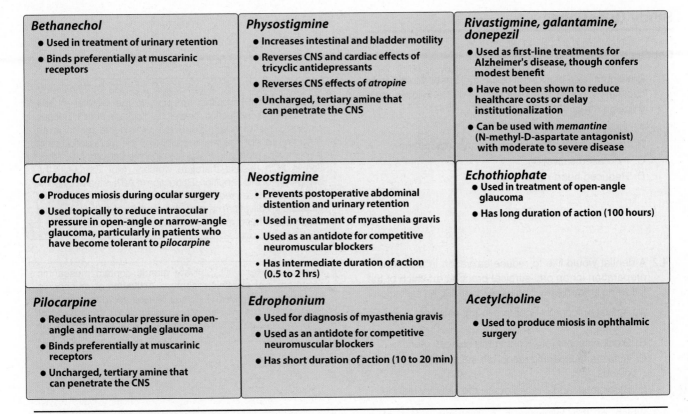

Figure 4.11
Summary of actions of some cholinergic agonists. CNS = central nervous system.

A. Reactivation of acetylcholinesterase

Pralidoxime [pral-i-DOX-eem] (2-PAM) can reactivate inhibited AChE. However, it is unable to penetrate into the CNS and therefore is not useful in treating the CNS effects of organophosphates. The presence of a charged group allows it to approach an anionic site on the enzyme, where it essentially displaces the phosphate group of the organophosphate and regenerates the enzyme. If given before aging of the alkylated enzyme occurs, it can reverse both muscarinic and nicotinic peripheral effects of organophosphates, but not the CNS effects. With the newer nerve agents that produce aging of the enzyme complex within seconds, *pralidoxime* is less effective. *Pralidoxime* is a weak AChE inhibitor and, at higher doses, may cause side effects similar to other AChE inhibitors (Figures 4.6 and 4.9). In addition, it cannot overcome toxicity of reversible AChE inhibitors (for example, *physostigmine*).

B. Other treatments

Atropine is administered to prevent muscarinic side effects of these agents. Such effects include increased bronchial and salivary secretion, bronchoconstriction, and bradycardia. *Diazepam* is also administered to reduce the persistent convulsion caused by these agents. General supportive measures, such as maintenance of patent airway, oxygen supply, and artificial respiration, may be necessary as well.

Study Questions

Choose the ONE best answer.

4.1 Botulinum toxin blocks the release of acetylcholine from cholinergic nerve terminals. Which of the following is a possible effect of botulinum toxin?

A. Skeletal muscle paralysis.
B. Improvement of myasthenia gravis symptoms.
C. Increased salivation.
D. Reduced heart rate.

Correct answer = A. Acetylcholine released by cholinergic neurons acts on nicotinic receptors in the skeletal muscle cells to cause contraction. Therefore, blockade of ACh release causes skeletal muscle paralysis. Myasthenia gravis is an autoimmune disease where antibodies are produced against nicotinic receptors and inactivate nicotinic receptors. A reduction in ACh release therefore worsens (not improves) the symptoms of this condition. Reduction in ACh release by botulinum toxin causes reduction in secretions including saliva (not increase in salivation) causing dry mouth and an increase (not reduction) in heart rate due to reduced vagal activity.

4.2 A dentist would like to reduce salivation in a patient in preparation for an oral surgical procedure. Which of the following strategies will be useful in reducing salivation?

A. Activate nicotinic receptors in the salivary glands.
B. Block nicotinic receptors in the salivary glands.
C. Activate muscarinic receptors in the salivary glands.
D. Block muscarinic receptors in the salivary glands.

Correct answer = D. Salivary glands contain muscarinic receptors, not nicotinic receptors. Activation of muscarinic receptors in the salivary glands causes secretion of saliva. Blocking muscarinic receptors, using drugs such as atropine, reduces salivary secretions and makes the mouth dry.

4.3 Which of the following is a systemic effect of a muscarinic agonist?

A. Reduced heart rate (bradycardia).
B. Increased blood pressure.
C. Mydriasis (dilation of the pupil).
D. Reduced urinary frequency.
E. Constipation.

Correct answer = A. A muscarinic agonist binds to and activates muscarinic receptors in the heart, endothelial cells (blood vessels), the gut, and iris sphincter (eye) and urinary bladder wall muscles, in addition to several other tissues. Activation of muscarinic receptors by an agonist causes a reduction in heart rate, constriction of circular muscles in the iris sphincter leading to constriction of the pupil (miosis), increased GI motility (hence, diarrhea, not constipation), and contraction of bladder muscles leading to an increase (not decrease) in urination frequency. In the endothelial cells of blood vessels, muscarinic activation produces release of nitric oxide that causes vasorelaxation and a reduction (not increase) in blood pressure.

4.4 If an ophthalmologist wants to dilate the pupils for an eye examination, which of the following drugs/classes of drugs could be theoretically useful?

A. Muscarinic receptor activator (agonist).
B. Muscarinic receptor inhibitor (antagonist).
C. Acetylcholine.
D. Pilocarpine.
E. Neostigmine.

Correct answer = B. Muscarinic agonists (for example, ACh, pilocarpine) contract the circular smooth muscles in the iris sphincter and constrict the pupil (miosis). Anticholinesterases (for example, neostigmine, physostigmine) also cause miosis by increasing the level of ACh. Muscarinic antagonists, on the other hand, relax the circular smooth muscles in the iris sphincter and cause dilation of the pupil (mydriasis).

4.5 In Alzheimer's disease, there is a deficiency of cholinergic neuronal function in the brain. Theoretically, which of the following strategies will be useful in treating the symptoms of Alzheimer's disease?

A. Inhibiting cholinergic receptors in the brain.
B. Inhibiting the release of acetylcholine in the brain.
C. Inhibiting the acetylcholinesterase enzyme in the brain.
D. Activating the acetylcholinesterase enzyme in the brain.

Correct answer = C. Since there is already a deficiency in brain cholinergic function in Alzheimer's disease, inhibiting cholinergic receptors or inhibiting the release of ACh will worsen the condition. Activating the acetylcholinesterase enzyme will increase the degradation of ACh, which will again worsen the condition. However, inhibiting the acetylcholinesterase enzyme will help to increase the levels of ACh in the brain and thereby help to relieve the symptoms of Alzheimer's disease.

4.6 An elderly female who lives in a farm house was brought to the emergency room in serious condition after ingesting a liquid from an unlabeled bottle found near her bed, apparently in a suicide attempt. She presented with diarrhea, frequent urination, convulsions, breathing difficulties, constricted pupils (miosis), and excessive salivation. Which of the following is correct regarding this patient?

A. She most likely consumed an organophosphate pesticide.
B. The symptoms are consistent with sympathetic activation.
C. Her symptoms can be treated using an anticholinesterase agent.
D. Her symptoms can be treated using a cholinergic agonist.

Correct answer = A. The symptoms are consistent with that of cholinergic crisis. Since the elderly female lives on a farm and since the symptoms are consistent with that of cholinergic crisis (usually caused by cholinesterase inhibitors), it may be assumed that she has consumed an organophosphate pesticide (irreversible cholinesterase inhibitor). Assuming that the symptoms are caused by organophosphate poisoning, administering an anticholinesterase agent or a cholinergic agonist will worsen the condition. The symptoms are not consistent with that of sympathetic activation, as sympathetic activation will cause symptoms opposite to that of cholinergic crisis seen in this patient.

4.7 Sarin is a volatile nerve agent that inhibits cholinesterase enzymes. Which of the following symptoms would you expect to see in a patient exposed to sarin?

A. Urinary retention.
B. Tachycardia.
C. Constriction of pupils (miosis).
D. Dilation of the pupils (mydriasis).
E. Dry mouth.

Correct answer = C. Sarin is an organophosphate nerve gas that inhibits cholinesterase enzymes and increases ACh levels. Therefore, symptoms of cholinergic crisis (increased urination, bradycardia, excessive secretions, constriction of pupils, etc.) should be expected in patients exposed to sarin. Urinary retention, tachycardia, mydriasis, and dry mouth are usually seen with muscarinic antagonists.

4.8 Head and neck irradiation in cancer patients can decrease salivary secretion and cause dry mouth. All of the following drugs or classes of drugs are theoretically useful in improving secretion of saliva in these patients *except*:

A. Muscarinic antagonists.
B. Muscarinic agonists.
C. Anticholinesterase agents.
D. Pilocarpine.
E. Neostigmine.

Correct answer = A. Activation of muscarinic receptors in the salivary glands causes secretion of saliva. This can be achieved in theory by using a muscarinic agonist such as pilocarpine or an anticholinesterase agent such as neostigmine (increases levels of ACh). Muscarinic antagonists (anticholinergic drugs) will reduce salivary secretion and worsen dry mouth.

4.9 Which of the following drugs or classes of drugs will be useful in treating the symptoms of myasthenia gravis?

A. Nicotinic antagonists.
B. Muscarinic agonists.
C. Muscarinic antagonists.
D. Anticholinesterase agents.

Correct answer = D. The function of nicotinic receptors in skeletal muscles is diminished in myasthenia gravis due to the development of antibodies to nicotinic receptors in the patient's body (autoimmune disease). Any drug that can increase the levels of ACh in the neuromuscular junction can improve symptoms in myasthenia gravis. Thus, cholinesterase inhibitors help to improve the symptoms of myasthenia gravis. Muscarinic drugs have no role in myasthenia gravis, and nicotinic antagonists will worsen the symptoms.

4.10 *Atropa belladonna* is a plant that contains atropine (a muscarinic antagonist). Which of the following drugs or classes of drugs will be useful in treating poisoning with belladonna?

A. Malathion.
B. Physostigmine.
C. Muscarinic antagonists.
D. Nicotinic antagonists.

Correct answer = B. Atropine is a competitive muscarinic receptor antagonist that causes anticholinergic effects. Muscarinic agonists or any other drugs that can increase the levels of ACh will be able to counteract the effects of atropine. Thus, anticholinesterases such as malathion and physostigmine can counteract the effects of atropine in theory. However, malathion being an irreversible inhibitor of acetylcholinesterase is not used for systemic treatment in patients. Muscarinic antagonists will worsen the toxicity of atropine. Nicotinic antagonists could worsen the toxicity by acting on parasympathetic ganglionic receptors and thus reducing the release of ACh.

Cholinergic Antagonists

5

Rajan Radhakrishnan and Thomas B. Whalen

I. OVERVIEW

Cholinergic antagonist is a general term for agents that bind to cholinoceptors (muscarinic or nicotinic) and prevent the effects of acetylcholine (ACh) and other cholinergic agonists. The most clinically useful of these agents are selective blockers of muscarinic receptors. They are commonly known as anticholinergic agents (a misnomer, as they antagonize only muscarinic receptors), antimuscarinic agents (more accurate terminology), or parasympatholytics. The effects of parasympathetic innervation are, thus, interrupted, and the actions of sympathetic stimulation are left unopposed. A second group of drugs, the ganglionic blockers, shows a preference for the nicotinic receptors of the sympathetic and parasympathetic ganglia. Clinically, they are the least important of the cholinergic antagonists. A third family of compounds, the neuromuscular-blocking agents (mostly nicotinic antagonists), interfere with transmission of efferent impulses to skeletal muscles. These agents are used as skeletal muscle relaxant adjuvants in anesthesia during surgery, intubation, and various orthopedic procedures. Figure 5.1 summarizes the cholinergic antagonists discussed in this chapter.

II. ANTIMUSCARINIC AGENTS

Commonly known as anticholinergic drugs, these agents (for example, *atropine* and *scopolamine*) block muscarinic receptors (Figure 5.2), causing inhibition of muscarinic functions. In addition, these drugs block the few exceptional sympathetic neurons that are cholinergic, such as those innervating the salivary and sweat glands. Because they do not block nicotinic receptors, the anticholinergic drugs (more precisely, antimuscarinic drugs) have little or no action at skeletal neuromuscular junctions (NMJs) or autonomic ganglia. The anticholinergic drugs are beneficial in a variety of clinical situations. [Note: A number of antihistamines and antidepressants (mainly tricyclic antidepressants) also have antimuscarinic activity.]

A. Atropine

Atropine [A-troe-peen] is a tertiary amine belladonna alkaloid with a high affinity for muscarinic receptors. It binds competitively and

ANTIMUSCARINIC AGENTS
Atropine ISOPTO ATROPINE
Benztropine COGENTIN
Cyclopentolate AK-PENTOLATE, CYCLOGYL
Darifenacin ENABLEX
Fesoterodine TOVIAZ
Ipratropium ATROVENT
Oxybutynin DITROPAN, GELNIQUE, OXYTROL
Scopolamine ISOPTO HYOSCINE, TRANSDERM SCŌP
Solifenacin VESICARE
Tiotropium SPIRIVA HANDIHALER
Tolterodine DETROL
Trihexyphenidyl ARTANE
Tropicamide MYDRIACYL, TROPICACYL
Trospium chloride SANCTURA
GANGLIONIC BLOCKERS
Nicotine NICODERM, NICORETTE, NICOTROL INHALER
NEUROMUSCULAR BLOCKERS
Cisatracurium NIMBEX
Pancuronium PAVULON
Rocuronium ZEMURON
Succinylcholine ANECTINE, QUELICIN
Vecuronium ONLY GENERIC

Figure 5.1
Summary of cholinergic antagonists.

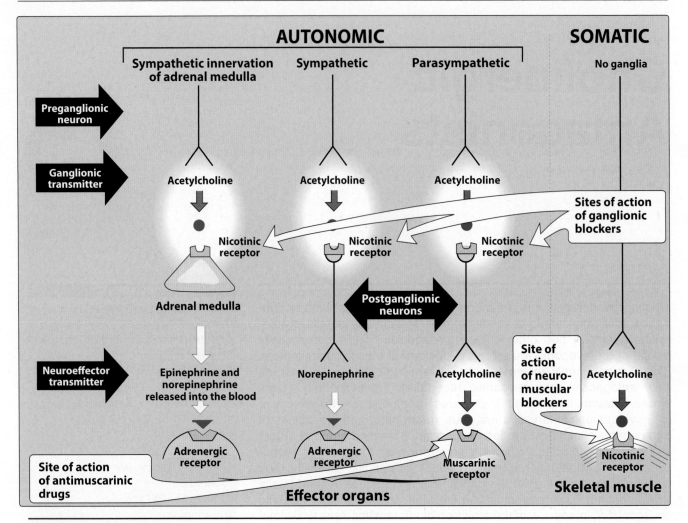

Figure 5.2
Sites of actions of cholinergic antagonists.

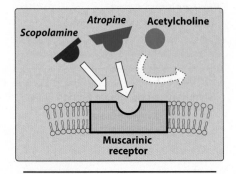

Figure 5.3
Competition of *atropine* and *scopolamine* with acetylcholine for the muscarinic receptor.

prevents ACh from binding to those sites (Figure 5.3). *Atropine* acts both centrally and peripherally. Its general actions last about 4 hours, except when placed topically in the eye, where the action may last for days. Neuroeffector organs have varying sensitivity to *atropine*. The greatest inhibitory effects are on bronchial tissue and the secretion of sweat and saliva (Figure 5.4).

1. Actions:

    a. Eye: *Atropine* blocks muscarinic activity in the eye, resulting in mydriasis (dilation of the pupil), unresponsiveness to light, and cycloplegia (inability to focus for near vision). In patients with angle-closure glaucoma, intraocular pressure may rise dangerously.

    b. Gastrointestinal (GI): *Atropine* (as the active isomer, L-hyoscyamine) can be used as an antispasmodic to reduce activity of the GI tract. *Atropine* and *scopolamine* (discussed below) are probably the most potent antispasmodic drugs available. Although gastric motility is reduced, hydrochloric acid production is not significantly affected. Thus, *atropine* is not effective for the treatment of peptic ulcer. [Note: *Pirenzepine*, an M_1 muscarinic antagonist, does reduce gastric acid secretion at doses that do not antagonize other systems.] Doses of *atropine* that reduce spasms also reduce saliva secretion, ocular accommodation, and urination. These effects decrease compliance with *atropine*.

c. **Cardiovascular:** *Atropine* produces divergent effects on the cardiovascular system, depending on the dose (Figure 5.4). At low doses, the predominant effect is a slight decrease in heart rate. This effect results from blockade of the M_1 receptors on the inhibitory prejunctional (or presynaptic) neurons, thus permitting increased ACh release. Higher doses of *atropine* cause a progressive increase in heart rate by blocking the M_2 receptors on the sinoatrial node.

d. **Secretions:** *Atropine* blocks muscarinic receptors in the salivary glands, producing dryness of the mouth (xerostomia). The salivary glands are exquisitely sensitive to *atropine*. Sweat and lacrimal glands are similarly affected. [Note: Inhibition of secretions by sweat glands can cause elevated body temperature, which can be dangerous in children and the elderly.]

2. **Therapeutic uses:**

a. **Ophthalmic:** Topical *atropine* exerts both mydriatic and cycloplegic effects, and it permits the measurement of refractive errors without interference by the accommodative capacity of the eye. Shorter-acting antimuscarinics (*cyclopentolate* and *tropicamide*) have largely replaced *atropine* due to prolonged mydriasis observed with *atropine* (7 to 14 days vs. 6 to 24 hours with other agents). [Note: *Phenylephrine* or similar α-adrenergic drugs are preferred for pupillary dilation if cycloplegia is not required.]

b. **Antispasmodic:** *Atropine* is used as an antispasmodic agent to relax the GI tract.

c. **Cardiovascular:** The drug is used to treat bradycardia of varying etiologies.

d. **Antisecretory:** *Atropine* is sometimes used as an antisecretory agent to block secretions in the upper and lower respiratory tracts prior to surgery.

e. **Antidote for cholinergic agonists:** *Atropine* is used for the treatment of organophosphate (insecticides, nerve gases) poisoning, of overdose of clinically used anticholinesterases such as *physostigmine*, and in some types of mushroom poisoning (certain mushrooms contain cholinergic substances that block cholinesterases). Massive doses of *atropine* may be required over a long period of time to counteract the poisons. The ability of *atropine* to enter the central nervous system (CNS) is of particular importance in treating central toxic effects of anticholinesterases.

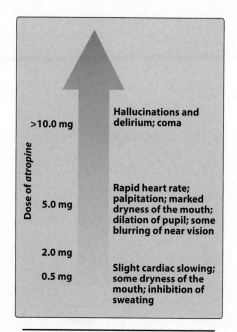

Figure 5.4
Dose-dependent effects of *atropine*.

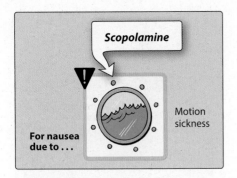

Figure 5.5
Scopolamine is an effective anti–motion sickness agent.

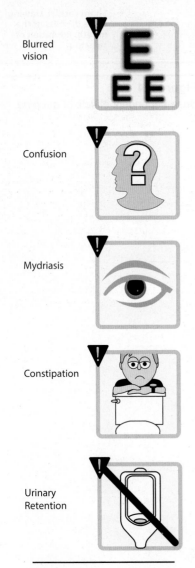

Blurred vision

Confusion

Mydriasis

Constipation

Urinary Retention

Figure 5.6
Adverse effects commonly observed with muscarinic antagonists.

3. **Pharmacokinetics:** *Atropine* is readily absorbed, partially metabolized by the liver, and eliminated primarily in urine. It has a half-life of about 4 hours.

4. **Adverse effects:** Depending on the dose, *atropine* may cause dry mouth, blurred vision, "sandy eyes," tachycardia, urinary retention, and constipation. Effects on the CNS include restlessness, confusion, hallucinations, and delirium, which may progress to depression, collapse of the circulatory and respiratory systems, and death. Low doses of cholinesterase inhibitors, such as *physostigmine*, may be used to overcome *atropine* toxicity. *Atropine* may also induce troublesome urinary retention. The drug may be dangerous in children, because they are sensitive to its effects, particularly to rapid increases in body temperature that it may elicit.

B. Scopolamine

Scopolamine [skoe-POL-a-meen], another tertiary amine plant alkaloid, produces peripheral effects similar to those of *atropine*. However, *scopolamine* has greater action on the CNS (unlike *atropine,* CNS effects are observed at therapeutic doses) and a longer duration of action as compared to *atropine*. It has some special actions as indicated below.

1. **Actions:** *Scopolamine* is one of the most effective anti–motion sickness drugs available (Figure 5.5). It also has the unusual effect of blocking short-term memory. In contrast to *atropine, scopolamine* produces sedation, but at higher doses, it can produce excitement. *Scopolamine* may produce euphoria and is susceptible to abuse.

2. **Therapeutic uses:** The therapeutic use of *scopolamine* is limited to prevention of motion sickness and postoperative nausea and vomiting. For motion sickness, it is available as a topical patch that provides effects for up to 3 days. [Note: As with all drugs used for motion sickness, it is much more effective prophylactically than for treating motion sickness once it occurs.]

3. **Pharmacokinetics and adverse effects:** These aspects are similar to those of *atropine*.

C. Ipratropium and tiotropium

Ipratropium [i-pra-TROE-pee-um] and *tiotropium* [ty-oh-TROPE-ee-um] are quaternary derivatives of *atropine*. These agents are approved as bronchodilators for maintenance treatment of bronchospasm associated with chronic obstructive pulmonary disease (COPD). *Ipratropium* is also used in the acute management of bronchospasm in asthma. Both agents are delivered via inhalation. Because of their positive charges, these drugs do not enter the systemic circulation or the CNS, isolating their effects to the pulmonary system. *Tiotropium* is administered once daily, a major advantage over *ipratropium*, which requires dosing up to four times daily. Important characteristics of the muscarinic antagonists are summarized in Figures 5.6 and 5.7.

D. Tropicamide and cyclopentolate

These agents are used as ophthalmic solutions for mydriasis and cycloplegia. Their duration of action is shorter than that of *atropine*. *Tropicamide* produces mydriasis for 6 hours and *cyclopentolate* for 24 hours.

E. Benztropine and trihexyphenidyl

Benztropine and *trihexyphenidyl* are useful as adjuncts with other antiparkinsonian agents to treat Parkinson's disease (see Chapter 8) and other types of parkinsonian syndromes, including antipsychotic-induced extrapyramidal symptoms.

F. Darifenacin, fesoterodine, oxybutynin, solifenacin, tolterodine, and trospium chloride

These synthetic *atropine*-like drugs are used to treat overactive bladder. By blocking muscarinic receptors in the bladder, intravesical pressure is lowered, bladder capacity is increased, and the frequency of bladder contractions is reduced. Side effects include dry mouth, constipation, and blurred vision, which limit tolerability of these agents if used continually. *Oxybutynin* [ox-i-BYOO-ti-nin] is available as a transdermal system (topical patch), which is better tolerated because it causes less dry mouth than oral formulations. The overall efficacies of these antimuscarinic drugs are similar.

III. GANGLIONIC BLOCKERS

Ganglionic blockers specifically act on the nicotinic receptors of both parasympathetic and sympathetic autonomic ganglia. Some also block the ion channels of the autonomic ganglia. These drugs show no selectivity toward the parasympathetic or sympathetic ganglia and are not effective as neuromuscular antagonists. Thus, these drugs block the entire output of the autonomic nervous system at the nicotinic receptor. Except for nicotine, the other drugs mentioned in this category are nondepolarizing, competitive antagonists. The responses of the nondepolarizing blockers are complex and mostly unpredictable. Therefore, ganglionic blockade is rarely used therapeutically, but often serves as a tool in experimental pharmacology.

A. Nicotine

A component of cigarette smoke, *nicotine* [NIK-oh-teen], is a poison with many undesirable actions. It is without therapeutic benefit and is deleterious to health. Depending on the dose, *nicotine* depolarizes autonomic ganglia, resulting first in stimulation and then in paralysis of all ganglia. The stimulatory effects are complex and result from increased release of neurotransmitters (Figure 5.8), due to effects on both sympathetic and parasympathetic ganglia. For example, enhanced release of dopamine and norepinephrine may be associated with pleasure as well as appetite suppression. The overall response of a physiologic system is a summation of the stimulatory and inhibitory effects of *nicotine*. These include increased blood pressure and cardiac rate (due to release of transmitter from

Drug	Therapeutic uses
Muscarinic blockers	
Trihexyphenidyl Benztropine	● Treatment of Parkinson's disease
Darifenacin Fesoterodine Oxybutynin Solifenacin Tolterodine Trospium	● Treatment of overactive urinary bladder
Cyclopentolate Tropicamide Atropine*	● In ophthalmology, to produce mydriasis and cycloplegia prior to refraction
Atropine*	● To treat spastic disorders of the GI tract ● To treat organophosphate poisoning ● To suppress respiratory secretions prior to surgery ● To treat bradycardia
Scopolamine	● To prevent motion sickness
Ipratropium Tiotropium	● Treatment of COPD
Ganglionic blockers	
Nicotine	● Smoking cessation

Figure 5.7
Summary of cholinergic antagonists. *Contraindicated in angle-closure glaucoma. GI = gastrointestinal; COPD = chronic obstructive pulmonary disease.

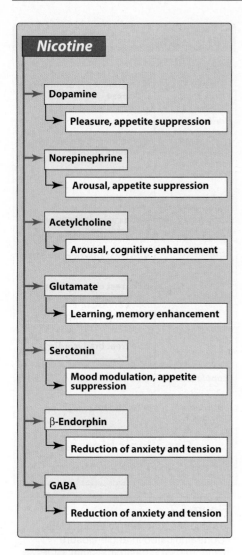

Figure 5.8
Neurochemical effects of *nicotine*.
GABA = γ-aminobutyric acid.

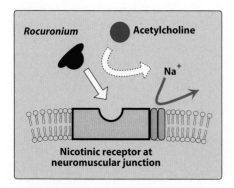

Figure 5.9
Mechanism of action of competitive
neuromuscular-blocking drugs.

adrenergic terminals and from the adrenal medulla) and increased peristalsis and secretions. At higher doses, the blood pressure falls because of ganglionic blockade, and activity in both the GI tract and bladder musculature ceases (see Chapter 16 for a full discussion of *nicotine*).

IV. NEUROMUSCULAR-BLOCKING AGENTS

These drugs block cholinergic transmission between motor nerve endings and the nicotinic receptors on the skeletal muscle (Figure 5.2). They possess some chemical similarities to ACh, and they act either as antagonists (nondepolarizing type) or as agonists (depolarizing type) at the receptors on the endplate of the NMJ. Neuromuscular blockers are clinically useful during surgery to facilitate tracheal intubation and provide complete muscle relaxation at lower anesthetic doses, allowing for more rapid recovery from anesthesia and reducing postoperative respiratory depression.

A. Nondepolarizing (competitive) blockers

The first drug known to block the skeletal NMJ was *curare* [kyoo-RAH-ree], which native South American hunters of the Amazon region used to paralyze prey. The development of the drug *tubocurarine* [too-boe-kyoo-AR-een] followed, but it has been replaced by other agents with fewer adverse effects, such as *cisatracurium* [cis-a-trah-CURE-ih-um], *pancuronium* [pan-kure-OH-nee-um], *rocuronium* [roe-kyoor-OH-nee-um], and *vecuronium* [ve-KYOO-roe-nee-um]. The neuromuscular-blocking agents have significantly increased the safety of anesthesia, because less anesthetic is required to produce muscle relaxation, allowing patients to recover quickly and completely after surgery. Neuromuscular blockers should not be used to substitute for inadequate depth of anesthesia.

1. Mechanism of action:

a. At low doses: Nondepolarizing agents competitively block ACh at the nicotinic receptors (Figure 5.9). That is, they compete with ACh at the receptor without stimulating it. Thus, these drugs prevent depolarization of the muscle cell membrane and inhibit muscular contraction. Their competitive action can be overcome by administration of cholinesterase inhibitors, such as *neostigmine* and *edrophonium*, which increase the concentration of ACh in the neuromuscular junction. Anesthesiologists employ this strategy to shorten the duration of the neuromuscular blockade. In addition, at low doses the muscle will respond to direct electrical stimulation from a peripheral nerve stimulator to varying degrees, allowing for monitoring of the extent of neuromuscular blockade.

b. At high doses: Nondepolarizing agents can block the ion channels of the motor endplate. This leads to further weakening of neuromuscular transmission, thereby reducing the ability of cholinesterase inhibitors to reverse the actions of the nondepolarizing blockers. With complete blockade, the muscle does not respond to direct electrical stimulation.

2. **Actions:** Not all muscles are equally sensitive to blockade by competitive agents. Small, rapidly contracting muscles of the face and eye are most susceptible and are paralyzed first, followed by the fingers, limbs, neck, and trunk muscles. Next, the intercostal muscles are affected and, lastly, the diaphragm. The muscles recover in the reverse manner.

3. **Pharmacokinetics:** All neuromuscular-blocking agents are injected intravenously or occasionally intramuscularly since they are not effective orally. These agents possess two or more quaternary amines in their bulky ring structure that prevent their absorption from the gut. They penetrate membranes very poorly and do not enter cells or cross the blood–brain barrier. Many of the drugs are not metabolized, and their actions are terminated by redistribution (Figure 5.10). For example, *pancuronium* is excreted unchanged in urine. *Cisatracurium* is degraded spontaneously in plasma and by ester hydrolysis. [Note: *Atracurium* has been replaced by its isomer, *cisatracurium*. *Atracurium* releases histamine and is metabolized to laudanosine, which can provoke seizures. *Cisatracurium*, which has the same pharmacokinetic properties as *atracurium*, is less likely to have these effects.] The amino steroid drugs *vecuronium* and *rocuronium* are deacetylated in the liver, and their clearance may be prolonged in patients with hepatic disease. These drugs are also excreted unchanged in bile. The choice of an agent depends on the desired onset and duration of the muscle relaxation. The onset, duration of action, and other characteristics of the neuromuscular-blocking drugs are shown in Figure 5.11.

4. **Adverse effects:** In general, these agents are safe with minimal side effects. The adverse effects of the specific neuromuscular blockers are shown in Figure 5.11.

5. **Drug interactions:**

   a. **Cholinesterase inhibitors:** Drugs such as *neostigmine, physostigmine, pyridostigmine,* and *edrophonium* can overcome the action of nondepolarizing neuromuscular blockers. However, with increased dosage, cholinesterase inhibitors can cause a depolarizing block as a result of elevated ACh concentrations at the endplate membrane. If the neuromuscular blocker has entered the ion channel, cholinesterase inhibitors are not as effective in overcoming blockade.

   b. **Halogenated hydrocarbon anesthetics:** Drugs such as *desflurane* act to enhance neuromuscular blockade by exerting a stabilizing action at the NMJ. These agents sensitize the NMJ to the effects of neuromuscular blockers.

   c. **Aminoglycoside antibiotics:** Drugs such as *gentamicin* and *tobramycin* inhibit ACh release from cholinergic nerves by competing with calcium ions. They synergize with *pancuronium* and other competitive blockers, enhancing the blockade.

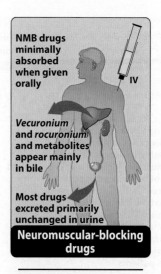

NMB drugs minimally absorbed when given orally

IV

Vecuronium and *rocuronium* and metabolites appear mainly in bile

Most drugs excreted primarily unchanged in urine

Neuromuscular-blocking drugs

Figure 5.10
Pharmacokinetics of the neuromuscular-blocking drugs. IV = intravenous.

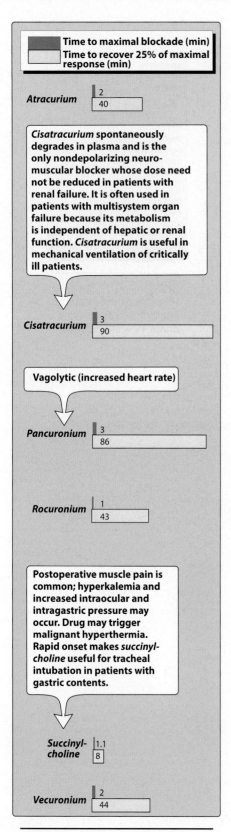

Figure 5.11

Onset and duration of action of neuromuscular-blocking drugs.

d. Calcium channel blockers: These agents may increase the neuromuscular blockade of competitive blockers.

B. Depolarizing agents

Depolarizing blocking agents work by depolarizing the plasma membrane of the muscle fiber, similar to the action of ACh. However, these agents are more resistant to degradation by acetylcholinesterase (AChE) and can thus more persistently depolarize the muscle fibers. *Succinylcholine* [suk-sin-il-KOE-leen] is the only depolarizing muscle relaxant in use today.

1. **Mechanism of action:** *Succinylcholine* attaches to the nicotinic receptor and acts like ACh to depolarize the junction (Figure 5.12). Unlike ACh, which is instantly destroyed by AChE, the depolarizing agent persists at high concentrations in the synaptic cleft, remaining attached to the receptor for a relatively longer time and providing constant stimulation of the receptor. [Note: The duration of action of *succinylcholine* is dependent on diffusion from the motor endplate and hydrolysis by plasma pseudocholinesterase. Genetic variants in which plasma pseudocholinesterase levels are low or absent lead to prolonged neuromuscular paralysis.] The depolarizing agent first causes the opening of the sodium channel associated with the nicotinic receptors, which results in depolarization of the receptor (Phase I). This leads to a transient twitching of the muscle (fasciculations). Continued binding of the depolarizing agent renders the receptor incapable of transmitting further impulses. With time, continuous depolarization gives way to gradual repolarization as the sodium channel closes or is blocked. This causes a resistance to depolarization (Phase II) and flaccid paralysis.

2. **Actions:** As with the competitive blockers, the respiratory muscles are paralyzed last. *Succinylcholine* initially produces brief muscle fasciculations that cause muscle soreness. This may be prevented by administering a small dose of nondepolarizing neuromuscular blocker prior to *succinylcholine*. Normally, the duration of action of *succinylcholine* is extremely short, due to rapid hydrolysis by plasma pseudocholinesterase. However, *succinylcholine* that gets to the NMJ is not metabolized by AChE, allowing the agent to bind to nicotinic receptors, and redistribution to plasma is necessary for metabolism (therapeutic benefits last only for a few minutes).

3. **Therapeutic uses:** Because of its rapid onset of action, *succinylcholine* is useful when rapid endotracheal intubation is required during the induction of anesthesia (a rapid action is essential if aspiration of gastric contents is to be avoided during intubation). It is also used during electroconvulsive shock treatment.

4. **Pharmacokinetics:** *Succinylcholine* is injected intravenously. Its brief duration of action results from redistribution and rapid hydrolysis by plasma pseudocholinesterase. Therefore, it is sometimes

given by continuous infusion to maintain a longer duration of effect. Drug effects rapidly disappear upon discontinuation.

5. **Adverse effects:**

a. **Hyperthermia:** *Succinylcholine* can potentially induce malignant hyperthermia in susceptible patients (see Chapter 13).

b. **Apnea:** Administration of *succinylcholine* to a patient who is deficient in plasma cholinesterase or who has an atypical form of the enzyme can lead to prolonged apnea due to paralysis of the diaphragm. The rapid release of potassium may also contribute to prolonged apnea in patients with electrolyte imbalances who receive this drug. In patients with electrolyte imbalances who are also receiving *digoxin* or diuretics (such as heart failure patients) *succinylcholine* should be used cautiously or not at all.

c. **Hyperkalemia:** *Succinylcholine* increases potassium release from intracellular stores. This may be particularly dangerous in burn patients and patients with massive tissue damage in which potassium has been rapidly lost from within cells.

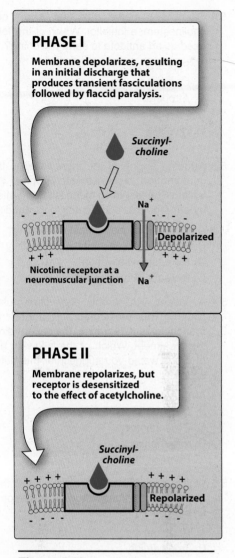

PHASE I

Membrane depolarizes, resulting in an initial discharge that produces transient fasciculations followed by flaccid paralysis.

Succinyl-choline

Na$^+$

Nicotinic receptor at a neuromuscular junction

Depolarized

Na$^+$

PHASE II

Membrane repolarizes, but receptor is desensitized to the effect of acetylcholine.

Succinyl-choline

Repolarized

Figure 5.12
Mechanism of action of depolarizing neuromuscular-blocking drugs.

Study Questions

Choose the ONE best answer.

5.1 During an ophthalmic surgical procedure, the surgeon wanted to constrict the pupil of the patient using a miotic drug. However, he accidentally used another drug that caused dilation of the pupil (mydriasis) instead. Most likely, which of the following drugs did he use?

A. Acetylcholine.
B. Pilocarpine.
C. Tropicamide.
D. Phentolamine.
E. Bethanechol.

Correct answer = C. Muscarinic agonists such as ACh, pilocarpine, and bethanechol contract the circular muscles of iris sphincter and cause constriction of the pupil (miosis), whereas muscarinic antagonists such as atropine and tropicamide prevent the contraction of the circular muscles of the iris and cause dilation of the pupil (mydriasis). α-Adrenergic antagonists such as phentolamine relax the radial muscles of the iris and cause miosis.

5.2 Sarin is a nerve gas that is an organophosphate cholinesterase inhibitor. Which of the following could be used as an antidote to sarin poisoning?

A. Pilocarpine.
B. Carbachol.
C. Atropine.
D. Physostigmine.
E. Nicotine.

Correct answer = C. Sarin is an organophosphate cholinesterase inhibitor. It causes an increase in ACh levels in tissues that leads to cholinergic crisis by the activation of muscarinic as well as nicotinic receptors. Most of the symptoms of cholinergic crisis are mediated by muscarinic receptors and, therefore, the muscarinic antagonist atropine is used as an antidote for sarin poisoning. Cholinergic agonists such as pilocarpine, carbachol, physostigmine (indirect agonists), and nicotine will worsen the symptoms of sarin poisoning.

5.3 Atropine is one of the ingredients in the antidiarrheal combination diphenoxylate/atropine available in the United States. Which of the following effects is produced by atropine that contributes to its antidiarrheal effect?

A. Increase in gastrointestinal motility.
B. Reduction in gastrointestinal motility.
C. Increase in salivation.
D. Increase in acid secretion.

Correct answer = B. Muscarinic agonists produce an increase in gastrointestinal motility, salivation, and acid secretion. Atropine is a muscarinic antagonist and therefore causes a reduction in gastrointestinal motility that contributes to its antidiarrheal effect.

5.4 A patient with chronic obstructive pulmonary disease (COPD) was prescribed a β_2 agonist for the relief of bronchospasm. However, the patient did not respond to this treatment. Which of the following drugs or classes of drugs would you suggest for this patient as the next option?

A. β_1 Agonist.
B. Muscarinic agonist.
C. Physostigmine.
D. Ipratropium.
E. Phentolamine.

Correct answer = D. Major receptors present in the bronchial tissues are muscarinic and adrenergic-β_2 receptors. Muscarinic activation causes bronchoconstriction, and β_2 receptor activation causes bronchodilation. Therefore, direct or indirect (physostigmine) muscarinic agonists will worsen bronchospasm. Ipratropium is a muscarinic antagonist that can relax bronchial smooth muscles and relieve bronchospasm in patients who are not responsive to β_2 agonists. α_1 and β_1 receptors are not commonly present in bronchial tissues and, therefore, β_1 agonists or α antagonists (phentolamine) do not have any significant effects on bronchospasm.

5.5 Which of the following drugs would be the most effective anti–motion sickness drug for a person planning to go on a cruise?

A. Atropine.
B. Tropicamide.
C. Scopolamine.
D. Darifenacin.
E. Tiotropium.

Correct answer = C. All muscarinic antagonists (anticholinergic drugs) listed above are theoretically useful as anti–motion sickness drugs; however, scopolamine is the most effective in preventing motion sickness in practice. Tropicamide mostly has ophthalmic uses, and tiotropium is used for respiratory disorders (COPD). Darifenacin is used for overactive bladder.

5.6 Which of the following is correct regarding ganglion-blocking drugs?

A. Blockade of sympathetic ganglia could result in reduced blood pressure.
B. Blockade of parasympathetic ganglia could result in reduced heart rate.
C. Nicotine is a nondepolarizing ganglion blocker.
D. Atropine is a nondepolarizing ganglion blocker.

Correct answer = A. Selective blockade (in theory) of the sympathetic ganglion causes reduction in norepinephrine release and therefore reduction in heart rate and blood pressure. Selective blockade (in theory) of the parasympathetic ganglion causes reduction in ACh release and therefore an increase in heart rate. Receptors at both sympathetic and parasympathetic ganglia are of the nicotinic type. Nicotine is an agonist at nicotinic receptors and produces a depolarizing block in the ganglia. Atropine is a muscarinic antagonist and has no effect on the nicotinic receptors found in the ganglia.

5.7 Which of the following is correct regarding the neuromuscular blockers (NMBs)?

A. Nondepolarizing NMBs are administered orally.

B. Cholinesterase inhibitors reduce the effects of nondepolarizing NMBs.

C. Nondepolarizing NMBs affect diaphragm muscles first.

D. Effects of depolarizing neuromuscular blockers can be reversed using cholinesterase inhibitors.

Correct answer = B. Nondepolarizing NMBs such as cisatracurium and vecuronium are highly polar compounds and are poorly absorbed from the GI tract. Therefore, they are administered parenterally, not orally. Nondepolarizing NMBs are competitive antagonists at nicotinic receptors. Therefore, increasing the levels of ACh at the neuromuscular junction reduces the effects of these agents. Cholinesterase inhibitors increase the levels of ACh at the neuromuscular junction and reduce the effects of nondepolarizing NMBs, but may enhance (not reverse) the effects of depolarizing NMBs. Nondepolarizing NMBs first affect rapidly contracting muscles seen in the face and eyes and affect the diaphragm muscles last.

5.8 Which of the following is correct regarding drug interactions with nondepolarizing neuromuscular blockers (NMBs)?

A. Desflurane reduces the effects of nondepolarizing NMBs.

B. Cholinesterase inhibitors increase the effects of nondepolarizing NMBs.

C. Aminoglycosides increase the effects of nondepolarizing NMBs.

D. Calcium channel blockers reduce the effects of nondepolarizing NMBs.

Correct answer = C. Halogenated hydrocarbon anesthetics such as desflurane enhance the effects of nondepolarizing NMBs by exerting a stabilization effect at the neuromuscular junction (NMJ). Acetylcholinesterase inhibitors increase the levels of ACh at the NMJ and reduce the effects of nondepolarizing NMBs. Aminoglycoside antibiotics increase the effects of nondepolarizing NMBs by reducing the release of ACh from the cholinergic neurons. Calcium channel blockers increase the effects of nondepolarizing NMBs, possibly by affecting ion transport at the NMJ.

5.9 A patient was administered a neuromuscular blocker (NMB) prior to a surgical procedure to produce skeletal muscle paralysis. This NMB drug affected small, rapidly contracting muscles of the face and eyes first and diaphragm muscles last. The effect of this drug was easily reversed with neostigmine. Which of the following neuromuscular blockers was most likely administered to this patient?

A. Rocuronium.

B. Succinylcholine.

C. Diazepam.

D. Tubocurarine.

Correct answer = A. There are two types of NMBs: depolarizing and nondepolarizing NMBs. Depolarizing NMBs are agonists at the nicotinic receptors, whereas nondepolarizing NMBs are antagonists at the nicotinic receptors. Both types of NMBs affect the rapidly contracting muscles (face, eye, etc.) first and diaphragm muscles last. However, cholinesterase inhibitors such as neostigmine increase ACh levels in the NMJ and reverse the effects of nondepolarizing NMBs, but not those of depolarizing NMBs. Therefore, the NMB administered to this patient is most probably rocuronium, which is a nondepolarizing NMB. Tubocurarine is also a nondepolarizing NMB, but it is not used in practice. Succinylcholine is a depolarizing NMB, and diazepam is a benzodiazepine that does not cause paralysis of skeletal muscles.

5.10 A patient was administered a neuromuscular blocker (NMB) prior to a surgical procedure to produce skeletal muscle paralysis. This NMB drug caused initial skeletal muscle fasciculations before the onset of paralysis. The effect of this drug could not be reversed with neostigmine. Which of the following neuromuscular blockers was most likely administered to this patient?

A. Cisatracurium.

B. Succinylcholine.

C. Diazepam.

D. Tubocurarine.

Correct answer = B. Depolarizing NMBs cause muscle fasciculations before causing paralysis, and their effects cannot be reversed using cholinesterase inhibitors such as neostigmine. Nondepolarizing NMBs do not cause muscle fasciculations, and their effects can be reversed using cholinesterase inhibitors. Therefore, the NMB used in this patient is succinylcholine, which is a depolarizing NMB. Cisatracurium and tubocurarine are nondepolarizing NMBs, and diazepam does not cause paralysis of skeletal muscles.

Adrenergic Agonists

6

Rajan Radhakrishnan

I. OVERVIEW

The adrenergic drugs affect receptors that are stimulated by norepinephrine (noradrenaline) or epinephrine (adrenaline). These receptors are known as adrenergic receptors or adrenoceptors. Adrenergic drugs that activate adrenergic receptors are termed sympathomimetics, and drugs that block the activation of adrenergic receptors are termed sympatholytics. Some sympathomimetics directly activate adrenergic receptors (direct-acting agonists), while others act indirectly by enhancing release or blocking reuptake of norepinephrine (indirect-acting agonists). This chapter describes agents that either directly or indirectly stimulate adrenoceptors (Figure 6.1). Sympatholytic drugs are discussed in Chapter 7.

II. THE ADRENERGIC NEURON

Adrenergic neurons release norepinephrine as the primary neurotransmitter. These neurons are found in the central nervous system (CNS) and also in the sympathetic nervous system, where they serve as links between ganglia and the effector organs. Adrenergic drugs act on adrenergic receptors, located either presynaptically on the neuron or postsynaptically on the effector organ (Figure 6.2).

A. Neurotransmission at adrenergic neurons

Neurotransmission in adrenergic neurons closely resembles that described for the cholinergic neurons (see Chapter 4), except that norepinephrine is the neurotransmitter instead of acetylcholine. Neurotransmission involves the following steps: synthesis, storage, release, and receptor binding of norepinephrine, followed by removal of the neurotransmitter from the synaptic gap (Figure 6.3).

1. **Synthesis of norepinephrine:** Tyrosine is transported by a carrier into the adrenergic neuron, where it is hydroxylated to dihydroxyphenylalanine (DOPA) by tyrosine hydroxylase. This is the rate-limiting step in the formation of norepinephrine. DOPA is then decarboxylated by the enzyme aromatic I-amino acid decarboxylase to form dopamine in the presynaptic neuron.

DIRECT-ACTING AGENTS

Albuterol ACCUNEB, PROAIR HFA, VENTOLIN HFA
Clonidine CATAPRES, DURACLON
Dobutamine* DOBUTREX
Dopamine*
Epinephrine* ADRENALIN, EPIPEN
Fenoldopam CORLOPAM
Formoterol FORADIL AEROLIZER, PERFOROMIST
Isoproterenol* ISUPREL
Mirabegron MYRBETRIQ
Norepinephrine * LEVOPHED
Phenylephrine NEO-SYNEPHRINE, SUDAFED PE
Salmeterol SEREVENT DISKUS
Terbutaline

INDIRECT-ACTING AGENTS

Amphetamine ADDERALL
Cocaine

DIRECT AND INDIRECT ACTING (mixed action) AGENTS

Ephedrine VARIOUS
Pseudoephedrine SUDAFED

Figure 6.1
Summary of adrenergic agonists. Agents marked with an *asterisk* (*) are catecholamines.

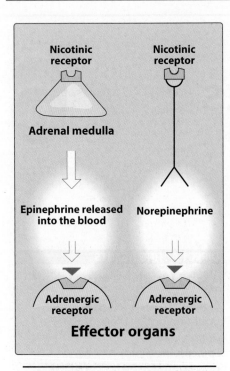

Figure 6.2
Sites of actions of adrenergic agonists.

2. **Storage of norepinephrine in vesicles:** Dopamine is then transported into synaptic vesicles by an amine transporter system. This carrier system is blocked by *reserpine* (see Chapter 7). Dopamine is next hydroxylated to form norepinephrine by the enzyme dopamine β-hydroxylase.

3. **Release of norepinephrine:** An action potential arriving at the nerve junction triggers an influx of calcium ions from the extracellular fluid into the cytoplasm of the neuron. The increase in calcium causes synaptic vesicles to fuse with the cell membrane and to undergo exocytosis to expel their contents into the synapse. Drugs such as *guanethidine* block this release.

4. **Binding to receptors:** Norepinephrine released from the synaptic vesicles diffuses into the synaptic space and binds to postsynaptic receptors on the effector organ or to presynaptic receptors on the nerve ending. Binding of norepinephrine to receptors triggers a cascade of events within the cell, resulting in the formation of intracellular second messengers that act as links (transducers) in the communication between the neurotransmitter and the action generated within the effector cell. Adrenergic receptors use both the cyclic adenosine monophosphate (cAMP) second messenger system and the phosphatidylinositol cycle to transduce the signal into an effect. Norepinephrine also binds to presynaptic receptors (mainly α_2 subtype) that modulate the release of the neurotransmitter.

5. **Removal of norepinephrine:** Norepinephrine may 1) diffuse out of the synaptic space and enter the systemic circulation; 2) be metabolized to inactive metabolites by catechol-*O*-methyltransferase (COMT) in the synaptic space; or 3) undergo reuptake back into the neuron. The reuptake by the neuronal membrane involves a sodium-chloride (Na^+/Cl^-)-dependent norepinephrine transporter (NET) that can be inhibited by tricyclic antidepressants (TCAs), such as *imipramine*, by serotonin–norepinephrine reuptake inhibitors such as *duloxetine*, or by *cocaine* (Figure 6.3). Reuptake of norepinephrine into the presynaptic neuron is the primary mechanism for termination of its effects.

6. **Potential fates of recaptured norepinephrine:** Once norepinephrine reenters the adrenergic neuron, it may be taken up into synaptic vesicles via the amine transporter system and be sequestered for release by another action potential, or it may persist in a protected pool in the cytoplasm. Alternatively, norepinephrine can be oxidized by monoamine oxidase (MAO) present in neuronal mitochondria.

B. Adrenergic receptors (adrenoceptors)

In the sympathetic nervous system, several classes of adrenoceptors can be distinguished pharmacologically. Two main families of receptors, designated α and β, are classified on the basis of their responses to the adrenergic agonists *epinephrine*, *norepinephrine*, and *isoproterenol*. Each of these main receptor types has a number of specific receptor subtypes that have been identified. Alterations in the primary structure of the receptors influence their affinity for various agents.

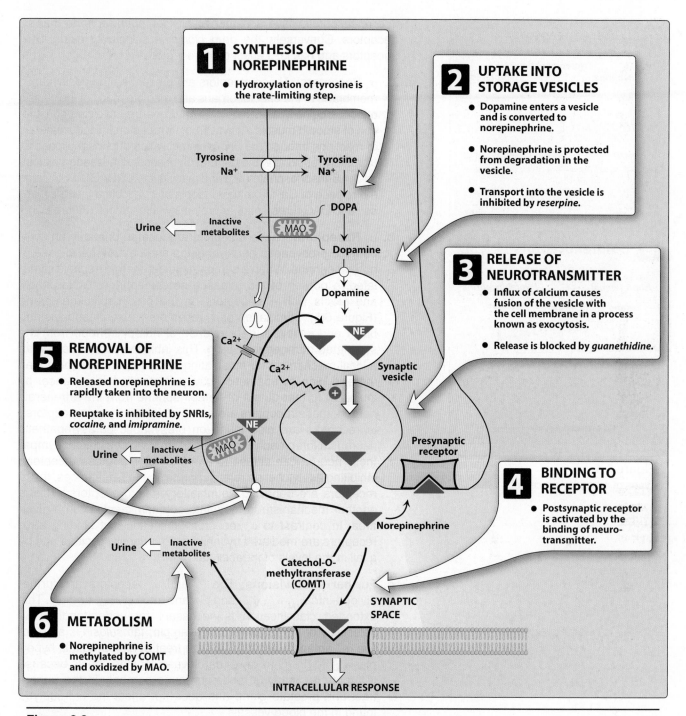

Figure 6.3
Synthesis and release of norepinephrine from the adrenergic neuron. MAO = monoamine oxidase, SNRI = serotonin-norepinephrine reuptake inhibitor.

1. **α-Adrenoceptors:** The α-adrenoceptors show a weak response to the synthetic agonist *isoproterenol*, but they are responsive to the naturally occurring catecholamines *epinephrine* and *norepinephrine* (Figure 6.4). For α receptors, the rank order of potency and affinity is *epinephrine ≥ norepinephrine >> isoproterenol*. The α-adrenoceptors are subdivided into two subgroups, α_1 and α_2, based on their affinities for α agonists and blocking drugs. For example,

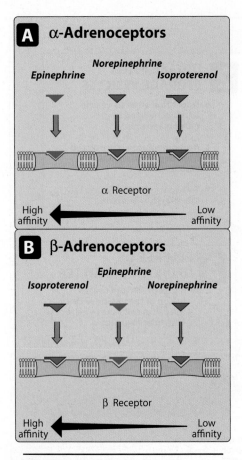

Figure 6.4
Types of adrenergic receptors.

the α_1 receptors have a higher affinity for *phenylephrine* than α_2 receptors. Conversely, the drug *clonidine* selectively binds to α_2 receptors and has less effect on α_1 receptors.

a. **α_1 Receptors:** These receptors are present on the postsynaptic membrane of the effector organs and mediate many of the classic effects, originally designated as α-adrenergic, involving constriction of smooth muscle. Activation of α_1 receptors initiates a series of reactions through the G protein activation of phospholipase C, ultimately resulting in the generation of second messengers inositol-1,4,5-trisphosphate (IP_3) and diacylglycerol (DAG). IP_3 initiates the release of Ca^{2+} from the endoplasmic reticulum into the cytosol, and DAG turns on other proteins within the cell (Figure 6.5).

b. **α_2 Receptors:** These receptors are located primarily on sympathetic presynaptic nerve endings and control the release of norepinephrine. When a sympathetic adrenergic nerve is stimulated, a portion of the released norepinephrine "circles back" and reacts with α_2 receptors on the presynaptic membrane (Figure 6.5). Stimulation of α_2 receptors causes feedback inhibition and inhibits further release of norepinephrine from the stimulated adrenergic neuron. This inhibitory action serves as a local mechanism for modulating norepinephrine output when there is high sympathetic activity. [Note: In this instance, by inhibiting further output of norepinephrine from the adrenergic neuron, these receptors are acting as inhibitory autoreceptors.] α_2 receptors are also found on presynaptic parasympathetic neurons. Norepinephrine released from a presynaptic sympathetic neuron can diffuse to and interact with these receptors, inhibiting acetylcholine release. [Note: In these instances, these receptors are behaving as inhibitory heteroreceptors.] This is another mechanism to modulate autonomic activity in a given area. In contrast to α_1 receptors, the effects of binding at α_2 receptors are mediated by inhibition of adenylyl cyclase and by a fall in the levels of intracellular cAMP.

c. **Further subdivisions:** The α_1 and α_2 receptors are further divided into α_{1A}, α_{1B}, α_{1C}, and α_{1D} and into α_{2A}, α_{2B}, and α_{2C}. This extended classification is necessary for understanding the selectivity of some drugs. For example, *tamsulosin* is a selective α_{1A} antagonist that is used to treat benign prostatic hyperplasia. The drug has fewer cardiovascular side effects because it targets α_{1A} subtype receptors found primarily in the urinary tract and prostate gland and does not affect the α_{1B} subtype found in the blood vessels.

2. **β-Adrenoceptors:** Responses of β receptors differ from those of α receptors and are characterized by a strong response to *isoproterenol*, with less sensitivity to *epinephrine* and *norepinephrine* (Figure 6.4). For β receptors, the rank order of potency is *isoproterenol > epinephrine > norepinephrine*. The β-adrenoceptors can be subdivided into three major subgroups, β_1, β_2, and β_3, based on their affinities for adrenergic agonists and antagonists. β_1 receptors have approximately equal affinities for *epinephrine* and *norepinephrine*, whereas β_2 receptors have a higher affinity for *epinephrine* than for *norepinephrine*. Thus, tissues with a

predominance of β_2 receptors (such as the vasculature of skeletal muscle) are particularly responsive to the effects of circulating epinephrine released by the adrenal medulla. β_3 receptors are involved in lipolysis and also have effects on the detrusor muscle of the bladder. Binding of a neurotransmitter at any of the three types of β receptors results in activation of adenylyl cyclase and increased concentrations of cAMP within the cell.

3. **Distribution of receptors:** Adrenergically innervated organs and tissues usually have a predominant type of receptor. For example, tissues such as the vasculature of skeletal muscle have both α_1 and β_2 receptors, but the β_2 receptors predominate. Other tissues may have one type of receptor almost exclusively. For example, the heart contains predominantly β_1 receptors.

4. **Characteristic responses mediated by adrenoceptors:** It is useful to organize the physiologic responses to adrenergic stimulation according to receptor type, because many drugs preferentially stimulate or block one type of receptor. Figure 6.6 summarizes the most prominent effects mediated by the adrenoceptors. As a generalization, stimulation of α_1 receptors characteristically produces vasoconstriction (particularly in skin and abdominal viscera) and an increase in total peripheral resistance and blood pressure. Stimulation of β_1 receptors characteristically causes cardiac stimulation (increase in heart rate and contractility), whereas stimulation of β_2 receptors produces vasodilation (in skeletal muscle vascular beds) and smooth muscle relaxation.

5. **Desensitization of receptors:** Prolonged exposure to the catecholamines reduces the responsiveness of these receptors, a phenomenon known as desensitization. Three mechanisms have been suggested to explain this phenomenon: 1) sequestration of the receptors so that they are unavailable for interaction with the ligand; 2) down-regulation, that is, a disappearance of the receptors either by destruction or by decreased synthesis; and 3) an inability to couple to G protein, because the receptor has been phosphorylated on the cytoplasmic side.

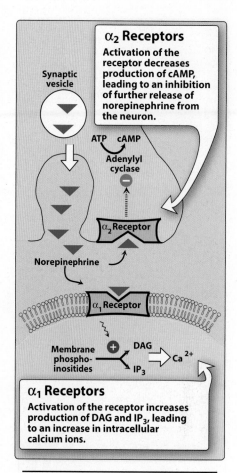

Figure 6.5
Second messengers mediate the effects of α receptors. DAG = diacylglycerol; IP_3 = inositol trisphosphate; ATP = adenosine triphosphate; cAMP = cyclic adenosine monophosphate.

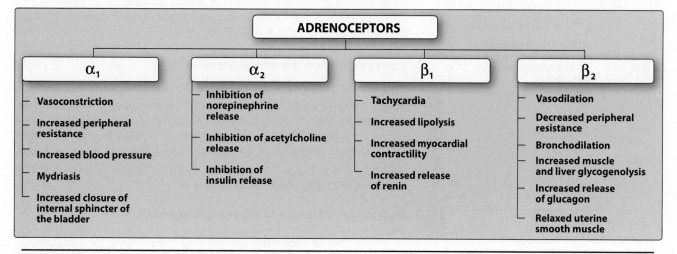

Figure 6.6
Major effects mediated by α- and β-adrenoceptors.

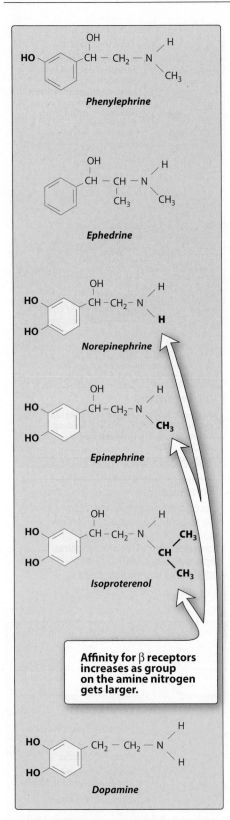

Figure 6.7
Structures of several important adrenergic agonists. Drugs containing the catechol ring are shown in *yellow*.

III. CHARACTERISTICS OF ADRENERGIC AGONISTS

Most of the adrenergic drugs are derivatives of β-phenylethylamine (Figure 6.7). Substitutions on the benzene ring or on the ethylamine side chains produce a variety of compounds with varying abilities to differentiate between α and β receptors and to penetrate the CNS. Two important structural features of these drugs are 1) the number and location of OH substitutions on the benzene ring and 2) the nature of the substituent on the amino nitrogen.

A. Catecholamines

Sympathomimetic amines that contain the 3,4-dihydroxybenzene group (such as *epinephrine*, *norepinephrine*, *isoproterenol*, and *dopamine*) are called catecholamines. These compounds share the following properties:

1. **High potency:** Catecholamines (with –OH groups in the 3 and 4 positions on the benzene ring) show the highest potency in directly activating α or β receptors.

2. **Rapid inactivation:** Catecholamines are metabolized by COMT postsynaptically and by MAO intraneuronally, as well as by COMT and MAO in the gut wall, and by MAO in the liver. Thus, catecholamines have only a brief period of action when given parenterally, and they are inactivated (ineffective) when administered orally.

3. **Poor penetration into the CNS:** Catecholamines are polar and, therefore, do not readily penetrate into the CNS. Nevertheless, most catecholamines have some clinical effects (anxiety, tremor, and headaches) that are attributable to action on the CNS.

B. Noncatecholamines

Compounds lacking the catechol hydroxyl groups have longer half-lives, because they are not inactivated by COMT. These include *phenylephrine*, *ephedrine*, and *amphetamine* (Figure 6.7). These agents are poor substrates for MAO (an important route of metabolism) and, thus, show a prolonged duration of action. Increased lipid solubility of many of the noncatecholamines (due to lack of polar hydroxyl groups) permits greater access to the CNS.

C. Substitutions on the amine nitrogen

The nature of the substituent on the amine nitrogen is important in determining β selectivity of the adrenergic agonist. For example, *epinephrine*, with a –CH$_3$ substituent on the amine nitrogen, is more potent at β receptors than *norepinephrine*, which has an unsubstituted amine. Similarly, *isoproterenol*, which has an isopropyl substituent –CH(CH$_3$)$_2$ on the amine nitrogen (Figure 6.7), is a strong β agonist with little α activity (Figure 6.4).

D. Mechanism of action of adrenergic agonists

1. **Direct-acting agonists:** These drugs act directly on α or β receptors, producing effects similar to those that occur following stimulation of sympathetic nerves or release of epinephrine from the adrenal

medulla (Figure 6.8). Examples of direct-acting agonists include *epinephrine*, *norepinephrine*, *isoproterenol*, and *phenylephrine*.

2. **Indirect-acting agonists:** These agents may block the reuptake of norepinephrine or cause the release of norepinephrine from the cytoplasmic pools or vesicles of the adrenergic neuron (Figure 6.8). The norepinephrine then traverses the synapse and binds to α or β receptors. Examples of reuptake inhibitors and agents that cause norepinephrine release include *cocaine* and *amphetamines*, respectively.

3. **Mixed-action agonists:** *Ephedrine* and its stereoisomer, *pseudoephedrine*, both stimulate adrenoceptors directly and release norepinephrine from the adrenergic neuron (Figure 6.8).

IV. DIRECT-ACTING ADRENERGIC AGONISTS

Direct-acting agonists bind to adrenergic receptors on effector organs without interacting with the presynaptic neuron. As a group, these agents are widely used clinically.

A. Epinephrine

Epinephrine [ep-i-NEF-rin] is one of the four catecholamines (*epinephrine*, *norepinephrine*, *dopamine*, and *dobutamine*) commonly used in therapy. The first three are naturally occurring neurotransmitters, and the latter is a synthetic compound. In the adrenal medulla, *norepinephrine* is methylated to yield *epinephrine*, which is stored in chromaffin cells along with *norepinephrine*. On stimulation, the adrenal medulla releases about 80% *epinephrine* and 20% *norepinephrine* directly into the circulation. *Epinephrine* interacts with both α and β receptors. At low doses, β effects (vasodilation) on the vascular system predominate, whereas at high doses, α effects (vasoconstriction) are the strongest.

1. Actions:

a. Cardiovascular: The major actions of *epinephrine* are on the cardiovascular system. *Epinephrine* strengthens the contractility of the myocardium (positive inotrope: β_1 action) and increases its rate of contraction (positive chronotrope: β_1 action). Therefore, cardiac output increases. These effects increase oxygen demands on the myocardium. *Epinephrine* activates β_1 receptors on the kidney to cause renin release. Renin is an enzyme involved in the production of angiotensin II, a potent vasoconstrictor. *Epinephrine* constricts arterioles in the skin, mucous membranes, and viscera (α effects), and it dilates vessels going to the liver and skeletal muscle (β_2 effects). Renal blood flow is decreased. Therefore, the cumulative effect is an increase in systolic blood pressure, coupled with a slight decrease in diastolic pressure due to β_2 receptor–mediated vasodilation in the skeletal muscle vascular bed (Figure 6.9).

b. Respiratory: *Epinephrine* causes powerful bronchodilation by acting directly on bronchial smooth muscle (β_2 action). It also inhibits the release of allergy mediators such as histamines from mast cells.

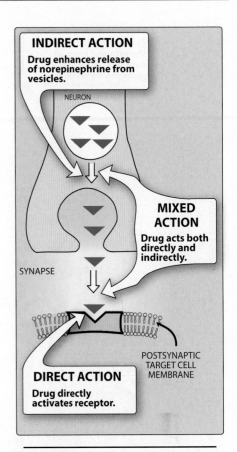

Figure 6.8
Sites of action of direct-, indirect-, and mixed-acting adrenergic agonists.

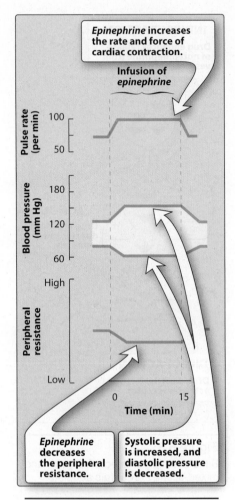

Figure 6.9
Cardiovascular effects of intravenous infusion of low doses of *epinephrine*.

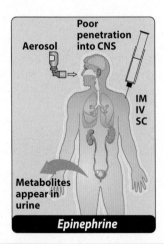

Figure 6.10
Pharmacokinetics of *epinephrine*.
CNS = central nervous system.

c. Hyperglycemia: *Epinephrine* has a significant hyperglycemic effect because of increased glycogenolysis in the liver (β_2 effect), increased release of glucagon (β_2 effect), and a decreased release of insulin (α_2 effect).

d. Lipolysis: *Epinephrine* initiates lipolysis through agonist activity on the β receptors of adipose tissue. Increased levels of cAMP stimulate a hormone-sensitive lipase, which hydrolyzes triglycerides to free fatty acids and glycerol.

2. Therapeutic uses:

a. Bronchospasm: *Epinephrine* is the primary drug used in the emergency treatment of respiratory conditions when bronchoconstriction has resulted in diminished respiratory function. Thus, in treatment of acute asthma and anaphylactic shock, *epinephrine* is the drug of choice and can be life saving in this setting. Within a few minutes after subcutaneous administration, respiratory function greatly improves. However, selective β_2 agonists, such as *albuterol*, are favored in the chronic treatment of asthma because of a longer duration of action and minimal cardiac stimulatory effects.

b. Anaphylactic shock: *Epinephrine* is the drug of choice for the treatment of type I hypersensitivity reactions (including anaphylaxis) in response to allergens.

c. Cardiac arrest: *Epinephrine* may be used to restore cardiac rhythm in patients with cardiac arrest.

d. Anesthetics: Local anesthetic solutions may contain low concentrations (for example, 1:100,000 parts) of *epinephrine*. *Epinephrine* greatly increases the duration of local anesthesia by producing vasoconstriction at the site of injection. This allows the local anesthetic to persist at the injection site before being absorbed into the systemic circulation. Very weak solutions of *epinephrine* can also be applied topically to vasoconstrict mucous membranes and control oozing of capillary blood.

3. Pharmacokinetics: *Epinephrine* has a rapid onset but a brief duration of action (due to rapid degradation). The preferred route is intramuscular (anterior thigh) due to rapid absorption. In emergency situations, *epinephrine* is given intravenously (IV) for the most rapid onset of action. It may also be given subcutaneously, by endotracheal tube, and by inhalation (Figure 6.10). It is rapidly metabolized by MAO and COMT, and the metabolites metanephrine and vanillylmandelic acid are excreted in urine.

4. Adverse effects: *Epinephrine* can produce adverse CNS effects that include anxiety, fear, tension, headache, and tremor. It can trigger cardiac arrhythmias, particularly if the patient is receiving *digoxin*. *Epinephrine* can also induce pulmonary edema. *Epinephrine* may have enhanced cardiovascular actions in patients with hyperthyroidism, and the dose must be reduced in these individuals. Patients with hyperthyroidism may have an increased production of adrenergic receptors in the vasculature, leading to a hypersensitive response. Inhalation anesthetics also sensitize the heart to the effects of *epinephrine*, which may lead to tachycardia. *Epinephrine* increases the release of endogenous stores of glucose. In diabetic patients, dosages of *insulin* may have to be increased. Nonselective β-blockers prevent vasodilatory effects of *epinephrine* on β_2 receptors, leaving α receptor stimulation unopposed. This may lead to increased peripheral resistance and increased blood pressure.

B. Norepinephrine

Because *norepinephrine* [nor-ep-ih-NEF-rin] is the neurotransmitter of adrenergic nerves, it should, theoretically, stimulate all types of adrenergic receptors. However, when administered in therapeutic doses, the α-adrenergic receptor is most affected.

1. Cardiovascular actions:

a. Vasoconstriction: *Norepinephrine* causes a rise in peripheral resistance due to intense vasoconstriction of most vascular beds, including the kidney (α_1 effect). Both systolic and diastolic blood pressures increase (Figure 6.11). [Note: *Norepinephrine* causes greater vasoconstriction than *epinephrine*, because it does not induce compensatory vasodilation via β_2 receptors on blood vessels supplying skeletal muscles. The weak β_2 activity of *norepinephrine* also explains why it is not useful in the treatment of asthma or anaphylaxis.]

b. Baroreceptor reflex: *Norepinephrine* increases blood pressure, and this stimulates the baroreceptors, inducing a rise in vagal activity. The increased vagal activity produces a reflex bradycardia, which is sufficient to counteract the local actions of *norepinephrine* on the heart, although the reflex compensation does not affect the positive inotropic effects of the drug (Figure 6.11). When *atropine*, which blocks the transmission of vagal effects, is given before *norepinephrine*, stimulation of the heart by *norepinephrine* is evident as tachycardia.

2. Therapeutic uses:
Norepinephrine is used to treat shock, because it increases vascular resistance and, therefore, increases blood pressure. It has no other clinically significant uses.

3. Pharmacokinetics:
Norepinephrine is given IV for rapid onset of action. The duration of action is 1 to 2 minutes, following the end of the infusion. It is rapidly metabolized by MAO and COMT, and inactive metabolites are excreted in the urine.

4. Adverse effects:
These are similar to *epinephrine*. In addition, *norepinephrine* is a potent vasoconstrictor and may cause blanching and sloughing of skin along an injected vein. If extravasation (leakage of drug from the vessel into tissues surrounding the injection site) occurs, it can cause tissue necrosis. It should not be administered in peripheral veins, if possible. Impaired circulation from *norepinephrine* may be treated with the α receptor antagonist *phentolamine*.

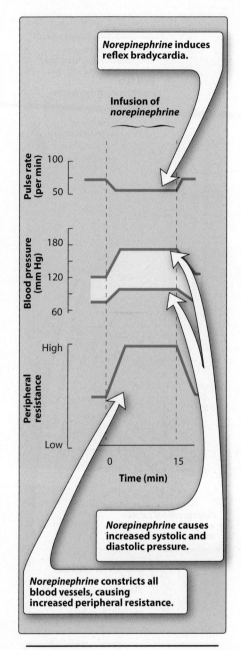

Figure 6.11
Cardiovascular effects of intravenous infusion of *norepinephrine*.

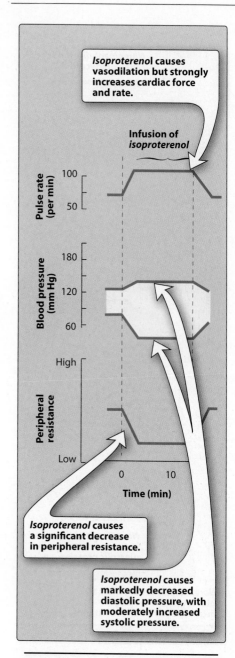

Figure 6.12
Cardiovascular effects of intravenous infusion of *isoproterenol.*

C. Isoproterenol

Isoproterenol [eye-soe-proe-TER-e-nole] is a direct-acting synthetic catecholamine that stimulates both β_1- and β_2-adrenergic receptors. Its nonselectivity is one of its drawbacks and the reason why it is rarely used therapeutically. Its action on α receptors is insignificant. *Isoproterenol* produces intense stimulation of the heart, increasing heart rate, contractility, and cardiac output (Figure 6.12). It is as active as *epinephrine* in this action. *Isoproterenol* also dilates the arterioles of skeletal muscle (β_2 effect), resulting in decreased peripheral resistance. Because of its cardiac stimulatory action, it may increase systolic blood pressure slightly, but it greatly reduces mean arterial and diastolic blood pressures (Figure 6.12). *Isoproterenol* is a potent bronchodilator (β_2 effect). The use of *isoproterenol* has largely been replaced with other drugs, but it may be useful in atrioventricular (AV) block. The adverse effects of *isoproterenol* are similar to those of *epinephrine.*

D. Dopamine

Dopamine [DOE-pa-meen], the immediate metabolic precursor of norepinephrine, occurs naturally in the CNS in the basal ganglia, where it functions as a neurotransmitter, as well as in the adrenal medulla. *Dopamine* can activate α- and β-adrenergic receptors. For example, at higher doses, it causes vasoconstriction by activating α_1 receptors, whereas at lower doses, it stimulates β_1 cardiac receptors. In addition, D_1 and D_2 dopaminergic receptors, distinct from the α- and β-adrenergic receptors, occur in the peripheral mesenteric and renal vascular beds, where binding of *dopamine* produces vasodilation. D_2 receptors are also found on presynaptic adrenergic neurons, where their activation interferes with norepinephrine release.

1. **Actions:**

   a. **Cardiovascular:** *Dopamine* exerts a stimulatory effect on the β_1 receptors of the heart, having both positive inotropic and chronotropic effects (Figure 6.13). At very high doses, *dopamine* activates α_1 receptors on the vasculature, resulting in vasoconstriction.

   b. **Renal and visceral:** *Dopamine* dilates renal and splanchnic arterioles by activating dopaminergic receptors, thereby increasing blood flow to the kidneys and other viscera (Figure 6.13). These receptors are not affected by α- or β-blocking drugs. Therefore, *dopamine* is clinically useful in the treatment of shock, in which significant increases in sympathetic activity might compromise renal function.

2. **Therapeutic uses:** *Dopamine* is the drug of choice for cardiogenic and septic shock and is given by continuous infusion. It raises blood pressure by stimulating the β_1 receptors on the heart to increase cardiac output and α_1 receptors on blood vessels to increase total peripheral resistance. In addition, it enhances perfusion to the kidney and splanchnic areas, as described above.

Increased blood flow to the kidney enhances the glomerular filtration rate and causes diuresis. In this regard, *dopamine* is far superior to *norepinephrine*, which diminishes blood supply to the kidney and may cause renal shutdown. It is also used to treat hypotension and severe heart failure, primarily in patients with low or normal peripheral vascular resistance and in patients who have oliguria.

3. **Adverse effects:** An overdose of *dopamine* produces the same effects as sympathetic stimulation. *Dopamine* is rapidly metabolized by MAO or COMT, and its adverse effects (nausea, hypertension, and arrhythmias) are, therefore, short-lived.

E. Fenoldopam

Fenoldopam [fen-OL-de-pam] is an agonist of peripheral dopamine D_1 receptors. It is used as a rapid-acting vasodilator to treat severe hypertension in hospitalized patients, acting on coronary arteries, kidney arterioles, and mesenteric arteries. *Fenoldopam* is a racemic mixture, and the R-isomer is the active component. It undergoes extensive first-pass metabolism and has a 10-minute elimination half-life after IV infusion. Headache, flushing, dizziness, nausea, vomiting, and tachycardia (due to vasodilation) may be observed with this agent.

F. Dobutamine

Dobutamine [doe-BYOO-ta-meen] is a synthetic, direct-acting catecholamine that is a β_1 receptor agonist. It increases cardiac rate and output with few vascular effects. *Dobutamine* is used to increase cardiac output in acute heart failure (see Chapter 19), as well as for inotropic support after cardiac surgery. The drug increases cardiac output and does not significantly elevate oxygen demands of the myocardium, a major advantage over other sympathomimetic drugs. *Dobutamine* should be used with caution in atrial fibrillation, because it increases AV conduction. Other adverse effects are similar to *epinephrine*. Tolerance may develop with prolonged use.

G. Oxymetazoline

Oxymetazoline [OX-ee-mee-TAZ-ih-leen] is a direct-acting synthetic adrenergic agonist that stimulates both α_1- and α_2-adrenergic receptors. *Oxymetazoline* is found in many over-the-counter short-term nasal spray decongestants, as well as in ophthalmic drops for the relief of redness of the eyes associated with swimming, colds, and contact lenses. *Oxymetazoline* directly stimulates α receptors on blood vessels supplying the nasal mucosa and conjunctiva, thereby producing vasoconstriction and decreasing congestion. It is absorbed in the systemic circulation regardless of the route of administration and may produce nervousness, headaches, and trouble sleeping. Local irritation and sneezing may occur with intranasal administration. Rebound congestion and dependence are observed with long-term use.

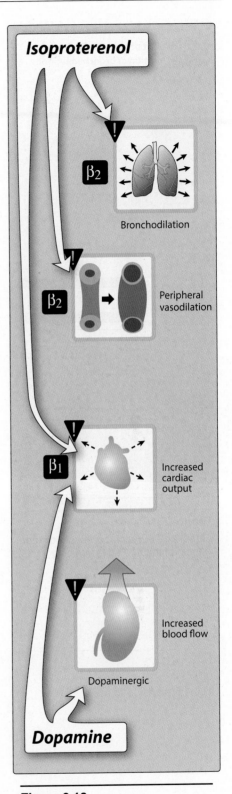

Figure 6.13
Clinically important actions of *isoproterenol* and *dopamine*.

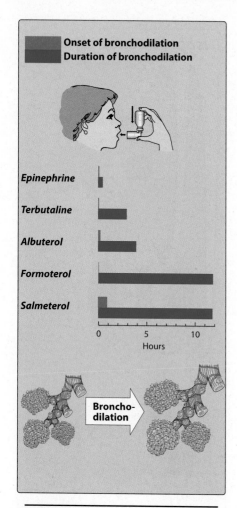

Figure 6.14
Onset and duration of bronchodilation effects of inhaled adrenergic agonists.

H. Phenylephrine

Phenylephrine [fen-ill-EF-reen] is a direct-acting, synthetic adrenergic drug that binds primarily to α_1 receptors. *Phenylephrine* is a vasoconstrictor that raises both systolic and diastolic blood pressures. It has no effect on the heart itself but, rather, induces reflex bradycardia when given parenterally. The drug is used to treat hypotension in hospitalized or surgical patients (especially those with a rapid heart rate). Large doses can cause hypertensive headache and cardiac irregularities. *Phenylephrine* acts as a nasal decongestant when applied topically or taken orally. *Phenylephrine* has replaced *pseudoephedrine* in many oral decongestants, since *pseudoephedrine* has been misused to make *methamphetamine*. *Phenylephrine* is also used in ophthalmic solutions for mydriasis.

I. Clonidine

Clonidine [KLOE-ni-deen] is an α_2 agonist that is used for the treatment of hypertension. It can also be used to minimize the symptoms that accompany withdrawal from opiates, tobacco smoking, and benzodiazepines. *Clonidine* acts centrally on presynaptic α_2 receptors to produce inhibition of sympathetic vasomotor centers, decreasing sympathetic outflow to the periphery. The most common side effects of *clonidine* are lethargy, sedation, constipation, and xerostomia. Abrupt discontinuance must be avoided to prevent rebound hypertension. *Clonidine* and another α_2 agonist *methyldopa* are discussed along with antihypertensives in Chapter 17.

J. Albuterol and terbutaline

Albuterol [al-BYOO-ter-ole] and *terbutaline* [ter-BYOO-te-leen] are short-acting β_2 agonists used primarily as bronchodilators and administered by a metered-dose inhaler (Figure 6.14). *Albuterol* is the short-acting β_2 agonist of choice for the management of acute asthma symptoms. Inhaled *terbutaline* is no longer available in the United States, but is still used in other countries. *Terbutaline* is also used off-label as a uterine relaxant to suppress premature labor. One of the most common side effects of these agents is tremor, but patients tend to develop tolerance to this effect. Other side effects include restlessness, apprehension, and anxiety. When these drugs are administered orally, they may cause tachycardia or arrhythmia (due to β_1 receptor activation), especially in patients with underlying cardiac disease. Monoamine oxidase inhibitors (MAOIs) also increase the risk of adverse cardiovascular effects, and concomitant use should be avoided.

K. Salmeterol and formoterol

Salmeterol [sal-ME-ter-ole] and *formoterol* [for-MOH-ter-ole] are long-acting β agonists (LABAs) that are β_2 selective. A single dose by a metered-dose inhalation device, such as a dry powder inhaler, provides sustained bronchodilation over 12 hours, compared with less than 3 hours for *albuterol*. Unlike *formoterol*, however, *salmeterol* has a somewhat delayed onset of action (Figure 6.14). These agents are not recommended as monotherapy, but are highly efficacious when combined with a corticosteroid. *Salmeterol* and *formoterol* are the agents of choice for treating nocturnal asthma in symptomatic patients taking other asthma medications. LABAs have been shown to increase the risk of asthma-related deaths.

L. Mirabegron

Mirabegron [mir-a-BEG-ron] is a β_3 agonist that relaxes the detrusor smooth muscle and increases bladder capacity. It is used for patients with overactive bladder. *Mirabegron* may increase blood pressure and should not be used in patients with uncontrolled hypertension. It increases levels of *digoxin* and also inhibits the CYP2D6 isozyme, which may enhance the effects of other medications metabolized by this pathway (for example, *metoprolol*).

V. INDIRECT-ACTING ADRENERGIC AGONISTS

Indirect-acting adrenergic agonists cause the release, inhibit the reuptake, or inhibit the degradation of epinephrine or norepinephrine (Figure 6.8). They potentiate the effects of epinephrine or norepinephrine produced endogenously, but do not directly affect postsynaptic receptors.

A. Amphetamine

The marked central stimulatory action of *amphetamine* [am-FET-a-meen] is often mistaken by drug abusers as its only action. However, the drug can also increase blood pressure significantly by α_1 agonist action on the vasculature, as well as β_1-stimulatory effects on the heart. Its actions are mediated primarily through an increase in nonvesicular release of catecholamines such as dopamine and norepinephrine from nerve terminals. Thus, *amphetamine* is an indirect-acting adrenergic drug. The actions and therapeutic uses of *amphetamine* and its derivatives are discussed under stimulants of the CNS (see Chapter 16).

B. Tyramine

Tyramine [TIE-ra-meen] is not a clinically useful drug, but it is important because it is found in fermented foods, such as aged cheese and Chianti wine. It is a normal by-product of tyrosine metabolism. Normally, it is oxidized by MAO in the gastrointestinal tract, but, if the patient is taking MAOIs, it can precipitate serious vasopressor episodes. Like *amphetamines*, *tyramine* can enter the nerve terminal and displace stored norepinephrine. The released catecholamine then acts on adrenoceptors.

C. Cocaine

Cocaine [koe-KANE] is unique among local anesthetics in having the ability to block the sodium-chloride (Na^+/Cl^-)-dependent norepinephrine transporter required for cellular uptake of norepinephrine into the adrenergic neuron. Consequently, norepinephrine accumulates in the synaptic space, resulting in enhanced sympathetic activity and potentiation of the actions of epinephrine and norepinephrine. Therefore, small doses of the catecholamines produce greatly magnified effects

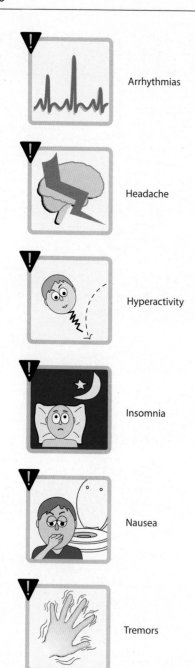

Arrhythmias

Headache

Hyperactivity

Insomnia

Nausea

Tremors

Figure 6.15
Some adverse effects observed with adrenergic agonists.

in an individual taking *cocaine*. In addition, the duration of action of epinephrine and norepinephrine is increased. Like *amphetamines*, it can increase blood pressure by α_1 agonist actions and β stimulatory effects. [Note: *Cocaine* as a drug of abuse is discussed in Chapter 15.]

VI. MIXED-ACTION ADRENERGIC AGONISTS

Ephedrine [eh-FED-rin] and *pseudoephedrine* [soo-doe-eh-FED-rin] are mixed-action adrenergic agents. They not only release stored norepinephrine from nerve endings (Figure 6.8) but also directly stimulate both α and β receptors. Thus, a wide variety of adrenergic actions ensue that are similar to those of *epinephrine*, although less potent. *Ephedrine* and *pseudoephedrine* are not catechols and are poor substrates for COMT and MAO. Therefore, these drugs have a long duration of action. *Ephedrine* and *pseudoephedrine* have excellent absorption orally and penetrate into the CNS, but *pseudoephedrine* has fewer CNS effects. *Ephedrine* is eliminated largely unchanged in urine, and *pseudoephedrine* undergoes incomplete hepatic metabolism before elimination in urine. *Ephedrine* raises systolic and diastolic blood pressures by vasoconstriction and cardiac stimulation and can be used to treat hypotension. *Ephedrine* produces bronchodilation, but it is less potent and slower acting than *epinephrine* or *isoproterenol*. It was previously used to prevent asthma attacks but has been replaced by more effective medications. *Ephedrine* produces a mild stimulation of the CNS. This increases alertness, decreases fatigue, and prevents sleep. It also improves athletic performance. [Note: The clinical use of *ephedrine* is declining because of the availability of better, more potent agents that cause fewer adverse effects. *Ephedrine*-containing herbal supplements (mainly ephedra-containing products) have been banned by the U.S. Food and Drug Administration because of life-threatening cardiovascular reactions.] *Pseudoephedrine* is primarily used orally to treat nasal and sinus congestion. *Pseudoephedrine* has been illegally used to produce *methamphetamine*. Therefore, products containing *pseudoephedrine* have certain restrictions and must be kept behind the sales counter in the United States. Important characteristics of the adrenergic agonists are summarized in Figures 6.15–6.17.

TISSUE	RECEPTOR TYPE	ACTION	OPPOSING ACTIONS
Heart			
• Sinus and AV	β_1	↑ Automaticity	Cholinergic receptors
• Conduction pathway	β_1	↑ Conduction velocity, automaticity	Cholinergic receptors
• Myofibrils	β_1	↑ Contractility, automaticity	
Vascular smooth muscle	β_2	Vasodilation	α-Adrenergic receptors
Bronchial smooth muscle	β_2	Bronchodilation	Cholinergic receptors
Kidneys	β_1	↑ Renin release	α_1-Adrenergic receptors
Liver	β_2, α_1	↑ Glycogenolysis and gluconeogenesis	—
Adipose tissue	β_3	↑ Lipolysis	α_2-Adrenergic receptors
Skeletal muscle	β_2	↑ Increased contractility Potassium uptake; glycogenolysis Dilates arteries to skeletal muscle Tremor	—
Eye-ciliary muscle	β_2	Relaxation	Cholinergic receptors
GI tract	β_2	↓ Motility	Cholinergic receptors
Gall bladder	β_2	Relaxation	Cholinergic receptors
Urinary bladder detrusor muscle	β_2	Relaxation	Cholinergic receptors
Uterus	β_2	Relaxation	Oxytocin

Figure 6.16
Summary of β-adrenergic receptors. AV = atrioventricular; GI = gastrointestinal.

	DRUG	RECEPTOR SPECIFICITY	THERAPEUTIC USES
	Epinephrine	α_1, α_2 β_1, β_2	Acute asthma Anaphylactic shock In local anesthetics to increase duration of action
	Norepinephrine	α_1, α_2 β_1	Treatment of shock
	Isoproterenol	β_1, β_2	As a cardiac stimulant
	Dopamine	Dopaminergic α_1, β_1	Treatment of shock Treatment of congestive heart failure Raise blood pressure
	Dobutamine	β_1	Treatment of acute heart failure
	Oxymetazoline	α_1	As a nasal decongestant
	Phenylephrine	α_1	As a nasal decongestant Raise blood pressure Treatment of paroxysmal supraventricular tachycardia
	Clonidine	α_2	Treatment of hypertension
	Albuterol *Terbutaline*	β_2	Treatment of bronchospasm (short acting)
	Salmeterol *Formoterol*	β_2	Treatment of bronchospasm (long acting)
	Amphetamine	α, β, CNS	As a CNS stimulant in treatment of children with attention deficit syndrome, narcolepsy, and for appetite control
	Ephedrine *Pseudoephedrine*	α, β, CNS	As a nasal decongestant Raise blood pressure

CATECHOLAMINES

- Rapid onset of action
- Brief duration of action
- Not administered orally
- Do not penetrate the blood-brain barrier

NONCATECHOL-AMINES

Compared to catecholamines:

- Longer duration of action
- All can be administered orally or via inhalation

Figure 6.17
Summary of the therapeutic uses of adrenergic agonists. CNS = central nervous system.

Study Questions

Choose the ONE best answer.

6.1 Which of the following is correct regarding adrenergic neurotransmission?

   A. Epinephrine is the major neurotransmitter released from sympathetic nerve terminals.

   B. Norepinephrine is mainly released from the adrenal glands.

   C. Tricyclic antidepressants and cocaine prevent reuptake of norepinephrine into the nerve terminals.

   D. Monoamine oxidase (MAO) converts dopamine to norepinephrine in the nerve terminal.

> Correct answer = C. Tricyclic antidepressants (TCAs) and cocaine inhibit the transporter protein that prevents the reuptake of norepinephrine into the sympathetic nerve terminals. Norepinephrine, not epinephrine, is the major neurotransmitter released from sympathetic nerve terminals. Epinephrine, not norepinephrine, is mainly released from the adrenal glands. Dopamine is converted to norepinephrine by dopamine β-hydroxylase, not by MAO.

6.2 All of the following are correct regarding adrenergic receptors, *except*:

   A. α_1 Receptors are primarily located on the postsynaptic membrane in the effector organs.

   B. α_2 Receptors are primarily located on the presynaptic sympathetic nerve terminals.

   C. β_1 Receptors are found mainly in the heart.

   D. β_2 Receptors are found mainly in adipose tissue.

> Correct answer = D. α_1 Receptors are located on the postsynaptic membrane in the effector organs such as blood vessels. α_2 Receptors are mainly found on the presynaptic sympathetic nerve terminals, where they inhibit the release of norepinephrine when activated. β_1 Receptors are found in the heart, in addition to some other tissues, and cause increase in heart rate and contractility when activated. β_2 receptors are found in the lungs, in addition to some other tissues, and cause relaxation of bronchial smooth muscles when activated. β_3 Receptors are found in adipose tissue and are involved in lipolysis.

6.3 A hypertensive patient was accidentally given an α_2 agonist instead of an α_1 blocker. Which of the following is correct in this situation?

   A. α_2 Agonists can increase the release of norepinephrine from sympathetic nerve terminals.

   B. α_2 Agonists can reduce blood pressure in this patient.

   C. α_2 Agonists can increase blood pressure in this patient.

   D. α_2 Agonists will not affect blood pressure in this patient.

> Correct answer = B. α_2 Agonists activate α_2 receptors located in the presynaptic terminal of sympathetic neurons and cause a reduction in the release of norepinephrine from sympathetic nerve terminals. This leads to a reduction in blood pressure. α_2 Agonists such as clonidine and methyldopa are therefore used as antihypertensive agents.

6.4 Which of the following is correct regarding responses mediated by adrenergic receptors?

   A. Stimulation of α_1 receptors increases blood pressure.

   B. Stimulation of α_1 receptors reduces blood pressure.

   C. Stimulation of sympathetic presynaptic α_2 receptors increases norepinephrine release.

   D. Stimulation of β_2 receptors increases heart rate (tachycardia).

   E. Stimulation of β_2 receptors causes bronchoconstriction.

> Correct answer = A. Stimulation of α_1 receptors, mostly found in the blood vessels, causes vasoconstriction and increase in blood pressure. Stimulation of α_2 receptors on the sympathetic presynaptic terminal reduces the release of norepinephrine. β_2 receptors are not found in the heart, so activation of β_2 receptors does not affect heart rate. Stimulation of β_2 receptors found in the bronchial tissues causes bronchodilation, not bronchoconstriction.

6.5 An asthma patient was given a nonselective β agonist to relieve bronchoconstriction. Which of the following adverse effects would you expect to see in this patient?

   A. Bradycardia.

   B. Tachycardia.

   C. Hypotension (reduction in blood pressure).

   D. Worsening bronchoconstriction.

> Correct answer = B. A nonselective β agonist activates both β_1 as well as β_2 receptors. β_1 activation causes an increase in heart rate (tachycardia), contractility, and subsequent increase in blood pressure. It relieves bronchoconstriction because of the β_2 receptor activation.

6.6 Which of the following adrenergic agonists is most likely to cause CNS side effects when administered systemically?

A. Epinephrine.

B. Norepinephrine.

C. Isoproterenol.

D. Dopamine.

E. Ephedrine.

Correct answer = E. Ephedrine is more lipophilic compared to the other drugs listed and therefore is more likely to cross the blood–brain barrier when administered systemically. Therefore, ephedrine is more likely to cause CNS side effects compared to other listed drugs.

6.7 A 12-year-old boy who is allergic to peanuts was brought to the emergency room after accidentally consuming peanuts contained in fast food. He is in anaphylactic shock. Which of the following drugs would be most appropriate to treat this patient?

A. Norepinephrine.

B. Phenylephrine.

C. Dobutamine.

D. Epinephrine.

Correct answer = D. Norepinephrine has more α agonistic effects and activates mainly α_1, α_2, and β_1 receptors. Epinephrine has more β agonistic effects and activates mainly α_1, α_2, β_1, and β_2 receptors. Phenylephrine has predominantly α effects and activates mainly α_1 receptors. Dobutamine mainly activates β_1 receptors and has no significant effects on β_2 receptors. Thus, epinephrine is the drug of choice in anaphylactic shock that can both stimulate the heart (β_1 activation) and dilate bronchioles (β_2 activation).

6.8 A 70-year-old patient was brought to the emergency room with a blood pressure of 76/60 mm Hg, tachycardia, and low cardiac output. He was diagnosed with acute heart failure. Which of the following drugs would be the most appropriate to improve his cardiac function?

A. Epinephrine.

B. Fenoldopam.

C. Dobutamine.

D. Isoproterenol.

Correct answer = C. Among the choices, the ideal drug to increase contractility of the heart in acute heart failure is dobutamine, since it is a selective β_1-adrenergic agonist. Fenoldopam is a dopamine agonist used to treat severe hypertension. Other drugs are nonselective adrenergic agonists that could cause unwanted side effects.

6.9 Which of the following adrenergic agonists is commonly present in nasal sprays available over-the-counter (OTC) to treat nasal congestion?

A. Clonidine.

B. Albuterol.

C. Oxymetazoline.

D. Dobutamine.

E. Norepinephrine.

Correct answer = C. Drugs with selective α_1 agonistic activity are commonly used as nasal decongestants because of their ability to cause vasoconstriction in the nasal vessels. Oxymetazoline is an α_1 agonist and therefore the preferred drug among the choices as a nasal decongestant. Clonidine is an α_2 agonist, albuterol is a β_2 agonist, dobutamine is a β_1 agonist, and norepinephrine is a nonselective adrenergic agonist.

6.10 One of your patients who is hypertensive and gets mild asthma attacks occasionally bought an herbal remedy online to help with his asthma. He is not on any asthma medications currently but is receiving a β_1-selective blocker for his hypertension. The herbal remedy seems to relieve his asthma attacks, but his blood pressure seems to increase despite the β-blocker therapy. Which of the following drugs is most likely present in the herbal remedy he is taking?

A. Phenylephrine.

B. Norepinephrine.

C. Dobutamine.

D. Ephedrine.

E. Salmeterol.

Correct answer = D. Two drugs among the choices that could relieve asthma are ephedrine and salmeterol, as they activate β_2 receptors in the bronchioles and cause bronchodilation. However, salmeterol is a selective β_2 agonist and should not cause an increase in blood pressure. Ephedrine on the other hand stimulates the release of norepinephrine and acts as a direct agonist at α- and β-adrenergic receptors, thus causing an increase in blood pressure. Phenylephrine (a nonselective α agonist) does not cause bronchodilation. Norepinephrine is a nonselective adrenergic agonist that does not have any stimulatory effects on β_2 receptors. Also, norepinephrine is not active when given orally.

Adrenergic Antagonists

7

Rajan Radhakrishnan

I. OVERVIEW

The adrenergic antagonists (also called adrenergic blockers or sympatholytics) bind to adrenoceptors but do not trigger the usual receptor-mediated intracellular effects. These drugs act by either reversibly or irreversibly attaching to the adrenoceptors, thus preventing activation by endogenous catecholamines. Like the agonists, the adrenergic antagonists are classified according to their relative affinities for α or β receptors in the sympathetic nervous system. Numerous adrenergic antagonists have important roles in clinical medicine, primarily to treat diseases associated with the cardiovascular system. [Note: Antagonists that block dopamine receptors are most important in the central nervous system (CNS) and are, therefore, considered in that section.] The adrenergic antagonists discussed in this chapter are summarized in Figure 7.1.

II. α-ADRENERGIC BLOCKING AGENTS

Drugs that block α adrenoceptors profoundly affect blood pressure. Because normal sympathetic control of the vasculature occurs in large part through agonist actions on α-adrenergic receptors, blockade of these receptors reduces the sympathetic tone of the blood vessels, resulting in decreased peripheral vascular resistance. This induces a reflex tachycardia resulting from the lowered blood pressure. The magnitude of the response depends on the sympathetic tone of the individual when the agent is given. [Note: β receptors, including β_1 adrenoceptors on the heart, are not affected by α blockade.] The α-adrenergic blocking agents, *phenoxybenzamine* and *phentolamine*, have limited clinical applications.

A. Phenoxybenzamine

Phenoxybenzamine [fen-ox-ee-BEN-za-meen] is nonselective, linking covalently to both α_1 and α_2 receptors (Figure 7.2). The block is irreversible and noncompetitive, and the only way the body can overcome the block is to synthesize new adrenoceptors, which requires a day or longer. Therefore, the actions of *phenoxybenzamine* last about 24 hours. After the drug is injected, a delay of a few hours occurs before a blockade develops.

α BLOCKERS
Alfuzosin UROXATRAL
Doxazosin CARDURA
Phenoxybenzamine DIBENZYLINE
Phentolamine REGITINE
Prazosin MINIPRESS
Tamsulosin FLOMAX
Terazosin HYTRIN
Yohimbine YOCON

β BLOCKERS
Acebutolol SECTRAL
Atenolol TENORMIN
Betaxolol BETOPTIC-S, KERLONE
Bisoprolol ZEBETA
Carteolol CARTROL
Carvedilol COREG, COREG CR
Esmolol BREVIBLOC
Labetalol TRANDATE
Metoprolol LOPRESSOR, TOPROL-XL
Nadolol CORGARD
Nebivolol BYSTOLIC
Penbutolol LEVATOL
Pindolol VISKEN
Propranolol INDERAL LA, INNOPRAN XL
Timolol BETIMOL, ISTALOL, TIMOPTIC

DRUGS AFFECTING NEURO-TRANSMITTER UPTAKE OR RELEASE
Reserpine SERPASIL

Figure 7.1
Summary of blocking agents and drugs affecting neurotransmitter uptake or release.

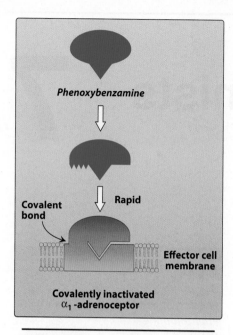

Figure 7.2
Covalent inactivation of α_1 adrenoceptor by *phenoxybenzamine*.

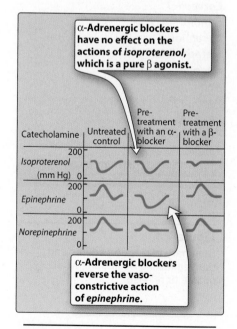

Figure 7.3
Summary of effects of adrenergic blockers on the changes in blood pressure induced by *isoproterenol*, *epinephrine*, and *norepinephrine*.

1. **Actions:**

   a. **Cardiovascular effects:** By blocking α receptors, *phenoxybenzamine* prevents vasoconstriction of peripheral blood vessels by endogenous catecholamines. The decreased peripheral resistance provokes a reflex tachycardia. Furthermore, the ability to block presynaptic inhibitory α_2 receptors in the heart can contribute to an increased cardiac output. [Note: Blocking these receptors results in more norepinephrine release, which stimulates β_1 receptors on the heart, increasing cardiac output.] Thus, the drug has been unsuccessful in maintaining lowered blood pressure in hypertension, and it is no longer used for this purpose.

   b. **Epinephrine reversal:** All α-adrenergic blockers reverse the α agonist actions of *epinephrine*. For example, the vasoconstrictive action of *epinephrine* is interrupted, but vasodilation of other vascular beds caused by stimulation of β_2 receptors is not blocked. Therefore, in the presence of *phenoxybenzamine*, the systemic blood pressure decreases in response to *epinephrine* (Figure 7.3). [Note: The actions of *norepinephrine* are not reversed but are diminished because *norepinephrine* lacks significant β agonist action on the vasculature.] *Phenoxybenzamine* has no effect on the actions of *isoproterenol*, which is a pure β agonist (Figure 7.3).

2. **Therapeutic uses:** *Phenoxybenzamine* is used in the treatment of pheochromocytoma, a catecholamine-secreting tumor of cells derived from the adrenal medulla. It may be used prior to surgical removal of the tumor to prevent a hypertensive crisis, and it is also useful in the chronic management of inoperable tumors. *Phenoxybenzamine* is sometimes effective in treating Raynaud disease and frostbite.

3. **Adverse effects:** *Phenoxybenzamine* can cause postural hypotension, nasal stuffiness, nausea, and vomiting. It may inhibit ejaculation. It may also induce reflex tachycardia, which is mediated by the baroreceptor reflex. *Phenoxybenzamine* should be used with caution in patients with cerebrovascular or cardiovascular disease.

B. Phentolamine

In contrast to *phenoxybenzamine*, *phentolamine* [fen-TOLE-a-meen] produces a competitive block of α_1 and α_2 receptors that lasts for approximately 4 hours after a single injection. Like *phenoxybenzamine*, it produces postural hypotension and causes *epinephrine* reversal. *Phentolamine*-induced reflex cardiac stimulation and tachycardia are mediated by the baroreceptor reflex and by blocking the α_2 receptors of the cardiac sympathetic nerves. The drug can also trigger arrhythmias and anginal pain, and *phentolamine* is contraindicated in patients with coronary artery disease. *Phentolamine* is used for the short-term management of pheochromocytoma. It is also used locally to prevent dermal necrosis following extravasation of *norepinephrine*. *Phentolamine* is useful to treat hypertensive crisis due to abrupt withdrawal of *clonidine* and from ingesting tyramine-containing foods in patients taking monoamine oxidase inhibitors.

C. Prazosin, terazosin, doxazosin, tamsulosin, and alfuzosin

Prazosin [PRAY-zoe-sin], *terazosin* [ter-AY-zoe-sin], and *doxazosin* [dox-AY-zoe-sin] are selective competitive blockers of the α_1 receptor.

In contrast to *phenoxybenzamine* and *phentolamine*, they are useful in the treatment of hypertension. *Tamsulosin* [tam-SUE-loh-sin] and *alfuzosin* [al-FYOO-zoe-sin] are examples of other selective α₁ antagonists indicated for the treatment of benign prostatic hyperplasia (BPH). Metabolism leads to inactive products that are excreted in urine except for those of *doxazosin*, which appear in feces. *Doxazosin* is the longest acting of these drugs.

1. **Mechanism of action:** All of these agents decrease peripheral vascular resistance and lower blood pressure by causing relaxation of both arterial and venous smooth muscle. These drugs, unlike *phenoxybenzamine* and *phentolamine*, cause minimal changes in cardiac output, renal blood flow, and glomerular filtration rate. *Tamsulosin* has the least effect on blood pressure because it is less selective for α_{1B} receptors found in the blood vessels and more selective for α_{1A} receptors in the prostate and bladder. Blockade of the α_{1A} receptors decreases tone in the smooth muscle of the bladder neck and prostate and improves urine flow.

2. **Therapeutic uses:** Individuals with elevated blood pressure treated with one of these drugs do not become tolerant to its action. However, the first dose of these drugs may produce an exaggerated orthostatic hypotensive response (Figure 7.4) that can result in syncope (fainting). This action, termed a "first-dose" effect, may be minimized by adjusting the first dose to one-third or one-fourth of the normal dose and by giving the drug at bedtime. These drugs may cause modest improvement in lipid profiles and glucose metabolism in hypertensive patients. Because of inferior cardiovascular outcomes as compared to other antihypertensives, α₁ antagonists are not used as monotherapy for the treatment of hypertension (see Chapter 17). The α₁ receptor antagonists have been used as an alternative to surgery in patients with symptomatic BPH (see Chapter 32).

3. **Adverse effects:** α₁-Blockers such as *prazosin* and *doxazosin* may cause dizziness, a lack of energy, nasal congestion, headache, drowsiness, and orthostatic hypotension (although to a lesser degree than that observed with *phenoxybenzamine* and *phentolamine*). An additive antihypertensive effect occurs when α₁ antagonists are given with vasodilators such as nitrates or PDE-5 inhibitors (for example, *sildenafil*), thereby necessitating cautious dose titration and use at the lowest possible doses. By blocking α receptors in the ejaculatory ducts and impairing smooth muscle contraction, α₁ antagonists may cause inhibition of ejaculation and retrograde ejaculation. These agents may cause "floppy iris syndrome," a condition in which the iris billows in response to intraoperative eye surgery. Figure 7.5 summarizes some adverse effects observed with α-blockers.

D. Yohimbine

Yohimbine [yo-HIM-bean] is a selective competitive α₂-blocker. It is found as a component of the bark of the yohimbe tree and has been used as a sexual stimulant and in the treatment of erectile dysfunction. Its use in the treatment of these disorders is not recommended, due to lack of demonstrated efficacy. *Yohimbine* works at the level of the CNS to increase sympathetic outflow to the periphery. It is contraindicated in cardiovascular disease, psychiatric conditions, and renal dysfunction because it may worsen these conditions.

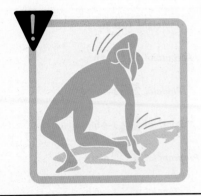

Figure 7.4
First dose of α₁ receptor blocker may produce an orthostatic hypotensive response that can result in syncope (fainting).

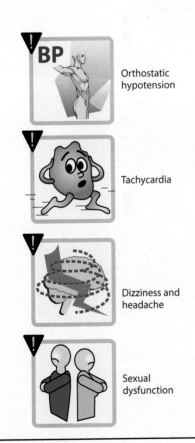

BP

Orthostatic hypotension

Tachycardia

Dizziness and headache

Sexual dysfunction

Figure 7.5
Some adverse effects commonly observed with nonselective α-adrenergic blocking agents.

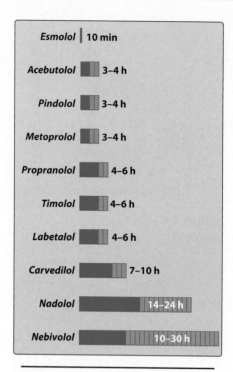

Figure 7.6
Elimination half-lives for some
β-blockers.

III. β-ADRENERGIC BLOCKING AGENTS

All of the clinically available β-blockers are competitive antagonists. Nonselective β-blockers act at both β_1 and β_2 receptors, whereas cardioselective β antagonists primarily block β_1 receptors. [Note: There are no clinically useful β_2 antagonists.] These drugs also differ in intrinsic sympathomimetic activity, CNS effects, blockade of sympathetic receptors, vasodilation, and pharmacokinetics (Figure 7.6). Although all β-blockers lower blood pressure, they do not induce postural hypotension, because the α adrenoceptors remain functional. Therefore, normal sympathetic control of the vasculature is maintained. β-Blockers are effective in treating hypertension, angina, cardiac arrhythmias, myocardial infarction, heart failure, hyperthyroidism, and glaucoma. They are also used for the prophylaxis of migraine headaches. [Note: The names of all β-blockers end in "-olol" except for *labetalol* and *carvedilol*.]

A. Propranolol: A nonselective β antagonist

Propranolol [proe-PRAN-oh-lole] is the prototype β-adrenergic antagonist and blocks both β_1 and β_2 receptors with equal affinity. Sustained-release preparations for once-a-day dosing are available.

1. Actions:

a. Cardiovascular: *Propranolol* diminishes cardiac output, having both negative inotropic and chronotropic effects (Figure 7.7). It directly depresses sinoatrial and atrioventricular nodal activity. The resulting bradycardia usually limits the dose of the drug. During exercise or stress, when the sympathetic nervous system is activated, β-blockers attenuate the expected increase in heart rate. Cardiac output, workload, and oxygen consumption are decreased by blockade of β_1 receptors, and these effects are useful in the treatment of angina (see Chapter 21). The β-blockers are effective in attenuating supraventricular cardiac arrhythmias, but generally are not effective against ventricular arrhythmias (except those induced by exercise).

b. Peripheral vasoconstriction: Nonselective blockade of β receptors prevents β_2-mediated vasodilation in skeletal muscles, increasing peripheral vascular resistance (Figure 7.7). The reduction in cardiac output produced by all β-blockers leads to decreased blood pressure, which triggers a reflex peripheral vasoconstriction that is reflected in reduced blood flow to the periphery. In patients with hypertension, total peripheral resistance returns to normal or decreases with long term use of *propranolol*. There is a gradual reduction of both systolic and diastolic blood pressures in hypertensive patients.

c. Bronchoconstriction: Blocking β_2 receptors in the lungs of susceptible patients causes contraction of the bronchiolar smooth muscle (Figure 7.7). This can precipitate an exacerbation in patients with chronic obstructive pulmonary disease (COPD) or asthma. Therefore, β-blockers, particularly, nonselective ones, are contraindicated in patients with COPD or asthma.

d. Disturbances in glucose metabolism: β blockade leads to decreased glycogenolysis and decreased glucagon secretion.

Therefore, if *propranolol* is given to a diabetic patient receiving *insulin*, careful monitoring of blood glucose is essential, because pronounced hypoglycemia may occur after *insulin* injection. β-blockers also attenuate the normal physiologic response to hypoglycemia.

e. **Blocked action of isoproterenol:** Nonselective β-blockers, including *propranolol*, have the ability to block the actions of *isoproterenol* (β_1, β_2 agonist) on the cardiovascular system. Thus, in the presence of a β-blocker, *isoproterenol* does not produce cardiac stimulation (β_1 mediated) or reductions in mean arterial pressure and diastolic pressure (β_2 mediated; Figure 7.3). [Note: In the presence of a nonselective β-blocker, *epinephrine* no longer lowers diastolic blood pressure or stimulates the heart, but its vasoconstrictive action (mediated by α receptors) remains unimpaired. The actions of *norepinephrine* on the cardiovascular system are mediated primarily by α receptors and are, therefore, unaffected.]

2. **Therapeutic uses:**

a. **Hypertension:** *Propranolol* does not reduce blood pressure in people with normal blood pressure. *Propranolol* lowers blood pressure in hypertension by several different mechanisms of action. Decreased cardiac output is the primary mechanism, but inhibition of renin release from the kidney, decrease in total peripheral resistance with long-term use, and decreased sympathetic outflow from the CNS also contribute to the antihypertensive effects (see Chapter 17).

b. **Angina pectoris:** *Propranolol* decreases the oxygen requirement of heart muscle and, therefore, is effective in reducing chest pain on exertion that is common in angina. *Propranolol* is, thus, useful in the chronic management of stable angina.

c. **Myocardial infarction:** *Propranolol* and other β-blockers have a protective effect on the myocardium. Thus, patients who have had one myocardial infarction appear to be protected against a second heart attack by prophylactic use of β-blockers. In addition, administration of a β-blocker immediately following a myocardial infarction reduces infarct size and hastens recovery. The mechanism for these effects may be a blocking of the actions of circulating catecholamines, which would increase the oxygen demand in an already ischemic heart muscle. *Propranolol* also reduces the incidence of sudden arrhythmic death after myocardial infarction.

d. **Migraine:** *Propranolol* is effective in reducing migraine episodes when used prophylactically (see Chapter 36). It is one of the more useful β-blockers for this indication, due to its lipophilic nature that allows it to penetrate the CNS. [Note: For the acute management of migraine, serotonin agonists such as *sumatriptan* are used, as well as other drugs.]

e. **Hyperthyroidism:** *Propranolol* and other β-blockers are effective in blunting the widespread sympathetic stimulation that occurs in hyperthyroidism. In acute hyperthyroidism (thyroid storm),

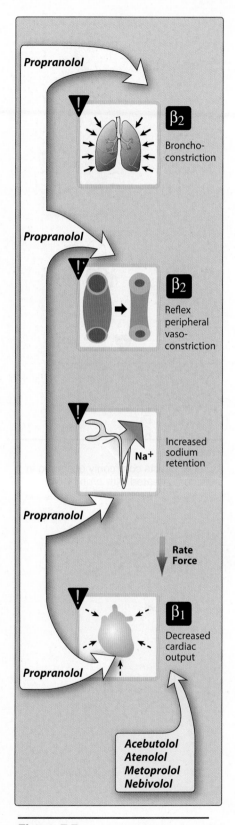

Figure 7.7
Actions of *propranolol* and other β-blockers.

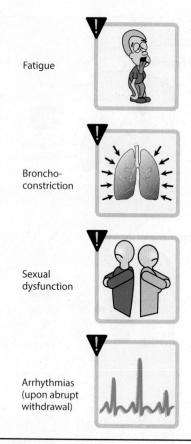

Fatigue

Broncho-constriction

Sexual dysfunction

Arrhythmias (upon abrupt withdrawal)

Figure 7.8
Adverse effects commonly observed in individuals treated with *propranolol*.

β-blockers may be lifesaving in protecting against serious cardiac arrhythmias.

3. **Pharmacokinetics:** After oral administration, *propranolol* is almost completely absorbed. It is subject to first-pass effect, and only about 25% of an administered dose reaches the circulation. The volume of distribution of *propranolol* is quite large (4 L/kg), and the drug readily crosses the blood–brain barrier due to its high lipophilicity. *Propranolol* is extensively metabolized, and most metabolites are excreted in the urine.

4. **Adverse effects:**

   a. **Bronchoconstriction:** *Propranolol* has the potential to cause significant bronchoconstriction due to blockade of β_2 receptors (Figure 7.8). Death by asphyxiation has been reported for patients with asthma whom were inadvertently administered the drug. Therefore, *propranolol* is contraindicated in patients with COPD or asthma.

   b. **Arrhythmias:** Treatment with β-blockers must never be stopped abruptly because of the risk of precipitating cardiac arrhythmias, which may be severe. The β-blockers must be tapered off gradually over a period of at least a few weeks. Long-term treatment with a β antagonist leads to up-regulation of the β receptor. On suspension of therapy, the increased receptors can worsen angina or hypertension.

   c. **Sexual impairment:** Because ejaculation in the male is mediated through α-adrenergic activation, β-blockers do not affect ejaculation or internal bladder sphincter function. On the other hand, some men do complain of impaired sexual activity. The reasons for this are not clear and may be independent of β receptor blockade.

   d. **Metabolic disturbances:** β Blockade leads to decreased glycogenolysis and decreased glucagon secretion. Fasting hypoglycemia may occur. In addition, β-blockers can prevent the counterregulatory effects of catecholamines during hypoglycemia. Thus, the perception of symptoms of hypoglycemia such as tremor, tachycardia, and nervousness are blunted by β-blockers. A major role of β receptors is to mobilize energy molecules such as free fatty acids. [Note: Lipases in fat cells are activated mainly by β_2 and β_3 receptor stimulation, leading to the metabolism of triglycerides into free fatty acids.] Patients administered nonselective β-blockers have increased low-density lipoprotein ("bad" cholesterol), increased triglycerides, and reduced high-density lipoprotein ("good" cholesterol). These effects on the serum lipid profile may be less pronounced with the use of β_1-selective antagonists such as *metoprolol*.

   e. **CNS effects:** *Propranolol* has numerous CNS-mediated effects, including depression, dizziness, lethargy, fatigue, weakness, visual disturbances, hallucinations, short-term memory loss, emotional lability, vivid dreams (including nightmares), and depression. Fewer CNS effects may be seen with more hydrophilic β-blockers (for example, *atenolol*), since they do not cross the blood–brain barrier as readily.

f. **Drug interactions:** Drugs that interfere with, or inhibit, the metabolism of *propranolol*, such as *cimetidine*, *fluoxetine*, *paroxetine*, and *ritonavir*, may potentiate its antihypertensive effects. Conversely, those that stimulate or induce its metabolism, such as barbiturates, *phenytoin*, and *rifampin*, can decrease its effects.

B. Nadolol and timolol: Nonselective β antagonists

Nadolol [NAH-doh-lole] and *timolol* [TIM-o-lole] also block β$_1$- and β$_2$-adrenoceptors and are more potent than *propranolol*. *Nadolol* has a very long duration of action (Figure 7.6). *Timolol* reduces the production of aqueous humor in the eye. It is used topically in the treatment of chronic open-angle glaucoma and, occasionally, for systemic treatment of hypertension.

1. **Treatment of glaucoma:** β-blockers, such as topically applied *timolol*, *betaxolol*, or *carteolol*, are effective in diminishing intraocular pressure in glaucoma. This occurs by decreasing the secretion of aqueous humor by the ciliary body. Unlike the cholinergic drugs, these agents neither affect the ability of the eye to focus for near vision nor change pupil size. When administered intraocularly, the onset is about 30 minutes, and the effects last for 12 to 24 hours. The β-blockers are only used for chronic management of glaucoma. In an acute attack of glaucoma, *pilocarpine* is still the drug of choice for emergency lowering of intraocular pressure. Other agents used in the treatment of glaucoma are summarized in Figure 7.9.

CLASS OF DRUG	DRUG NAMES	MECHANISM OF ACTION	SIDE EFFECTS
β-Adrenergic antagonists (topical)	*Betaxolol, carteolol, levobunolol, metipranolol, timolol*	Decrease of aqueous humor production	Ocular irritation; contraindicated in patients with asthma, obstructive airway disease, bradycardia, and congestive heart failure.
α-Adrenergic agonists (topical)	*Apraclonidine, brimonidine*	Decrease of aqueous humor production and increase of aqueous outflow	Red eye and ocular irritation, allergic reactions, malaise, and headache.
Cholinergic agonists (topical)	*Pilocarpine, carbachol*	Increase of aqueous outflow	Eye or brow pain, increased myopia, and decreased vision.
Prostaglandin-like analogues (topical)	*Latanoprost, travoprost, bimatoprost*	Increase of aqueous humor outflow	Red eye and ocular irritation, increased iris pigmentation, and excessive hair growth of eye lashes.
Carbonic anhydrase inhibitors (topical and systemic)	*Dorzolamide* and *brinzolamide* (topical), *acetazolamide*, and *methazolamide* (oral)	Decrease of aqueous humor production	Transient myopia, nausea, diarrhea, loss of appetite and taste, and renal stones (oral drugs).

Figure 7.9
Classes of drugs used to treat glaucoma.

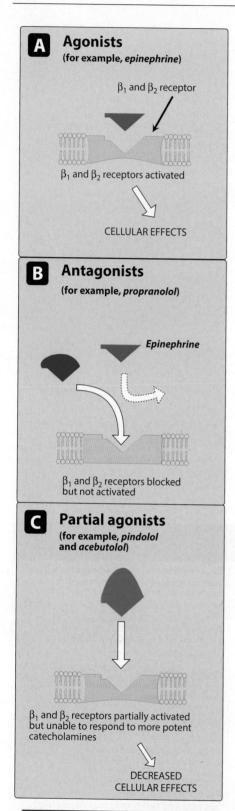

Figure 7.10
Comparison of agonists, antagonists, and partial agonists of β adrenoceptors.

C. Acebutolol, atenolol, betaxolol, bisoprolol, esmolol, metoprolol, and nebivolol: Selective β₁ antagonists

Drugs that preferentially block the β₁ receptors minimize the unwanted bronchoconstriction (β₂ effect) seen with *propranolol* use in asthma patients. Cardioselective β-blockers, such as *acebutolol* [a-se-BYOO-toe-lole], *atenolol* [a-TEN-oh-lole], and *metoprolol* [me-TOE-proe-lole], antagonize β₁ receptors at doses 50- to 100-fold less than those required to block β₂ receptors. This cardioselectivity is most pronounced at low doses and is lost at high doses. [Note: Since β₁ selectivity of these agents is lost at high doses, they may antagonize β₂ receptors.]

1. **Actions:** These drugs lower blood pressure in hypertension and increase exercise tolerance in angina (Figure 7.7). *Esmolol* [EZ-moe-lole] has a very short half-life (Figure 7.6) due to metabolism of an ester linkage. It is only available intravenously and is used to control blood pressure or heart rhythm during surgery or diagnostic procedures. In contrast to *propranolol*, the cardioselective β-blockers have fewer effects on pulmonary function, peripheral resistance, and carbohydrate metabolism. Nevertheless, asthma patients treated with these agents must be carefully monitored to make certain that respiratory activity is not compromised. In addition to its cardioselective β blockade, *nebivolol* releases nitric oxide from endothelial cells and causes vasodilation.

2. **Therapeutic uses:** The cardioselective β-blockers are useful in hypertensive patients with impaired pulmonary function. These agents are also first-line therapy for chronic stable angina. *Bisoprolol* and the extended-release formulation of *metoprolol* are indicated for the management of chronic heart failure. Because these drugs have less effect on peripheral vascular β₂ receptors, coldness of extremities (Raynaud phenomenon), a common side effect of β-blockers, is less frequent.

D. Acebutolol and pindolol: Antagonists with partial agonist activity

1. **Actions:**

a. **Cardiovascular:** *Acebutolol* (β₁-selective antagonist) and *pindolol* (nonselective β-blocker) [PIN-doe-lole] are not pure antagonists. These drugs also have the ability to weakly stimulate both β₁ and β₂ receptors (Figure 7.10) and are said to have intrinsic sympathomimetic activity (ISA). These partial agonists stimulate the β receptor to which they are bound, yet they inhibit stimulation by the more potent endogenous catecholamines, epinephrine and norepinephrine. The result of these opposing actions is a diminished effect on cardiac rate and cardiac output compared to that of β-blockers without ISA.

b. **Decreased metabolic effects:** β-blockers with ISA minimize the disturbances of lipid and carbohydrate metabolism that are seen with other β-blockers. For example, these agents do not decrease plasma HDL levels.

2. **Therapeutic use in hypertension:** β-blockers with ISA are effective in hypertensive patients with moderate bradycardia, because a further decrease in heart rate is less pronounced with these drugs. [Note: β-blockers with ISA are not used for stable angina or arrhythmias due to their partial agonist effect.] Figure 7.11 summarizes some of the indications for β-blockers.

E. Labetalol and carvedilol: Antagonists of both α and β adrenoceptors

1. **Actions:** *Labetalol* [lah-BET-a-lole] and *carvedilol* [CAR-ve-dil-ol] are nonselective β-blockers with concurrent α_1-blocking actions that produce peripheral vasodilation, thereby reducing blood pressure. They contrast with the other β-blockers that produce initial peripheral vasoconstriction, and these agents are, therefore, useful in treating hypertensive patients for whom increased peripheral vascular resistance is undesirable. *Carvedilol* also decreases lipid peroxidation and vascular wall thickening, effects that have benefit in heart failure.

2. **Therapeutic use in hypertension and heart failure:** *Labetalol* is employed as an alternative to *methyldopa* in the treatment of pregnancy-induced hypertension. Intravenous *labetalol* is also used to treat hypertensive emergencies, because it can rapidly lower blood pressure (see Chapter 17). β-blockers should not be given to patients with an acute exacerbation of heart failure, as they can worsen the condition. However, *carvedilol* as well as *metoprolol* and *bisoprolol* are beneficial in patients with stable chronic heart failure. These agents work by blocking the effects of sympathetic stimulation on the heart, which causes worsening heart failure over time (see Chapter 19).

3. **Adverse effects:** Orthostatic hypotension and dizziness are associated with α_1 blockade. Figure 7.12 summarizes the receptor specificities and uses of the β-adrenergic antagonists.

IV. DRUGS AFFECTING NEUROTRANSMITTER RELEASE OR UPTAKE

Some agents act on the adrenergic neuron, either to interfere with neurotransmitter release from storage vesicles or to alter the uptake of the neurotransmitter into the adrenergic neuron. However, due to the advent of newer and more effective agents with fewer side effects, these agents are seldom used therapeutically. *Reserpine* [re-SER-peen] is one of the remaining agents in this category.

Reserpine, a plant alkaloid, blocks the Mg^{2+}/adenosine triphosphate–dependent transport of biogenic amines (norepinephrine, dopamine, and serotonin) from the cytoplasm into storage vesicles in the adrenergic nerve terminals in all body tissues. This causes the ultimate depletion of biogenic amines. Sympathetic function, in general, is impaired because of decreased release of norepinephrine. *Reserpine* has a slow onset, a long duration of action, and effects that persist for many days after discontinuation. It has been used for the management of hypertension but has largely been replaced with newer agents with better side effect profiles and fewer drug interactions.

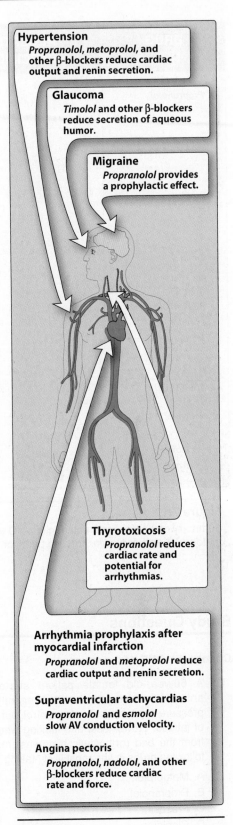

Hypertension
Propranolol, metoprolol, and other β-blockers reduce cardiac output and renin secretion.

Glaucoma
Timolol and other β-blockers reduce secretion of aqueous humor.

Migraine
Propranolol provides a prophylactic effect.

Thyrotoxicosis
Propranolol reduces cardiac rate and potential for arrhythmias.

Arrhythmia prophylaxis after myocardial infarction
Propranolol and *metoprolol* reduce cardiac output and renin secretion.

Supraventricular tachycardias
Propranolol and *esmolol* slow AV conduction velocity.

Angina pectoris
Propranolol, nadolol, and other β-blockers reduce cardiac rate and force.

Figure 7.11
Some clinical applications of β-blockers. AV = atrioventricular.

DRUG	RECEPTOR SPECIFICITY	THERAPEUTIC USES
Propranolol	β_1, β_2	**Hypertension** **Migraine** **Hyperthyroidism** **Angina pectoris** **Myocardial infarction**
Nadolol *Pindolol*[1]	β_1, β_2	**Hypertension**
Timolol	β_1, β_2	**Glaucoma, hypertension**
Atenolol *Bisoprolol*[2] *Esmolol* *Metoprolol*[2]	β_1	**Hypertension** **Angina** **Myocardial infarction**
Acebutolol[1]	β_1	**Hypertension**
Nebivolol	β_1, NO ↑	**Hypertension**
Carvedilol[2] *Labetalol*	$\alpha_1, \beta_1, \beta_2$	**Hypertension**

Figure 7.12

Summary of β-adrenergic antagonists. NO = nitric oxide. [1]*Acebutolol* and *pindolol* are partial agonists, as well. [2]*Bisoprolol*, *metoprolol*, and *carvedilol* are also used for the treatment of heart failure.

Study Questions

Choose the ONE best answer.

7.1 A 60-year-old female patient started on a new antihypertensive medication recently. Her blood pressure seems to be under control, but she complains of fatigue, drowsiness, and fainting when she gets up from the bed (orthostatic hypotension). Which of the following drugs is she most likely taking?

A. Metoprolol.
B. Propranolol.
C. Prazosin.
D. Clonidine.

Correct answer = C. α-Blockers (prazosin) are more likely to cause orthostatic hypotension compared to β-blockers (metoprolol, propranolol) and α_2 agonists (clonidine).

7.2 A 30-year-old male patient was brought to the ER with amphetamine overdose. He presented with high blood pressure and arrhythmia. Which of the following is correct regarding this patient?

    A. Amphetamine can activate all types of adrenergic receptors.

    B. β-Blockers are the ideal antidotes for amphetamine poisoning.

    C. α-Blockers can normalize the blood pressure in this patient.

    D. Miosis could be a possible symptom of amphetamine poisoning.

Correct answer = A. Amphetamine is an indirect adrenergic agonist that mainly enhances the release of norepinephrine from peripheral sympathetic neurons. Therefore, it activates all types of adrenergic receptors (that is, α and β receptors) and causes an increase in blood pressure. Since both α and β receptors are activated by amphetamine, α-blockers or β-blockers alone cannot relieve the symptoms of amphetamine poisoning. Since amphetamine causes sympathetic activation, it causes mydriasis, not miosis.

7.3 A new antihypertensive drug was tested in an animal model of hypertension. The drug when given alone reduces blood pressure in the animal. Norepinephrine when given in the presence of this drug did not cause any significant change in blood pressure or heart rate in the animal. The new drug is similar to which of the following drugs in terms of its pharmacological mechanism of action?

    A. Prazosin.

    B. Clonidine.

    C. Propranolol.

    D. Metoprolol.

    E. Carvedilol.

Correct answer = E. Norepinephrine activates both α_1 and β_1 receptors and causes an increase in heart rate and blood pressure. A drug that prevents the increase in blood pressure caused by norepinephrine should be similar to carvedilol that antagonizes both α_1 and β_1 receptors. Prazosin is an α_1 antagonist, clonidine is an α_2 agonist, and propranolol and metoprolol are β antagonists, and these drugs cannot completely prevent the cardiovascular effects of norepinephrine.

7.4 A β-blocker was prescribed for hypertension in a female asthma patient. After about a week of treatment, the asthma attacks got worse, and the patient was asked to stop taking the β-blocker. Which of the following β-blockers would you suggest as an alternative in this patient that is less likely to worsen her asthma?

    A. Propranolol.

    B. Metoprolol.

    C. Labetalol.

    D. Carvedilol.

Correct answer = B. The patient was most likely given a nonselective β-blocker (antagonizes both β_1 and β_2 receptors) that made her asthma worse due to β_2 antagonism. An alternative is to prescribe a cardioselective (antagonizes only β_1) β-blocker that does not antagonize β_2 receptors in the bronchioles. Metoprolol is a cardioselective β-blocker. Propranolol, labetalol, and carvedilol are nonselective β-blockers and could worsen the asthma.

7.5 A 70-year-old male needs to be treated with an α-blocker for overflow incontinence due to his enlarged prostate. Which of the following drugs would you suggest in this patent that will not affect his blood pressure significantly?

    A. Prazosin.

    B. Doxazosin.

    C. Phentolamine.

    D. Tamsulosin.

    E. Terazosin.

Correct answer = D. Tamsulosin is an α_1 antagonist that is more selective to the α_1 receptor subtype (α_{1A}) present in the prostate and less selective to the α_1 receptor subtype (α_{1B}) present in the blood vessels. Therefore, tamsulosin does not affect blood pressure significantly. Prazosin, doxazosin, terazosin, and phentolamine antagonize both these subtypes and cause significant hypotension as a side effect.

7.6 A 50-year-old male was brought to the emergency room after being stung by a hornet. The patient was found to be in anaphylactic shock, and the medical team tried to reverse the bronchoconstriction and hypotension using epinephrine. However, the patient did not fully respond to the epinephrine treatment. The patient's wife mentioned that he is taking a prescription medication for his blood pressure, the name of which she does not remember. Which of the following medications is he most likely taking that could have prevented the effects of epinephrine?

A. Doxazosin.
B. Propranolol.
C. Metoprolol.
D. Acebutolol.

Correct answer = B. Epinephrine reverses hypotension by activating β_1 receptors and relieves bronchoconstriction by activating β_2 receptors in anaphylaxis. Since epinephrine was not effective in reversing hypotension or bronchoconstriction in this patient, it could be assumed that the patient was on a nonselective β-blocker (propranolol). Doxazosin (α_1-blocker), metoprolol, or acebutolol (both β_1-selective blockers) would not have completely prevented the effects of epinephrine.

7.7 Which of the following is correct regarding α-adrenergic blockers?

A. α-Adrenergic blockers are used in the treatment of hypotension in anaphylactic shock.
B. α-Adrenergic blockers are used in the treatment of benign prostatic hyperplasia (BPH).
C. α-Adrenergic blockers may cause bradycardia.
D. α-Adrenergic blockers are used in the treatment of asthma.
E. α-Adrenergic blockers reduce the frequency of urination.

Correct answer = B. α-Adrenergic blockers are used in the treatment of BPH because of their relaxant effect on prostate smooth muscles. Being antihypertensive agents, they are not useful in treating hypotension in anaphylaxis. α-Adrenergic blockers generally cause reflex tachycardia (not bradycardia) due to the significant drop in blood pressure caused by them. α-Adrenergic blockers have no significant effects on bronchial tissues and are not useful in treating asthma. They increase (not reduce) the frequency of urination by relaxing the internal sphincter of the urinary bladder, which is controlled by α_1 receptors.

7.8 Which of the following is correct regarding β-blockers?

A. Treatment with β-blockers should not be stopped abruptly.
B. Propranolol is a cardioselective β-blocker.
C. β-Blockers may cause orthostatic hypotension.
D. Cardioselective β-blockers worsen asthma.
E. β-Blockers decrease peripheral resistance by causing vasorelaxation.

Correct answer = A. If β-blocker therapy is stopped abruptly, that could cause angina and rebound hypertension. This could be due to the up-regulation of β receptors in the body. β-Blockers do not cause direct vasorelaxation. Therefore, they do not decrease peripheral resistance and are less likely to cause orthostatic hypotension. Propranolol is a nonselective β-blocker (not cardioselective). Cardioselective β-blockers antagonize only β_1 receptors and do not worsen asthma as they do not antagonize β_2 receptors.

7.9 Which of the following drugs is commonly used topically in the treatment of glaucoma?

A. Atropine.
B. Timolol.
C. Tropicamide.
D. Scopolamine.

Correct answer = B. β-Blockers reduce the formation of aqueous humor in the eye and therefore reduce intraocular pressure, thus relieving glaucoma. Timolol is a nonselective β-blocker that is commonly used topically to treat glaucoma. Atropine, tropicamide, and scopolamine are anticholinergic drugs that might worsen glaucoma.

7.10 Which of the following is correct regarding carvedilol?

A. Carvedilol is a cardioselective β-blocker.
B. Carvedilol is safe for use in asthma patients.
C. Carvedilol has α_1-blocking activity.
D. Carvedilol is contraindicated in the treatment of stable chronic heart failure.

Correct answer = C. Carvedilol is a nonselective β-blocker with α_1-blocking activity. Since it also blocks β_2 receptors in the lungs, carvedilol could exacerbate asthma. Carvedilol is not used in patients with acute exacerbation of heart failure but is used in the treatment of stable, chronic heart failure.

Drugs for Neurodegenerative Diseases

8

Jose A. Rey

I. OVERVIEW

Most drugs that affect the central nervous system (CNS) act by altering some step in the neurotransmission process. Drugs affecting the CNS may act presynaptically by influencing the production, storage, release, or termination of action of neurotransmitters. Other agents may activate or block postsynaptic receptors. This chapter provides an overview of the CNS, with a focus on those neurotransmitters that are involved in the actions of the clinically useful CNS drugs. These concepts are useful in understanding the etiology and treatment strategies for the neurodegenerative disorders that respond to drug therapy: Parkinson's disease, Alzheimer's disease, multiple sclerosis (MS), and amyotrophic lateral sclerosis (ALS) (Figure 8.1).

II. NEUROTRANSMISSION IN THE CNS

In many ways, the basic functioning of neurons in the CNS is similar to that of the autonomic nervous system (ANS) described in Chapter 3. For example, transmission of information in both the CNS and in the periphery involves the release of neurotransmitters that diffuse across the synaptic space to bind to specific receptors on the postsynaptic neuron. In both systems, the recognition of the neurotransmitter by the membrane receptor of the postsynaptic neuron triggers intracellular changes. However, several major differences exist between neurons in the peripheral ANS and those in the CNS. The circuitry of the CNS is much more complex than that of the ANS, and the number of synapses in the CNS is far greater. The CNS, unlike the peripheral ANS, contains powerful networks of inhibitory neurons that are constantly active in modulating the rate of neuronal transmission. In addition, the CNS communicates

ANTI-PARKINSON DRUGS
Amantadine SYMMETREL
Apomorphine APOKYN
Benztropine COGENTIN
Biperiden AKINETON
Bromocriptine PARLODEL
Carbidopa LODOSYN
Entacapone COMTAN
Levodopa (w/Carbidopa) SINEMET, PARCOPA
Pramipexole MIRAPEX
Procyclidine KEMADRIN
Rasagiline AZILECT
Ropinirole REQUIP
Rotigotine NEUPRO
Selegiline (Deprenyl) ELDEPRYL, ZELAPAR
Tolcapone TASMAR
Trihexyphenidyl ARTANE

ANTI-ALZHEIMER DRUGS
Donepezil ARICEPT
Galantamine RAZADYNE
Memantine NAMENDA
Rivastigmine EXELON

Figure 8.1
Summary of agents used in the treatment of Parkinson's disease, Alzheimer's disease, multiple sclerosis, and amyotrophic lateral sclerosis. (Figure continues on next page.)

ANTI-MULTIPLE SCLEROSIS DRUGS

Azathioprine AZASAN, IMURAN
Cyclophosphamide CYTOXAN
Dalfampridine AMPYRA
Dexamethasone BAYCADRON, DECADRON
Dimethyl fumarate TECFIDERA
Fingolimod GILENYA
Glatiramer COPAXONE
Interferon β1a AVONEX, REBIF
Interferon β1b BETASERON, EXTAVIA
Mitoxantrone NOVANTRONE
Natalizumab TYSABRI
Prednisone DELTASONE
Teriflunomide AUBAGIO

ANTI-ALS DRUGS

Riluzole RILUTEK

Figure 8.1 (continued)
Summary of agents used in the treatment of Parkinson's disease, Alzheimer's disease, multiple sclerosis, and amyotrophic lateral sclerosis (ALS).

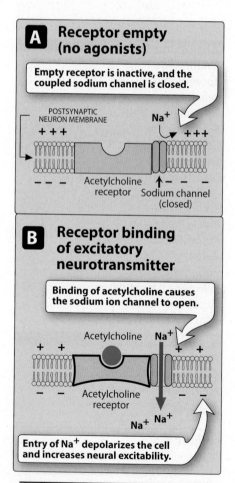

Figure 8.2
Binding of the excitatory neurotransmitter, acetylcholine, causes depolarization of the neuron.

through the use of multiple neurotransmitters, whereas the ANS uses only two primary neurotransmitters, acetylcholine and norepinephrine.

III. SYNAPTIC POTENTIALS

In the CNS, receptors at most synapses are coupled to ion channels. Binding of the neurotransmitter to the postsynaptic membrane receptors results in a rapid but transient opening of ion channels. Open channels allow specific ions inside and outside the cell membrane to flow down their concentration gradients. The resulting change in the ionic composition across the membrane of the neuron alters the postsynaptic potential, producing either depolarization or hyperpolarization of the postsynaptic membrane, depending on the specific ions and the direction of their movement.

A. Excitatory pathways

Neurotransmitters can be classified as either excitatory or inhibitory, depending on the nature of the action they elicit. Stimulation of excitatory neurons causes a movement of ions that results in a depolarization of the postsynaptic membrane. These excitatory postsynaptic potentials (EPSP) are generated by the following: 1) Stimulation of an excitatory neuron causes the release of neurotransmitter molecules, such as glutamate or acetylcholine, which bind to receptors on the postsynaptic cell membrane. This causes a transient increase in the permeability of sodium (Na^+) ions. 2) The influx of Na^+ causes a weak depolarization, or EPSP, that moves the postsynaptic potential toward its firing threshold. 3) If the number of stimulated excitatory neurons increases, more excitatory neurotransmitter is released. This ultimately causes the EPSP depolarization of the postsynaptic cell to pass a threshold, thereby generating an all-or-none action potential. [Note: The generation of a nerve impulse typically reflects the activation of synaptic receptors by thousands of excitatory neurotransmitter molecules released from many nerve fibers.] Figure 8.2 shows an example of an excitatory pathway.

B. Inhibitory pathways

Stimulation of inhibitory neurons causes movement of ions that results in a hyperpolarization of the postsynaptic membrane. These inhibitory postsynaptic potentials (IPSP) are generated by the following: 1) Stimulation of inhibitory neurons releases neurotransmitter molecules, such as γ-aminobutyric acid (GABA) or glycine, which bind to receptors on the postsynaptic cell membrane. This causes a transient increase in the permeability of specific ions, such as potassium (K^+) and chloride (Cl^-). 2) The influx of Cl^- and efflux of K^+ cause a weak hyperpolarization, or IPSP, that moves the postsynaptic potential away from its firing threshold. This diminishes the generation of action potentials. Figure 8.3 shows an example of an inhibitory pathway.

C. Combined effects of the EPSP and IPSP

Most neurons in the CNS receive both EPSP and IPSP input. Thus, several different types of neurotransmitters may act on the same neuron, but each binds to its own specific receptor. The overall action is the summation of the individual actions of the various neurotransmitters on the neuron. The neurotransmitters are not uniformly distributed in the CNS but are localized in specific clusters of neurons, the axons of which may synapse with specific regions of the brain. Many neuronal tracts, thus, seem to be chemically coded, and this may offer greater opportunity for selective modulation of certain neuronal pathways.

IV. NEURODEGENERATIVE DISEASES

Neurodegenerative diseases of the CNS include Parkinson's disease, Alzheimer's disease, MS, and ALS. These devastating illnesses are characterized by the progressive loss of selected neurons in discrete brain areas, resulting in characteristic disorders of movement, cognition, or both.

V. OVERVIEW OF PARKINSON'S DISEASE

Parkinsonism is a progressive neurological disorder of muscle movement, characterized by tremors, muscular rigidity, bradykinesia (slowness in initiating and carrying out voluntary movements), and postural and gait abnormalities. Most cases involve people over the age of 65, among whom the incidence is about 1 in 100 individuals.

A. Etiology

The cause of Parkinson's disease is unknown for most patients. The disease is correlated with destruction of dopaminergic neurons in the substantia nigra with a consequent reduction of dopamine actions in the corpus striatum, parts of the basal ganglia system that are involved in motor control.

1. **Substantia nigra:** The substantia nigra, part of the extrapyramidal system, is the source of dopaminergic neurons (shown in red in Figure 8.4) that terminate in the neostriatum. Each dopaminergic neuron makes thousands of synaptic contacts within the neostriatum and, therefore, modulates the activity of a large number of cells. These dopaminergic projections from the substantia nigra fire tonically rather than in response to specific muscular movements or sensory input. Thus, the dopaminergic system appears to serve as a tonic, sustaining influence on motor activity, rather than participating in specific movements.

2. **Neostriatum:** Normally, the neostriatum is connected to the substantia nigra by neurons (shown in orange in Figure 8.4) that secrete the inhibitory transmitter GABA at their termini. In turn, cells of the substantia nigra send neurons back to the neostriatum, secreting the inhibitory transmitter dopamine at their termini. This mutual inhibitory pathway normally maintains a degree of inhibition of both areas. In Parkinson's disease, destruction of cells in the substantia nigra results in the degeneration of the nerve terminals that secrete dopamine in the neostriatum. Thus, the normal inhibitory influence of dopamine on cholinergic neurons

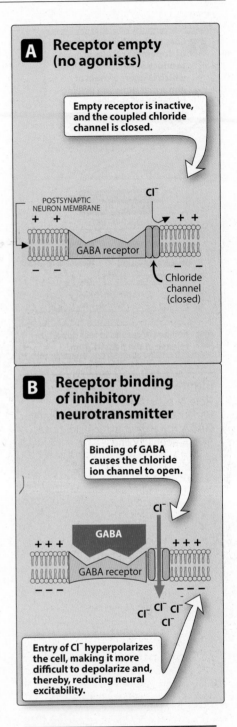

A Receptor empty (no agonists)

Empty receptor is inactive, and the coupled chloride channel is closed.

POSTSYNAPTIC NEURON MEMBRANE

Cl⁻

GABA receptor

Chloride channel (closed)

B Receptor binding of inhibitory neurotransmitter

Binding of GABA causes the chloride ion channel to open.

Cl⁻

GABA

GABA receptor

Cl⁻ Cl⁻ Cl⁻ Cl⁻

Entry of Cl⁻ hyperpolarizes the cell, making it more difficult to depolarize and, thereby, reducing neural excitability.

Figure 8.3
Binding of the inhibitory neurotransmitter, γ-aminobutyric acid (GABA), causes hyperpolarization of the neuron.

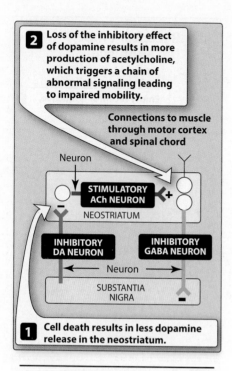

2 Loss of the inhibitory effect of dopamine results in more production of acetylcholine, which triggers a chain of abnormal signaling leading to impaired mobility.

Connections to muscle through motor cortex and spinal chord

Neuron

STIMULATORY ACh NEURON

NEOSTRIATUM

INHIBITORY DA NEURON

INHIBITORY GABA NEURON

Neuron

SUBSTANTIA NIGRA

1 Cell death results in less dopamine release in the neostriatum.

Figure 8.4
Role of substantia nigra in Parkinson's disease. DA = dopamine; GABA = γ-aminobutyric acid; ACh = acetylcholine.

in the neostriatum is significantly diminished, resulting in over-production or a relative overactivity of acetylcholine by the stim-ulatory neurons (shown in green in Figure 8.4). This triggers a chain of abnormal signaling, resulting in loss of the control of muscle movements.

3. **Secondary parkinsonism:** Drugs such as the phenothiazines and *haloperidol,* whose major pharmacologic action is blockade of dopamine receptors in the brain, may produce parkinsonian symp-toms (also called pseudoparkinsonism). These drugs should be used with caution in patients with Parkinson's disease.

B. Strategy of treatment

In addition to an abundance of inhibitory dopaminergic neurons, the neostriatum is also rich in excitatory cholinergic neurons that oppose the action of dopamine (Figure 8.4). Many of the symptoms of parkinsonism reflect an imbalance between the excitatory cho-linergic neurons and the greatly diminished number of inhibitory dopaminergic neurons. Therapy is aimed at restoring dopamine in the basal ganglia and antagonizing the excitatory effect of choliner-gic neurons, thus reestablishing the correct dopamine/acetylcholine balance.

VI. DRUGS USED IN PARKINSON'S DISEASE

Many currently available drugs aim to maintain CNS dopamine levels as constant as possible. These agents offer temporary relief from the symptoms of the disorder, but they do not arrest or reverse the neuronal degeneration caused by the disease.

A. Levodopa and carbidopa

Levodopa [lee-voe-DOE-pa] is a metabolic precursor of dopamine (Figure 8.5). It restores dopaminergic neurotransmission in the neostriatum by enhancing the synthesis of dopamine in the surviv-ing neurons of the substantia nigra. In early disease, the number of residual dopaminergic neurons in the substantia nigra (typically about 20% of normal) is adequate for conversion of *levodopa* to dopamine. Thus, in new patients, the therapeutic response to *levodopa* is consis-tent, and the patient rarely complains that the drug effects "wear off." Unfortunately, with time, the number of neurons decreases, and fewer cells are capable of converting exogenously administered *levodopa* to dopamine. Consequently, motor control fluctuation develops. Relief provided by *levodopa* is only symptomatic, and it lasts only while the drug is present in the body. The effects of *levodopa* on the CNS can be greatly enhanced by coadministering *carbidopa* [kar-bi-DOE-pa], a dopamine decarboxylase inhibitor that does not cross the blood–brain barrier.

1. **Mechanism of action:**

   a. **Levodopa:** Dopamine does not cross the blood–brain barrier, but its immediate precursor, *levodopa,* is actively transported into the CNS and converted to dopamine (Figure 8.5). *Levodopa*

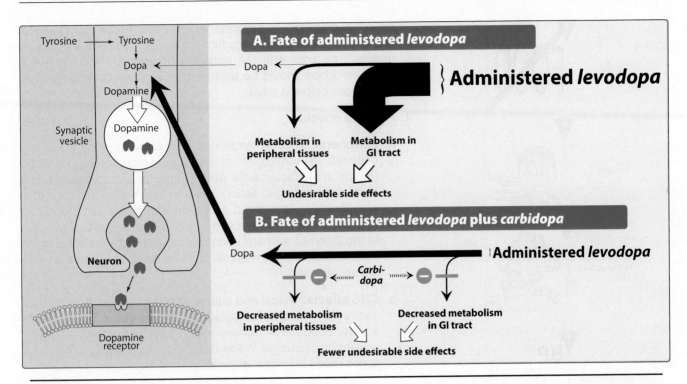

Figure 8.5
Synthesis of dopamine from *levodopa* in the absence and presence of *carbidopa,* an inhibitor of dopamine decarboxylase in the peripheral tissues. GI = gastrointestinal.

must be administered with *carbidopa*. Without *carbidopa*, much of the drug is decarboxylated to dopamine in the periphery, resulting in nausea, vomiting, cardiac arrhythmias, and hypotension.

b. **Carbidopa:** *Carbidopa,* a dopamine decarboxylase inhibitor, diminishes the metabolism of *levodopa* in the periphery, thereby increasing the availability of *levodopa* to the CNS. The addition of *carbidopa* lowers the dose of *levodopa* needed by four- to fivefold and, consequently, decreases the severity of the side effects arising from peripherally formed dopamine.

2. **Therapeutic uses:** *Levodopa* in combination with *carbidopa* is an efficacious drug regimen for the treatment of Parkinson's disease. It decreases rigidity, tremors, and other symptoms of parkinsonism. In approximately two-thirds of patients with Parkinson's disease, *levodopa–carbidopa* substantially reduces the severity of symptoms for the first few years of treatment. Patients typically experience a decline in response during the 3rd to 5th year of therapy. Withdrawal from the drug must be gradual.

3. **Absorption and metabolism:** The drug is absorbed rapidly from the small intestine (when empty of food). *Levodopa* has an extremely short half-life (1 to 2 hours), which causes fluctuations in plasma concentration. This may produce fluctuations in motor response, which generally correlate with the plasma concentration of *levodopa,* or perhaps give rise to the more troublesome "on–off" phenomenon, in which the motor fluctuations are not related to plasma levels in a simple way. Motor fluctuations may cause the

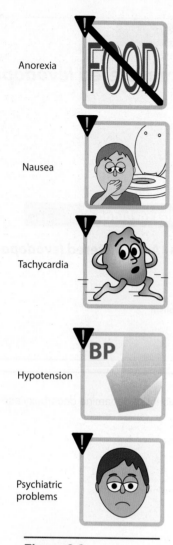

Figure 8.6
Adverse effects of
levodopa.

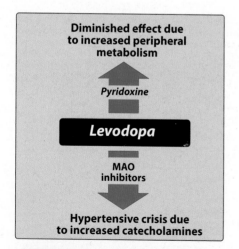

Figure 8.7

Some drug interactions observed
with *levodopa.* MAO = monoamine
oxidase.

patient to suddenly lose normal mobility and experience tremors, cramps, and immobility. Ingestion of meals, particularly if high in protein, interferes with the transport of *levodopa* into the CNS. Thus, *levodopa* should be taken on an empty stomach, typically 30 minutes before a meal.

4. **Adverse effects:**

a. **Peripheral effects:** Anorexia, nausea, and vomiting occur because of stimulation of the chemoreceptor trigger zone (Figure 8.6). Tachycardia and ventricular extrasystoles result from dopaminergic action on the heart. Hypotension may also develop. Adrenergic action on the iris causes mydriasis. In some individuals, blood dyscrasias and a positive reaction to the Coombs test are seen. Saliva and urine are a brownish color because of the melanin pigment produced from catecholamine oxidation.

b. **CNS effects:** Visual and auditory hallucinations and abnormal involuntary movements (dyskinesias) may occur. These effects are the opposite of parkinsonian symptoms and reflect overactivity of dopamine in the basal ganglia. *Levodopa* can also cause mood changes, depression, psychosis, and anxiety.

5. **Interactions:** The vitamin pyridoxine (B_6) increases the peripheral breakdown of *levodopa* and diminishes its effectiveness (Figure 8.7). Concomitant administration of *levodopa* and non-selective monoamine oxidase inhibitors (MAOIs), such as *phenelzine*, can produce a hypertensive crisis caused by enhanced catecholamine production. Therefore, concomitant administration of these agents is contraindicated. In many psychotic patients, *levodopa* exacerbates symptoms, possibly through the buildup of central catecholamines. Cardiac patients should be carefully monitored for the possible development of arrhythmias. Antipsychotic drugs are generally contraindicated in Parkinson's disease, because they potently block dopamine receptors and may augment parkinsonian symptoms. However, low doses of atypical antipsychotics are sometimes used to treat *levodopa*-induced psychotic symptoms.

B. Selegiline and rasagiline

Selegiline [seh-LEDGE-ah-leen], also called *deprenyl* [DE-pre-nill], selectively inhibits monoamine oxidase (MAO) type B (metabolizes dopamine) at low to moderate doses. It does not inhibit MAO type A (metabolizes norepinephrine and serotonin) unless given above recommended doses, where it loses its selectivity. By decreasing the metabolism of dopamine, *selegiline* increases dopamine levels in the brain (Figure 8.8). When *selegiline* is administered with *levodopa*, it enhances the actions of *levodopa* and substantially reduces the required dose. Unlike nonselective MAOIs, *selegiline* at recommended doses has little potential for causing hypertensive crises. However, the drug loses selectivity at high doses, and there is a risk for severe hypertension. *Selegiline* is metabolized to *methamphetamine* and *amphetamine,* whose stimulating properties may produce insomnia if the drug is administered later than mid-afternoon. *Rasagiline* [ra-SA-gi-leen], an irreversible and selective inhibitor of brain MAO type B, has five times the potency of *selegiline*. Unlike *selegiline, rasagiline* is not metabolized to an *amphetamine*-like substance.

C. Catechol-*O*-methyltransferase inhibitors

Normally, the methylation of *levodopa* by catechol-*O*-methyltransferase (COMT) to 3-*O*-methyldopa is a minor pathway for *levodopa* metabolism. However, when peripheral dopamine decarboxylase activity is inhibited by *carbidopa,* a significant concentration of 3-*O*-methyldopa is formed that competes with *levodopa* for active transport into the CNS (Figure 8.9). *Entacapone* [en-TAK-a-pone] and *tolcapone* [TOLE-ka-pone] selectively and reversibly inhibit COMT. Inhibition of COMT by these agents leads to decreased plasma concentrations of 3-*O*-methyldopa, increased central uptake of *levodopa,* and greater concentrations of brain dopamine. Both of these agents reduce the symptoms of "wearing-off" phenomena seen in patients on *levodopa–carbidopa.* The two drugs differ primarily in their pharmacokinetic and adverse effect profiles.

1. **Pharmacokinetics:** Oral absorption of both drugs occurs readily and is not influenced by food. They are extensively bound to plasma albumin, with a limited volume of distribution. *Tolcapone* has a relatively long duration of action (probably due to its affinity for the enzyme) compared to *entacapone,* which requires more frequent dosing. Both drugs are extensively metabolized and eliminated in feces and urine. The dosage may need to be adjusted in patients with moderate or severe cirrhosis.

2. **Adverse effects:** Both drugs exhibit adverse effects that are observed in patients taking *levodopa–carbidopa,* including diarrhea, postural hypotension, nausea, anorexia, dyskinesias, hallucinations, and sleep disorders. Most seriously, fulminating hepatic necrosis is associated with *tolcapone* use. Therefore, it should be used, along with appropriate hepatic function monitoring, only in patients in whom other modalities have failed. *Entacapone* does not exhibit this toxicity and has largely replaced *tolcapone.*

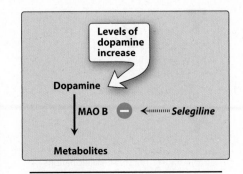

Figure 8.8
Action of *selegiline* (*deprenyl*) in dopamine metabolism. MAO B = monoamine oxidase type B.

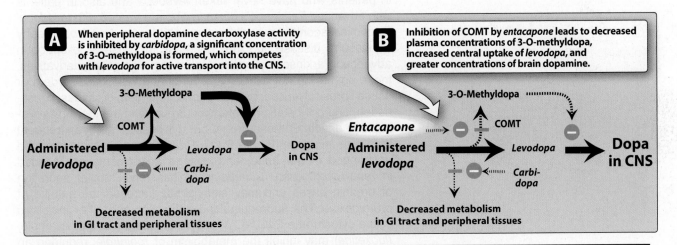

Figure 8.9
Effect of *entacapone* on dopa concentration in the central nervous system (CNS). COMT = catechol-*O*-methyltransferase.

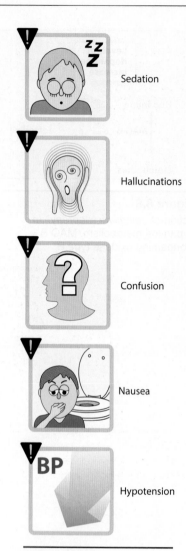

Sedation

Hallucinations

Confusion

Nausea

Hypotension

Figure 8.10
Some adverse effects of
dopamine agonists.

D. Dopamine receptor agonists

This group of antiparkinsonian compounds includes *bromocriptine*, an ergot derivative, the nonergot drugs, *ropinirole* [roe-PIN-i-role], *pramipexole* [pra-mi-PEX-ole], *rotigotine* [ro-TIG-oh-teen], and the newer agent, *apomorphine* [A-poe-more-feen]. These agents have a longer duration of action than that of *levodopa* and are effective in patients exhibiting fluctuations in response to *levodopa*. Initial therapy with these drugs is associated with less risk of developing dyskinesias and motor fluctuations as compared to patients started on *levodopa*. *Bromocriptine, pramipexole,* and *ropinirole* are effective in patients with Parkinson's disease complicated by motor fluctuations and dyskinesias. However, these drugs are ineffective in patients who have not responded to *levodopa*. *Apomorphine* is an injectable dopamine agonist that is used in severe and advanced stages of the disease to supplement oral medications. Side effects severely limit the utility of the dopamine agonists (Figure 8.10).

1. **Bromocriptine:** The actions of the ergot derivative *bromocriptine* [broe-moe-KRIP-teen] are similar to those of *levodopa,* except that hallucinations, confusion, delirium, nausea, and orthostatic hypotension are more common, whereas dyskinesia is less prominent. In psychiatric illness, *bromocriptine* may cause the mental condition to worsen. It should be used with caution in patients with a history of myocardial infarction or peripheral vascular disease. Because *bromocriptine* is an ergot derivative, it has the potential to cause pulmonary and retroperitoneal fibrosis.

2. **Apomorphine, pramipexole, ropinirole, and rotigotine:** These are nonergot dopamine agonists that are approved for the treatment of Parkinson's disease. *Pramipexole* and *ropinirole* are orally active agents. *Apomorphine* and *rotigotine* are available in injectable and transdermal delivery systems, respectively. *Apomorphine* is used for acute management of the hypomobility "off" phenomenon in advanced Parkinson's disease. *Rotigotine* is administered as a once-daily transdermal patch that provides even drug levels over 24 hours. These agents alleviate the motor deficits in patients who have never taken *levodopa* and also in patients with advanced Parkinson's disease who are treated with *levodopa*. Dopamine agonists may delay the need to use *levodopa* in early Parkinson's disease and may decrease the dose of *levodopa* in advanced Parkinson's disease. Unlike the ergotamine derivatives, these agents do not exacerbate peripheral vascular disorders or cause fibrosis. Nausea, hallucinations, insomnia, dizziness, constipation, and orthostatic hypotension are among the more distressing side effects of these drugs, but dyskinesias are less frequent than with *levodopa* (Figure 8.11). *Pramipexole* is mainly excreted unchanged in the urine, and dosage adjustments are needed in renal dysfunction. *Cimetidine* inhibits renal tubular secretion of organic bases and may significantly increase the half-life of *pramipexole*. The fluoroquinolone antibiotics and other inhibitors of the cytochrome P450 (CYP450) 1A2 isoenzyme (for example, *fluoxetine*) may inhibit the metabolism of *ropinirole*, requiring an adjustment in *ropinirole* dosage. Figure 8.12 summarizes some properties of dopamine agonists.

E. Amantadine

It was accidentally discovered that the antiviral drug *amantadine* [a-MAN-ta-deen], used to treat influenza, has an antiparkinsonian action. *Amantadine* has several effects on a number of neurotransmitters implicated in parkinsonism, including increasing the release of dopamine, blocking cholinergic receptors, and inhibiting the *N*-methyl-D-aspartate (NMDA) type of glutamate receptors. Current evidence supports action at NMDA receptors as the primary action at therapeutic concentrations. [Note: If dopamine release is already at a maximum, *amantadine* has no effect.] The drug may cause restlessness, agitation, confusion, and hallucinations, and, at high doses, it may induce acute toxic psychosis. Orthostatic hypotension, urinary retention, peripheral edema, and dry mouth also may occur. *Amantadine* is less efficacious than *levodopa,* and tolerance develops more readily. However, *amantadine* has fewer side effects.

F. Antimuscarinic agents

The antimuscarinic agents are much less efficacious than *levodopa* and play only an adjuvant role in antiparkinsonism therapy. The actions of *benztropine* [BENZ-troe-peen], *trihexyphenidyl* [tri-hex-ee-FEN-i-dill], *procyclidine* [pro-SYE-kli-deen], and *biperiden* [bi-PER-i-den] are similar, although individual patients may respond more favorably to one drug. Blockage of cholinergic transmission produces effects similar to augmentation of dopaminergic transmission, since it helps to correct the imbalance in the dopamine/acetylcholine ratio (Figure 8.4). These agents can induce mood changes and produce xerostomia (dryness of the mouth), constipation, and visual problems typical of muscarinic blockers (see Chapter 5). They interfere with gastrointestinal peristalsis and are contraindicated in patients with glaucoma, prostatic hyperplasia, or pyloric stenosis.

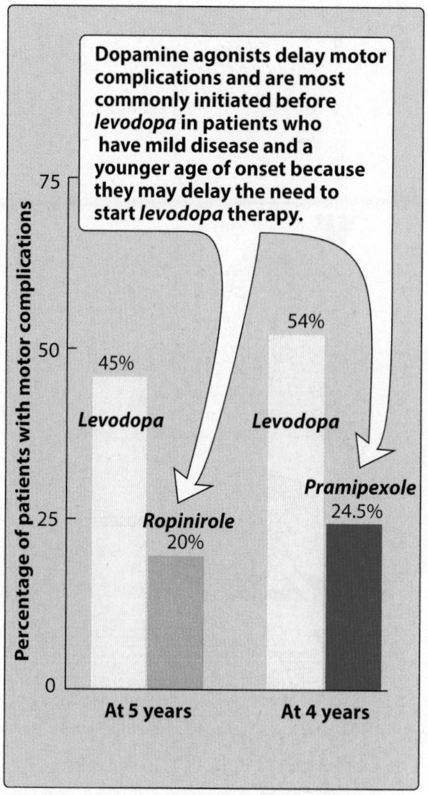

Figure 8.11

Motor complications in patients treated with *levodopa* or dopamine agonists.

VII. DRUGS USED IN ALZHEIMER'S DISEASE

Dementia of the Alzheimer type has three distinguishing features: 1) accumulation of senile plaques (β-amyloid accumulations), 2) formation of numerous neurofibrillary tangles, and 3) loss of cortical neurons, particularly cholinergic neurons. Current therapies aim to either improve cholinergic transmission within the CNS or prevent excitotoxic actions resulting from overstimulation of NMDA-glutamate receptors in

Characteristic	Pramipexole	Ropinirole	Rotigotine
Bioavailability	>90%	55%	45%
V_d	7 L/kg	7.5 L/kg	84 L/kg
Half-life	8 hours[1]	6 hours	7 hours[3]
Metabolism	Negligible	Extensive	Extensive
Elimination	Renal	Renal[2]	Renal[2]

Figure 8.12

Pharmacokinetic properties of dopamine agonists *pramipexole, ropinirole,* and *rotigotine.* Vd = volume of distribution. [1]Increases to 12 hours in patients older than 65 years; [2]Less than 10% excreted unchanged; [3]Administered as a once-daily transdermal patch.

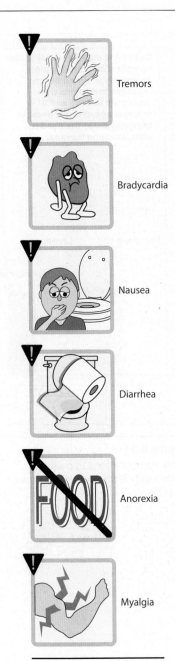

Figure 8.13
Adverse effects of AChE inhibitors.

selected areas of the brain. Pharmacologic intervention for Alzheimer's disease is only palliative and provides modest short-term benefit. None of the available therapeutic agents alter the underlying neurodegenerative process.

A. Acetylcholinesterase inhibitors

Numerous studies have linked the progressive loss of cholinergic neurons and, presumably, cholinergic transmission within the cortex to the memory loss that is a hallmark symptom of Alzheimer's disease. It is postulated that inhibition of acetylcholinesterase (AChE) within the CNS will improve cholinergic transmission, at least at those neurons that are still functioning. The reversible AChE inhibitors approved for the treatment of mild to moderate Alzheimer's disease include *donepezil* [doe-NE-peh-zil], *galantamine* [ga-LAN-ta-meen], and *rivastigmine* [ri-va-STIG-meen]. All of them have some selectivity for AChE in the CNS, as compared to the periphery. *Galantamine* may also augment the action of acetylcholine at nicotinic receptors in the CNS. At best, these compounds provide a modest reduction in the rate of loss of cognitive functioning in Alzheimer patients. *Rivastigmine* is the only agent approved for the management of dementia associated with Parkinson's disease and also the only AChE inhibitor available as a transdermal formulation. *Rivastigmine* is hydrolyzed by AChE to a carbamylate metabolite and has no interactions with drugs that alter the activity of CYP450 enzymes. The other agents are substrates for CYP450 and have a potential for such interactions. Common adverse effects include nausea, diarrhea, vomiting, anorexia, tremors, bradycardia, and muscle cramps (Figure 8.13).

B. NMDA receptor antagonist

Stimulation of glutamate receptors in the CNS appears to be critical for the formation of certain memories. However, overstimulation of glutamate receptors, particularly of the NMDA type, may result in excitotoxic effects on neurons and is suggested as a mechanism for neurodegenerative or apoptotic (programmed cell death) processes. Binding of glutamate to the NMDA receptor assists in the opening of an ion channel that allows Ca^{2+} to enter the neuron. Excess intracellular Ca^{2+} can activate a number of processes that ultimately damage neurons and lead to apoptosis. *Memantine* [meh-MAN-teen] is an NMDA receptor antagonist indicated for moderate to severe Alzheimer's disease. It acts by blocking the NMDA receptor and limiting Ca^{2+} influx into the neuron, such that toxic intracellular levels are not achieved. *Memantine* is well tolerated, with few dose-dependent adverse events. Expected side effects, such as confusion, agitation, and restlessness, are indistinguishable from the symptoms of Alzheimer's disease. Given its different mechanism of action and possible neuroprotective effects, *memantine* is often given in combination with an AChE inhibitor.

VIII. DRUGS USED IN MULTIPLE SCLEROSIS

Multiple sclerosis is an autoimmune inflammatory demyelinating disease of the CNS. The course of MS is variable. For some, MS may consist of one or two acute neurologic episodes. In others, it is a chronic, relapsing, or progressive disease that may span 10 to 20 years. Historically, corticosteroids (for example, *dexamethasone* and *prednisone*) have been used to treat acute exacerbations of the disease. Chemotherapeutic agents, such as *cyclophosphamide* and *azathioprine*, have also been used.

A. Disease-modifying therapies

Drugs currently approved for MS are indicated to decrease relapse rates or in some cases to prevent accumulation of disability. The major target of these medications is to modify the immune response through inhibition of white blood cell–mediated inflammatory processes that eventually lead to myelin sheath damage and decreased or inappropriate axonal communication between cells.

1. **Interferon β_{1a} and interferon β_{1b}:** The immunomodulatory effects of *interferon* [in-ter-FEER-on] help to diminish the inflammatory responses that lead to demyelination of the axon sheaths. Adverse effects of these medications may include depression, local injection site reactions, hepatic enzyme increases, and flu-like symptoms.

2. **Glatiramer:** *Glatiramer* [gluh-TEER-a-mur] is a synthetic polypeptide that resembles myelin protein and may act as a decoy to T-cell attack. Some patients experience a postinjection reaction that includes flushing, chest pain, anxiety, and itching. It is usually self-limiting.

3. **Fingolimod:** *Fingolimod* [fin-GO-li-mod] is an oral drug that alters lymphocyte migration, resulting in fewer lymphocytes in the CNS. *Fingolimod* may cause first-dose bradycardia and is associated with an increased risk of infection and macular edema.

4. **Teriflunomide:** *Teriflunomide* [te-ree-FLOO-no-mide] is an oral pyrimidine synthesis inhibitor that leads to a lower concentration of active lymphocytes in the CNS. *Teriflunomide* may cause elevated liver enzymes. It should be avoided in pregnancy.

5. **Dimethyl fumarate:** *Dimethyl fumarate* [dye-METH-il FOO-ma-rate] is an oral agent that may alter the cellular response to oxidative stress to reduce disease progression. Flushing and abdominal pain are the most common adverse events.

6. **Natalizumab:** *Natalizumab* [na-ta-LIZ-oo-mab] is a monoclonal antibody indicated for MS in patients who have failed first-line therapies.

7. **Mitoxantrone:** *Mitoxantrone* [my-toe-ZAN-trone] is a cytotoxic anthracycline analog that kills T cells and may also be used for MS.

B. Symptomatic treatment

Many different classes of drugs are used to manage symptoms of MS such as spasticity, constipation, bladder dysfunction, and depression. *Dalfampridine* [DAL-fam-pre-deen], an oral potassium channel blocker, improves walking speeds in patients with MS. It is the first drug approved for this use.

IX. DRUGS USED IN AMYOTROPHIC LATERAL SCLEROSIS

ALS is characterized by progressive degeneration of motor neurons, resulting in the inability to initiate or control muscle movement. *Riluzole* [RIL-ue-zole], an NMDA receptor antagonist, is currently the only drug indicated for the management of ALS. It is believed to act by inhibiting glutamate release and blocking sodium channels. *Riluzole* may improve survival time and delay the need for ventilator support in patients suffering from ALS.

Study Questions

Choose the ONE best answer.

8.1 Which one of the following combinations of antiparkinsonian drugs is an appropriate treatment plan?

    A. Amantadine, carbidopa, and entacapone.

    B. Levodopa, carbidopa, and entacapone.

    C. Pramipexole, carbidopa, and entacapone.

    D. Ropinirole, selegiline, and entacapone.

    E. Ropinirole, carbidopa, and selegiline.

Correct answer = B. To reduce the dose of levodopa and its peripheral side effects, the peripheral decarboxylase inhibitor, carbidopa, is coadministered. As a result of this combination, more levodopa is available for metabolism by catechol-O-methyltransferase (COMT) to 3-O-methyldopa, which competes with levodopa for the active transport processes into the CNS. By administering entacapone (an inhibitor of COMT), the competing product is not formed, and more levodopa enters the brain. The other choices are not appropriate, because neither peripheral decarboxylase nor COMT nor monoamine oxidase metabolizes amantadine or the direct-acting dopamine agonists, ropinirole and pramipexole.

8.2 Peripheral adverse effects of levodopa, including nausea, hypotension, and cardiac arrhythmias, can be diminished by including which of the following drugs in the therapy?

    A. Amantadine.

    B. Ropinirole.

    C. Carbidopa.

    D. Tolcapone.

    E. Pramipexole.

Correct answer = C. Carbidopa inhibits the peripheral decarboxylation of levodopa to dopamine, thereby diminishing the gastrointestinal and cardiovascular side effects of levodopa. The other agents listed do not ameliorate adverse effects of levodopa.

8.3 Which of the following antiparkinsonian drugs may cause vasospasm?

    A. Amantadine.

    B. Bromocriptine.

    C. Carbidopa.

    D. Entacapone.

    E. Ropinirole.

Correct answer = B. Bromocriptine is a dopamine receptor agonist that may cause vasospasm. It is contraindicated in patients with peripheral vascular disease. Ropinirole directly stimulates dopamine receptors, but it does not cause vasospasm. The other drugs do not act directly on dopamine receptors.

8.4 Modest improvement in the memory of patients with Alzheimer's disease may occur with drugs that increase transmission at which of the following receptors?

    A. Adrenergic.

    B. Cholinergic.

    C. Dopaminergic.

    D. GABAergic.

    E. Serotonergic.

Correct answer = B. AChE inhibitors, such as rivastigmine, increase cholinergic transmission in the CNS and may cause a modest delay in the progression of Alzheimer's disease. Increased transmission at the other types of receptors listed does not result in improved memory.

8.5 Which medication is a glutamate receptor antagonist that can be used in combination with an acetylcholinesterase inhibitor to manage the symptoms of Alzheimer's disease?

A. Rivastigmine.
B. Ropinirole.
C. Fluoxetine.
D. Memantine.
E. Donepezil.

Correct answer = D. When combined with an acetylcholinesterase inhibitor, memantine has modest efficacy in keeping patients with Alzheimer's disease at or above baseline for at least 6 months and may delay disease progression.

8.6 Which of the following agents is available as a patch for once-daily use and is likely to provide steady drug levels to treat Alzheimer's disease?

A. Rivastigmine.
B. Donepezil.
C. Memantine.
D. Galantamine.
E. Glatiramer.

Correct answer = A. Rivastigmine is the only agent available as a transdermal delivery system for the treatment of Alzheimer's disease. It may also be used for dementia associated with Parkinson's disease.

8.7 Which of the following is the only medication that is approved for the management of amyotrophic lateral sclerosis?

A. Pramipexole.
B. Selegiline.
C. Galantamine.
D. Riluzole.
E. Glatiramer.

Correct answer = D. Riluzole continues to be the only agent FDA approved for the debilitating and lethal illness of ALS. It is used to, ideally, delay the progression and need for ventilator support in severe patients.

8.8 Which of the following medications reduces immune system–mediated inflammation via inhibition of pyrimidine synthesis to reduce the number of activated lymphocytes in the CNS?

A. Riluzole.
B. Rotigotine.
C. Teriflunomide.
D. Dexamethasone.

Correct answer = C. Teriflunomide is believed to exert its disease modifying and anti-inflammatory effects by inhibiting the enzyme dihydro-orotate dehydrogenase to reduce pyrimidine synthesis.

8.9 Which of the following agents may cause tremors as a side effect and, thus, should be used with caution in patients with Parkinson's disease, even though it is also indicated for the treatment of dementia associated with Parkinson's disease?

A. Benztropine.
B. Rotigotine.
C. Rivastigmine.
D. Dimethyl fumarate.

Correct answer = C. Though rivastigmine is an acetylcholinesterase inhibitor, which can cause tremors as an adverse effect, its use is not contraindicated in patients with Parkinson's disease, as this agent is also the only medication approved for dementia associated with Parkinson's disease. It should be used with caution, as it may worsen the parkinsonian-related tremors. A risk–benefit discussion should occur with the patient and the caregiver before rivastigmine is used.

8.10 Which of the following agents exerts its therapeutic effect in multiple sclerosis via potassium channel blockade?

A. Dalfampridine.
B. Donepezil.
C. Riluzole.
D. Bromocriptine.

Correct answer = A. Dalfampridine is a potassium channel blocker and is the only agent that is indicated to improve walking speed in patients with MS.

Anxiolytic and Hypnotic Drugs

9

Jose A. Rey

I. OVERVIEW

Disorders involving anxiety are among the most common mental disorders. Anxiety is an unpleasant state of tension, apprehension, or uneasiness (a fear that arises from either a known or an unknown source). The physical symptoms of severe anxiety are similar to those of fear (such as tachycardia, sweating, trembling, and palpitations) and involve sympathetic activation. Episodes of mild anxiety are common life experiences and do not warrant treatment. However, severe, chronic, debilitating anxiety may be treated with antianxiety drugs (sometimes called anxiolytics) and/or some form of psychotherapy. Because many antianxiety drugs also cause some sedation, they may be used clinically as both anxiolytic and hypnotic (sleep-inducing) agents. Figure 9.1 summarizes the anxiolytic and hypnotic agents. Some antidepressants are also indicated for certain anxiety disorders; however, they are discussed with other antidepressants (see Chapter 10).

II. BENZODIAZEPINES

Benzodiazepines are widely used anxiolytic drugs. They have largely replaced barbiturates and *meprobamate* in the treatment of anxiety and insomnia, because benzodiazepines are generally considered to be safer and more effective (Figure 9.2). Though benzodiazepines are commonly used, they are not necessarily the best choice for anxiety or insomnia. Certain antidepressants with anxiolytic action, such as the selective serotonin reuptake inhibitors, are preferred in many cases, and nonbenzodiazepine hypnotics and antihistamines may be preferable for insomnia.

A. Mechanism of action

The targets for benzodiazepine actions are the γ-aminobutyric acid ($GABA_A$) receptors. [Note: GABA is the major inhibitory neurotransmitter in the central nervous system (CNS).] The $GABA_A$ receptors are composed of a combination of five α, β, and γ subunits that span the postsynaptic membrane (Figure 9.3). For each subunit, many subtypes exist (for example, there are six subtypes of the α subunit). Binding of GABA to its receptor triggers an opening of the central ion channel, allowing chloride through the pore (Figure 9.3). The influx of chloride ions causes hyperpolarization of the neuron and decreases neurotransmission by inhibiting the formation of action potentials.

BENZODIAZEPINES

Alprazolam XANAX
Chlordiazepoxide LIBRIUM
Clonazepam KLONOPIN
Clorazepate TRANXENE
Diazepam VALIUM, DIASTAT
Estazolam
Flurazepam DALMANE
Lorazepam ATIVAN
Midazolam VERSED
Oxazepam
Quazepam DORAL
Temazepam RESTORIL
Triazolam HALCION

BENZODIAZEPINE ANTAGONIST

Flumazenil ROMAZICON

OTHER ANXIOLYTIC DRUGS

Antidepressants VARIOUS (SEE CHAPTER 10)
Buspirone BUSPAR

BARBITURATES

Amobarbital AMYTAL
Pentobarbital NEMBUTAL
Phenobarbital LUMINAL SODIUM
Secobarbital SECONAL
Thiopental PENTOTHAL

OTHER HYPNOTIC AGENTS

Antihistamines VARIOUS (SEE CHAPTER 30)
Doxepin SILENOR
Eszopiclone LUNESTA
Ramelteon ROZEREM
Zaleplon SONATA
Zolpidem AMBIEN, INTERMEZZO, ZOLPIMIST

Figure 9.1

Summary of anxiolytic and hypnotic drugs.

121

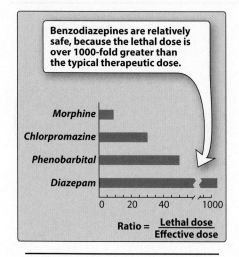

Figure 9.2
Ratio of lethal dose to effective dose for *morphine* (an opioid, see Chapter 14), *chlorpromazine* (an antipsychotic, see Chapter 11), and the anxiolytic, hypnotic drugs, *phenobarbital* and *diazepam*.

Benzodiazepines modulate GABA effects by binding to a specific, high-affinity site (distinct from the GABA-binding site) located at the interface of the α subunit and the γ subunit on the GABA$_A$ receptor (Figure 9.3). [Note: These binding sites are sometimes labeled "benzodiazepine (BZ) receptors." Common BZ receptor subtypes in the CNS are designated as BZ$_1$ or BZ$_2$ depending on whether the binding site includes an α_1 or α_2 subunit, respectively.] Benzodiazepines increase the frequency of channel openings produced by GABA. [Note: Binding of a benzodiazepine to its receptor site increases the affinity of GABA for the GABA-binding site (and vice versa).] The clinical effects of the various benzodiazepines correlate well with the binding affinity of each drug for the GABA receptor–chloride ion channel complex.

B. Actions

All benzodiazepines exhibit the following actions to some extent:

1. **Reduction of anxiety:** At low doses, the benzodiazepines are anxiolytic. They are thought to reduce anxiety by selectively enhancing GABAergic transmission in neurons having the α_2 subunit in their GABA$_A$ receptors, thereby inhibiting neuronal circuits in the limbic system of the brain.

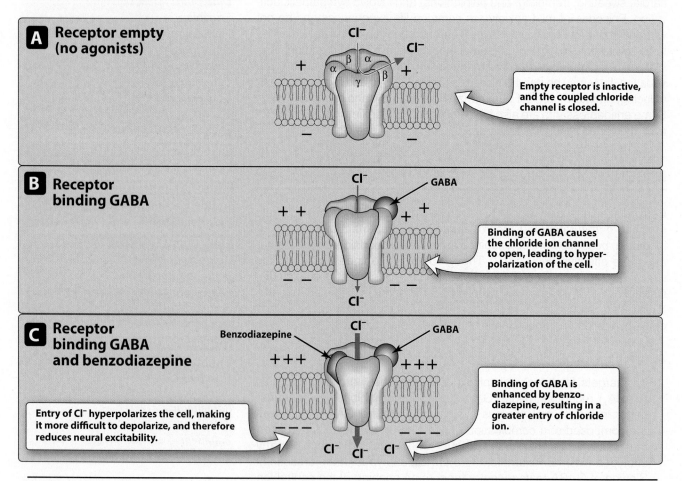

Figure 9.3
Schematic diagram of benzodiazepine–GABA–chloride ion channel complex. GABA = γ-aminobutyric acid.

2. **Sedative/hypnotic:** All benzodiazepines have sedative and calming properties, and some can produce hypnosis (artificially produced sleep) at higher doses. The hypnotic effects are mediated by the α_1-GABA$_A$ receptors.

3. **Anterograde amnesia:** Temporary impairment of memory with use of the benzodiazepines is also mediated by the α_1-GABA$_A$ receptors. The ability to learn and form new memories is also impaired.

4. **Anticonvulsant:** Several benzodiazepines have anticonvulsant activity. This effect is partially, although not completely, mediated by α_1-GABA$_A$ receptors.

5. **Muscle relaxant:** At high doses, the benzodiazepines relax the spasticity of skeletal muscle, probably by increasing presynaptic inhibition in the spinal cord, where the α_2-GABA$_A$ receptors are largely located. *Baclofen* [BAK-loe-fen] is a muscle relaxant that is believed to affect GABA receptors at the level of the spinal cord.

C. Therapeutic uses

The individual benzodiazepines show small differences in their relative anxiolytic, anticonvulsant, and sedative properties. However, the duration of action varies widely among this group, and pharmacokinetic considerations are often important in choosing one benzodiazepine over another.

1. **Anxiety disorders:** Benzodiazepines are effective for the treatment of the anxiety symptoms secondary to panic disorder, generalized anxiety disorder (GAD), social anxiety disorder, performance anxiety, posttraumatic stress disorder, obsessive–compulsive disorder, and extreme anxiety associated with phobias, such as fear of flying. The benzodiazepines are also useful in treating anxiety related to depression and schizophrenia. These drugs should be reserved for severe anxiety only and not used to manage the stress of everyday life. Because of their addiction potential, they should only be used for short periods of time. The longer-acting agents, such as *clonazepam* [kloe-NAZ-e-pam], *lorazepam* [lor-AZ-e-pam], and *diazepam* [dye-AZ-e-pam], are often preferred in those patients with anxiety that may require prolonged treatment. The antianxiety effects of the benzodiazepines are less subject to tolerance than the sedative and hypnotic effects. [Note: Tolerance (that is, decreased responsiveness to repeated doses of the drug) occurs when used for more than 1 to 2 weeks. Tolerance is associated with a decrease in GABA receptor density. Cross-tolerance exists between the benzodiazepines and *ethanol*.] For panic disorders, *alprazolam* [al-PRAY-zoe-lam] is effective for short- and long-term treatment, although it may cause withdrawal reactions in about 30% of patients.

2. **Sleep disorders:** A few of the benzodiazepines are useful as hypnotic agents. These agents decrease the latency to sleep onset and increase stage II of non–rapid eye movement (REM) sleep. Both REM sleep and slow-wave sleep are decreased. In the treatment of insomnia, it is important to balance the sedative effect needed at bedtime with the residual sedation ("hangover") upon

awakening. Commonly prescribed benzodiazepines for sleep disorders include intermediate-acting *temazepam* [te-MAZ-e-pam] and short-acting *triazolam* [try-AY-zoe-lam]. Long-acting *flurazepam* [flure-AZ-e-pam] is rarely used, due to its extended half-life, which may result in excessive daytime sedation and accumulation of the drug, especially in the elderly. *Estazolam* [eh-STAY-zoe-lam] and *quazepam* [QUAY-ze-pam] are considered intermediate- and long-acting agents, respectively.

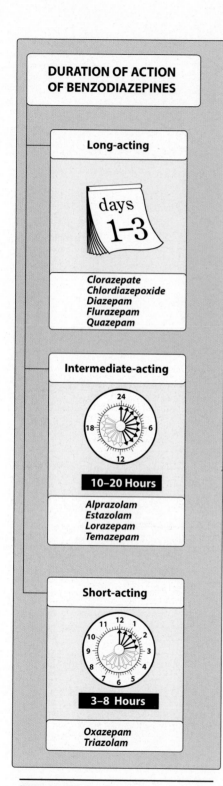

Figure 9.4
Comparison of the durations of action of the benzodiazepines.

   a. Temazepam: This drug is useful in patients who experience frequent wakening. However, because the peak sedative effect occurs 1 to 3 hours after an oral dose, it should be given 1 to 2 hours before bedtime.

   b. Triazolam: Whereas *temazepam* is useful for insomnia caused by the inability to stay asleep, short-acting *triazolam* is effective in treating individuals who have difficulty in going to sleep. Tolerance frequently develops within a few days, and withdrawal of the drug often results in rebound insomnia. Therefore, this drug is not a preferred agent, and it is best used intermittently. In general, hypnotics should be given for only a limited time, usually less than 2 to 4 weeks.

3. Amnesia: The shorter-acting agents are often employed as premedication for anxiety-provoking and unpleasant procedures, such as endoscopy, dental procedures, and angioplasty. They cause a form of conscious sedation, allowing the person to be receptive to instructions during these procedures. *Midazolam* [mi-DAY-zoe-lam] is a benzodiazepine used to facilitate amnesia while causing sedation prior to anesthesia.

4. Seizures: *Clonazepam* is occasionally used as an adjunctive therapy for certain types of seizures, whereas *lorazepam* and *diazepam* are the drugs of choice in terminating status epilepticus (see Chapter 12). Due to cross-tolerance, *chlordiazepoxide* [klor-di-az-e-POX-ide], *clorazepate* [klor-AZ-e-pate], *diazepam, lorazepam,* and *oxazepam* [ox-AZ-e-pam] are useful in the acute treatment of alcohol withdrawal and reduce the risk of withdrawal-related seizures.

5. Muscular disorders: *Diazepam* is useful in the treatment of skeletal muscle spasms, such as occur in muscle strain, and in treating spasticity from degenerative disorders, such as multiple sclerosis and cerebral palsy.

D. Pharmacokinetics

1. Absorption and distribution: The benzodiazepines are lipophilic. They are rapidly and completely absorbed after oral administration, distribute throughout the body and penetrate into the CNS.

2. Duration of action: The half-lives of the benzodiazepines are important clinically, because the duration of action may determine the therapeutic usefulness. The benzodiazepines can be roughly divided into short-, intermediate-, and long-acting groups (Figure 9.4). The longer-acting agents form active metabolites with long half-lives. However, with some benzodiazepines, the clinical duration of action does not correlate with the actual half-life (otherwise, a dose of *diazepam* could conceivably be given only every other day, given its active metabolites). This may be due to receptor dissociation rates in the CNS and subsequent redistribution to fatty tissues and other areas.

3. **Fate:** Most benzodiazepines, including *chlordiazepoxide* and *diazepam,* are metabolized by the hepatic microsomal system to compounds that are also active. For these benzodiazepines, the apparent half-life of the drug represents the combined actions of the parent drug and its metabolites. Drug effects are terminated not only by excretion but also by redistribution. The benzodiazepines are excreted in the urine as glucuronides or oxidized metabolites. All benzodiazepines cross the placenta and may depress the CNS of the newborn if given before birth. The benzodiazepines are not recommended for use during pregnancy. Nursing infants may also be exposed to the drugs in breast milk.

E. Dependence

Psychological and physical dependence on benzodiazepines can develop if high doses of the drugs are given for a prolonged period. All benzodiazepines are controlled substances. Abrupt discontinuation of the benzodiazepines results in withdrawal symptoms, including confusion, anxiety, agitation, restlessness, insomnia, tension, and (rarely) seizures. Benzodiazepines with a short elimination half-life, such as *triazolam,* induce more abrupt and severe withdrawal reactions than those seen with drugs that are slowly eliminated such as *flurazepam* (Figure 9.5).

F. Adverse effects

Drowsiness and confusion are the most common side effects of the benzodiazepines. Ataxia occurs at high doses and precludes activities that require fine motor coordination, such as driving an automobile. Cognitive impairment (decreased long-term recall and retention of new knowledge) can occur with use of benzodiazepines. *Triazolam* often shows a rapid development of tolerance, early morning insomnia, and daytime anxiety, as well as amnesia and confusion.

Benzodiazepines should be used cautiously in patients with liver disease. These drugs should be avoided in patients with acute angle-closure glaucoma. Alcohol and other CNS depressants enhance the sedative–hypnotic effects of the benzodiazepines. Benzodiazepines are, however, considerably less dangerous than the older anxiolytic and hypnotic drugs. As a result, a drug overdose is seldom lethal unless other central depressants, such as alcohol, are taken concurrently.

III. BENZODIAZEPINE ANTAGONIST

Flumazenil [floo-MAZ-eh-nill] is a GABA receptor antagonist that can rapidly reverse the effects of benzodiazepines. The drug is available for intravenous (IV) administration only. Onset is rapid, but the duration is short, with a half-life of about 1 hour. Frequent administration may be necessary

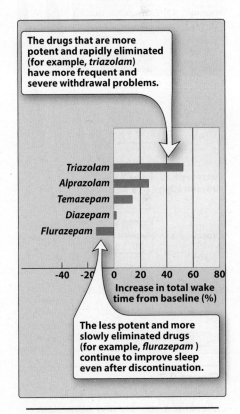

Figure 9.5
Frequency of rebound insomnia resulting from discontinuation of benzodiazepine therapy.

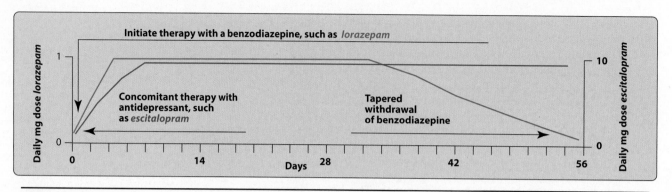

Figure 9.6
Treatment guideline for persistent anxiety.

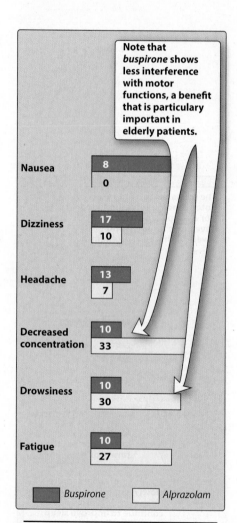

Figure 9.7
Comparison of common adverse effects of *buspirone* and *alprazolam*. Results are expressed as the percentage of patients showing each symptom.

to maintain reversal of a long-acting benzodiazepine. Administration of *flumazenil* may precipitate withdrawal in dependent patients or cause seizures if a benzodiazepine is used to control seizure activity. Seizures may also result if the patient has a mixed ingestion with tricyclic antidepressants or antipsychotics. Dizziness, nausea, vomiting, and agitation are the most common side effects.

IV. OTHER ANXIOLYTIC AGENTS

A. Antidepressants

Many antidepressants are effective in the treatment of chronic anxiety disorders and should be considered as first-line agents, especially in patients with concerns for addiction or dependence. Selective serotonin reuptake inhibitors (SSRIs, such as *escitalopram* or *paroxetine*) or serotonin/norepinephrine reuptake inhibitors (SNRIs), such as *venlafaxine* or *duloxetine*) may be used alone or prescribed in combination with a low dose of a benzodiazepine during the first weeks of treatment (Figure 9.6). After 4 to 6 weeks, when the antidepressant begins to produce an anxiolytic effect, the benzodiazepine dose can be tapered. SSRIs and SNRIs have a lower potential for physical dependence than the benzodiazepines and have become first-line treatment for GAD. While only certain SSRIs or SNRIs have been approved for the treatment of GAD, the efficacy of these drugs for GAD is most likely a class effect. Thus, the choice among these antidepressants should be based upon side effects and cost. Long-term use of antidepressants and benzodiazepines for anxiety disorders is often required to maintain ongoing benefit and prevent relapse.

B. Buspirone

Buspirone [byoo-SPYE-rone] is useful for the chronic treatment of GAD and has an efficacy comparable to that of the benzodiazepines. It has a slow onset of action and is not effective for short-term or "as-needed" treatment of acute anxiety states. The actions of *buspirone* appear to be mediated by serotonin ($5-HT_{1A}$) receptors, although it also displays some affinity for D_2 dopamine receptors and $5-HT_{2A}$

serotonin receptors. Thus, its mode of action differs from that of the benzodiazepines. In addition, *buspirone* lacks the anticonvulsant and muscle-relaxant properties of the benzodiazepines. The frequency of adverse effects is low, with the most common effects being headaches, dizziness, nervousness, nausea, and light-headedness. Sedation and psychomotor and cognitive dysfunction are minimal, and dependence is unlikely. *Buspirone* does not potentiate the CNS depression of alcohol. Figure 9.7 compares some common adverse effects of *buspirone* and the benzodiazepine *alprazolam.*

V. BARBITURATES

The barbiturates were formerly the mainstay of treatment to sedate patients or to induce and maintain sleep. Today, they have been largely replaced by the benzodiazepines, primarily because barbiturates induce tolerance and physical dependence and are associated with very severe withdrawal symptoms. All barbiturates are controlled substances. Certain barbiturates, such as the very short-acting *thiopental,* have been used to induce anesthesia but are infrequently used today due to the advent of newer agents with fewer adverse effects.

A. Mechanism of action

The sedative–hypnotic action of the barbiturates is due to their interaction with GABA$_A$ receptors, which enhances GABAergic transmission. The binding site of barbiturates on the GABA receptor is distinct from that of the benzodiazepines. Barbiturates potentiate GABA action on chloride entry into the neuron by prolonging the duration of the chloride channel openings. In addition, barbiturates can block excitatory glutamate receptors. Anesthetic concentrations of *pentobarbital* also block high-frequency sodium channels. All of these molecular actions lead to decreased neuronal activity.

B. Actions

Barbiturates are classified according to their duration of action (Figure 9.8). For example, ultra–short-acting *thiopental* [thye-oh-PEN-tal] acts within seconds and has a duration of action of about 30 minutes. In contrast, long-acting *phenobarbital* [fee-noe-BAR-bi-tal] has a duration of action greater than a day. *Pentobarbital* [pen-toe-BAR-bi-tal], *secobarbital* [see-koe-BAR-bi-tal], *amobarbital* [am-oh-BAR-bi-tal], and *butalbital* [bu-TAL-bi-tal] are short-acting barbiturates.

1. **Depression of CNS:** At low doses, the barbiturates produce sedation (have a calming effect and reduce excitement). At higher doses, the drugs cause hypnosis, followed by anesthesia (loss of feeling or sensation), and, finally, coma and death. Thus, any degree of depression of the CNS is possible, depending on the dose. Barbiturates do not raise the pain threshold and have no analgesic properties. They may even exacerbate pain. Chronic use leads to tolerance.

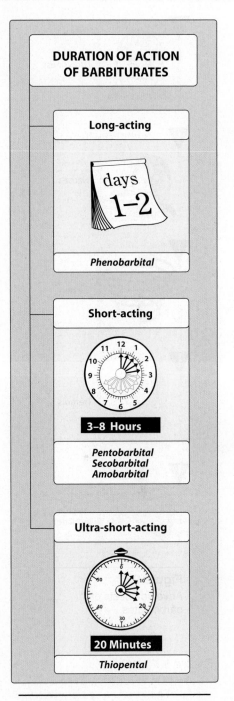

Figure 9.8
Barbiturates classified according to their durations of action.

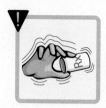

Potential for addiction

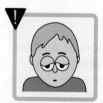

Drowsiness

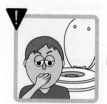

Nausea

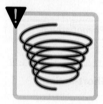

Vertigo

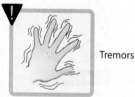

Tremors

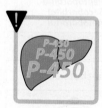

Enzyme induction

Figure 9.9
Adverse effects of barbiturates.

2. Respiratory depression: Barbiturates suppress the hypoxic and chemoreceptor response to CO_2, and overdosage is followed by respiratory depression and death.

C. Therapeutic uses

1. Anesthesia: The ultra–short-acting barbiturates, such as *thiopental,* have been used intravenously to induce anesthesia but have largely been replaced by other agents.

2. Anticonvulsant: *Phenobarbital* has specific anticonvulsant activity that is distinguished from the nonspecific CNS depression. It is used in long-term management of tonic–clonic seizures. However, *phenobarbital* can depress cognitive development in children and decrease cognitive performance in adults, and it should be used only if other therapies have failed. Similarly, *phenobarbital* may be used for the treatment of refractory status epilepticus.

3. Sedative/hypnotic: Barbiturates have been used as mild sedatives to relieve anxiety, nervous tension, and insomnia. When used as hypnotics, they suppress REM sleep more than other stages. However, the use of barbiturates for insomnia is no longer generally accepted, given their adverse effects and potential for tolerance. *Butalbital* is commonly used in combination products (with *acetaminophen* and *caffeine* or *aspirin* and *caffeine*) as a sedative to assist in the management of tension-type or migraine headaches.

D. Pharmacokinetics

Barbiturates are well absorbed after oral administration and distribute throughout the body. All barbiturates redistribute from the brain to the splanchnic areas, to skeletal muscle, and, finally, to adipose tissue. This movement is important in causing the short duration of action of *thiopental* and similar short-acting derivatives. Barbiturates readily cross the placenta and can depress the fetus. These agents are metabolized in the liver, and inactive metabolites are excreted in urine.

E. Adverse effects

Barbiturates cause drowsiness, impaired concentration, and mental and physical sluggishness (Figure 9.9). The CNS depressant effects of barbiturates synergize with those of *ethanol.*

Hypnotic doses of barbiturates produce a drug "hangover" that may lead to impaired ability to function normally for many hours after waking. Occasionally, nausea and dizziness occur. Barbiturates induce cytochrome P450 (CYP450) microsomal enzymes in the liver. Therefore, chronic barbiturate administration diminishes the action of many drugs that are metabolized by the CYP450 system. Barbiturates are contraindicated in patients with acute intermittent porphyria. Abrupt withdrawal from barbiturates may cause tremors, anxiety, weakness, restlessness, nausea and vomiting, seizures, delirium, and cardiac arrest. Withdrawal is much more severe than that associated with opiates and can result in death. Death may also result from overdose. Severe depression of respiration is coupled with central cardiovascular depression and results in a shock-like condition with shallow, infrequent breathing. Treatment includes supportive care and gastric decontamination for recent ingestions.

VI. OTHER HYPNOTIC AGENTS

A. Zolpidem

The hypnotic *zolpidem* [ZOL-pi-dem] is not structurally related to benzo-diazepines, but it selectively binds to the benzodiazepine receptor sub-type BZ_1. *Zolpidem* has no anticonvulsant or muscle-relaxing properties. It shows few withdrawal effects, exhibits minimal rebound insomnia, and little tolerance occurs with prolonged use. *Zolpidem* is rapidly absorbed from the gastrointestinal (GI) tract, and it has a rapid onset of action and short elimination half-life (about 2 to 3 hours). It provides a hypnotic effect for approximately 5 hours (Figure 9.10). [Note: A lingual spray and an extended-release formulation are also available. A sublingual tablet formulation may be used for middle-of-the-night awakening.] *Zolpidem* undergoes hepatic oxidation by the CYP450 system to inactive products. Thus, drugs such as *rifampin,* which induce this enzyme system, shorten the half-life of *zolpidem,* and drugs that inhibit the CYP3A4 isoenzyme may increase the half-life. Adverse effects of *zolpidem* include night-mares, agitation, anterograde amnesia, headache, GI upset, dizziness, and daytime drowsiness. Unlike the benzodiazepines, at usual hypnotic doses, the nonbenzodiazepine drugs, *zolpidem, zaleplon,* and *eszopi-clone,* do not significantly alter the various sleep stages and, hence, are often the preferred hypnotics. This may be due to their relative selectivity for the BZ_1 receptor. All three agents are controlled substances.

B. Zaleplon

Zaleplon [ZAL-e-plon] is an oral nonbenzodiazepine hypnotic similar to *zolpidem*; however, *zaleplon* causes fewer residual effects on psychomo-tor and cognitive function compared to *zolpidem* or the benzodiazepines. This may be due to its rapid elimination, with a half-life of approximately 1 hour. The drug is metabolized by CYP3A4.

C. Eszopiclone

Eszopiclone [es-ZOE-pi-clone] is an oral nonbenzodiazepine hyp-notic that also acts on the BZ_1 receptor. It has been shown to be effective for insomnia for up to 6 months. *Eszopiclone* is rapidly absorbed (time to peak, 1 hour), extensively metabolized by oxidation and demethylation via the CYP450 system, and mainly excreted in urine. Elimination half-life is approximately 6 hours. Adverse events with *eszopiclone* include anxiety, dry mouth, headache, peripheral edema, somnolence, and unpleasant taste.

D. Ramelteon

Ramelteon [ram-EL-tee-on] is a selective agonist at the MT_1 and MT_2 subtypes of melatonin receptors. Melatonin is a hormone secreted by the pineal gland that helps to maintain the circadian rhythm underly-ing the normal sleep–wake cycle. Stimulation of MT_1 and MT_2 recep-tors by *ramelteon* is thought to induce and promote sleep. *Ramelteon* is indicated for the treatment of insomnia characterized by difficulty falling asleep (increased sleep latency). It has minimal potential for abuse, and no evidence of dependence or withdrawal effects has been observed. Therefore, *ramelteon* can be administered long term. Common adverse effects of *ramelteon* include dizziness, fatigue, and somnolence. *Ramelteon* may also increase prolactin levels.

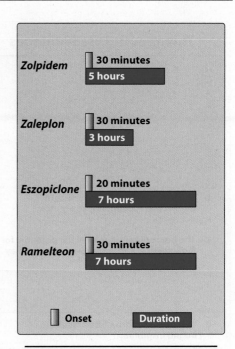

Figure 9.10
Onset and duration of action of the commonly used nonbenzodiazepine hypnotic agents.

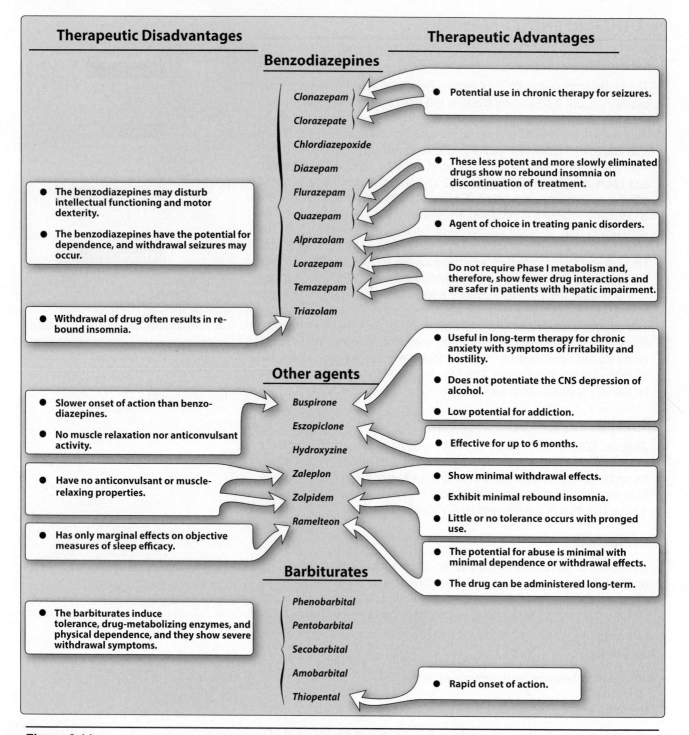

Figure 9.11
Therapeutic disadvantages and advantages of some anxiolytic and hypnotic agents. CNS = central nervous system.

E. Antihistamines

Some antihistamines with sedating properties, such as *diphenhydramine, hydroxyzine,* and *doxylamine,* are effective in treating mild types of situational insomnia. However, they have undesirable side effects (such as anticholinergic effects) that make them less useful than the benzodiazepines and the nonbenzodiazepines. Some sedative antihistamines are marketed in numerous over-the-counter products.

F. Antidepressants

The use of sedating antidepressants with strong antihistamine profiles has been ongoing for decades. *Doxepin* [DOX-e-pin], an older tricyclic agent with SNRI mechanisms of antidepressant and anxiolytic action, was recently approved at low doses for the management of insomnia. Other antidepressants, such as *trazodone* [TRAZ-oh-done], *mirtazapine* [mir-TAZ-a-pine], and other older tricyclic antidepressants with strong antihistamine properties are used off-label for the treatment of insomnia (see Chapter 10).

Figure 9.11 summarizes the therapeutic disadvantages and advantages of some of the anxiolytic and hypnotic drugs.

Study Questions

Choose the ONE best answer.

9.1 Which one of the following statements is correct regarding benzodiazepines?

  A. Benzodiazepines directly open chloride channels.

  B. Benzodiazepines show analgesic actions.

  C. Clinical improvement of anxiety requires 2 to 4 weeks of treatment with benzodiazepines.

  D. All benzodiazepines have some sedative effects.

  E. Benzodiazepines, like other CNS depressants, readily produce general anesthesia.

Correct answer = D. Although all benzodiazepines can cause sedation, the drugs labeled "benzodiazepines" in Figure 9.1 are promoted for the treatment of sleep disorder. Benzodiazepines enhance the binding of $GABA_A$ to its receptor, which increases the permeability of chloride. The benzodiazepines do not relieve pain but may reduce the anxiety associated with pain. Unlike the tricyclic antidepressants and the monoamine oxidase inhibitors, the benzodiazepines are effective within hours of administration. Benzodiazepines do not produce general anesthesia and, therefore, are relatively safe drugs with a high therapeutic index.

9.2 Which one of the following is a short-acting hypnotic?

  A. Phenobarbital.

  B. Diazepam.

  C. Chlordiazepoxide.

  D. Triazolam.

  E. Flurazepam.

Correct answer = D. Triazolam is a short-acting drug. It has little daytime sedation. The other drugs listed are longer acting.

9.3 Which one of the following statements is correct regarding the anxiolytic and hypnotic agents?

  A. Phenobarbital shows analgesic properties.

  B. Diazepam and phenobarbital induce the cytochrome P450 enzyme system.

  C. Phenobarbital is useful in the treatment of acute intermittent porphyria.

  D. Phenobarbital induces respiratory depression, which is enhanced by the consumption of ethanol.

  E. Buspirone has actions similar to those of the benzodiazepines.

Correct answer = D. Barbiturates and ethanol are a potentially lethal combination. Phenobarbital is unable to alter the pain threshold. Only phenobarbital strongly induces the synthesis of the hepatic cytochrome P450 drug-metabolizing system. Phenobarbital is contraindicated in the treatment of acute intermittent porphyria. Buspirone lacks the anticonvulsant and muscle-relaxant properties of the benzodiazepines and causes only minimal sedation.

9.4 A 45-year-old man who has been injured in a car accident is brought into the emergency room. His blood alcohol level on admission is 275 mg/dL. Hospital records show a prior hospitalization for alcohol-related seizures. His wife confirms that he has been drinking heavily for 3 weeks. What treatment should be provided to the patient if he goes into withdrawal?

A. None.
B. Lorazepam.
C. Pentobarbital.
D. Phenytoin.
E. Buspirone.

Correct answer = B. It is important to treat the seizures associated with alcohol withdrawal. Benzodiazepines, such as chlordiazepoxide, diazepam, or the shorter-acting lorazepam, are effective in controlling this problem. They are less sedating than pentobarbital or phenytoin.

9.5 Which one of the following is a short-acting hypnotic and better for sleep induction compared to sleep maintenance?

A. Temazepam.
B. Flurazepam.
C. Zaleplon.
D. Buspirone.
E. Escitalopram.

Correct answer = C. Zaleplon has the shortest half-life and duration of action. Buspirone and escitalopram are not effective hypnotic agents. Temazepam and flurazepam have longer durations of action and will reduce nighttime awakenings but will have a greater risk of daytime sedation or hangover effect compared to zaleplon.

9.6 Which of the following agents has a rapid anxiolytic effect and would be best for the acute management of anxiety?

A. Buspirone.
B. Venlafaxine.
C. Lorazepam.
D. Escitalopram.
E. Duloxetine.

Correct answer = C. The benzodiazepines have same-dose, first-dose efficacy for anxiety, whereas the other agents require 2 to 8 weeks for clinically significant improvement in anxiety.

9.7 Which of the following sedative–hypnotic agents utilizes melatonin receptor agonism as the mechanism of action to induce sleep?

A. Zolpidem.
B. Eszopiclone.
C. Estazolam.
D. Ramelteon.
E. Diphenhydramine.

Correct answer = D. Ramelteon is the only melatonin receptor agonist to promote sleep, especially in sleep-phase disrupted sleep. Zolpidem, eszopiclone, and estazolam all utilize the benzodiazepine receptor, and diphenhydramine is a histamine receptor antagonist.

9.8 All of the following agents for the management of insomnia are controlled substances and may have a risk for addiction or dependence except:

A. Zaleplon.
B. Flurazepam.
C. Doxepin.
D. Zolpidem.
E. Triazolam.

Correct answer = C. Only doxepin, a tricyclic agent with significant antihistaminergic properties, is considered to have no risk of addiction or dependence, whereas the other agents listed all have DEA schedule IV designations with some risk for addiction or dependence, especially when used for extended periods.

9.9 All of the following agents may cause cognitive impairment, including memory problems when used at recommended doses except:

A. Diphenhydramine.
B. Zolpidem.
C. Alprazolam.
D. Phenobarbital.
E. Ramelteon.

Correct answer = E. All of the above listed agents, except ramelteon, have been associated with cognitive impairments, including memory impairment. Diphenhydramine likely causes its cognitive problems from its anticholinergic and antihistaminergic effects. Zolpidem, alprazolam, and phenobarbital are well-known causes of cognitive impairment, including anterograde amnesia. Ramelteon has safety data extending to 6 months and is a noncontrolled hypnotic agent acting as a melatonin receptor agonist. It is not considered to have a risk for cognitive impairment as compared to the other agents listed.

9.10 Which agent is best used in the Emergency Room setting for patients who are believed to have received too much of a benzodiazepine drug or taken an overdose of benzodiazepines?

   A. Diazepam.
   B. Ramelteon.
   C. Flumazenil.
   D. Doxepin.
   E. Naloxone.

Correct answer = C. Flumazenil is only indicated to reverse the effects of benzodiazepines via antagonizing the benzodiazepine receptor. It should be used with caution due to a risk of seizures if the patient has been a long time recipient of benzodiazepines or if the overdose attempt was with mixed drugs. Naloxone is an opioid receptor antagonist. The other agents are not efficacious in reversing effects of benzodiazepines.

Antidepressants

Jose A. Rey

10

I. OVERVIEW

The symptoms of depression are feelings of sadness and hopelessness, as well as the inability to experience pleasure in usual activities, changes in sleep patterns and appetite, loss of energy, and suicidal thoughts. Mania is characterized by the opposite behavior: enthusiasm, anger, rapid thought and speech patterns, extreme self-confidence, and impaired judgment. This chapter provides an overview of drugs used for the treatment of depression and mania.

II. MECHANISM OF ANTIDEPRESSANT DRUGS

Most clinically useful antidepressant drugs (Figure 10.1) potentiate, either directly or indirectly, the actions of norepinephrine and/or serotonin (5-HT) in the brain. This, along with other evidence, led to the biogenic amine theory, which proposes that depression is due to a deficiency of monoamines, such as norepinephrine and serotonin, at certain key sites in the brain. Conversely, the theory proposes that mania is caused by an overproduction of these neurotransmitters. However, the biogenic amine theory of depression and mania is overly simplistic. It fails to explain the pharmacological effects of any of the antidepressant and antimania drugs on neurotransmission, which often occur immediately; however, the time course for a therapeutic response occurs over several weeks. This suggests that decreased reuptake of neurotransmitters is only an initial effect of the drugs, which may not be directly responsible for the antidepressant effects.

III. SELECTIVE SEROTONIN REUPTAKE INHIBITORS

The selective serotonin reuptake inhibitors (SSRIs) are a group of antidepressant drugs that specifically inhibit serotonin reuptake, having 300- to 3000-fold greater selectivity for the serotonin transporter, as compared to the norepinephrine transporter. This contrasts with the tricyclic antidepressants (TCAs) and serotonin/norepinephrine reuptake inhibitors (SNRIs) that nonselectively inhibit the reuptake of norepinephrine and serotonin (Figure 10.2). Moreover, the SSRIs have little blocking activity at muscarinic, α-adrenergic, and histaminic H_1 receptors. Therefore, common side effects associated with TCAs, such as orthostatic hypotension, sedation, dry mouth, and blurred vision, are not commonly seen with

SELECTIVE SEROTONIN REUPTAKE INHIBITORS (SSRIs)
Citalopram CELEXA
Escitalopram LEXAPRO
Fluoxetine PROZAC
Fluvoxamine LUVOX CR
Paroxetine PAXIL
Sertraline ZOLOFT

SEROTONIN/NOREPINEPHRINE REUPTAKE INHIBITORS (SNRIs)
Desvenlafaxine PRISTIQ
Duloxetine CYMBALTA
Levomilnacipran FETZIMA
Venlafaxine EFFEXOR

ATYPICAL ANTIDEPRESSANTS
Bupropion WELLBUTRIN, ZYBAN
Mirtazapine REMERON
Nefazodone
Trazodone DESYREL
Vilazodone VIIBRYD
Vortioxetine BRINTELLIX

TRICYCLIC ANTIDEPRESSANTS (TCAs)
Amitriptyline
Amoxapine
Clomipramine ANAFRANIL
Desipramine NORPRAMIN
Doxepin SINEQUAN
Imipramine TOFRANIL
Maprotiline LUDIOMIL
Nortriptyline PAMELOR
Protriptyline VIVACTIL
Trimipramine SURMONTIL

MONOAMINE OXIDASE INHIBITORS (MAOIs)
Isocarboxazid MARPLAN
Phenelzine NARDIL
Selegiline EMSAM
Tranylcypromine PARNATE

Figure 10.1
Summary of antidepressants.

**DRUGS USED TO TREAT MANIA
and BIPOLAR DISORDER**

Carbamazepine TEGRETOL, EQUETRO, CARBATROL

Lamotrigine LAMICTAL

Lithium

Valproic acid DEPAKENE, DEPAKOTE

Figure 10.1 (Continued)

DRUG	UPTAKE INHIBITION	
	Nor-epinephrine	Serotonin
Selective serotonin reuptake inhibitor		
Fluoxetine	0	++++
Selective serotonin/ norepinephrine reuptake inhibitors		
Venlafaxine	++*	++++
Duloxetine	++++	++++
Tricyclic antidepressants		
Imipramine	++++	+++
Nortriptyline	++++	++

Figure 10.2
Relative receptor specificity of some antidepressant drugs. *Venlafaxine* inhibits norepinephrine reuptake only at high doses. ++++ = very strong affinity; +++ = strong affinity; ++ = moderate affinity; + = weak affinity; 0 = little or no affinity.

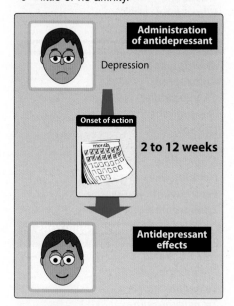

Figure 10.3
Onset of therapeutic effects of the major antidepressant drugs requires several weeks.

---

the SSRIs. Because they have different adverse effects and are relatively safe even in overdose, the SSRIs have largely replaced TCAs and monoamine oxidase inhibitors (MAOIs) as the drugs of choice in treating depression. The SSRIs include *fluoxetine* [floo-OX-e-teen] (the prototypic drug), *citalopram* [sye-TAL-oh-pram], *escitalopram* [es-sye-TAL-oh-pram], *fluvoxamine* [floo-VOX-e-meen], *paroxetine* [pa-ROX-e-teen], and *sertraline* [SER-tra-leen]. *Escitalopram* is the pure S-enantiomer of *citalopram*.

A. Actions

The SSRIs block the reuptake of serotonin, leading to increased concentrations of the neurotransmitter in the synaptic cleft. Antidepressants, including SSRIs, typically take at least 2 weeks to produce significant improvement in mood, and maximum benefit may require up to 12 weeks or more (Figure 10.3). Patients who do not respond to one antidepressant may respond to another, and approximately 80% or more will respond to at least one antidepressant drug.

B. Therapeutic uses

The primary indication for SSRIs is depression, for which they are as effective as the TCAs. A number of other psychiatric disorders also respond favorably to SSRIs, including obsessive–compulsive disorder, panic disorder, generalized anxiety disorder, posttraumatic stress disorder, social anxiety disorder, premenstrual dysphoric disorder, and bulimia nervosa (only *fluoxetine* is approved for bulimia).

C. Pharmacokinetics

All of the SSRIs are well absorbed after oral administration. Peak levels are seen in approximately 2 to 8 hours on average. Food has little effect on absorption (except with *sertraline*, for which food increases its absorption). The majority of SSRIs have plasma half-lives that range between 16 and 36 hours. Metabolism by cytochrome P450 (CYP450)–dependent enzymes and glucuronide or sulfate conjugation occur extensively. *Fluoxetine* differs from the other members of the class by having a much longer half-life (50 hours), and the half-life of its active metabolite *S*-norfluoxetine is quite long, averaging 10 days. It is available as a sustained-release preparation allowing once-weekly dosing. *Fluoxetine* and *paroxetine* are potent inhibitors of a CYP450 isoenzyme (CYP2D6) responsible for the elimination of TCAs, antipsychotic drugs, and some antiarrhythmic and β-adrenergic antagonist drugs. Other CYP450 isoenzymes (CYP2C9/19, CYP3A4, CYP1A2) are involved with SSRI metabolism and may also be inhibited to various degrees by the SSRIs. Dosages of the SSRIs should be reduced in patients with hepatic impairment.

D. Adverse effects

Although the SSRIs are considered to have fewer and less severe adverse effects than the TCAs and MAOIs, the SSRIs are not without adverse effects, such as headache, sweating, anxiety and agitation, gastrointestinal (GI) effects (nausea, vomiting, diarrhea), weakness and fatigue, sexual dysfunction, changes in weight, sleep disturbances (insomnia and somnolence), and the above-mentioned potential for drug–drug interactions (Figure 10.4). Additionally, SSRIs have been associated with hyponatremia, especially in the elderly and patients who are volume depleted or taking diuretics.

1. **Sleep disturbances:** *Paroxetine* and *fluvoxamine* are generally more sedating than activating, and they may be useful in patients who have difficulty sleeping. Conversely, patients who are fatigued or complaining of excessive somnolence may benefit from one of the more activating SSRIs, such as *fluoxetine* or *sertraline.*

2. **Sexual dysfunction:** Sexual dysfunction, which may include loss of libido, delayed ejaculation, and anorgasmia, is common with the SSRIs. One option for managing SSRI-induced sexual dysfunction is to change the antidepressant to one with fewer sexual side effects, such as *bupropion* or *mirtazapine.* Alternatively, the dose of the drug may be reduced.

3. **Use in children and teenagers:** Antidepressants should be used cautiously in children and teenagers, because about 1 out of 50 children report suicidal ideation as a result of SSRI treatment. Pediatric patients should be observed for worsening depression and suicidal thinking with initiation or dosage change of any antidepressant. *Fluoxetine, sertraline,* and *fluvoxamine* are approved for use in children to treat obsessive–compulsive disorder, and *fluoxetine* and *escitalopram* are approved to treat childhood depression.

4. **Overdose:** Overdose with SSRIs does not usually cause cardiac arrhythmias, with the exception of *citalopram*, which may cause QT prolongation. [Note: The TCAs have a significant risk for arrhythmias in overdose.] Seizures are a possibility because all antidepressants may lower the seizure threshold. All SSRIs have the potential to cause serotonin syndrome, especially when used in the presence of a MAOI or other highly serotonergic drug. Serotonin syndrome may include the symptoms of hyperthermia, muscle rigidity, sweating, myoclonus (clonic muscle twitching), and changes in mental status and vital signs.

5. **Discontinuation syndrome:** All of the SSRIs have the potential to cause a discontinuation syndrome after their abrupt withdrawal, particularly the agents with shorter half-lives and inactive metabolites. *Fluoxetine* has the lowest risk of causing an SSRI discontinuation syndrome due to its longer half-life and active metabolite. Possible signs and symptoms of SSRI discontinuation syndrome include headache, malaise, and flu-like symptoms, agitation and irritability, nervousness, and changes in sleep pattern.

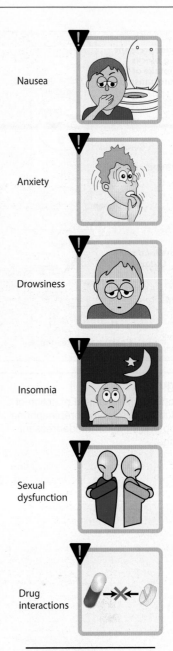

Nausea

Anxiety

Drowsiness

Insomnia

Sexual dysfunction

Drug interactions

Figure 10.4
Some commonly observed adverse effects of selective serotonin reuptake inhibitors.

IV. SEROTONIN/NOREPINEPHRINE REUPTAKE INHIBITORS

Venlafaxine [VEN-la-fax-een], *desvenlafaxine* [dez-VEN-la-fax-een], *levomilnacipran* [leevo-mil-NA-si-pran], and *duloxetine* [doo-LOX-e-teen] inhibit the reuptake of both serotonin and norepinephrine (Figure 10.5). These agents, termed SNRIs, may be effective in treating depression in patients in whom SSRIs are ineffective. Furthermore, depression is often accompanied by chronic painful symptoms, such as backache and muscle aches, against which SSRIs are also relatively ineffective. This

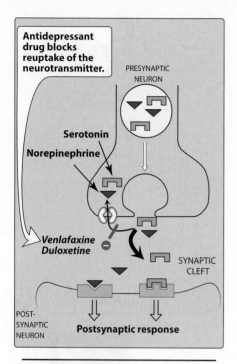

Figure 10.5
Proposed mechanism of action of selective serotonin/norepinephrine reuptake inhibitor antidepressant drugs.

pain is, in part, modulated by serotonin and norepinephrine pathways in the central nervous system (CNS). Both SNRIs and the TCAs, with their dual inhibition of both serotonin and norepinephrine reuptake, are sometimes effective in relieving pain associated with diabetic peripheral neuropathy, postherpetic neuralgia, fibromyalgia, and low back pain. The SNRIs, unlike the TCAs, have little activity at α-adrenergic, muscarinic, or histamine receptors and, thus, have fewer of these receptor-mediated adverse effects than the TCAs. The SNRIs may precipitate a discontinuation syndrome if treatment is abruptly stopped.

A. Venlafaxine and desvenlafaxine

Venlafaxine is a potent inhibitor of serotonin reuptake and, at medium to higher doses, is an inhibitor of norepinephrine reuptake. *Venlafaxine* has minimal inhibition of the CYP450 isoenzymes and is a substrate of the CYP2D6 isoenzyme. *Desvenlafaxine* is the active, demethylated metabolite of *venlafaxine*. The most common side effects of *venlafaxine* are nausea, headache, sexual dysfunction, dizziness, insomnia, sedation, and constipation. At high doses, there may be an increase in blood pressure and heart rate. The clinical activity and adverse effect profile of *desvenlafaxine* are similar to that of *venlafaxine.*

B. Duloxetine

Duloxetine inhibits serotonin and norepinephrine reuptake at all doses. It is extensively metabolized in the liver to inactive metabolites and should be avoided in patients with liver dysfunction. GI side effects are common with *duloxetine*, including nausea, dry mouth, and constipation. Insomnia, dizziness, somnolence, sweating, and sexual dysfunction are also seen. *Duloxetine* may increase blood pressure or heart rate. *Duloxetine* is a moderate inhibitor of CYP2D6 isoenzymes and may increase concentrations of drugs metabolized by this pathway, such as antipsychotics.

C. Levomilnacipran

Levomilnacipran is an enantiomer of *milnacipran* (an older SNRI used for the treatment of depression in Europe and fibromyalgia in the United States). The adverse effect profile of *levomilnacipran* is similar to other SNRIs. It is primarily metabolized by CYP3A4, and, thus, activity may be altered by inducers or inhibitors of this enzyme system.

V. ATYPICAL ANTIDEPRESSANTS

The atypical antidepressants are a mixed group of agents that have actions at several different sites. This group includes *bupropion* [byoo-PROE-pee-on], *mirtazapine* [mir-TAZ-a-peen], *nefazodone* [ne-FAZ-oh-done], *trazodone* [TRAZ-oh-done], *vilazodone* [vil-AZ-oh-done], and *vortioxetine* [vor-TEE-ox-e-teen].

A. Bupropion

Bupropion is a weak dopamine and norepinephrine reuptake inhibitor that is used to alleviate the symptoms of depression. *Bupropion* is also useful for decreasing cravings and attenuating withdrawal symptoms of nicotine in patients trying to quit smoking. Side effects may include dry mouth, sweating, nervousness, tremor, and a dose-dependent increased risk for seizures. It has a very low incidence of sexual dysfunction. *Bupropion* is metabolized by the CYP2B6 pathway and has a relatively low risk for drug–drug interactions, given the few agents that inhibit/induce this enzyme. However, *bupropion* may inhibit CYP2D6 and, thus, increase exposure to substrates of this isoenzyme. Use of *bupropion* should be avoided in patients at risk for seizures or those who have eating disorders such as bulimia.

B. Mirtazapine

Mirtazapine enhances serotonin and norepinephrine neurotransmission by serving as an antagonist at presynaptic α_2 receptors. Additionally, some of the antidepressant activity may be related to antagonism at 5-HT$_2$ receptors. It is sedating because of its potent antihistaminic activity, but it does not cause the antimuscarinic side effects of the TCAs, or interfere with sexual function like the SSRIs. Increased appetite and weight gain frequently occur (Figure 10.6). *Mirtazapine* is markedly sedating, which may be an advantage in depressed patients having difficulty sleeping.

C. Nefazodone and trazodone

These drugs are weak inhibitors of serotonin reuptake. Their therapeutic benefit appears to be related to their ability to block postsynaptic 5-HT$_{2a}$ receptors. Both agents are sedating, probably because of their potent histamine H$_1$-blocking activity. *Trazodone* is commonly used off-label for the management of insomnia. *Trazodone* has been associated with priapism, and *nefazodone* has been associated with a risk for hepatotoxicity. Both agents also have mild to moderate α_1 receptor antagonism, contributing to orthostasis and dizziness.

D. Vilazodone

Vilazodone is a serotonin reuptake inhibitor and a 5-HT$_{1a}$ partial agonist. Although the extent to which the 5-HT$_{1a}$ receptor activity contributes to its therapeutic effects is unknown, this possible mechanism of action renders it unique from that of the SSRIs. The adverse effect profile of *vilazodone* is similar to the SSRIs, including a risk for discontinuation syndrome if abruptly stopped.

E. Vortioxetine

Vortioxetine utilizes a combination of serotonin reuptake inhibition, 5-HT$_{1a}$ agonism, and 5-HT$_3$ and 5-HT$_7$ antagonism as its suggested mechanisms of action to treat depression. It is unclear to what extent the activities other than inhibition of serotonin reuptake influence the overall effects of *vortioxetine*. The common adverse effects include nausea, vomiting, and constipation, which may be expected due to its serotonergic mechanisms.

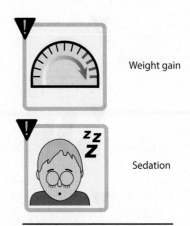

Weight gain

Sedation

Figure 10.6
Some commonly observed adverse effects of *mirtazapine*.

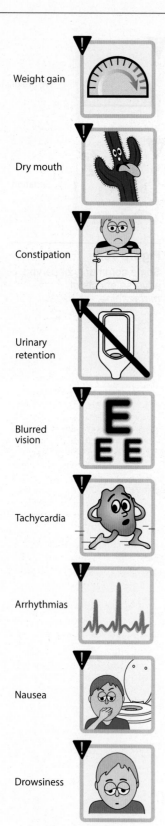

Weight gain

Dry mouth

Constipation

Urinary retention

Blurred vision

Tachycardia

Arrhythmias

Nausea

Drowsiness

Figure 10.7
Some commonly observed adverse effects of tricyclic antidepressants.

VI. TRICYCLIC ANTIDEPRESSANTS

The TCAs block norepinephrine and serotonin reuptake into the presynaptic neuron and, thus, if discovered today, might have been referred to as SNRIs, except for their differences in adverse effects relative to this newer class of antidepressants. The TCAs include the tertiary amines *imipramine* [ee-MIP-ra-meen] (the prototype drug), *amitriptyline* [a-mee-TRIP-ti-leen], *clomipramine* [kloe-MIP-ra-meen], *doxepin* [DOX-e-pin], and *trimipramine* [trye-MIP-ra-meen], and the secondary amines *desipramine* [dess-IP-ra-meen] and *nortriptyline* [nor-TRIP-ti-leen] (the *N*-demethylated metabolites of *imipramine* and *amitriptyline*, respectively) and *protriptyline* [proe-TRIP-ti-leen]. *Maprotiline* [ma-PROE-ti-leen] and *amoxapine* [a-MOX-a-peen] are related "tetracyclic" antidepressant agents and are commonly included in the general class of TCAs. Patients who do not respond to one TCA may benefit from a different drug in this group.

A. Mechanism of action

1. **Inhibition of neurotransmitter reuptake:** TCAs and *amoxapine* are potent inhibitors of the neuronal reuptake of norepinephrine and serotonin into presynaptic nerve terminals. *Maprotiline* and *desipramine* are relatively selective inhibitors of norepinephrine reuptake.

2. **Blocking of receptors:** TCAs also block serotonergic, α-adrenergic, histaminic, and muscarinic receptors. It is not known if any of these actions produce the therapeutic benefit of the TCAs. However, actions at these receptors are likely responsible for many of their adverse effects. *Amoxapine* also blocks 5-HT$_2$ and dopamine D$_2$ receptors.

B. Actions

The TCAs elevate mood, improve mental alertness, increase physical activity, and reduce morbid preoccupation in 50% to 70% of individuals with major depression. The onset of the mood elevation is slow, requiring 2 weeks or longer (Figure 10.3). Patient response can be used to adjust dosage. After a therapeutic response, the dosage can be gradually reduced to improve tolerability, unless relapse occurs. Physical and psychological dependence have been rarely reported. This necessitates slow withdrawal to minimize discontinuation syndromes and cholinergic rebound effects.

C. Therapeutic uses

The TCAs are effective in treating moderate to severe depression. Some patients with panic disorder also respond to TCAs. *Imipramine* has been used to control bed-wetting in children older than 6 years of age; however, it has largely been replaced by *desmopressin* and nonpharmacologic treatments (enuresis alarms). The TCAs, particularly *amitriptyline*, have been used to help prevent migraine headache and treat chronic pain syndromes (for example, neuropathic pain) in a number of conditions for which the cause of pain is unclear. Low doses of TCAs, especially *doxepin*, can be used to treat insomnia.

D. Pharmacokinetics

TCAs are well absorbed upon oral administration. Because of their lipophilic nature, they are widely distributed and readily penetrate into the CNS. As a result of their variable first-pass metabolism in the liver, TCAs have low and inconsistent bioavailability. These drugs are metabolized by the hepatic microsomal system (and, thus, may be sensitive to agents that induce or inhibit the CYP450 isoenzymes) and conjugated with glucuronic acid. Ultimately, the TCAs are excreted as inactive metabolites via the kidney.

E. Adverse effects

Blockade of muscarinic receptors leads to blurred vision, xerostomia (dry mouth), urinary retention, sinus tachycardia, constipation, and aggravation of angle-closure glaucoma (Figure 10.7). These agents affect cardiac conduction similarly to *quinidine* and may precipitate life-threatening arrhythmias in an overdose situation. The TCAs also block α-adrenergic receptors, causing orthostatic hypotension, dizziness, and reflex tachycardia. *Imipramine* is the most likely, and *nortriptyline* the least likely, to cause orthostatic hypotension. Sedation may be prominent, especially during the first several weeks of treatment, and is related to the ability of these drugs to block histamine H_1 receptors. Weight gain is a common adverse effect of the TCAs. Sexual dysfunction occurs in a minority of patients, and the incidence is lower than that associated with the SSRIs.

TCAs (like all antidepressants) should be used with caution in patients with bipolar disorder, even during their depressed state, because antidepressants may cause a switch to manic behavior. The TCAs have a narrow therapeutic index (for example, five- to sixfold the maximal daily dose of *imipramine* can be lethal). Depressed patients who are suicidal should be given only limited quantities of these drugs and be monitored closely. Drug interactions with the TCAs are shown in Figure 10.8. The TCAs may exacerbate certain medical conditions, such as benign prostatic hyperplasia, epilepsy, and preexisting arrhythmias.

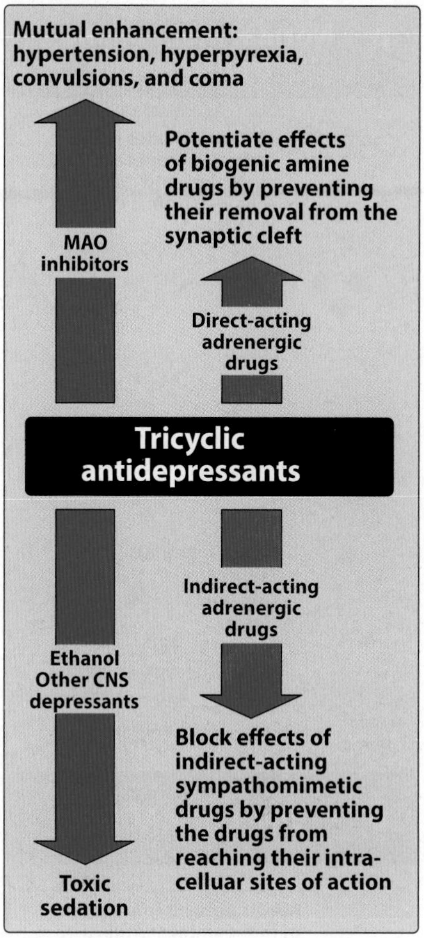

Figure 10.8
Drugs interacting with tricyclic antidepressants. CNS = central nervous system; MAO = monoamine oxidase.

VII. MONOAMINE OXIDASE INHIBITORS

Monoamine oxidase (MAO) is a mitochondrial enzyme found in nerve and other tissues, such as the gut and liver. In the neuron, MAO functions as a "safety valve" to oxidatively deaminate and inactivate any excess neurotransmitters (for example, norepinephrine, dopamine, and serotonin) that may leak out of synaptic vesicles when the neuron is at rest. The MAOIs may irreversibly or reversibly inactivate the enzyme, permitting neurotransmitters to escape degradation and, therefore, to accumulate within the presynaptic neuron and leak into the synaptic space. The four MAOIs currently available for treatment of depression include *phenelzine* [FEN-el-zeen], *tranylcypromine* [tran-il-SIP-roe-meen], *isocarboxazid* [eye-soe-car-BOX-ih-zid], and *selegiline* [seh-LEDGE-ah-leen]. [Note: *Selegiline* is also used for the treatment of Parkinson's disease. It is the only antidepressant available in a transdermal delivery system.] Use of MAOIs is limited due to the complicated dietary restrictions required while taking these agents.

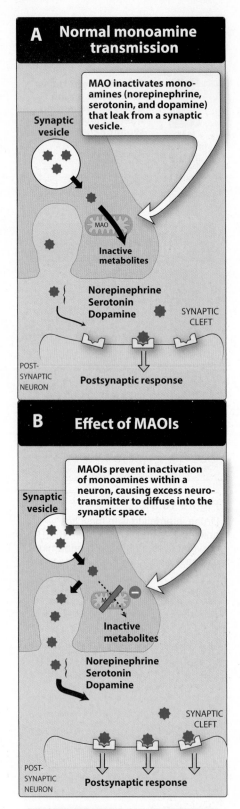

A **Normal monoamine transmission**

MAO inactivates monoamines (norepinephrine, serotonin, and dopamine) that leak from a synaptic vesicle.

Synaptic vesicle

MAO

Inactive metabolites

Norepinephrine
Serotonin
Dopamine

SYNAPTIC CLEFT

POST-SYNAPTIC NEURON

Postsynaptic response

B **Effect of MAOIs**

MAOIs prevent inactivation of monoamines within a neuron, causing excess neurotransmitter to diffuse into the synaptic space.

Synaptic vesicle

MAO

Inactive metabolites

Norepinephrine
Serotonin
Dopamine

SYNAPTIC CLEFT

POST-SYNAPTIC NEURON

Postsynaptic response

Figure 10.9
Mechanism of action of monoamine oxidase inhibitors (MAOIs).

A. Mechanism of action

Most MAOIs, such as *phenelzine,* form stable complexes with the enzyme, causing irreversible inactivation. This results in increased stores of norepinephrine, serotonin, and dopamine within the neuron and subsequent diffusion of excess neurotransmitter into the synaptic space (Figure 10.9). These drugs inhibit not only MAO in the brain but also MAO in the liver and gut that catalyzes oxidative deamination of drugs and potentially toxic substances, such as tyramine, which is found in certain foods. The MAOIs, therefore, show a high incidence of drug–drug and drug–food interactions. *Selegiline* administered as the transdermal patch may produce less inhibition of gut and hepatic MAO at low doses because it avoids first-pass metabolism.

B. Actions

Although MAO is fully inhibited after several days of treatment, the antidepressant action of the MAOIs, like that of the SSRIs, SNRIs, and TCAs, is delayed several weeks. *Selegiline* and *tranylcypromine* have an amphetamine-like stimulant effect that may produce agitation or insomnia.

C. Therapeutic uses

The MAOIs are indicated for depressed patients who are unresponsive or allergic to TCAs and SSRIs or who experience strong anxiety. A special subcategory of depression, called atypical depression, may respond preferentially to MAOIs. Because of their risk for drug–drug and drug–food interactions, the MAOIs are considered last-line agents in many treatment settings.

D. Pharmacokinetics

These drugs are well absorbed after oral administration. Enzyme regeneration, when irreversibly inactivated, varies, but it usually occurs several weeks after termination of the drug. Thus, when switching antidepressant agents, a minimum of 2 weeks of delay must be allowed after termination of MAOI therapy and the initiation of another antidepressant from any other class. MAOIs are hepatically metabolized and excreted rapidly in urine.

E. Adverse effects

Severe and often unpredictable side effects, due to drug–food and drug–drug interactions, limit the widespread use of MAOIs. For example, tyramine, which is contained in foods, such as aged cheeses and meats, chicken liver, pickled or smoked fish, and red wines, is normally inactivated by MAO in the gut. Individuals receiving a MAOI are unable to degrade tyramine obtained from the diet. Tyramine causes the release of large amounts of stored catecholamines from nerve terminals, resulting in a hypertensive crisis, with signs and symptoms such as occipital headache, stiff neck, tachycardia, nausea, hypertension, cardiac arrhythmias, seizures, and, possibly, stroke. Patients must, therefore, be educated to avoid tyramine-containing foods. *Phentolamine* and *prazosin* are helpful in the management of tyramine-induced hypertension. Other possible side effects of treatment with MAOIs include drowsiness, orthostatic hypotension, blurred vision, dry mouth, and constipation. Due to the risk of serotonin syndrome, the use of MAOIs with other antidepressants is contraindicated. For example, SSRIs should not be coadministered with MAOIs. Both SSRIs and MAOIs require a washout period of at least 2 weeks before the other type is administered, with the exception of *fluoxetine*, which should be discontinued at least 6 weeks before a MAOI is initiated. In addition, the MAOIs have many other critical drug interactions, and caution is required when administering these agents concurrently with other drugs. Figure 10.10 summarizes the side effects of the antidepressant drugs.

VIII. TREATMENT OF MANIA AND BIPOLAR DISORDER

The treatment of bipolar disorder has increased in recent years, due to increased recognition of the disorder and also an increase in the number of available medications for the treatment of mania.

A. Lithium

Lithium salts are used acutely and prophylactically for managing bipolar patients. *Lithium* is effective in treating 60% to 80% of patients exhibiting mania and hypomania. Although many cellular processes are altered by treatment with *lithium salts*, the mode of action is unknown. The therapeutic index of *lithium* is extremely low, and *lithium salts* can be toxic. Common adverse effects may include headache, dry mouth, polydipsia, polyuria, polyphagia, GI distress (give *lithium* with food), fine hand tremor, dizziness, fatigue, dermatologic reactions, and sedation. Adverse effects due to higher plasma levels may indicate toxicity and include ataxia, slurred speech, coarse tremors, confusion, and convulsions. Thyroid function may be decreased and should be monitored. Unlike other mood stabilizers, *lithium* is renally eliminated, and though caution should be used when dosing this drug in renally impaired patients, it may be the best choice in patients with hepatic impairment.

B. Other drugs

Several antiepileptic drugs, including *carbamazepine, valproic acid,* and *lamotrigine*, have been approved as mood stabilizers for bipolar disorder. Other agents that may improve manic symptoms include the older (*chlorpromazine and haloperidol*) and newer antipsychotics. The atypical antipsychotics *risperidone, olanzapine, ziprasidone, aripiprazole, asenapine,* and *quetiapine* (see Chapter 11) are also used for the management of mania. *Quetiapine, lurasidone,* and the combination of *olanzapine* and *fluoxetine* have been approved for bipolar depression.

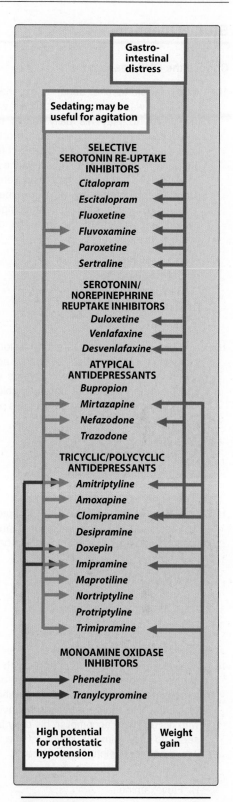

Figure 10.10
Side effects of some drugs used to treat depression.

Study Questions

Choose the ONE best answer.

10.1 A 55-year-old teacher began to experience changes in mood. He was losing interest in his work and lacked the desire to play his daily tennis match. He was preoccupied with feelings of guilt, worthlessness, and hopelessness. In addition to the psychiatric symptoms, the patient complained of muscle aches throughout his body. Physical and laboratory tests were unremarkable. After 6 weeks of therapy with fluoxetine, his symptoms resolved. However, the patient complains of sexual dysfunction. Which of the following drugs might be useful in this patient?

A. Fluvoxamine.
B. Sertraline.
C. Citalopram.
D. Mirtazapine.
E. Lithium.

Correct answer = D. Mirtazapine is largely free from sexual side effects. However, sexual dysfunction commonly occurs with SSRIs (fluvoxamine, sertraline, and citalopram), as well as with TCAs, and SNRIs. Lithium is used for the treatment of mania and bipolar disorder.

10.2 A 25-year-old woman has a long history of depressive symptoms accompanied by body aches and pain secondary to a car accident 2 years earlier. Physical and laboratory tests are unremarkable. Which of the following drugs might be useful in this patient?

A. Fluoxetine.
B. Sertraline.
C. Phenelzine.
D. Mirtazapine.
E. Duloxetine.

Correct answer = E. Duloxetine is a SNRI that can be used for depression accompanied by symptoms of pain. SSRIs (fluoxetine and sertraline), MAOIs (phenelzine), and atypical antidepressants (mirtazapine) have little activity against pain syndromes.

10.3 A 51-year-old woman with symptoms of major depression also has angle-closure glaucoma. Which of the following antidepressants should be avoided in this patient?

A. Amitriptyline.
B. Sertraline.
C. Bupropion.
D. Mirtazapine.
E. Fluvoxamine.

Correct answer = A. Because of its potent antimuscarinic activity, amitriptyline should not be given to patients with glaucoma because of the risk of acute increases in intraocular pressure. The other antidepressants all lack antagonist activity at the muscarinic receptor.

10.4 A 36-year-old man presents with symptoms of compulsive behavior. If anything is out of order, he feels that "work will not be accomplished effectively or efficiently." He realizes that his behavior is interfering with his ability to accomplish his daily tasks but cannot seem to stop himself. Which of the following drugs would be most helpful to this patient?

A. Imipramine.
B. Fluvoxamine.
C. Amitriptyline.
D. Tranylcypromine.
E. Lithium.

Correct answer = B. SSRIs are particularly effective in treating obsessive–compulsive disorder, and fluvoxamine is approved for this condition. The other drugs are less effective in the treatment of obsessive–compulsive disorder.

10.5 Which antidepressant has, as its two proposed principle mechanisms of action, 5-HT$_{1a}$ receptor partial agonism and 5-HT reuptake inhibition?

A. Fluoxetine.

B. Aripiprazole.

C. Maprotiline.

D. Vilazodone.

E. Mirtazapine.

Correct answer = D. In addition to inhibition of serotonin reuptake, the antidepressant activity of vilazodone may be related to its 5-HT$_{1a}$ receptor agonism. Though aripiprazole is also proposed to have 5-HT$_{1a}$ partial agonism, it is not a serotonin reuptake inhibitor.

10.6 Which antidepressant is the most sedating?

A. Fluoxetine.

B. Duloxetine.

C. Nortriptyline.

D. Citalopram.

E. Venlafaxine.

Correct answer = C. Nortriptyline is the most sedating of the list due to its histamine-blocking activity. (See Figure 10.10.)

10.7 Which mood stabilizer is completely renally eliminated and may be beneficial for patients with hepatic impairment?

A. Valproic acid.

B. Carbamazepine.

C. Lithium.

D. Risperidone.

E. Aripiprazole.

Correct answer = C. Lithium is the only agent for bipolar disorder that does not require hepatic metabolism and, thus, may be dosed without issue in a hepatically impaired patient. However, if the patient had renal impairment, the lithium dosage would have to be adjusted.

10.8 Which antidepressant has, as its two principle mechanisms of action, 5-HT$_{2A}$ receptor antagonism and α_2 receptor antagonism?

A. Fluoxetine.

B. Doxepin.

C. Maprotiline.

D. Mirtazapine.

E. Selegiline.

Correct answer = D. Mirtazapine is the only antidepressant with this combination of mechanisms of action that are believed to contribute to its therapeutic effects. The other agents listed are reuptake inhibitors of either serotonin (fluoxetine) or norepinephrine (maprotiline), or both (doxepin), or act as a MAOI (selegiline).

10.9 Which agent is *best known* to have the side effect of decreasing the thyroid function of the patient being chronically treated with this agent?

A. Carbamazepine.

B. Lithium.

C. Valproic acid.

D. Chlorpromazine.

E. Lurasidone.

Correct answer = B. Lithium is best known for causing a drug-induced hypothyroidism in patients after long-term use. Though it is possible with other mood stabilizers, lithium has the most reported cases, and thus, thyroid function tests should be performed at baseline and during follow-up to monitor for this possible effect. Also, since hypothyroidism may present with symptoms of depression, it is important to differentiate a patient's observed depressive symptoms from the psychopathology of the bipolar disorder or depression versus symptoms of hypothyroidism.

10.10 Which agent would be a poor choice in a 70-year-old elderly female with depressive symptoms due to the drug having significant α_1 receptor antagonism and thus a higher risk for falls due to orthostatic hypotension?

A. Lithium.

B. Bupropion.

C. Escitalopram.

D. Imipramine.

E. Sertraline.

Correct answer = D. Lithium should not be used for depression in an elderly patient without first trying first-line antidepressants, and even then, it is used as an adjunct. Bupropion, sertraline, and escitalopram have very little effect on blood pressure (no α_1 receptor antagonism) and are considered acceptable choices for the treatment of depression in the elderly. Imipramine is associated with a high risk for orthostasis in the elderly and should be avoided due to its adverse effect profile and risk for falls.

Antipsychotic Drugs

11

Jose A. Rey

I. OVERVIEW

The antipsychotic drugs (also called neuroleptics or major tranquilizers) are used primarily to treat schizophrenia, but they are also effective in other psychotic and manic states. The use of antipsychotic medications involves a difficult trade-off between the benefit of alleviating psychotic symptoms and the risk of a wide variety of troubling adverse effects. Antipsychotic drugs (Figure 11.1) are not curative and do not eliminate chronic thought disorders, but they often decrease the intensity of hallucinations and delusions and permit the person with schizophrenia to function in a supportive environment.

II. SCHIZOPHRENIA

Schizophrenia is a type of chronic psychosis characterized by delusions, hallucinations (often in the form of voices), and thinking or speech disturbances. The onset of illness is often during late adolescence or early adulthood. It occurs in about 1% of the population and is a chronic and disabling disorder. Schizophrenia has a strong genetic component and probably reflects some fundamental biochemical abnormality, possibly a dysfunction of the mesolimbic or mesocortical dopaminergic neuronal pathways.

III. ANTIPSYCHOTIC DRUGS

The antipsychotic drugs are divided into first- and second-generation agents. The first-generation drugs are further classified as "low potency" or "high potency." This classification does not indicate clinical effectiveness of the drugs, but rather specifies affinity for the dopamine D_2 receptor, which, in turn, may influence the adverse effect profile of the drug.

A. First-generation antipsychotics

The first-generation antipsychotic drugs (also called conventional, typical, or traditional antipsychotics) are competitive inhibitors at a variety of receptors, but their antipsychotic effects reflect competitive blocking of dopamine D_2 receptors. First-generation antipsychotics are more likely to be associated with movement disorders known as extrapyramidal symptoms (EPS), particularly drugs that bind tightly to dopaminergic neuroreceptors, such as *haloperidol* [HAL-oh-PER-i-dol].

FIRST-GENERATION ANTIPSYCHOTIC (low potency)
Chlorpromazine THORAZINE
Thioridazine

FIRST-GENERATION ANTIPSYCHOTIC (high potency)
Fluphenazine PROLIXIN
Haloperidol HALDOL
Loxapine LOXITANE
Perphenazine
Pimozide ORAP
Prochlorperazine COMPAZINE
Thiothixene NAVANE
Trifluoperazine STELAZINE

SECOND-GENERATION ANTIPSYCHOTIC
Aripiprazole ABILIFY
Asenapine SAPHRIS
Clozapine CLOZARIL
Iloperidone FANAPT
Lurasidone LATUDA
Olanzapine ZYPREXA
Paliperidone INVEGA
Quetiapine SEROQUEL
Risperidone RISPERDAL
Ziprasidone GEODON

Figure 11.1
Summary of antipsychotic agents.

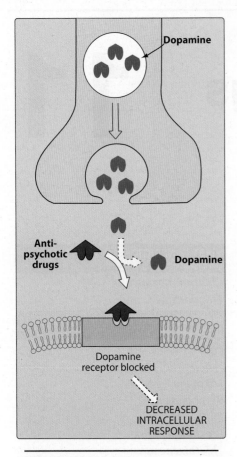

Figure 11.2
Dopamine-blocking actions of
antipsychotic drugs.

Movement disorders are less likely with medications that bind weakly, such as *chlorpromazine* [klor-PROE-ma-zeen]. No one drug is clinically more effective than another.

B. Second-generation antipsychotic drugs

The second-generation antipsychotic drugs (also called "atypical" antipsychotics) have a lower incidence of EPS than the first-generation agents but are associated with a higher risk of metabolic side effects, such as diabetes, hypercholesterolemia, and weight gain. The second-generation drugs appear to owe their unique activity to blockade of both serotonin and dopamine and, perhaps, other receptors.

1. **Drug selection:** Second-generation agents are generally used as first-line therapy for schizophrenia to minimize the risk of debilitating EPS associated with the first-generation drugs that act primarily at the dopamine D_2 receptor. The second-generation antipsychotics exhibit an efficacy that is equivalent to, and occasionally exceeds, that of the first-generation antipsychotic agents. However, consistent differences in therapeutic efficacy among the second-generation drugs have not been established, and individual patient response and comorbid conditions must often be used to guide drug selection.

2. **Refractory patients:** Approximately 10% to 20% of patients with schizophrenia have an insufficient response to all first- and second-generation antipsychotics. For these patients, *clozapine* [KLOE-za-peen] has shown to be an effective antipsychotic with a minimal risk of EPS. However, its clinical use is limited to refractory patients because of serious adverse effects. *Clozapine* can produce bone marrow suppression, seizures, and cardiovascular side effects, such as orthostasis. The risk of severe agranulocytosis necessitates frequent monitoring of white blood cell counts.

C. Mechanism of action

1. **Dopamine antagonism:** All of the first-generation and most of the second-generation antipsychotic drugs block D_2 dopamine receptors in the brain and the periphery (Figure 11.2).

2. **Serotonin receptor–blocking activity:** Most of the second-generation agents appear to exert part of their unique action through inhibition of serotonin receptors (5-HT), particularly 5-HT_{2A} receptors. *Clozapine* has high affinity for D_1, D_4, 5-HT_2, muscarinic, and α-adrenergic receptors, but it is also a weak dopamine D_2 receptor antagonist (Figure 11.3). *Risperidone* [ris-PEAR-ih-dohn] blocks 5-HT_{2A} receptors to a greater extent than it does D_2 receptors, as does *olanzapine* [oh-LANZ-ah-peen]. The second-generation antipsychotic *aripiprazole* [a-rih-PIP-ra-zole] is a partial agonist at D_2 and 5-HT_{1A} receptors, as well as an antagonist of 5-HT_{2A} receptors. *Quetiapine* [qwe-TY-uh-peen] blocks D_2 receptors more potently than 5-HT_{2A} receptors but is relatively weak at blocking either receptor. Its low risk for EPS may also be related to the relatively short period of time it binds to the D_2 receptor.

D. Actions

The clinical effects of antipsychotic drugs appear to reflect a blockade at dopamine and/or serotonin receptors. However, many of these agents also block cholinergic, adrenergic, and histaminergic receptors (Figure 11.4). It is unknown what role, if any, these actions have in alleviating the symptoms of psychosis. However, the undesirable side effects of antipsychotic drugs often result from pharmacological actions at these other receptors.

1. **Antipsychotic effects:** All antipsychotic drugs can reduce hallucinations and delusions associated with schizophrenia (known as "positive" symptoms) by blocking D_2 receptors in the mesolimbic system of the brain. The "negative" symptoms, such as blunted affect, apathy, and impaired attention, as well as cognitive impairment, are not as responsive to therapy, particularly with the first-generation antipsychotics. Many second-generation agents, such as *clozapine*, can ameliorate the negative symptoms to some extent.

2. **Extrapyramidal effects:** Dystonias (sustained contraction of muscles leading to twisting, distorted postures), Parkinson-like symptoms, akathisia (motor restlessness), and tardive dyskinesia (involuntary movements, usually of the tongue, lips, neck, trunk, and limbs) can occur with both acute and chronic treatment. Blockade of dopamine receptors in the nigrostriatal pathway probably causes these unwanted movement symptoms. The second-generation antipsychotics exhibit a lower incidence of EPS.

3. **Antiemetic effects:** With the exception of *aripiprazole*, most of the antipsychotic drugs have antiemetic effects that are mediated by blocking D_2 receptors of the chemoreceptor trigger zone of the medulla (see Chapter 31). Figure 11.5 summarizes the antiemetic uses of antipsychotic agents, as well as other drugs that combat nausea.

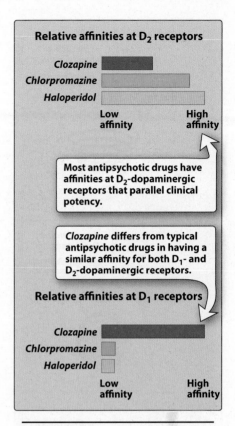

Most antipsychotic drugs have affinities at D_2-dopaminergic receptors that parallel clinical potency.

Clozapine differs from typical antipsychotic drugs in having a similar affinity for both D_1- and D_2-dopaminergic receptors.

Figure 11.3
Relative affinity of *clozapine, chlorpromazine*, and *haloperidol* at D_1 and D_2 dopaminergic receptors.

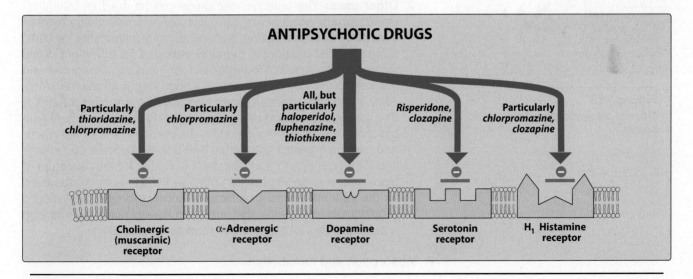

Figure 11.4
Antipsychotic drugs block at dopaminergic and serotonergic receptors as well as at adrenergic, cholinergic, and histamine-binding receptors.

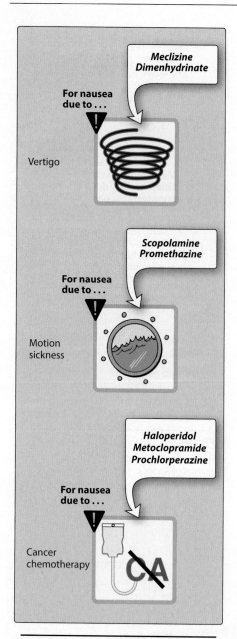

Figure 11.5
Therapeutic application of antiemetic agents.

4. **Anticholinergic effects:** Some of the antipsychotics, particularly *thioridazine, chlorpromazine, clozapine,* and *olanzapine,* produce anticholinergic effects. These effects include blurred vision, dry mouth (the exception is *clozapine,* which increases salivation), confusion, and inhibition of gastrointestinal and urinary tract smooth muscle, leading to constipation and urinary retention. The anticholinergic effects may actually assist in reducing the risk of EPS with these agents.

5. **Other effects:** Blockade of α-adrenergic receptors causes orthostatic hypotension and light-headedness. The antipsychotics also alter temperature-regulating mechanisms and can produce poikilothermia (condition in which body temperature varies with the environment). In the pituitary, antipsychotics block D_2 receptors, leading to an increase in prolactin release. Sedation occurs with those drugs that are potent antagonists of the H_1-histamine receptor, including *chlorpromazine, olanzapine, quetiapine,* and *clozapine.* Sexual dysfunction may also occur with the antipsychotics due to various receptor-binding characteristics.

E. **Therapeutic uses**

1. **Treatment of schizophrenia:** The antipsychotics are considered the only efficacious pharmacological treatment for schizophrenia. The first-generation antipsychotics are most effective in treating positive symptoms of schizophrenia. The atypical antipsychotics with 5-HT_{2A} receptor–blocking activity may be effective in many patients who are resistant to the traditional agents, especially in treating the negative symptoms of schizophrenia.

2. **Prevention of nausea and vomiting:** The older antipsychotics (most commonly, *prochlorperazine* [PROE-clor-PEAR-a-zeen]) are useful in the treatment of drug-induced nausea.

3. **Other uses:** The antipsychotic drugs can be used as tranquilizers to manage agitated and disruptive behavior secondary to other disorders. *Chlorpromazine* is used to treat intractable hiccups. *Pimozide* [PIM-oh-zide] is primarily indicated for treatment of the motor and phonic tics of Tourette disorder. However, *risperidone* and *haloperidol* are also commonly prescribed for this tic disorder. Also, *risperidone* and *aripiprazole* are approved for the management of disruptive behavior and irritability secondary to autism. Many antipsychotic agents are approved for the management of the manic and mixed symptoms associated with bipolar disorder. *Lurasidone* [loo-RAS-i-done] and *quetiapine* are indicated for the treatment of bipolar depression. *Paliperidone* [pal-ee-PEAR-i-dohn] is approved for the treatment of schizoaffective disorder. Some antipsychotics (*aripiprazole* and *quetiapine*) are used as adjunctive agents with antidepressants for treatment of refractory depression.

F. **Absorption and metabolism**

After oral administration, the antipsychotics show variable absorption that is unaffected by food (except for *ziprasidone* [zi-PRAS-i-done] and *paliperidone,* the absorption of which is increased with food). These agents readily pass into the brain and have a large volume of distribution. They are metabolized to many different metabolites, usually by the cytochrome P450 system in the liver, particularly the CYP2D6, CYP1A2, and CYP3A4 isoenzymes. Some metabolites are active and have been developed as pharmacological agents themselves (for example, *paliperidone* is the active metabolite of *risperidone*, and the antidepressant *amoxapine* is the active metabolite of *loxapine*). *Fluphenazine decanoate, haloperidol decanoate, risperidone* microspheres, *paliperidone palmitate, aripiprazole monohydrate*, and *olanzapine pamoate* are long-acting injectable (LAI) formulations of antipsychotics. These formulations have a therapeutic duration of action of up to 2 to 4 weeks and, therefore, are often used to treat outpatients and individuals who are nonadherent with oral medications.

G. Adverse effects

Adverse effects of the antipsychotic drugs can occur in practically all patients and are significant in about 80% (Figure 11.6).

1. **Extrapyramidal effects:** The inhibitory effects of dopaminergic neurons are normally balanced by the excitatory actions of cholinergic neurons in the striatum. Blocking dopamine receptors alters this balance, causing a relative excess of cholinergic influence, which results in extrapyramidal motor effects. The appearance of the movement disorders is generally time and dose dependent, with dystonias occurring within a few hours to days of treatment, followed by akathisias occurring within days to weeks. Parkinson-like symptoms of bradykinesia, rigidity, and tremor usually occur within weeks to months of initiating treatment. Tardive dyskinesia (see below), which can be irreversible, may occur after months or years of treatment.

   If cholinergic activity is also blocked, a new, more nearly normal balance is restored, and extrapyramidal effects are minimized. This can be achieved by administration of an anticholinergic drug, such as *benztropine*. The therapeutic trade-off is a lower incidence of EPS in exchange for the side effect of muscarinic receptor blockade. Those antipsychotic drugs that exhibit strong anticholinergic activity, such as *thioridazine* [THYE-oh-RID-a-zeen], show fewer extrapyramidal disturbances, because the cholinergic activity is already strongly dampened. This contrasts with *haloperidol* and *fluphenazine* [floo-FEN-a-zeen], which have low anticholinergic activity and produce extrapyramidal effects more frequently because of the preferential blocking of dopaminergic transmission. Akathisia may respond better to β blockers (for example, *propranolol*) or benzodiazepines, rather than anticholinergic medications.

2. **Tardive dyskinesia:** Long-term treatment with antipsychotics can cause this motor disorder. Patients display involuntary movements, including bilateral and facial jaw movements and "fly-catching" motions of the tongue. A prolonged holiday from antipsychotics may cause the symptoms to diminish or disappear within a few months. However, in many individuals, tardive dyskinesia is irreversible and persists after discontinuation of therapy. Tardive dyskinesia is postulated to result from an increased number of dopamine receptors that are synthesized as a compensatory response to long-term

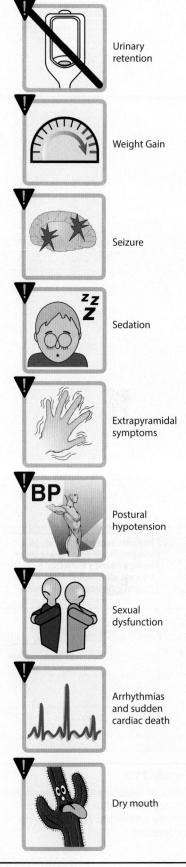

Urinary retention

Weight Gain

Seizure

Sedation

Extrapyramidal symptoms

Postural hypotension

Sexual dysfunction

Arrhythmias and sudden cardiac death

Dry mouth

Figure 11.6
Adverse effects observed in individuals treated with antipsychotic drugs.

dopamine receptor blockade. This makes the neuron supersensitive to the actions of dopamine, and it allows the dopaminergic input to this structure to overpower the cholinergic input, causing excess movement in the patient. Traditional anti-EPS medications may actually worsen this condition.

3. **Neuroleptic malignant syndrome:** This potentially fatal reaction to antipsychotic drugs is characterized by muscle rigidity, fever, altered mental status and stupor, unstable blood pressure, and myoglobinemia. Treatment necessitates discontinuation of the antipsychotic agent and supportive therapy. Administration of *dantrolene* or *bromocriptine* may be helpful.

4. **Other effects:** Drowsiness occurs due to CNS depression and antihistaminic effects, usually during the first few weeks of treatment. Confusion sometimes results. Those antipsychotic agents with potent antimuscarinic activity often produce dry mouth, urinary retention, constipation, and loss of visual accommodation. Others may block α-adrenergic receptors, resulting in lowered blood pressure and orthostatic hypotension. The antipsychotics depress the hypothalamus, affecting thermoregulation and causing amenorrhea, galactorrhea, gynecomastia, infertility, and erectile dysfunction. Significant weight gain is often a reason for nonadherence. Glucose and lipid profiles should be monitored in patients taking antipsychotics due to the potential for the second-generation agents to increase these laboratory parameters and the possible exacerbation of preexisting diabetes or hyperlipidemia. Some antipsychotics have been associated with mild to significant QT prolongation. *Thioridazine* has the highest risk, and *ziprasidone* and *iloperidone* [eye-low-PEAR-ee-dohn] also have cautions with their use due to this effect. Other antipsychotics have a general precaution regarding QT prolongation, even if the risk is relatively low.

5. **Cautions and contraindications:** All antipsychotics may lower the seizure threshold and should be used cautiously in patients with seizure disorders or those with an increased risk for seizures, such as withdrawal from alcohol. These agents also carry the warning of increased risk for mortality when used in elderly patients with dementia-related behavioral disturbances and psychosis. Antipsychotics used in patients with mood disorders should also be monitored for worsening of mood and suicidal ideation or behaviors.

H. Maintenance treatment

Patients who have had two or more psychotic episodes secondary to schizophrenia should receive maintenance therapy for at least 5 years, and some experts prefer indefinite therapy. Low doses of antipsychotic drugs are not as effective as higher-dose maintenance therapy in preventing relapse. The rate of relapse may be lower with second-generation drugs (Figure 11.7). Figure 11.8 summarizes the therapeutic uses of some of the antipsychotic drugs.

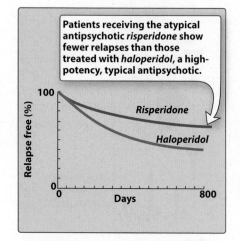

Figure 11.7
Rates of relapse among patients with schizophrenia after maintenance therapy with either *risperidone* or *haloperidol*.

DRUG	THERAPEUTIC NOTES
First generation	
Chlorpromazine	Moderate to high potential for EPS; moderate to high potential for weight gain, orthostasis, sedation, anti-muscarinic effects.
Fluphenazine	Oral formulation has a high potential for EPS; low potential for weight gain, sedation, and orthostasis; low to moderate potential for antimuscarinic effects; common use is in the LAI formulation administered every 2–3 weeks in patients with schizophrenia and a history of noncompliance with oral antipsychotic regimens.
Haloperidol	High potential for EPS; low potential for anti-adrenergic (orthostasis) or antimuscarinic adverse events; low potential for weight gain or sedation; available in a LAI formulation administered every 4 weeks.
Second generation	
Aripiprazole	Low potential for EPS; low potential for weight gain; low potential for sedation and antimuscarinic effects; also approved for the treatment of bipolar disorder; also approved for autistic disorder in children, and as an adjunctive treatment for major depression.
Asenapine	Low potential for EPS; low potential for weight gain; low to moderate potential for sedation; low potential for orthostasis; also approved for the treatment of bipolar disorder; available as a sublingual formulation.
Clozapine	Very low potential for EPS; risk for blood dyscrasias (for example, agranulocytosis = ~1%); risk for seizures; risk for myo-carditis; high potential for the following: sialorrhea, weight gain, antimuscarinic effects, orthostasis, and sedation.
Olanzapine	Low potential for EPS; moderate to high potential for weight gain and sedation; low potential for orthostasis; also approved for the treatment of bipolar disorder; available as a LAI formulation administered every 2–4 weeks.
Paliperidone	Low to moderate potential for EPS; low potential for weight gain; low potential for sedation; available as a LAI formulation administered every 4 weeks; also approved for use in schizoaffective disorder.
Quetiapine	Low potential for EPS; moderate potential for weight gain; moderate potential for orthostasis; moderate to high potential for sedation; also approved for the treatment of bipolar disorder and as an adjunctive treatment for major depression.
Risperidone	Low to moderate potential for EPS; low to moderate potential for weight gain; low to moderate potential for orthostasis; low to moderate potential for sedation; also approved for the treatment of bipolar disorder; also approved for autistic disorder in children; available as a LAI formulation administered every 2 weeks.
Ziprasidone	Low potential for extrapyramidal effects; contraindicated in patients with history of cardiac arrhythmias; minimal weight gain. Used in treatment of bipolar depression.

Figure 11.8
Summary of antipsychotic agents commonly used to treat schizophrenia. EPS = extrapyramidal effects; LAI = long-acting injectable.

Study Questions

Choose the ONE best answer.

11.1 An adolescent male is newly diagnosed with schizophrenia. Which of the following antipsychotic agents may have the best chance to improve his apathy and blunted affect?

A. Chlorpromazine.
B. Fluphenazine.
C. Haloperidol.
D. Risperidone.
E. Thioridazine.

Correct answer = D. Risperidone is the only antipsychotic on the list that has some reported benefit in improving the negative symptoms of schizophrenia. It is a second-generation antipsychotic, and the other drugs listed are first-generation antipsychotic agents. All of the agents have the potential to diminish the hallucinations and delusional thought processes (positive symptoms).

11.2 Which one of the following antipsychotics has been shown to be a partial agonist at the dopamine D_2 receptor?

A. Aripiprazole.
B. Clozapine.
C. Haloperidol.
D. Risperidone.
E. Thioridazine.

Correct answer = A. Aripiprazole is the agent that acts as a partial agonist at D_2 receptors. Theoretically, the drug would enhance action at these receptors when there is a low concentration of dopamine and would block the actions of high concentrations of dopamine. All of the other drugs are only antagonistic at D_2 receptors, with haloperidol being particularly potent.

11.3 A 21-year-old male has recently begun pimozide therapy for Tourette disorder. His parents bring him to the emergency department. They describe that he has been having "different-appearing tics" than before, such as prolonged contraction of the facial muscles. While being examined, he experiences opisthotonos (type of extrapyramidal spasm of the body in which the head and heels are bent backward and the body is bowed forward). Which of the following drugs would be beneficial in reducing these symptoms?

A. Benztropine.
B. Bromocriptine.
C. Lithium.
D. Prochlorperazine.
E. Risperidone.

Correct answer = A. The patient is experiencing EPS due to pimozide, and a muscarinic antagonist such as benztropine would be effective in reducing the symptoms. The other drugs would have no effect or, in the case of prochlorperazine and risperidone, might increase the symptoms.

11.4 A 28-year-old woman with schizoaffective disorder (combination of mood and psychotic symptoms) reports difficulty falling asleep. Which of the following would be most beneficial in this patient?

A. Lithium.
B. Chlorpromazine.
C. Haloperidol.
D. Paliperidone.
E. Ziprasidone.

Correct answer = D. Paliperidone is the only agent that is FDA approved for schizoaffective disorder. Chlorpromazine has significant sedative activity as well as antipsychotic properties and is the drug most likely to alleviate this patient's major complaint of insomnia. Although other antipsychotics may benefit this patient's disorder, paliperidone has the indication for this disorder, and if the underlying disorder is improved, then the symptom of insomnia may also improve without risking other, unwanted adverse effects, such as the anticholinergic effects of chlorpromazine.

11.5 Which of the following antipsychotic agents is considered to be the *most potent* and, thus, have the highest risk of extrapyramidal symptoms?

A. Thioridazine.
B. Fluphenazine.
C. Quetiapine.
D. Chlorpromazine.
E. Clozapine.

Correct answer = B. Among the older, conventional, or typical antipsychotics on this list, fluphenazine is the most potent and would thus be expected to have the highest incidence of EPS. The atypical antipsychotics listed (quetiapine and clozapine) could be considered low potency based on their common dosing and are considered to have the lowest risk for EPS.

11.6 Which antipsychotic has the most sedative potential and is sometimes questionably used as a hypnotic agent in certain clinical settings?

A. Fluphenazine.
B. Thiothixene.
C. Quetiapine.
D. Haloperidol.
E. Iloperidone.

Correct answer = C. Quetiapine has strong antihistaminergic effects causing sedation and is sometimes used at low doses as a sedative–hypnotic, even though this use is considered off-label. The other antipsychotic agents listed are weaker at blocking the histamine receptor and therefore are not as sedating.

11.7 A 30-year-old male patient who is treated with haloperidol for his diagnosis of schizophrenia is considered to be well-managed symptomatically for his psychotic symptoms. However, he is reporting restlessness, the inability to sit still at the dinner table, and his family notices that he is pacing up and down the hallway frequently. Of the following, which is the best medication to treat this antipsychotic-induced akathisia?

A. Benztropine.
B. Dantrolene.
C. Amoxapine.
D. Bromocriptine.
E. Propranolol.

Correct answer = E. Propranolol, a β-blocker, is considered the drug of choice for the management of antipsychotic-induced akathisia. Benztropine is more effective for pseudoparkinsonism and acute dystonias. Amoxapine is an antidepressant that has been associated with EPS. Bromocriptine is more effective for Parkinson-like symptoms, and dantrolene is a muscle relaxant that is best reserved for managing some symptoms of neuroleptic malignant syndrome.

11.8 Which of the following antipsychotic agents is available in a LAI formulation that may be useful for patients with difficulty adhering to therapy?

A. Asenapine.
B. Chlorpromazine.
C. Clozapine.
D. Quetiapine.
E. Risperidone.

Correct answer = E. Risperidone is available in a LAI formulation containing risperidone microspheres. The other agents listed do not have LAI formulations. Aripiprazole, fluphenazine, haloperidol, olanzapine, and paliperidone are other antipsychotics that are available in LAI formulations.

11.9 Which of the following antipsychotic agents is most associated with the possibility of a hematological dyscrasia such as agranulocytosis in a patient being treated for schizophrenia?

A. Chlorpromazine.
B. Buspirone.
C. Lithium.
D. Clozapine.
E. Asenapine.

Correct answer = D. Clozapine is the only antipsychotic medication that has a black box warning and a risk of agranulocytosis in approximately 1% of the patients treated. This requires regular monitoring of white blood cell counts. Although other antipsychotics have case reports of blood dyscrasias, clozapine is considered to have the highest risk.

11.10 Which antipsychotic agent has been most associated with significant QT interval prolongation and should be used with caution in patients with preexisting arrhythmias or patients taking other drugs associated with QT prolongation?

A. Thioridazine.
B. Risperidone.
C. Asenapine.
D. Lurasidone.
E. Aripiprazole.

Correct answer = A. Of the antipsychotic drugs listed, thioridazine has the highest risk for causing QT interval prolongation. Although this is a general warning for all antipsychotics, thioridazine has been issued a "black box warning," suggesting that it is associated with the greatest risk.

Drugs for Epilepsy

12

Jeannine M. Conway and Angela K. Birnbaum

I. OVERVIEW

Approximately 10% of the population will have at least one seizure in their lifetime. Globally, epilepsy is the third most common neurologic disorder after cerebrovascular and Alzheimer's disease. Epilepsy is not a single entity but an assortment of different seizure types and syndromes originating from several mechanisms that have in common the sudden, excessive, and synchronous discharge of cerebral neurons. This abnormal electrical activity may result in a variety of events, including loss of consciousness, abnormal movements, atypical or odd behavior, and distorted perceptions that are of limited duration but recur if untreated. The site of origin of the abnormal neuronal firing determines the symptoms that are produced. For example, if the motor cortex is involved, the patient may experience abnormal movements or a generalized convulsion. Seizures originating in the parietal or occipital lobe may include visual, auditory, and olfactory hallucinations. Medications are the most widely used mode of treatment for patients with epilepsy. In general, seizures can be controlled with one medication in approximately 75% of patients. Patients may require more than one medication in order to optimize seizure control, and some patients may never obtain total seizure control. A summary of antiepilepsy medications is shown in Figure 12.1.

II. ETIOLOGY OF SEIZURES

In most cases, epilepsy has no identifiable cause. Focal areas that are functionally abnormal may be triggered into activity by changes in physiologic factors, such as an alteration in blood gases, pH, electrolytes, and blood glucose and changes in environmental factors, such as sleep deprivation, alcohol intake, and stress. The neuronal discharge in epilepsy results from the firing of a small population of neurons in a specific area of the brain referred to as the "primary focus." Neuroimaging techniques, such as magnetic resonance imaging, positron emission tomography scans, and single photon emission coherence tomography, may identify areas of concern (Figure 12.2). Epilepsy can be due to an underlying genetic, structural, or metabolic cause or an unknown cause. Though multiple specific epilepsy syndromes that include symptoms other than seizures have been classified, a discussion of these syndromes is beyond the scope of this chapter.

APPROVED BEFORE 1990
Carbamazepine TEGRETOL
Diazepam VALIUM
Divalproex DEPAKOTE
Ethosuximide ZARONTIN
Lorazepam ATIVAN
Phenobarbital LUMINAL
Phenytoin DILANTIN
Primidone MYSOLINE

APPROVED AFTER 1990
Clobazam ONFI
Eslicarbazepine APTIOM
Ezogabine POTIGA
Felbamate FELBATOL
Fosphenytoin CEREBYX
Gabapentin NEURONTIN
Lacosamide VIMPAT
Lamotrigine LAMICTAL
Levetiracetam KEPPRA
Oxcarbazepine TRILEPTAL
Perampanel FYCOMPA
Pregabalin LYRICA
Rufinamide BANZEL
Tiagabine GABITRIL
Topiramate TOPAMAX
Vigabatrin SABRIL
Zonisamide ZONEGRAN

Figure 12.1
Summary of agents used in the treatment of epilepsy. Drugs arranged alphabetically.

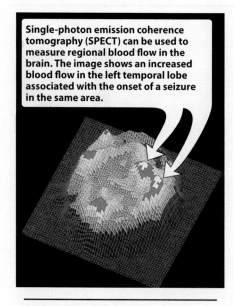

Single-photon emission coherence tomography (SPECT) can be used to measure regional blood flow in the brain. The image shows an increased blood flow in the left temporal lobe associated with the onset of a seizure in the same area.

Figure 12.2
Region of the brain in a person with epilepsy showing increased blood flow during a seizure.

A. Genetic epilepsy

These seizures result from an inherited abnormality in the central nervous system (CNS). Some genetic mutations have been identified in epilepsy syndromes. Obtaining a detailed family history may provide important information for assessing the possibility of a genetic link to seizures.

B. Structural/metabolic epilepsy

A number of causes, such as illicit drug use, tumor, head injury, hypoglycemia, meningeal infection, and the rapid withdrawal of alcohol from an alcoholic, can precipitate seizures. In cases when the cause of a seizure can be determined and corrected, medication may not be necessary. For example, a seizure that is caused by a drug reaction is not epilepsy and does not require chronic therapy. In other situations, antiepilepsy medications may be needed when the primary cause of the seizures cannot be corrected.

C. Unknown cause

When no specific anatomic cause for the seizure, such as trauma or neoplasm, is evident, a patient may be diagnosed with seizures where the underlying cause is unknown. Most cases of epilepsy are due to an unknown cause. Patients can be treated chronically with antiepilepsy medications or vagal nerve stimulation.

III. CLASSIFICATION OF SEIZURES

It is important to correctly classify seizures to determine appropriate treatment. Seizures have been categorized by site of origin, etiology, electrophysiologic correlation, and clinical presentation. The nomenclature developed by the International League Against Epilepsy is considered the standard way to classify seizures and epilepsy syndromes (Figure 12.3). Seizures have been classified into two broad groups: focal and generalized.

A. Focal

Focal seizures involve only a portion of the brain, typically part of one lobe of one hemisphere. The symptoms of each seizure type depend on the site of neuronal discharge and on the extent to which the electrical activity spreads to other neurons in the brain. Focal seizures may progress to become generalized tonic–clonic seizures.

1. **Simple partial:** These seizures are caused by a group of hyperactive neurons exhibiting abnormal electrical activity and are confined to a single locus in the brain. The electrical discharge does not spread, and the patient does not lose consciousness or awareness. The patient often exhibits abnormal activity of a single limb or muscle group that is controlled by the region of the brain experiencing the disturbance. The patient may also show sensory distortions. This activity may spread. Simple partial seizures may occur at any age.

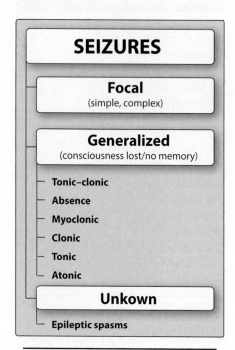

Figure 12.3
Classification of epilepsy.

2. **Complex partial:** These seizures exhibit complex sensory hallucinations and mental distortion. Motor dysfunction may involve chewing movements, diarrhea, and/or urination. Consciousness is altered. Simple partial seizure activity may spread to become complex and then spread to a secondarily generalized convulsion. Complex partial seizures may occur at any age.

B. Generalized

Generalized seizures may begin locally and then progress to include abnormal electrical discharges throughout both hemispheres of the brain. Primary generalized seizures may be convulsive or nonconvulsive, and the patient usually has an immediate loss of consciousness.

1. **Tonic–clonic:** These seizures result in loss of consciousness, followed by tonic (continuous contraction) and clonic (rapid contraction and relaxation) phases. The seizure may be followed by a period of confusion and exhaustion due to the depletion of glucose and energy stores.

2. **Absence:** These seizures involve a brief, abrupt, and self-limiting loss of consciousness. The onset generally occurs in patients at 3 to 5 years of age and lasts until puberty or beyond. The patient stares and exhibits rapid eye-blinking, which lasts for 3 to 5 seconds. An absence seizure has a very distinct three-per-second spike and wave discharge seen on electroencephalogram.

3. **Myoclonic:** These seizures consist of short episodes of muscle contractions that may recur for several minutes. They generally occur after wakening and exhibit as brief jerks of the limbs. Myoclonic seizures occur at any age but usually begin around puberty or early adulthood.

4. **Clonic:** These seizures consist of short episodes of muscle contractions that may closely resemble myoclonic seizures. Consciousness is more impaired with clonic seizures as compared to myoclonic.

5. **Tonic:** These seizures involve increased tone in the extension muscles and are generally less than 60 seconds long.

6. **Atonic:** These seizures are also known as drop attacks and are characterized by a sudden loss of muscle tone.

C. Mechanism of action of antiepilepsy medications

Drugs reduce seizures through such mechanisms as blocking voltage-gated channels (Na^+ or Ca^{2+}), enhancing inhibitory γ-aminobutyric acid (GABA)-ergic impulses and interfering with excitatory glutamate transmission. Some antiepilepsy medications appear to have multiple targets within the CNS, whereas the mechanism of action for some agents is poorly defined. Antiepilepsy medications suppress seizures but do not "cure" or "prevent" epilepsy.

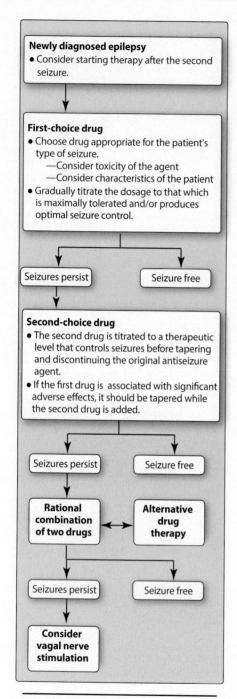

Figure 12.4
Therapeutic strategies for managing newly diagnosed epilepsy.

IV. DRUG SELECTION

Choice of drug treatment is based on the classification of the seizures, patient-specific variables (for example, age, comorbid medical conditions, lifestyle, and personal preference), and characteristics of the drug (such as cost and drug interactions). For example, focal-onset seizures are treated with a different set of medications than primary generalized seizures, although the list of effective agents overlaps. The toxicity of the agent and characteristics of the patient are major considerations in drug selection. In newly diagnosed patients, monotherapy is instituted with a single agent until seizures are controlled or toxicity occurs (Figure 12.4). Compared to those receiving combination therapy, patients receiving monotherapy exhibit better medication adherence and fewer side effects. If seizures are not controlled with the first medication, monotherapy with an alternate medication or the addition of medications should be considered (Figure 12.5). Failing that, other medical management (vagal nerve stimulation, surgery, etc.) should be considered. Awareness of the antiepilepsy medications available and their mechanisms of action, pharmacokinetics, potential for drug–drug interactions, and adverse effects is essential for successful treatment of the patient.

V. ANTIEPILEPSY MEDICATIONS

During the past 20 years, the Food and Drug Administration has approved many new antiepilepsy medications (Figure 12.1). Some of these agents are thought to have potential advantages over drugs approved prior to 1990 in terms of pharmacokinetics, tolerability, and reduced risk for drug–drug interactions. However, studies have failed to demonstrate that the newer drugs are significantly more efficacious than the older agents. For that reason, the antiepilepsy medications are described below in alphabetical order, rather than attempting to rank them by efficacy. Figure 12.6 summarizes pharmacokinetic properties of the antiepilepsy medications, and Figure 12.7 shows common adverse effects. Suicidal behavior and suicidal ideation have been identified as a risk with antiepilepsy medications. In addition, virtually, all antiepilepsy medications have been associated with multiorgan hypersensitivity reactions, a rare idiosyncratic reaction characterized by rash, fever, and systemic organ involvement.

A. Benzodiazepines

Benzodiazepines bind to GABA inhibitory receptors to reduce firing rate. Most benzodiazepines are reserved for emergency or acute seizure treatment due to tolerance. However, *clonazepam* [kloe-NAY-ze-pam] and *clobazam* [KLOE-ba-zam] may be prescribed as adjunctive therapy for particular types of seizures. *Diazepam* [dye-AZ-e-pam] is also available for rectal administration to avoid or interrupt prolonged generalized tonic–clonic seizures or clusters when oral administration is not possible.

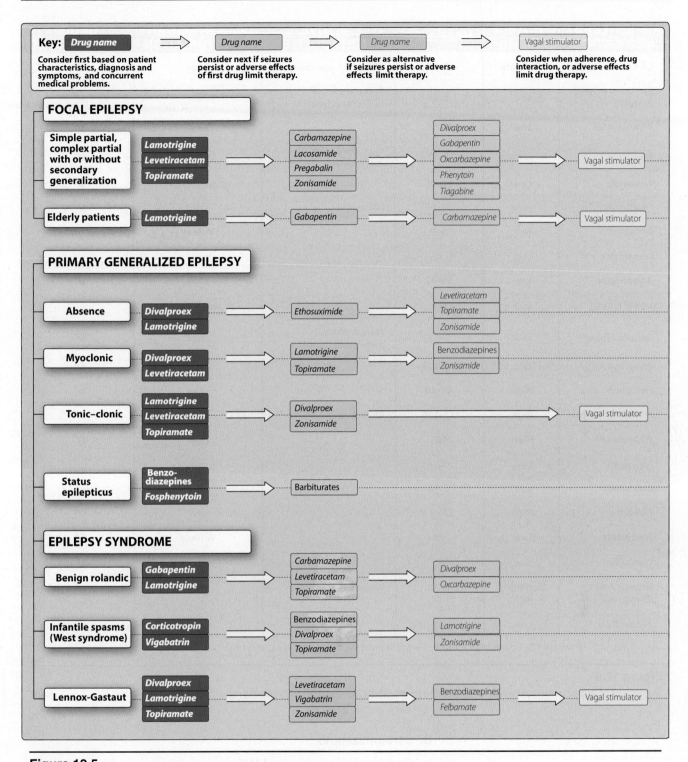

Figure 12.5
Therapeutic indications for the anticonvulsant agents. Benzodiazepines = *diazepam* and *lorazepam*.

ANTIEPILEPSY MEDICATION	PROTEIN BINDING*	HALF-LIFE	ACTIVE METABOLITE	MAJOR ORGAN OF ELIMINATION	DRUG INTERACTIONS
Carbamazepine	Moderate	6–15	CBZ-10,11-epoxide	Liver	✔
Eslicarbazepine acetate **^	Low	8–24	Eslicarbazepine (S-licarbazepine)	Kidney	✔
Ethosuximide	Low	25–26		Liver	✔
Ezogabine	Moderate	7–11	monoacetylated metabolite	Liver	✔
Felbamate	Low	20–23		Kidney/Liver	✔
Fosphenytoin**	High	12–60	phenytoin	Liver	✔
Gabapentin	Low	5–9		Kidney	
Lacosamide	Low	13		Various	
Lamotrigine	Low	25–32		Liver	✔
Levetiracetam	Low	6–8		Hydrolysis	
Oxcarbazepine**	Low	5–13	Monohydroxy metabolite (MHD)	Liver	✔
Phenobarbital	Low	72–124		Liver	✔
Phenytoin	High	12–60		Liver	✔
Primidone	High	72–124	Phenobarbital, PEMA	Liver	✔
Perampanel^	High	105		Liver	✔
Pregabalin	Low	5–6.5		Kidney	
Rufinamide	Low	6–10		Liver	✔
Tiagabine	High	7–9		Liver	✔
Topiramate	Low	21		Various	✔
Vigabatrin	Low	7.5		Kidney	✔
Valproic Acid (Divalproex)	Moderate/ High	6–18	Various	Liver	✔
Zonisamide	Low	63		Liver	✔

*Low = 60% or less, Moderate = 61%-85%, High = >85%; ^Newly approved. Limited data in patients available. **Prodrug.

Figure 12.6
Summary of the pharmacokinetics of antiepilepsy medications used as chronic therapy.

B. Carbamazepine

Carbamazepine [kar-ba-MAZ-a-peen] blocks sodium channels, thereby inhibiting the generation of repetitive action potentials in the epileptic focus and preventing their spread. Carbamazepine is effective for treatment of focal seizures and, additionally generalized tonic–clonic seizures, trigeminal neuralgia, and bipolar disorder. Carbamazepine is absorbed slowly and erratically following oral administration and may vary from generic to generic, resulting in large variations in serum concentrations of the drug. It induces its own metabolism, resulting in lower total *carbamazepine* blood concentrations at higher doses. *Carbamazepine* is an inducer of the CYP1A2, CYP2C, and CYP3A and UDP glucuronosyltransferase (UGT) enzymes, which increases the clearance of other drugs (Figure 12.8). Hyponatremia may be noted in some patients, especially the elderly, and may necessitate a change in medication. *Carbamazepine* should not be prescribed for patients with absence seizures because it may cause an increase in seizures.

C. Eslicarbazepine

Eslicarbazepine [es-li-kar-BAZ-a-peen] *acetate* is a prodrug that is converted to the active metabolite *eslicarbazepine* (S-licarbazepine) by hydrolysis. S-licarbazepine is the active metabolite of *oxcarbazepine* (see below). It is a voltage-gated sodium channel blocker and is approved for partial-onset seizures in adults. *Eslicarbazepine* exhibits linear pharmacokinetics and is eliminated via glucuronidation. The side effect profile includes dizziness, somnolence, diplopia, and headache. Serious adverse reactions such as rash, psychiatric side effects, and hyponatremia occur rarely.

D. Ethosuximide

Ethosuximide [eth-oh-SUX-i-mide] reduces propagation of abnormal electrical activity in the brain, most likely by inhibiting T-type calcium channels. It is only effective in treating absence seizures.

E. Ezogabine

Ezogabine [e-ZOG-a-been] is thought to open voltage-gated M-type potassium channels leading to stabilization of the resting membrane potential. *Ezogabine* exhibits linear pharmacokinetics and no drug interactions at lower doses. Possible unique side effects are urinary retention, QT interval prolongation, blue skin discoloration, and retinal abnormalities.

F. Felbamate

Felbamate [FEL-ba-mate] has a broad spectrum of anticonvulsant action with multiple proposed mechanisms including the blocking of voltage-dependent sodium channels, competing with the glycine coagonist binding site on the *N*-methyl-D-aspartate (NMDA) glutamate receptor, blocking of calcium channels, and potentiating GABA action. It is an inhibitor of drugs metabolized by CYP2C19 and induces drugs metabolized by CYP3A4. It is reserved for use in refractory epilepsies (particularly Lennox-Gastaut syndrome) because of the risk of aplastic anemia (about 1:4000) and hepatic failure.

G. Gabapentin

Gabapentin [GA-ba-pen-tin] is an analog of GABA. However, it does not act at GABA receptors, enhance GABA actions or convert to GABA. Its precise mechanism of action is not known. It is approved as adjunct therapy for focal seizures and treatment of postherpetic neuralgia. *Gabapentin* exhibits nonlinear pharmacokinetics (see Chapter 1) due to its uptake by a saturable transport system from the gut. *Gabapentin* does not bind to plasma proteins

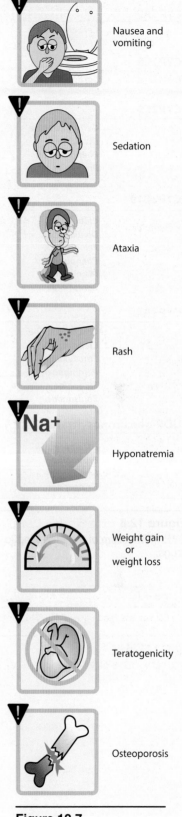

Figure 12.7
Notable adverse effects of antiseizure medications.

- Nausea and vomiting
- Sedation
- Ataxia
- Rash
- Na+ Hyponatremia
- Weight gain or weight loss
- Teratogenicity
- Osteoporosis

CYP1A2
Carbamazepine

CYP2C8
Carbamazepine

CYP2C9
Carbamazepine
Divalproex
Phenobarbital
Phenytoin

CYP2C19
Clobazam
Divalproex
Felbamate
Phenobarbital
Phenytoin
Zonisamide

CYP3A4
Carbamazepine
Clobazam
Ethosuximide
Perampanel
Tiagabine
Zonisamide

UDP-glucuronosyltransferase
Divalproex
Ezogabine
Lamotrigine
Lorazepam

Figure 12.8
CYP metabolism of the antiepileptic
drugs.

and is excreted unchanged through the kidneys. Reduced dosing is required in renal disease. *Gabapentin* is well tolerated by the elderly population with partial seizures due to its relatively mild adverse effects. It may also be a good choice for the older patient because there are few drug interactions.

H. Lacosamide

Lacosamide [la-KOE-sa-mide] in <u>vitro</u> affects voltage-gated sodium channels, resulting in stabilization of hyperexcitable neuronal membranes and inhibition of repetitive neuronal firing. *Lacosamide* binds to collapsin response mediator protein-2 (CRMP-2), a phosphoprotein involved in neuronal differentiation and control of axonal outgrowth. The role of CRMP-2 binding in seizure control is unknown. *Lacosamide* is approved for adjunctive treatment of focal seizures. It is available in an injectable formulation. The most common adverse events that limit treatment include dizziness, headache, and fatigue.

I. Lamotrigine

Lamotrigine [la-MOE-tri-jeen] blocks sodium channels, as well as high voltage-dependent calcium channels. *Lamotrigine* is effective in a wide variety of seizure types, including focal, generalized, absence seizures, and Lennox-Gastaut syndrome. It is also used to treat bipolar disorder. *Lamotrigine* is metabolized primarily to the 2-N-glucuronide metabolite through the UGT1A4 pathway. As with other antiepilepsy medications, general inducers increase *lamotrigine* clearance leading to lower *lamotrigine* concentrations, whereas *divalproex* results in a significant decrease in *lamotrigine* clearance (higher *lamotrigine* concentrations). *Lamotrigine* dosages should be reduced when adding *valproate* to therapy. Slow titration is necessary with *lamotrigine* (particularly when adding *lamotrigine* to a regimen that includes *valproate*) due to risk of rash, which may progress to a serious, life-threatening reaction.

J. Levetiracetam

Levetiracetam [lee-ve-tye-RA-se-tam] is approved for adjunct therapy of focal onset, myoclonic, and primary generalized tonic–clonic seizures in adults and children. The exact mechanism of anticonvulsant action is unknown. It demonstrates high affinity for a synaptic vesicle protein (SV2A). The drug is well absorbed orally and excreted in urine mostly unchanged, resulting in few to no drug interactions. *Levetiracetam* can cause mood alterations that may require a dose reduction or a change of medication.

K. Oxcarbazepine

Oxcarbazepine [ox-kar-BAY-zeh-peen] is a prodrug that is rapidly reduced to the 10-monohydroxy (MHD) metabolite responsible for its anticonvulsant activity. MHD blocks sodium channels, preventing the spread of the abnormal discharge. It is also thought to modulate calcium channels. It is approved for use in adults and children with partial-onset seizures. *Oxcarbazepine* is a less potent inducer of CYP3A4 and UGT than *carbamazepine*. The adverse effect of hyponatremia limits its use in the elderly.

L. Perampanel

Perampanel [per-AM-pa-nel] is a selective α-amino-3-hydroxy-5-methyl-4-isoxazolepropionic acid antagonist resulting in reduced excitatory activity. *Perampanel* has a long half-life enabling once-daily dosing. It is approved for adjunctive treatment of partial-onset seizures in patients 12 years or older. *Perampanel* is a newer antiepileptic agent, and limited data are available in patients.

M. Phenobarbital and primidone

The primary mechanism of action of *phenobarbital* [fee-noe-BAR-bih-tal] is enhancement of the inhibitory effects of GABA-mediated neurons (see Chapter 9). *Primidone* is metabolized to *phenobarbital* (major) and phenylethylmalonamide, both with anticonvulsant activity. *Phenobarbital* is used primarily in the treatment of status epilepticus when other agents fail.

N. Phenytoin and fosphenytoin

Phenytoin [FEN-i-toin] blocks voltage-gated sodium channels by selectively binding to the channel in the inactive state and slowing its rate of recovery. It is effective for treatment of focal and generalized tonic–clonic seizures and in the treatment of status epilepticus. *Phenytoin* induces drugs metabolized by the CYP2C and CYP3A families and the UGT enzyme system. *Phenytoin* exhibits saturable enzyme metabolism resulting in nonlinear pharmacokinetic properties (small increases in the daily dose can produce large increases in plasma concentration, resulting in drug-induced toxicity; Figure 12.9). Depression of the CNS occurs particularly in the cerebellum and vestibular system, causing nystagmus and ataxia. The elderly are highly susceptible to this effect. Gingival hyperplasia may cause the gums to grow over the teeth (Figure 12.10). Long-term use may lead to development of peripheral neuropathies and osteoporosis. Although *phenytoin* is advantageous due to its low cost, the actual cost of therapy may be much higher, considering the potential for serious toxicity and adverse effects.

Fosphenytoin [FOS-phen-i-toin] is a prodrug that is rapidly converted to *phenytoin* in the blood within minutes. Whereas *fosphenytoin* may be administered intramuscularly (IM), *phenytoin sodium* should never be given IM, as it causes tissue damage and necrosis. *Fosphenytoin* is the drug of choice and standard of care for IV and IM administration of *phenytoin*. Because of sound-alike and look-alike trade names, there is a risk for prescribing errors. The trade name of *fosphenytoin* is Cerebyx®, which is easily confused with Celebrex®, the cyclooxygenase-2 inhibitor, and Celexa®, the antidepressant.

O. Pregabalin

Pregabalin [pree-GA-ba-lin] binds to the α_2-δ site, an auxiliary subunit of voltage-gated calcium channels in the CNS, inhibiting excitatory neurotransmitter release. The exact role this plays in treatment is not known, but the drug has proven effects on focal-onset seizures, diabetic peripheral neuropathy, postherpetic neuralgia, and fibromyalgia. More than 90% of *pregabalin* is eliminated renally. Dosage adjustments are needed in renal dysfunction. It has no significant metabolism and few drug interactions. Weight gain and peripheral edema have been reported.

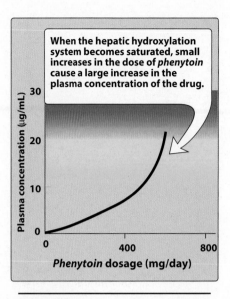

When the hepatic hydroxylation system becomes saturated, small increases in the dose of *phenytoin* cause a large increase in the plasma concentration of the drug.

Plasma concentration (µg/mL)

30

20

10

0

0   400   800

Phenytoin dosage (mg/day)

Figure 12.9
Nonlinear effect of *phenytoin* dosage on the plasma concentration of the drug.

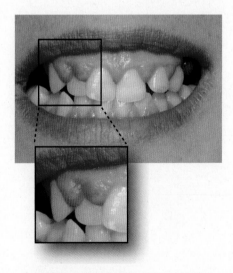

Figure 12.10
Gingival hyperplasia in patient treated with *phenytoin*.

P. Rufinamide

Rufinamide [roo-FIN-a-mide] acts at sodium channels. It is approved for the adjunctive treatment of seizures associated with Lennox-Gastaut syndrome in children over age 4 years and in adults. *Rufinamide* is a weak inhibitor of CYP2E1 and a weak inducer of CYP3A4 enzymes. Food increases absorption and peak serum concentrations. Serum concentrations of *rufinamide* are affected by other antiepilepsy medications. As with other antiepilepsy medications, it is induced by *carbamazepine* and *phenytoin* and inhibited when given with *valproate*. Adverse effects include the potential for shortened QT intervals. Patients with familial short QT syndrome should not be treated with *rufinamide*.

Q. Tiagabine

Tiagabine [ty-AG-a-been] blocks GABA uptake into presynaptic neurons permitting more GABA to be available for receptor binding, and therefore, it enhances inhibitory activity. *Tiagabine* is effective as adjunctive treatment in partial-onset seizures. In postmarketing surveillance, seizures have occurred in patients using *tiagabine* who did not have epilepsy. *Tiagabine* should not be used for indications other than epilepsy.

R. Topiramate

Topiramate [toe-PEER-a-mate] has multiple mechanisms of action. It blocks voltage-dependent sodium channels, reduces high-voltage calcium currents (L type), is a carbonic anhydrase inhibitor, and may act at glutamate (NMDA) sites. *Topiramate* is effective for use in partial and primary generalized epilepsy. It is also approved for prevention of migraine. It inhibits CYP2C19 and is induced by *phenytoin* and *carbamazepine*. Adverse effects include somnolence, weight loss, and paresthesias. Renal stones, glaucoma, oligohidrosis (decreased sweating), and hyperthermia have also been reported.

S. Valproic acid and divalproex

Possible mechanisms of action include sodium channel blockade, blockade of GABA transaminase, and action at the T-type calcium channels. These varied mechanisms provide a broad spectrum of activity against seizures. It is effective for the treatment of focal and primary generalized epilepsies. *Valproic acid* [val-PRO-ik A-sid] is available as a free acid. *Divalproex* [dye-val-PRO-ex] *sodium* is a combination of *sodium valproate* [val-PROE-ate] and *valproic acid* that is converted to *valproate* when it reaches the gastrointestinal tract. It was developed to improve gastrointestinal tolerance of *valproic acid*. All of the available salt forms are equivalent in efficacy (*valproic acid* and *sodium valproate*). Commercial products are available in multiple-salt dosage forms and extended-release formulations. Therefore, the risk for medication errors is high, and it is essential to be familiar with all preparations. *Valproate* inhibits metabolism of the CYP2C9, UGT, and epoxide hydrolase systems (Figure 12.8). Rare hepatotoxicity may cause a rise in liver enzymes, which should be monitored frequently. Teratogenicity is also of great concern.

T. Vigabatrin

Vigabatrin [vye-GA-ba-trin] acts as an irreversible inhibitor of γ-aminobutyric acid transaminase (GABA-T). GABA-T is the enzyme responsible for metabolism of GABA. *Vigabatrin* is associated with visual field loss ranging from mild to severe in 30% or more of patients. *Vigabatrin* is only available through physicians and pharmacies that participate in the restricted distribution SHARE program.

U. Zonisamide

Zonisamide [zoe-NIS-a-mide] is a sulfonamide derivative that has a broad spectrum of action. The compound has multiple effects, including blockade of both voltage-gated sodium channels and T-type calcium currents. It has a limited amount of carbonic anhydrase activity. *Zonisamide* is approved for use in patients with focal epilepsy. It is metabolized by the CYP3A4 isozyme and may, to a lesser extent, be affected by CYP3A5 and CYP2C19. In addition to typical CNS adverse effects, *zonisamide* may cause kidney stones. Oligohidrosis has been reported, and patients should be monitored for increased body temperature and decreased sweating. *Zonisamide* is contraindicated in patients with sulfonamide or carbonic anhydrase inhibitor hypersensitivity.

VI. STATUS EPILEPTICUS

In status epilepticus, two or more seizures occur without recovery of full consciousness in between episodes. These may be focal or primary generalized, convulsive or nonconvulsive. Status epilepticus is life threatening and requires emergency treatment usually consisting of administration of a fast-acting medication such as a benzodiazepine, followed by a slower-acting medication such as *phenytoin*.

VII. WOMEN'S HEALTH AND EPILEPSY

Women of childbearing potential with epilepsy require assessment of their antiepilepsy medications in regard to contraception and pregnancy planning. Several antiepilepsy medications increase the metabolism of hormonal contraceptives, potentially rendering them ineffective. These include *phenytoin*, *phenobarbital*, *carbamazepine*, *topiramate*, *oxcarbazepine*, *rufinamide*, and *clobazam*. These medications increase the metabolism of contraceptives regardless of the delivery system used (for example, patch, ring, implants, and oral tablets). Pregnancy planning is vital, as many antiepilepsy medications have the potential to affect fetal development and cause birth defects. All women considering pregnancy should be on high doses (1 to 5 mg) of folic acid prior to conception. *Divalproex* and barbiturates should be avoided. If possible, women already taking *divalproex* should be placed on other therapies prior to pregnancy and counseled about the potential for birth defects, including cognitive (Figure 12.11) and behavioral abnormalities and neural tube defects. The pharmacokinetics of antiepilepsy medications and the frequency and severity of seizures may change during pregnancy. Regular monitoring by both an obstetrician and a neurologist is important. All women with epilepsy should be encouraged to register with the Antiepileptic Drug Pregnancy Registry. Figure 12.12 summarizes important characteristics of the antiepilepsy medications.

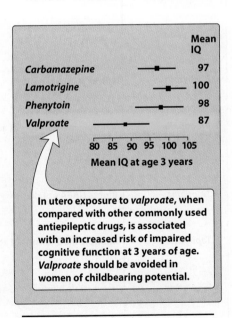

In utero exposure to *valproate*, when compared with other commonly used antiepileptic drugs, is associated with an increased risk of impaired cognitive function at 3 years of age. *Valproate* should be avoided in women of childbearing potential.

Figure 12.11
Cognitive function at 3 years of age after fetal exposure to doses of antiepileptic drugs. The means (black squares) and 95% confidence intervals (horizontal lines) are given for the children's IQ as a function of the antiepileptic drugs.

DRUG	MECHANISM OF ACTION	ADVERSE EFFECTS AND COMMENTS
Carbamazepine	Blocks Na+ channels	Hyponatremia, drowsiness, fatigue, dizziness, and blurred vision. Drug use has also been associated with Stevens-Johnson syndrome. Blood dyscrasias: neutropenia, leukopenia, thrombocytopenia, pancytopenia, and anemias.
Divalproex	Multiple mechanisms of action	Weight gain, easy bruising, nausea, tremor, hair loss, GI upset, liver damage, alopecia, and sedation. Hepatic failure, pancreatitis, and teratogenic effects have been observed. Broad spectrum of antiseizure activity.
Eslicarbazepine acetate	Blocks Na+ channels	Nausea, rash, hyponatremia, headache, sedation, dizziness, vertigo, ataxia, and diplopia.
Ethosuximide	Blocks Ca2+ channels	Drowsiness, hyperactivity, nausea, sedation, GI upset, weight gain, lethargy, SLE, and rash. Blood dyscrasias can occur; periodic CBCs should be done. Abrupt discontinuance of drug may cause seizures.
Ezogabine	Enhances K+ channels	Urinary retention, neuropsychiatric symptoms, dizziness, somnolence, QT prolongation, reports of blue skin discoloration, and retina changes.
Felbamate	Multiple mechanisms of action	Insomnia, dizziness, headache, ataxia, weight gain, and irritability. Aplastic anemia and hepatic failure. Broad spectrum of antiseizure activity. Requires patient to sign informed consent at dispensing.
Gabapentin	Unknown	Mild drowsiness, dizziness, ataxia, weight gain, and diarrhea. Few drug interactions. One hundred percent renal elimination.
Lacosamide	Multiple mechanisms of action	Dizziness, fatigue, and headache. Few drug interactions; Schedule V.
Lamotrigine	Multiple mechanisms of action	Nausea, drowsiness, dizziness, headache, and diplopia. Rash (Stevens-Johnson syndrome—potentially life threatening). Broad spectrum of antiseizure activity.
Levetiracetam	Multiple mechanisms of action	Sedation, dizziness, headache, anorexia, fatigue, infections, and behavioral symptoms. Few drug interactions. Broad spectrum of antiseizure activity.
Oxcarbazepine	Blocks Na+ channels	Nausea, rash, hyponatremia, headache, sedation, dizziness, vertigo, ataxia, and diplopia.
Perampanel	Blocks AMPA glutamate receptors	Serious psychiatric and behavioral reactions, dizziness, somnolence, fatigue, gait disturbance, and falls, long half-life.
Phenytoin	Blocks Na+ channels	Gingival hyperplasia, confusion, slurred speech, double vision, ataxia, sedation, dizziness, and hirsutism. Stevens-Johnson syndrome—potentially life threatening. Not recommended for chronic use. Primary treatment for status epilepticus (fosphenytoin).
Pregabalin	Multiple mechanisms of action	Weight gain, somnolence, dizziness, headache, diplopia, and ataxia. One hundred percent renal elimination.
Rufinamide	Unknown	Shortened QT interval. Multiple drug interactions.
Tiagabine	Blocks GABA uptake	Sedation, weight gain, fatigue, headache, tremor, dizziness, and anorexia. Multiple drug interactions.
Topiramate	Multiple mechanisms of action	Paresthesia, weight loss, nervousness, depression, anorexia, anxiety, tremor, cognitive complaints, headache, and oligohidrosis. Few drug interactions. Broad spectrum of antiseizure activity.
Vigabatrin	Irreversible binding of GABA-T	Vision loss, anemia, somnolence, fatigue, peripheral neuropathy, weight gain. Available only through SHARE pharmacies.
Zonisamide	Multiple mechanisms of action	Nausea, anorexia, ataxia, confusion, difficulty concentrating, sedation, paresthesia, and oligohidrosis. Broad spectrum of antiseizure activity.

Figure 12.12

Summary of antiepileptic drugs. AMPA = α-amino-3-hydroxy-5-methyl-4-isoxazolepropionic acid; CBC = complete blood count; GABA = γ-aminobutyric acid; GABA-T = γ-aminobutyric acid transaminase; GI = gastrointestinal; SLE = systemic lupus erythematosus.

Study Questions

Choose the ONE best answer.

12.1 A 9-year-old boy is sent for neurologic evaluation because of episodes of apparent inattention. Over the past year, the child has experienced episodes during which he develops a blank look on his face and his eyes blink for 15 seconds. He immediately resumes his previous activity. Which one the following best describes this patient's seizures?

A. Simple partial.
B. Complex partial.
C. Tonic–clonic.
D. Absence.
E. Myoclonic.

Correct answer = D. The patient is experiencing episodes of absence seizures. Consciousness is impaired briefly and they generally begin in children aged 4 to 12 years. Diagnosis includes obtaining an EEG that shows generalized 3-Hz waves.

12.2 A child is experiencing absence seizures that interrupt his ability to pay attention during school and activities. Which of the following therapies would be most appropriate for this patient?

A. Ethosuximide.
B. Carbamazepine.
C. Diazepam.
D. Carbamazepine plus primidone.
E. Watchful waiting.

Correct answer = A. The patient has had many seizures that interrupt his ability to pay attention during school and activities, so therapy is justified. Monotherapy with primary agents is preferred for most patients. The advantages of monotherapy include reduced frequency of adverse effects, fewer interactions between antiepileptic drugs, lower cost, and improved compliance. Carbamazepine and diazepam are not indicated for absence seizures.

12.3 Which of the following drugs is most useful for the treatment of absence seizures?

A. Topiramate.
B. Tiagabine.
C. Levetiracetam.
D. Lamotrigine.
E. Zonisamide.

Correct answer = D. Of the drugs listed, lamotrigine has the best data for use in absence seizures and would be the best choice. Tiagabine is only used for focal-onset seizures. Topiramate, levetiracetam, and zonisamide may be options if the lamotrigine does not work.

12.4 A 25-year-old woman with myoclonic seizures is well controlled on valproate. She indicates that she is interested in becoming pregnant in the next year. With respect to her antiepilepsy medication, which of the following should be considered?

A. Leave her on her current therapy.
B. Consider switching to lamotrigine.
C. Consider adding a second antiepilepsy medication.
D. Decrease her valproate dose.

Correct answer = B. Valproate is a poor choice in women of child-bearing age. A review of the medication history of this patient is warranted. If she has not tried any other antiepilepsy medication, then consideration of another antiepilepsy medication may be beneficial. Studies show that valproate taken during pregnancy can have a detrimental effect on cognitive abilities in children.

12.5 A woman with myoclonic seizures is well controlled with lamotrigine. She becomes pregnant and begins to have breakthrough seizures. What is most likely happening?

A. Her epilepsy is getting worse.
B. Lamotrigine concentrations are increasing.
C. Lamotrigine concentrations are decreasing.
D. Lamotrigine is no longer efficacious for this patient.

Correct answer = C. Pregnancy alters the pharmacokinetics of lamotrigine. As pregnancy progresses, most women require increased dosages to maintain blood concentrations and seizure control.

12.6 A 42-year-old man undergoes a neurologic evaluation because of episodes of apparent confusion. Over the past year, the man has experienced episodes during which he develops a blank look on his face and fails to respond to questions. Moreover, it appears to take several minutes before the man recovers from the episodes. Which one of the following best describes this type of seizure?

A. Focal (simple partial).
B. Focal (complex partial).
C. Tonic–clonic.
D. Absence.
E. Myoclonic.

Correct answer = B. The patient is experiencing episodes of complex partial seizures. Complex partial seizures impair consciousness and can occur in all age groups. Typically, staring is accompanied by impaired consciousness and recall. If asked a question, the patient might respond with an inappropriate or unintelligible answer. Automatic movements are associated with most complex partial seizures and involve the mouth and face (lip-smacking, chewing, tasting, and swallowing movements), upper extremities (fumbling, picking, tapping, or clasping movements), vocal apparatus (grunts or repetition of words and phrases), as are complex acts (such as walking or mixing foods in a bowl).

12.7 A 52-year-old man has had several focal complex partial seizures over the last year. Which one of the following therapies would be the most appropriate initial therapy for this patient?

A. Ethosuximide.
B. Levetiracetam.
C. Diazepam.
D. Carbamazepine plus primidone.
E. Watchful waiting.

Correct answer = B. The patient has had many seizures, and the risks of not starting drug therapy would be substantially greater than the risks of treating his seizures. Because the patient has impaired consciousness during the seizure, he is at risk for injury during an attack. Monotherapy with primary agents is preferred for most patients. The advantages of monotherapy include reduced frequency of adverse effects, absence of interactions between antiepileptic drugs, lower cost, and improved compliance. Ethosuximide and diazepam are not indicated for complex partial seizures.

12.8 A patient with focal complex partial seizures has been treated for 6 months with carbamazepine but, recently, has been experiencing breakthrough seizures on a more frequent basis. You are considering adding a second drug to the antiseizure regimen. Which of the following drugs is least likely to have a pharmacokinetic interaction with carbamazepine?

A. Topiramate.
B. Tiagabine.
C. Levetiracetam.
D. Lamotrigine.
E. Zonisamide.

Correct answer = C. Of the drugs listed, all of which are approved as adjunct therapy for refractory focal complex partial seizures, only levetiracetam does not affect the pharmacokinetics of other antiepileptic drugs, and other drugs do not significantly alter its pharmacokinetics. However, any of the listed drugs could be added depending on the plan and the patient characteristics. Treatment of epilepsy is complex, and diagnosis is based on history and may need to be reevaluated when drug therapy fails or seizures increase.

12.9 Which of the following is a first-line medication for generalized tonic–clonic seizures?

A. Ethosuximide.
B. Felbamate.
C. Vigabatrin.
D. Ezogabine.
E. Topiramate.

Correct answer = E. Topiramate is a broad spectrum antiepilepsy medication that is indicated for primary generalized tonic–clonic seizures. Ethosuximide should only be used for absence seizures. Felbamate is reserved for refractory seizures due to the risk of aplastic anemia and liver failure. Vigabatrin is not indicated for generalized seizures and is associated with visual field defects. Ezogabine is indicated for focal seizures and has been implicated in retinal abnormalities.

12.10 A 75-year-old woman had a stroke approximately 1 month ago. She is continuing to have small focal seizures where she fails to respond appropriately while talking. Which of the following is the most appropriate treatment for this individual?

A. Phenytoin.
B. Oxcarbazepine.
C. Levetiracetam.
D. Phenobarbital.

Correct answer = C. Levetiracetam is renally cleared and prone to very few drug interactions. Elderly patients usually have more comorbidities and are taking more medications than younger patients. Oxcarbazepine may cause hyponatremia, which is more symptomatic in the elderly. Phenytoin and phenobarbital have many drug interactions and a side effect profile that may be especially troublesome in the elderly age group including dizziness that may lead to falls, cognitive issues, and bone health issues.

Anesthetics

13

Thomas B. Whalen

I. OVERVIEW

General anesthesia is a reversible state of central nervous system (CNS) depression, causing loss of response to and perception of stimuli. For patients undergoing surgical or medical procedures, anesthesia provides five important benefits:

- Sedation and reduced anxiety
- Lack of awareness and amnesia
- Skeletal muscle relaxation
- Suppression of undesirable reflexes
- Analgesia

Because no single agent provides all desirable properties, several categories of drugs are combined to produce optimal anesthesia (Figure 13.1). Preanesthetics help calm patients, relieve pain, and prevent side effects of subsequently administered anesthetics or the procedure itself. Neuromuscular blockers facilitate tracheal intubation and surgery. Potent general anesthetics are delivered via inhalation and/or intravenous (IV) injection. Except for *nitrous oxide*, inhaled anesthetics are volatile, halogenated hydrocarbons. IV anesthetics consist of several chemically unrelated drug types commonly used to rapidly induce anesthesia.

II. PATIENT FACTORS IN SELECTION OF ANESTHESIA

Drugs are chosen to provide safe and efficient anesthesia based on the type of procedure and patient characteristics such as organ function, medical conditions, and concurrent medications.

A. Status of organ systems

1. **Cardiovascular system:** Anesthetic agents suppress cardiovascular function to varying degrees. This is an important consideration in patients with coronary artery disease, heart failure, dysrhythmias, valvular disease, and other cardiovascular disorders. Hypotension may develop during anesthesia, resulting in reduced perfusion pressure and ischemic injury to tissues. Treatment with vasoactive agents may be necessary. Some anesthetics, such as *halothane*, sensitize the heart to arrhythmogenic effects of sympathomimetic agents.

PREANESTHETIC MEDICATIONS
Antacids
Anticholinergics
Antiemetics
Antihistamines
Benzodiazepines
Opioids

GENERAL ANESTHETICS: INHALED
Desflurane SUPRANE
Halothane FLUOTHANE
Isoflurane FORANE
Nitrous oxide NITROUS OXIDE
Sevoflurane ULTANE

GENERAL ANESTHETICS: INTRAVENOUS
Barbiturates
Benzodiazepines
Dexmedetomidine PRECEDEX
Etomidate AMIDATE
Ketamine KETALAR
Opioids
Propofol DIPRIVAN

NEUROMUSCULAR BLOCKERS (see Chapter 5)
Cisatracurium, pancuronium, rocuronium, succinylcholine, vecuronium

LOCAL ANESTHETICS: AMIDES
Bupivacaine MARCAINE
Lidocaine XYLOCAINE
Mepivacaine CARBOCAINE
Ropivacaine NAROPIN

LOCAL ANESTHETICS: ESTERS
Chloroprocaine NESACAINE
Procaine NOVOCAINE
Tetracaine PONTOCAINE

Figure 13.1
Summary of common drugs used for anesthesia. See Chapter 5 for summary of neuromuscular-blocking agents.

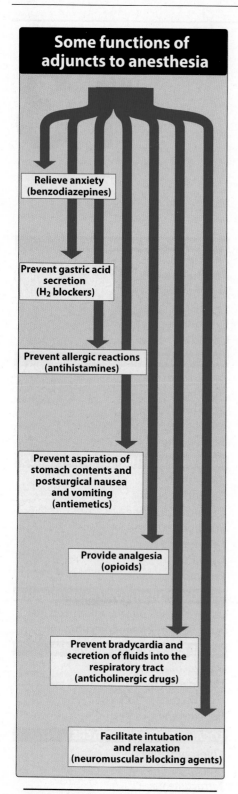

Some functions of adjuncts to anesthesia

Relieve anxiety (benzodiazepines)

Prevent gastric acid secretion (H₂ blockers)

Prevent allergic reactions (antihistamines)

Prevent aspiration of stomach contents and postsurgical nausea and vomiting (antiemetics)

Provide analgesia (opioids)

Prevent bradycardia and secretion of fluids into the respiratory tract (anticholinergic drugs)

Facilitate intubation and relaxation (neuromuscular blocking agents)

Figure 13.2
Actions of anesthesia adjunct drugs.

2. **Respiratory system:** Respiratory function must be considered for all anesthetics. Asthma and ventilation or perfusion abnormalities complicate control of inhalation anesthetics. Inhaled agents depress respiration but also act as bronchodilators. IV anesthetics and opioids suppress respiration. These effects may influence the ability to provide adequate ventilation and oxygenation during and after surgery.

3. **Liver and kidney:** The liver and kidneys influence long-term distribution and clearance of drugs and are also target organs for toxic effects. Release of fluoride, bromide, and other metabolites of halogenated hydrocarbons can affect these organs, especially if they accumulate with frequently repeated administration of anesthetics.

4. **Nervous system:** The presence of neurologic disorders (for example, epilepsy, myasthenia gravis, neuromuscular disease, compromised cerebral circulation) influences the selection of anesthetic.

5. **Pregnancy:** Special precautions should be observed when anesthetics and adjunctive agents are administered during pregnancy. Effects on fetal organogenesis are a major concern in early pregnancy. Transient use of *nitrous oxide* may cause aplastic anemia in the fetus. Oral clefts have occurred in fetuses when mothers received benzodiazepines in early pregnancy. Benzodiazepines should not be used during labor because of resultant temporary hypotonia and altered thermoregulation in the newborn.

B. Concomitant use of drugs

1. **Multiple adjunct agents:** Commonly, patients receive one or more of these preanesthetic medications: H₂ blockers (*famotidine, ranitidine*) to reduce gastric acidity; benzodiazepines (*midazolam, diazepam*) to allay anxiety and facilitate amnesia; nonopioids (*acetaminophen, celecoxib*) or opioids (*fentanyl*) for analgesia; antihistamines (*diphenhydramine*) to prevent allergic reactions; antiemetics (*ondansetron*) to prevent nausea; and/or anticholinergics (*glycopyrrolate*) to prevent bradycardia and secretion of fluids into the respiratory tract (Figure 13.2). Premedications facilitate smooth induction of anesthesia and lower required anesthetic doses. However, they can also enhance undesirable anesthetic effects (hypoventilation) and, when coadministered, may produce negative effects not observed when given individually.

2. **Concomitant use of other drugs:** Patients may take medications for underlying diseases or abuse drugs that alter response to anesthetics. For example, alcoholics have elevated levels of liver enzymes that metabolize anesthetics, and drug abusers may be tolerant to opioids.

III. STAGES AND DEPTH OF ANESTHESIA

General anesthesia has three stages: induction, maintenance, and recovery. Induction is the time from administration of a potent anesthetic to development of effective anesthesia. Maintenance provides sustained anesthesia. Recovery is the time from discontinuation of anesthetic until consciousness and protective reflexes return. Induction of anesthesia depends on how fast effective concentrations of anesthetic reach the brain. Recovery is essentially the reverse of induction and depends on how fast the anesthetic diffuses from the brain. Depth of anesthesia is the degree to which the CNS is depressed.

A. Induction

General anesthesia in adults is normally induced with an IV agent like *propofol*, producing unconsciousness in 30 to 40 seconds. Additional inhalation and/or IV drugs may be given to produce the desired depth of anesthesia. [Note: This often includes an IV neuromuscular blocker such as *rocuronium*, *vecuronium*, or *succinylcholine* to facilitate tracheal intubation and muscle relaxation.] For children without IV access, nonpungent agents, such as *sevoflurane*, are inhaled to induce general anesthesia.

B. Maintenance of anesthesia

After administering the anesthetic, vital signs and response to stimuli are monitored continuously to balance the amount of drug inhaled and/or infused with the depth of anesthesia. Maintenance is commonly provided with volatile anesthetics, which offer good control over the depth of anesthesia. Opioids such as *fentanyl* are used for analgesia along with inhalation agents, because the latter are not good analgesics. IV infusions of various drugs may be used during the maintenance phase.

C. Recovery

Postoperatively, the anesthetic admixture is withdrawn, and the patient is monitored for return of consciousness. For most anesthetic agents, recovery is the reverse of induction. Redistribution from the site of action (rather than metabolism of the drug) underlies recovery. If neuromuscular blockers have not been fully metabolized, reversal agents may be used. The patient is monitored to assure full recovery, with normal physiologic functions (spontaneous respiration, acceptable blood pressure and heart rate, intact reflexes, and no delayed reactions such as respiratory depression).

D. Depth of anesthesia

The depth of anesthesia has four sequential stages characterized by increasing CNS depression as the anesthetic accumulates in the brain (Figure 13.3). [Note: These stages were defined for the original anesthetic *ether*, which produces a slow onset of anesthesia. With modern anesthetics, the stages merge because of the rapid onset of stage III.]

1. **Stage I—Analgesia:** Loss of pain sensation results from interference with sensory transmission in the spinothalamic tract. The patient progresses from conscious and conversational to drowsy. Amnesia and reduced awareness of pain occur as stage II is approached.

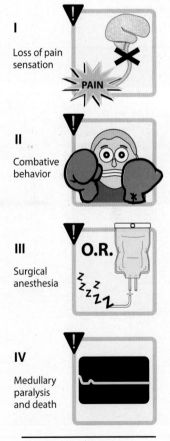

I
Loss of pain sensation

PAIN

II
Combative behavior

III
Surgical anesthesia

O.R.

z z z z z

IV
Medullary paralysis and death

Figure 13.3
Stages of anesthesia.
O.R. = operating room.

2. **Stage II—Excitement:** The patient displays delirium and possibly combative behavior. A rise and irregularity in blood pressure and respiration occur, as well as a risk of laryngospasm. To shorten or eliminate this stage, rapid-acting IV agents are given before inhalation anesthesia is administered.

3. **Stage III—Surgical anesthesia:** There is gradual loss of muscle tone and reflexes as the CNS is further depressed. Regular respiration and relaxation of skeletal muscles with eventual loss of spontaneous movement occur. This is the ideal stage for surgery. Careful monitoring is needed to prevent undesired progression to stage IV.

4. **Stage IV—Medullary paralysis:** Severe depression of the respiratory and vasomotor centers occurs. Ventilation and/or circulation must be supported to prevent death.

IV. INHALATION ANESTHETICS

Inhaled gases are used primarily for maintenance of anesthesia after administration of an IV agent (Figure 13.4). Depth of anesthesia can be rapidly altered by changing the inhaled concentration. Inhalational agents have very steep dose–response curves and very narrow therapeutic indices, so the difference in concentrations causing surgical anesthesia and

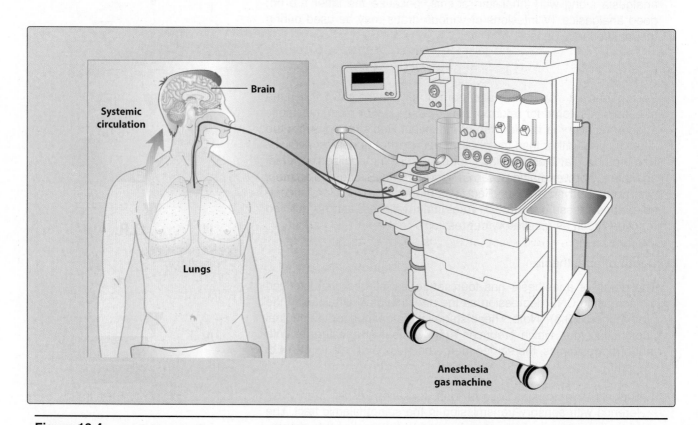

Figure 13.4
Volatile anesthetics delivered to the patient are absorbed via the lungs into the systemic circulation causing dose-dependent CNS depression.

severe cardiac and respiratory depression is small. No antagonists exist. To minimize waste, potent inhaled agents are delivered in a recirculation system containing absorbents that remove carbon dioxide and allow rebreathing of the agent.

A. Common features of inhalation anesthetics

Modern inhalation anesthetics are nonflammable, nonexplosive agents, including *nitrous oxide* and volatile, halogenated hydrocarbons. These agents decrease cerebrovascular resistance, resulting in increased brain perfusion. They cause bronchodilation but also decrease both spontaneous ventilation and hypoxic pulmonary vasoconstriction (increased pulmonary vascular resistance in poorly aerated regions of the lungs, redirecting blood flow to more oxygenated regions). Movement of these agents from the lungs to various body compartments depends upon their solubility in blood and tissues, as well as on blood flow. These factors play a role in induction and recovery.

B. Potency

Potency is defined quantitatively as the minimum alveolar concentration (MAC), the end-tidal concentration of inhaled anesthetic needed to eliminate movement in 50% of patients stimulated by a standardized incision. MAC is the median effective dose (ED_{50}) of the anesthetic, expressed as the percentage of gas in a mixture required to achieve that effect. Numerically, MAC is small for potent anesthetics such as *sevoflurane* and large for less potent agents such as *nitrous oxide*. The inverse of MAC is, thus, an index of potency. MAC values are used to compare pharmacologic effects of different anesthetics (high MAC equals low potency; Figure 13.5). *Nitrous oxide* alone cannot produce complete anesthesia, because an admixture with sufficient oxygen cannot approach its MAC value. The more lipid soluble an anesthetic, the lower the concentration needed to produce anesthesia and, thus, the higher the potency. Factors that can increase MAC (make the patient less sensitive) include hyperthermia, drugs that increase CNS catecholamines, and chronic ethanol abuse. Factors that can decrease MAC (make the patient more sensitive) include increased age, hypothermia, pregnancy, sepsis, acute intoxication, concurrent IV anesthetics, and α_2-adrenergic receptor agonists (for example, *clonidine*, *dexmedetomidine*).

C. Uptake and distribution of inhalation anesthetics

The principal objective of inhalation anesthesia is a constant and optimal brain partial pressure (P_{br}) of inhaled anesthetic (partial pressure equilibrium between alveoli [P_{alv}] and brain [P_{br}]). Thus, the alveoli are the "windows to the brain" for inhaled anesthetics. The partial pressure of an anesthetic gas at the origin of the respiratory pathway is the driving force moving the anesthetic into the alveolar space and, thence, into the blood (P_a), which delivers the drug to the brain and other body compartments. Because gases move from one body compartment to another according to partial pressure gradients, steady state is achieved when the partial pressure in each of these

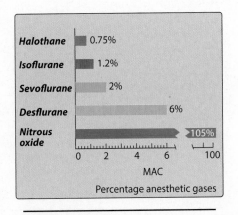

Figure 13.5

Minimal alveolar concentrations (MAC) for anesthetic gases.

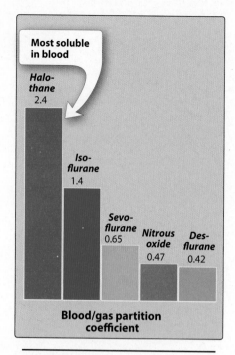

Figure 13.6
Blood/gas partition coefficients for some inhalation anesthetics.

compartments is equivalent to that in the inspired mixture. [Note: At equilibrium, $P_{alv} = P_a = P_{br}$.] The time course for attaining this steady state is determined by the following factors:

1. **Alveolar wash-in:** This refers to replacement of normal lung gases with the inspired anesthetic mixture. The time required for this process is directly proportional to the functional residual capacity of the lung (volume of gas remaining in the lungs at the end of a normal expiration) and inversely proportional to ventilatory rate. It is independent of the physical properties of the gas. As the partial pressure builds within the lung, anesthetic transfer from the lung begins.

2. **Anesthetic uptake (removal to peripheral tissues other than the brain):** Uptake is the product of gas solubility in the blood, cardiac output (CO), and the gradient between alveolar and blood anesthetic partial pressures.

   a. **Solubility in blood:** This is determined by a physical property of the anesthetic called the blood/gas partition coefficient (the ratio of the concentration of anesthetic in the blood phase to the concentration of anesthetic in the gas phase when the anesthetic is in equilibrium between the two phases; Figure 13.6). For inhaled anesthetics, think of the blood as a pharmacologically inactive reservoir. Drugs with low versus high solubility in blood differ in their speed of induction of anesthesia. When an anesthetic gas with low blood solubility such as *nitrous oxide* diffuses from the alveoli into the circulation, little anesthetic dissolves in the blood. Therefore, equilibrium between inhaled anesthetic and arterial blood occurs rapidly, and relatively few additional molecules of anesthetic are required to raise arterial anesthetic partial pressure. Agents with low solubility in blood, thus, quickly saturate the blood. In contrast, anesthetic gases with high blood solubility, such as *halothane*, dissolve more completely in the blood, and greater amounts of anesthetic and longer periods of time are required to raise blood partial pressure. This results in increased times of induction and recovery and slower changes in depth of anesthesia in response to changes in the concentration. The solubility in blood is ranked as follows: *halothane > isoflurane > sevoflurane > nitrous oxide > desflurane.*

   b. **Cardiac output:** CO affects removal of anesthetic to peripheral tissues, which are not the site of action. For inhaled anesthetics, higher CO removes anesthetic from the alveoli faster (due to increased blood flow through the lungs) and thus slows the rate of rise in alveolar concentration of gas. It therefore takes longer for the gas to reach equilibrium between the alveoli and the site of action in the brain. For inhaled anesthetics, higher CO equals slower induction. Again, for inhaled anesthetics, think of the blood as a pharmacologically inactive reservoir. Low CO (shock) speeds the rate of rise of the alveolar concentration of gas, since there is less removal to peripheral tissues. [Note: See section on Intravenous Anesthetics for effects of CO on IV anesthetics.]

c. **Alveolar-to-venous partial pressure gradient of anesthetic:** This is the driving force of anesthetic delivery. For all practical purposes, pulmonary end-capillary anesthetic partial pressure may be considered equal to alveolar anesthetic partial pressure if the patient does not have severe lung diffusion disease. The arterial circulation distributes the anesthetic to various tissues, and the pressure gradient drives free anesthetic gas into tissues. As venous circulation returns blood depleted of anesthetic to the lung, more gas moves into the blood from the lung according to the partial pressure difference. The greater the difference in anesthetic concentration between alveolar (arterial) and venous blood, the higher the uptake and the slower the induction. Over time, the partial pressure in venous blood closely approximates that in the inspired mixture, and no further net anesthetic uptake from the lung occurs.

3. **Effect of different tissue types on anesthetic uptake:** The time required for a particular tissue to achieve steady state with the partial pressure of an anesthetic gas in the inspired mixture is inversely proportional to the blood flow to that tissue (greater flow results in a more rapidly achieved steady state). It is also directly proportional to the capacity of that tissue to store anesthetic (a larger capacity results in a longer time required to achieve steady state). Capacity, in turn, is directly proportional to the tissue's volume and the tissue/blood solubility coefficient of the anesthetic. Four major tissue compartments determine the time course of anesthetic uptake:

a. **Brain, heart, liver, kidney, and endocrine glands:** These highly perfused tissues rapidly attain steady state with the partial pressure of anesthetic in the blood.

b. **Skeletal muscles:** These are poorly perfused during anesthesia and have a large volume, which prolongs the time required to achieve steady state.

c. **Fat:** Fat is also poorly perfused. However, potent volatile anesthetics are very lipid soluble, so fat has a large capacity to store them. Slow delivery to a high-capacity compartment prolongs the time required to achieve steady state in fat tissue.

d. **Bone, ligaments, and cartilage:** These are poorly perfused and have a relatively low capacity to store anesthetic. Therefore, these tissues have minimal impact on the time course of anesthetic distribution in the body.

4. **Washout:** When an inhalation anesthetic is discontinued, the body becomes the "source" that drives the anesthetic back into the alveolar space. The same factors that influence attainment of steady state with an inspired anesthetic determine the time course of its clearance from the body. Thus, *nitrous oxide* exits the body faster than *halothane* (Figure 13.7).

D. Mechanism of action

No specific receptor has been identified as the locus of general anesthetic action. The fact that chemically unrelated compounds produce anesthesia argues against the existence of a single receptor.

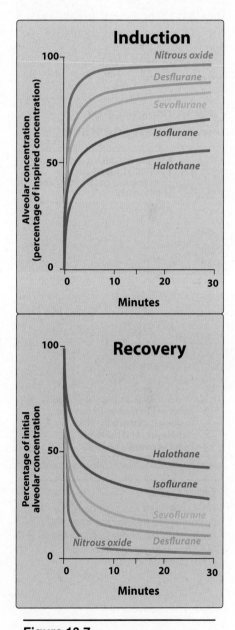

Figure 13.7
Changes in the alveolar blood concentrations of some inhalation anesthetics over time.

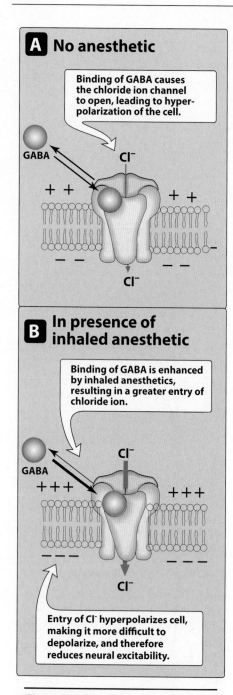

A No anesthetic

Binding of GABA causes the chloride ion channel to open, leading to hyperpolarization of the cell.

GABA   Cl⁻

+ +   + +

Cl⁻

B In presence of inhaled anesthetic

Binding of GABA is enhanced by inhaled anesthetics, resulting in a greater entry of chloride ion.

Cl⁻

GABA

+++   +++

Cl⁻

Entry of Cl⁻ hyperpolarizes cell, making it more difficult to depolarize, and therefore reduces neural excitability.

Figure 13.8
An example of modulation of a ligand-gated membrane channel modulated by inhaled anesthetics. GABA = γ-aminobutyric acid; Cl⁻ = chloride ion.

It appears that a variety of molecular mechanisms may contribute to the activity of general anesthetics. At clinically effective concentrations, general anesthetics increase the sensitivity of the γ-aminobutyric acid (GABA$_A$) receptors to the inhibitory neurotransmitter GABA. This increases chloride ion influx and hyperpolarization of neurons. Postsynaptic neuronal excitability and, thus, CNS activity are diminished (Figure 13.8). Unlike other anesthetics, *nitrous oxide* and *ketamine* do not have actions on GABA$_A$ receptors. Their effects are likely mediated via inhibition of the *N*-methyl-D-aspartate (NMDA) receptors. [Note: The NMDA receptor is a glutamate receptor. Glutamate is the body's main excitatory neurotransmitter.] Other receptors are also affected by volatile anesthetics. For example, the activity of the inhibitory glycine receptors in the spinal motor neurons is increased. In addition, inhalation anesthetics block excitatory postsynaptic currents of nicotinic receptors. The mechanism by which anesthetics perform these modulatory roles is not fully understood.

E. Halothane

Halothane is the prototype to which newer inhalation anesthetics are compared. When *halothane* [HAL-oh-thane] was introduced, its rapid induction and quick recovery made it an anesthetic of choice. Due to adverse effects and the availability of other anesthetics with fewer complications, *halothane* has been replaced in most countries.

1. **Therapeutic uses:** *Halothane* is a potent anesthetic but a relatively weak analgesic. Thus, it is usually coadministered with *nitrous oxide*, opioids, or local anesthetics. It is a potent bronchodilator. *Halothane* relaxes both skeletal and uterine muscles and can be used in obstetrics when uterine relaxation is indicated. *Halothane* is not hepatotoxic in children (unlike its potential effect on adults). Combined with its pleasant odor, it is suitable in pediatrics for inhalation induction, although *sevoflurane* is now the agent of choice.

2. **Pharmacokinetics:** *Halothane* is oxidatively metabolized in the body to tissue-toxic hydrocarbons (for example, trifluoroethanol) and bromide ion. These substances may be responsible for toxic reactions that some adults (especially females) develop after *halothane* anesthesia. This begins as a fever, followed by anorexia, nausea, and vomiting, and possibly signs of hepatitis. Although the incidence is low (approximately 1 in 10,000), half of affected patients may die of hepatic necrosis. To avoid this condition, *halothane* is not administered at intervals of less than 2 to 3 weeks. All halogenated inhalation anesthetics have been associated with hepatitis, but at a much lower incidence than with *halothane*.

3. **Adverse effects:**

   a. **Cardiac effects:** Halogenated hydrocarbons are vagomimetic and may cause *atropine*-sensitive bradycardia. In addition, *halothane* has the undesirable property of causing cardiac arrhythmias. [Note: *Halothane* can sensitize the heart to effects of catecholamines such as norepinephrine.] Halogenated anesthetics produce concentration-dependent hypotension. This is best treated with a direct-acting vasoconstrictor, such as *phenylephrine*.

b. **Malignant hyperthermia:** In a very small percentage of susceptible patients, exposure to halogenated hydrocarbon anesthetics or the neuromuscular blocker *succinylcholine* may induce malignant hyperthermia (MH), a rare life-threatening condition. MH causes a drastic and uncontrolled increase in skeletal muscle oxidative metabolism, overwhelming the body's capacity to supply oxygen, remove carbon dioxide, and regulate temperature, eventually leading to circulatory collapse and death if not treated immediately. Strong evidence indicates that MH is due to an excitation–contraction coupling defect. Burn victims and individuals with muscular dystrophy, myopathy, myotonia, and osteogenesis imperfecta are susceptible to MH. Susceptibility to MH is often inherited as an autosomal dominant disorder. Should a patient exhibit symptoms of MH, *dantrolene* is given as the anesthetic mixture is withdrawn, and measures are taken to rapidly cool the patient. *Dantrolene* [DAN-tro-lean] blocks release of Ca^{2+} from the sarcoplasmic reticulum of muscle cells, reducing heat production and relaxing muscle tone. It should be available whenever triggering agents are administered. In addition, the patient must be monitored and supported for respiratory, circulatory, and renal problems. Use of *dantrolene* and avoidance of triggering agents such as halogenated anesthetics in susceptible individuals have markedly reduced mortality from MH.

F. Isoflurane

This agent undergoes little metabolism and is, therefore, not toxic to the liver or kidney. *Isoflurane* [eye-so-FLOOR-ane] does not induce cardiac arrhythmias or sensitize the heart to catecholamines. However, like other halogenated gases, it produces dose-dependent hypotension. It has a pungent odor and stimulates respiratory reflexes (for example, breath holding, salivation, coughing, laryngospasm) and is therefore not used for inhalation induction. With higher blood solubility than *desflurane* and *sevoflurane*, *isoflurane* is typically used only when cost is a factor.

G. Desflurane

Desflurane [DES-floor-ane] provides very rapid onset and recovery due to low blood solubility. This makes it a popular anesthetic for outpatient procedures. However, it has a low volatility, requiring administration via a special heated vaporizer. Like *isoflurane*, it decreases vascular resistance and perfuses all major tissues very well. Because it stimulates respiratory reflexes, *desflurane* is not used for inhalation induction. It is relatively expensive and thus rarely used for maintenance during extended anesthesia. Its degradation is minimal and tissue toxicity is rare.

H. Sevoflurane

Sevoflurane [see-voe-FLOOR-ane] has low pungency, allowing rapid induction without irritating the airways. This makes it suitable for inhalation induction in pediatric patients. It has a rapid onset and recovery due to low blood solubility. *Sevoflurane* is metabolized by the liver, and compounds formed in the anesthesia circuit may be nephrotoxic if fresh gas flow is too low.

I. Nitrous oxide

Nitrous oxide [NYE-truss OX-ide] ("laughing gas") is a nonirritating potent analgesic but a weak general anesthetic. It is frequently used at concentrations of 30 to 50% in combination with oxygen for analgesia, particularly in dentistry. *Nitrous oxide* alone cannot produce surgical anesthesia, but it is commonly combined with other more potent agents. *Nitrous oxide* is poorly soluble in blood and other tissues, allowing it to move very rapidly in and out of the body. Within closed body compartments, *nitrous oxide* can increase the volume (for example, causing a pneumothorax) or pressure (for example, in the sinuses), because it replaces nitrogen in various air spaces faster than the nitrogen leaves. Its speed of movement allows *nitrous oxide* to retard oxygen uptake during recovery, thereby causing "diffusion hypoxia," which can be overcome by significant concentrations of inspired oxygen during recovery. *Nitrous oxide* does not depress respiration and does not produce muscle relaxation. When coadministered with other anesthetics, it has moderate to no effect on the cardiovascular system or on increasing cerebral blood flow, and it is the least hepatotoxic of the inhalation agents. Therefore, it is probably the safest of these anesthetics, provided that sufficient oxygen is administered simultaneously. Some characteristics of the inhalation anesthetics are summarized in Figure 13.9.

V. INTRAVENOUS ANESTHETICS

IV anesthetics cause rapid induction often occurring within one "arm–brain circulation time," or the time it takes to travel from the site of injection (usually the arm) to the brain, where it has its effect. Anesthesia may then be maintained with an inhalation agent. IV anesthetics may be used as sole agents for short procedures or administered as infusions to help maintain anesthesia during longer cases. In lower doses, they may be used for sedation.

A. Induction

After entering the blood, a percentage of drug binds to plasma proteins, and the rest remains unbound or "free." The degree of protein binding depends upon the physical characteristics of the drug, such as the degree of ionization and lipid solubility. The drug is carried by venous blood to the right side of the heart, through the pulmonary circulation, and via the left heart into the systemic circulation. The majority of CO flows to the brain, liver, and kidney ("vessel-rich organs"). Thus, a high proportion of initial drug bolus is delivered to the cerebral circulation and then passes along a concentration gradient from blood into the brain. The rate of this transfer is dependent on the arterial concentration of the unbound free drug, the lipid solubility of the drug, and the degree of ionization. Unbound, lipid-soluble, nonionized molecules cross into the brain most quickly. Once the drug has penetrated the CNS, it exerts its effects. Like inhalation anesthetics, the exact mode of action of IV anesthetics is unknown.

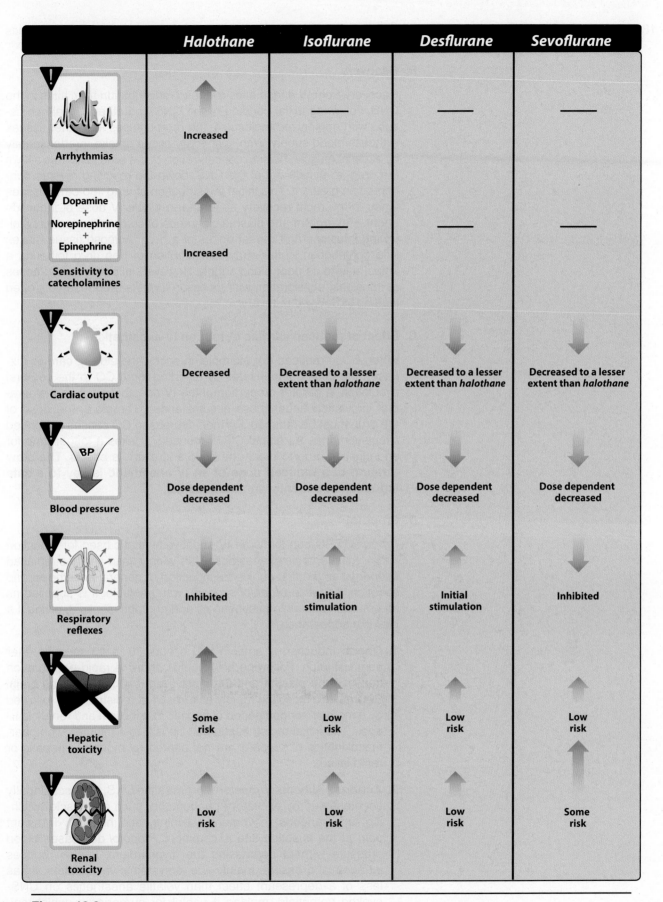

	Halothane	Isoflurane	Desflurane	Sevoflurane
Arrhythmias	Increased	—	—	—
Sensitivity to catecholamines (Dopamine + Norepinephrine + Epinephrine)	Increased	—	—	—
Cardiac output	Decreased	Decreased to a lesser extent than *halothane*	Decreased to a lesser extent than *halothane*	Decreased to a lesser extent than *halothane*
Blood pressure	Dose dependent decreased	Dose dependent decreased	Dose dependent decreased	Dose dependent decreased
Respiratory reflexes	Inhibited	Initial stimulation	Initial stimulation	Inhibited
Hepatic toxicity	Some risk	Low risk	Low risk	Low risk
Renal toxicity	Low risk	Low risk	Low risk	Some risk

Figure 13.9
Characteristics of some inhalation anesthetics.

B. Recovery

Recovery from IV anesthetics is due to redistribution from sites in the CNS. Following initial flooding of the CNS and other vessel-rich tissues with nonionized molecules, the drug diffuses into other tissues with less blood supply. With secondary tissue uptake, predominantly by skeletal muscle, plasma concentration of the drug falls. This allows the drug, to diffuse out of the CNS, down the resulting reverse concentration gradient. This initial redistribution of drug into other tissues leads to the rapid recovery seen after a single IV dose of induction agent. Metabolism and plasma clearance become important only following infusions and repeat doses of a drug. Adipose tissue makes little contribution to the early redistribution of free drug following a bolus, due to its poor blood supply. However, following repeat doses or infusions, equilibration with fat tissue forms a drug reservoir, often leading to delayed recovery.

C. Effect of reduced cardiac output on IV anesthetics

When CO is reduced (for example, in shock, the elderly, cardiac disease), the body compensates by diverting more CO to the cerebral circulation. A greater proportion of the IV anesthetic enters the cerebral circulation under these circumstances. Therefore, the dose of the drug must be reduced. Further, decreased CO causes prolonged circulation time. As global CO is reduced, it takes a longer time for an induction drug to reach the brain and exert its effects. **The slow titration of a reduced dose of an IV anesthetic is key to a safe induction in patients with reduced CO.**

D. Propofol

Propofol [PRO-puh-fol] is an IV sedative/hypnotic used for induction and/or maintenance of anesthesia. It is widely used and has replaced *thiopental* as the first choice for induction of general anesthesia and sedation. Because *propofol* is poorly water soluble, it is supplied as an emulsion containing soybean oil and egg phospholipid, giving it a milk-like appearance.

1. **Onset:** Induction is smooth and occurs 30 to 40 seconds after administration. Following an IV bolus, there is rapid equilibration between the plasma and the highly perfused tissue of the brain. Plasma levels decline rapidly as a result of redistribution, followed by a more prolonged period of hepatic metabolism and renal clearance. The initial redistribution half-life is 2 to 4 minutes. The pharmacokinetics of *propofol* are not altered by moderate hepatic or renal failure.

2. **Actions:** Although *propofol* depresses the CNS, it is occasionally accompanied by excitatory phenomena, such as muscle twitching, spontaneous movement, yawning, and hiccups. Transient pain at the injection site is common. *Propofol* decreases blood pressure without depressing the myocardium. It also reduces intracranial pressure, mainly due to systemic vasodilation. It has less of a depressant effect than volatile anesthetics on CNS-evoked potentials, making it useful for surgeries in which spinal cord function is monitored. It does not provide analgesia, so

supplementation with narcotics is required. *Propofol* is commonly infused in lower doses to provide sedation. The incidence of postoperative nausea and vomiting is very low, as this agent has some antiemetic effects.

E. Barbiturates

Thiopental [thigh-oh-PEN-tahl] is an ultra–short-acting barbiturate with high lipid solubility. It is a potent anesthetic but a weak analgesic. Barbiturates require supplementary analgesic administration during anesthesia. When given IV, agents such as *thiopental* and *methohexital* [meth-oh-HEX-uh-tall] quickly enter the CNS and depress function, often in less than 1 minute. However, diffusion out of the brain can also occur very rapidly because of redistribution to other tissues (Figure 13.10). These drugs may remain in the body for relatively long periods, because only about 15% of a dose entering the circulation is metabolized by the liver per hour. Thus, metabolism of *thiopental* is much slower than its redistribution. *Thiopental* has minor effects on the normal cardiovascular system, but may contribute to severe hypotension in patients with hypovolemia or shock. All barbiturates can cause apnea, coughing, chest wall spasm, laryngospasm, and bronchospasm (of particular concern for asthmatics). These agents have largely been replaced with newer agents that are better tolerated. *Thiopental* is no longer available in many countries, including the United States.

F. Benzodiazepines

The benzodiazepines are used in conjunction with anesthetics for sedation. The most commonly used is *midazolam* [my-DAZ-o-lam]. *Diazepam* [dye-AZ-uh-pam] and *lorazepam* [lore-AZ-uh-pam] are alternatives. All three facilitate amnesia while causing sedation, enhancing the inhibitory effects of various neurotransmitters, particularly GABA. Minimal cardiovascular depressant effects are seen, but all are potential respiratory depressants (especially when administered IV). They are metabolized by the liver with variable elimination half-lives, and *erythromycin* may prolong their effects. Benzodiazepines can induce a temporary form of anterograde amnesia in which the patient retains memory of past events, but new information is not transferred into long-term memory. Therefore, important treatment information should be repeated to the patient after the effects of the drug have worn off.

G. Opioids

Because of their analgesic property, opioids are commonly combined with other anesthetics. The choice of opioid is based primarily on the duration of action needed. The most commonly used opioids are *fentanyl* [FEN-ta-nil] and its congeners, *sufentanil* [SOO-fen-ta-nil] and *remifentanil* [REMI-fen-ta-nil], because they induce analgesia more rapidly than *morphine*. They may be administered intravenously, epidurally, or intrathecally (into the cerebrospinal fluid). Opioids are not good amnesics, and they can all cause hypotension, respiratory depression, and muscle rigidity, as well as postanesthetic nausea and vomiting. Opioid effects can be antagonized by *naloxone*.

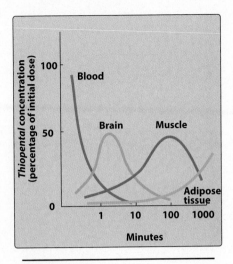

Figure 13.10
Redistribution of *thiopental* from the brain to muscle and adipose tissue.

H. Etomidate

Etomidate [ee-TOM-uh-date] is a hypnotic agent used to induce anesthesia, but it lacks analgesic activity. Its water solubility is poor, so it is formulated in a propylene glycol solution. Induction is rapid, and the drug is short-acting. Among its benefits are little to no effect on the heart and circulation. *Etomidate* is usually only used for patients with coronary artery disease or cardiovascular dysfunction. Its adverse effects include decreased plasma cortisol and aldosterone levels, which can persist up to 8 hours. *Etomidate* should not be infused for an extended time, because prolonged suppression of these hormones is hazardous. Injection site reaction and involuntary skeletal muscle movements are not uncommon. The latter are managed by administration of benzodiazepines and opioids.

I. Ketamine

Ketamine [KET-uh-meen], a short-acting, nonbarbiturate anesthetic, induces a dissociated state in which the patient is unconscious (but may appear to be awake) and does not feel pain. This dissociative anesthesia provides sedation, amnesia, and immobility. *Ketamine* stimulates central sympathetic outflow, causing stimulation of the heart with increased blood pressure and CO. It is also a potent bronchodilator. Therefore, it is beneficial in patients with hypovolemic or cardiogenic shock and in asthmatics. Conversely, it is contraindicated in hypertensive or stroke patients. The drug is lipophilic and enters the brain very quickly. Like the barbiturates, it redistributes to other organs and tissues. *Ketamine* is used mainly in children and elderly adults for short procedures. It is not widely used, because it increases cerebral blood flow and may induce hallucinations, particularly in young adults. *Ketamine* may be used illicitly, since it causes a dream-like state and hallucinations similar to *phencyclidine* (PCP).

J. Dexmedetomidine

Dexmedetomidine [dex-med-eh-TOM-uh-deen] is a sedative used in intensive care settings and surgery. It is relatively unique in its ability to provide sedation without respiratory depression. Like *clonidine*, it is an α_2 receptor agonist in certain parts of the brain. *Dexmedetomidine* has sedative, analgesic, sympatholytic, and anxiolytic effects that blunt many cardiovascular responses. It reduces volatile anesthetic, sedative, and analgesic requirements without causing significant respiratory depression. Some therapeutic advantages and disadvantages of the anesthetic agents are summarized in Figure 13.11.

VI. NEUROMUSCULAR BLOCKERS

Neuromuscular blockers are used to abolish reflexes to facilitate tracheal intubation and provide muscle relaxation as needed for surgery. Their mechanism of action is blockade of nicotinic acetylcholine receptors in the neuromuscular junction. These agents, which include *cisatracurium*, *pancuronium*, *rocuronium*, *succinylcholine*, and *vecuronium*, are described in Chapter 5.

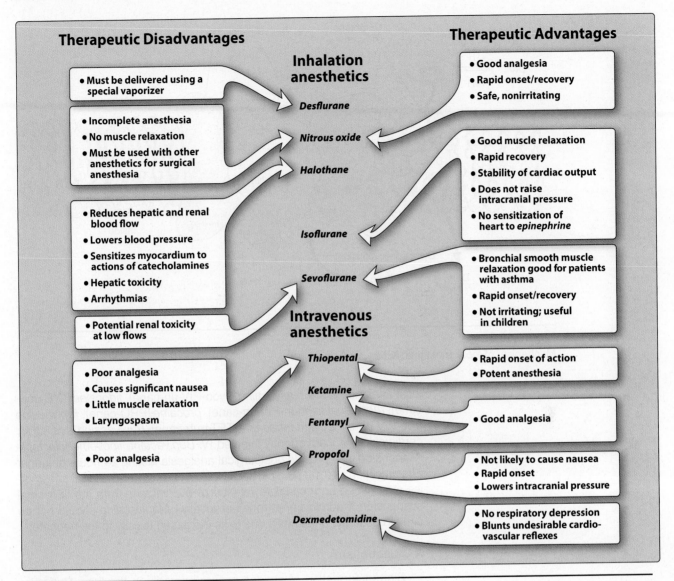

Figure 13.11
Therapeutic disadvantages and advantages of some anesthetic agents.

VII. LOCAL ANESTHETICS

Local anesthetics block nerve conduction of sensory impulses and, in higher concentrations, motor impulses from the periphery to the CNS. Na^+ ion channels are blocked to prevent the transient increase in permeability of the nerve membrane to Na^+ that is required for an action potential (Figure 13.12). When propagation of action potentials is prevented, sensation cannot be transmitted from the source of stimulation to the brain. Delivery techniques include topical administration, infiltration, peripheral nerve blocks, and neuraxial (spinal, epidural, or caudal) blocks. Small, unmyelinated nerve fibers for pain, temperature, and autonomic activity are most sensitive. Structurally, local anesthetics all include a lipophilic group joined by an amide or ester linkage to a carbon chain, which, in turn, is joined to a hydrophilic group (Figure 13.13). The most widely used

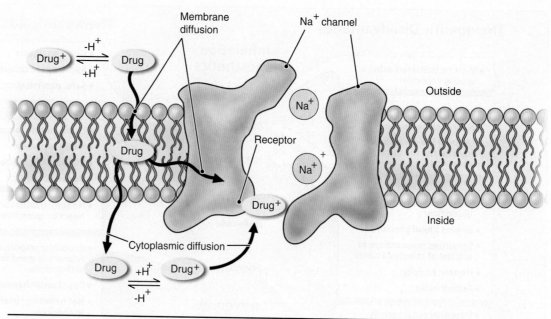

Figure 13.12
Mechanism of local anesthetic action.

local anesthetics are *bupivacaine* [byoo-PIV-uh-cane], *lidocaine* [LYE-doe-cane], *mepivacaine* [muh-PIV-uh-cane], *procaine* [PRO-cane], *ropivacaine* [roe-PIV-uh-cane], and *tetracaine* [TET-truh-cane]. *Bupivacaine* is noted for cardiotoxicity if inadvertently injected IV. *Bupivacaine liposome injectable suspension* may provide postsurgical analgesia lasting 24 hours or longer after injection into the surgical site. [Note: Non-*bupivacaine* local anesthetics may cause an immediate release of *bupivacaine* from the liposomal suspension if administered together locally.] *Mepivacaine* should not be used in obstetric anesthesia due to its increased toxicity to the neonate.

A. Metabolism

Biotransformation of amides occurs primarily in the liver. *Prilocaine* [PRY-low-cane], a dental anesthetic, is also metabolized in the plasma and kidney, and one of its metabolites may lead to methemoglobinemia. Esters are biotransformed by plasma cholinesterase (pseudocholinesterase). Patients with pseudocholinesterase deficiency may metabolize ester local anesthetics more slowly. At normal doses, this has little clinical effect. Reduced hepatic function predisposes patients to toxic effects, but should not significantly increase the duration of action of local anesthetics.

B. Onset and duration of action

The onset and duration of action of local anesthetics are influenced by several factors including tissue pH, nerve morphology, concentration, pKa, and lipid solubility of the drug. Of these, the pH of the tissue and pKa are most important. At physiologic pH, these compounds are charged. The ionized form interacts with the protein receptor of the Na^+ channel to inhibit its function and achieve local anesthesia. The pH may drop in infected sites, causing onset to be delayed or even prevented. Within limits, higher concentration and greater lipid solubility

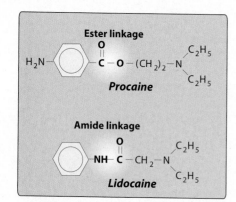

Figure 13.13
Representative structures of ester and amide anesthetics.

improve onset somewhat. Duration of action depends on the length of time the drug can stay near the nerve to block sodium channels.

C. Actions

Local anesthetics cause vasodilation, leading to rapid diffusion away from the site of action and shorter duration when these drugs are administered alone. By adding the vasoconstrictor *epinephrine*, the rate of local anesthetic absorption and diffusion is decreased. This minimizes systemic toxicity and increases the duration of action. Hepatic function does not affect the duration of action of local anesthesia, which is determined by redistribution and not biotransformation. Some local anesthetics have other therapeutic uses (for example, *lidocaine* is an IV antiarrhythmic).

D. Allergic reactions

Patient reports of allergic reactions to local anesthetics are fairly common, but often times reported "allergies" are actually side effects from *epinephrine* added to the local anesthetic. Psychogenic reactions to injections may be misdiagnosed as allergic reactions and may also mimic them with signs such as urticaria, edema, and bronchospasm. True allergy to an amide local anesthetic is exceedingly rare, whereas the ester *procaine* is somewhat more allergenic. Allergy to one ester rules out use of another ester, because the allergenic component is the metabolite para-aminobenzoic acid, produced by all esters. In contrast, allergy to one amide does not rule out the use of another amide. A patient may be allergic to other compounds in the local anesthetic, such as preservatives in multidose vials.

E. Administration to children and the elderly

Before administering local anesthetic to a child, the maximum dose based on weight should be calculated to prevent accidental overdose. There are no significant differences in response to local anesthetics between younger and older adults. It is prudent to stay well below maximum recommended doses in elderly patients who often have some compromise in liver function. Because some degree of cardiovascular compromise may be expected in elderly patients, reducing the dose of *epinephrine* may be prudent. Local anesthetics are safe for patients who are susceptible to MH.

F. Systemic local anesthetic toxicity

Toxic blood levels of the drug may be due to repeated injections or could result from a single inadvertent IV injection. Aspiration before every injection is imperative. The signs, symptoms, and timing of local anesthetic systemic toxicity are unpredictable. One must consider the diagnosis in any patient with altered mental status or cardiovascular instability following injection of local anesthetic. CNS symptoms (either excitation or depression) may be apparent but may also be subtle, nonspecific, or absent. Treatment for systemic local anesthetic toxicity includes airway management, support of breathing and circulation, seizure suppression and, if needed, cardiopulmonary resuscitation. Administering a 20% lipid emulsion infusion (lipid rescue therapy) is a valuable asset. Figure 13.14 summarizes pharmacologic properties of some local anesthetics.

CHARACTERISTIC	ESTERS	• Procaine • Tetracaine • Chloroprocaine • Cocaine	AMIDES	• Lidocaine • Mepivacaine • Bupivacaine • Prilocaine • Ropivacaine
Metabolism		Rapid by plasma cholinesterase		Slow, hepatic
Systemic toxicity		Less likely		More likely
Allergic reaction		Possible- PABA derivatives form		Very rare
Stability in solution		Breaks down in ampules (heat, sun)		Very stable chemically
Onset of action		Slow as a general rule		Moderate to fast
pK$_a$'s		Higher than physiologic pH (8.5–8.9)		Close to physiologic pH (7.6–8.1)

DRUG	POTENCY	ONSET	DURATION
Procaine	Low	Rapid	Short
Chloroprocaine	Low	Rapid	Short
Tetracaine	High	Slow	Long (spinal)
Lidocaine	Low	Rapid	Intermediate
Mepivacaine	Low	Moderate	Intermediate
Bupivacaine	High	Slow	Long
Ropivacaine	High	Moderate	Long

Figure 13.14

Summary of pharmacologic properties of some local anesthetics. PABA = para-aminobenzoic acid.

Study Questions

Choose the ONE best answer.

13.1 Which of the following is a potent analgesic but a weak anesthetic?

A. Etomidate.
B. Halothane.
C. Midazolam.
D. Nitrous oxide.
E. Thiopental.

Correct answer = D. Etomidate is a hypnotic agent but lacks analgesic activity. Midazolam is a common sedative/amnestic. Halothane and thiopental are potent anesthetics with weak analgesic properties. Nitrous oxide provides good analgesia but is a weak anesthetic that must be combined with other agents to provide complete anesthesia.

13.2 The potency of inhaled anesthetics is defined quantitatively as:

A. Blood/gas partition coefficient.
B. Cerebrovascular resistance.
C. Minimum alveolar concentration.
D. Diffusion hypoxia.

Correct answer = C. Potency of inhaled anesthetics is defined by MAC, equivalent to the median effective dose (ED$_{50}$) of the anesthetic. Blood/gas partition coefficient determines solubility of the gas in blood. Cerebrovascular resistance is decreased by inhalation anesthetics. Diffusion hypoxia is associated with nitrous oxide.

13.3 Which of the following determines the speed of recovery from intravenous anesthetics used for induction?

A. Liver metabolism of the drug.
B. Protein binding of the drug.
C. Ionization of the drug.
D. Redistribution of the drug from sites in the CNS.
E. Plasma clearance of the drug.

Correct answer = D. Following initial flooding of the CNS with nonionized molecules, the drug diffuses into other tissues. With secondary tissue uptake, the plasma concentration falls, allowing the drug to diffuse out of the CNS. This initial redistribution of drug into other tissues leads to the rapid recovery seen after a single dose of an IV induction drug. Protein binding, ionization, and lipid solubility affect the rate of transfer.

13.4 Which one of the following is a potent intravenous anesthetic but a weak analgesic?

A. Propofol.
B. Benzodiazepines.
C. Ketamine.
D. Fentanyl.
E. Isoflurane.

Correct answer = A. Propofol is a potent anesthetic but a weak analgesic. It is the most widely used intravenously administered general anesthetic. It has a high lipid solubility. The other choices do not fit this profile.

13.5 Which of the following is correct regarding local anesthetics?

A. They affect only small, unmyelinated nerve fibers.
B. They have either a lipophilic or a hydrophilic group.
C. They have either an amide or an ester linkage.
D. They are unaffected by pH of the tissue and pKa of the drug.
E. In their ionized form, they interact with the protein receptor of calcium channels.

Correct answer = C. The small, unmyelinated nerve fibers that conduct impulses for pain, temperature, and autonomic activity are most sensitive to the action of local anesthetics, but other nerve fibers are affected also. Local anesthetics have a lipophilic group, joined by either an amide or ester linkage to a carbon chain that, in turn, is joined to a hydrophilic group. Onset and duration of action of local anesthetics are influenced by both pH of the tissue and pK_a of the drug. Local anesthetics work by blocking sodium ion channels.

13.6 Which of the following is correct regarding malignant hyperthermia?

A. It is triggered by dantrolene.
B. It is triggered by local anesthetics.
C. It is generally mild and clinically insignificant.
D. It has no familial component.
E. It involves increased skeletal muscle oxidative metabolism.

Correct answer = E. Malignant hyperthermia involves increased skeletal muscle oxidative metabolism and is a life-threatening condition. Dantrolene is the specific pharmacologic treatment. Local anesthetics have been shown to be safe. Triggering agents include *succinylcholine* and halogenated hydrocarbon volatile anesthetic agents in susceptible individuals. Susceptibility to malignant hyperthermia is inherited in an autosomal dominant fashion.

13.7 A patient with heart failure and significantly reduced cardiac output requires surgical anesthesia. Which of the following would you expect to see in this patient?

A. Slower induction time with IV anesthetics.
B. Need for increased dosage of IV anesthetics.
C. Slower induction time with inhaled anesthetics.
D. Enhanced removal of inhaled anesthetics to peripheral tissues.

Correct answer = A. When cardiac output is reduced, the body compensates by diverting more cardiac output to the cerebral circulation. A greater proportion of the IV anesthetic enters the cerebral circulation under these circumstances. Therefore, the dose of the IV drug must be reduced (not increased). Also, with reduced cardiac output, it takes a longer time for an IV induction drug to reach the brain, resulting in a slower induction time. For inhaled anesthetics, lower cardiac output removes anesthetic from the alveoli to the peripheral tissues more slowly and thus enhances the rate of rise in alveolar concentration of gas. Therefore, the gas reaches equilibrium between the alveoli and the site of action in the brain more quickly.

13.8 An 80-year-old patient with asthma and low blood pressure requires anesthesia for an emergency surgical procedure. Which of the following agents would be most appropriate for inducing anesthesia in this patient?

A. Desflurane.
B. Ketamine.
C. Propofol.
D. Thiopental.

Correct answer = B. Ketamine may be beneficial since it is a potent bronchodilator and may not lower blood pressure like other agents. Desflurane is an inhaled anesthetic that may stimulate respiratory reflexes. It is used for maintenance, not induction, and may lower blood pressure. Propofol may also decrease blood pressure. Thiopental is a short-acting barbiturate that can cause bronchospasm.

13.9 A 52-year-old woman will be undergoing sedation with propofol for a brief diagnostic procedure. Which of the following is an advantage of propofol for this patient?

A. Rapid analgesia.

B. Sustained duration.

C. Decreased incidence of nausea and vomiting.

D. Less pain at the injection site.

Correct answer = C. Propofol has some antiemetic effect, so it does not cause postoperative nausea and vomiting. It has a short duration of action (which makes it good for brief procedures), but does not produce analgesia. Pain at the injection site is common.

13.10 A 32-year-old woman requests an epidural to ease labor pains. She reports that she had an allergic reaction to Novocain (procaine) at the dentist's office. Which of the following local anesthetics would be appropriate for use in an epidural for this patient?

A. Chloroprocaine.

B. Mepivacaine.

C. Ropivacaine.

D. Tetracaine.

Correct answer = C. Procaine is an ester local anesthetic. Since this patient has an allergy to procaine, other ester anesthetics (chloroprocaine, tetracaine) should not be used. Mepivacaine, an amide local anesthetic, should not be used due to the potential for increased toxicity to the neonate. Ropivacaine is an amide anesthetic.

Opioids

14

Robin Moorman Li

I. OVERVIEW

Management of pain is one of clinical medicine's greatest challenges. Pain is defined as an unpleasant sensation that can be either acute or chronic and is a consequence of complex neurochemical processes in the peripheral and central nervous systems (CNS). It is subjective, and the clinician must rely on the patient's perception and description of pain. Alleviation of pain depends on the specific type of pain, nociceptive or neuropathic pain. For example, with mild to moderate arthritic pain (nociceptive pain), nonopioid analgesics such as nonsteroidal anti-inflammatory agents (NSAIDs, see Chapter 36) are often effective. Neuropathic pain can be treated with opioids (some situations require higher doses) but responds best to anticonvulsants, tricyclic antidepressants, or serotonin/norepinephrine reuptake inhibitors. However, for severe or chronic malignant or nonmalignant pain, opioids are considered part of the treatment plan in select patients (Figure 14.1). Opioids are natural, semisynthetic, or synthetic compounds that produce *morphine*-like effects (Figure 14.2). These agents are divided into chemical classes based on their chemical structure (Figure 14.3). Clinically this is helpful in identifying opioids that have a greater chance of cross-sensitivity in a patient with an allergy to a particular opioid. All opioids act by binding to specific opioid receptors in the CNS to produce effects that mimic the action of endogenous peptide neurotransmitters (for example, endorphins, enkephalins, and dynorphins). Although the opioids have a broad range of effects, their primary use is to relieve intense pain, whether that pain results from surgery, injury, or chronic disease. Unfortunately, widespread availability of opioids has led to abuse of those agents with euphoric properties. Antagonists that reverse the actions of opioids are also clinically important for use in cases of overdose (Figure 14.1).

II. OPIOID RECEPTORS

The major effects of the opioids are mediated by three receptor families, which are commonly designated as μ (mu), κ (kappa), and δ (delta). Each receptor family exhibits a different specificity for the drug(s) it binds. The analgesic properties of the opioids are primarily mediated by the μ receptors that modulate responses to thermal, mechanical, and chemical nociception. The κ receptors in the dorsal horn also contribute to analgesia by modulating the response to chemical and thermal nociception.

STRONG AGONISTS
Alfentanil ALFENTA
Fentanyl ABSTRAL, ACTIQ, DURAGESIC, FENTORA, LAZANDA, SUBSYS
Heroin
Hydrocodone LORTAB, VICODIN, VARIOUS
Hydromorphone DILAUDID, EXALGO
Meperidine DEMEROL
Methadone DOLOPHINE
Morphine AVINZA, KADIAN, MS CONTIN, ORAMORPH
Oxycodone OXYCONTIN
Oxymorphone OPANA
Remifentanil ULTIVA
Sufentanil SUFENTA

MODERATE/LOW AGONISTS
Codeine

MIXED AGONIST–ANTAGONIST AND PARTIAL AGONISTS
Buprenorphine BUPRENEX, SUBUTEX
Butorphanol
Nalbuphine NUBAIN
Pentazocine TALWIN

ANTAGONISTS
Naloxone NARCAN
Naltrexone REVIA, VIVITROL

OTHER ANALGESICS
Tapentadol NUCYNTA
Tramadol ULTRAM

Figure 14.1
Summary of opioid analgesics and antagonists.

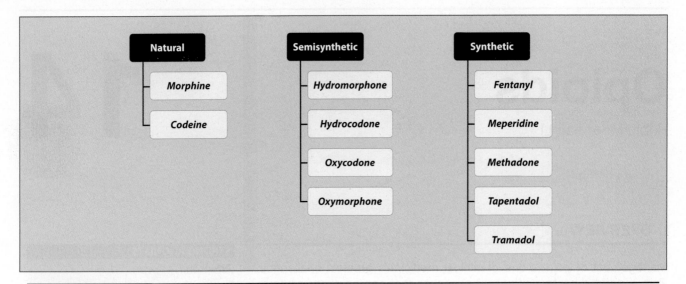

Figure 14.2
Summary of chemical classes of opioid agonists.

Phenanthrenes	Action on Opioid Receptors
Morphine	Agonist
Codeine	Agonist
Oxycodone	Agonist
Oxymorphone	Agonist
Hydromorphone	Agonist
Hydrocodone	Agonist
Buprenorphine	Partial agonist
Nalbuphine	Mixed Agonist/Antagonist
Butorphanol	Mixed Agonist/Antagonist
Benzmorphan	
Pentazocine	Mixed Agonist/Antagonist
Phenylpiperidines	
Fentanyl	Agonist
Alfentanil	Agonist
Sufentanil	Agonist
Meperidine	Agonist
Diphenylheptane	
Methadone	Agonist

Figure 14.3
Origin of opioids: natural, semisynthetic, or synthetic.

The enkephalins interact more selectively with δ receptors in the periphery. All three opioid receptors are members of the G protein–coupled receptor family and inhibit adenylyl cyclase. They are also associated with ion channels, increasing postsynaptic K^+ efflux (hyperpolarization) or reducing presynaptic Ca^{2+} influx, thus impeding neuronal firing and transmitter release (Figure 14.4).

III. OPIOID AGONISTS

Morphine [MOR-feen] is the major analgesic drug contained in crude opium and is the prototype strong μ receptor agonist. *Codeine* is present in crude opium in lower concentrations and is inherently less potent, making *codeine* the prototype of the weak opioid agonists. The currently available opioids have various differences in receptor affinity, pharmacokinetic profiles, available routes of administration, and adverse effect profiles. Comparing other available opioids to *morphine* is helpful in identifying the unique differences to guide the selection of a safe and effective pain management regimen (Figure 14.5).

A. Morphine

1. **Mechanism of action:** *Morphine* and other opioids exert their major effects by interacting stereospecifically with opioid receptors on the membranes of certain cells in the CNS and other anatomic structures, such as the gastrointestinal (GI) tract and the urinary bladder. *Morphine also* acts at κ receptors in lamina I and II of the dorsal horn of the spinal cord. It decreases the release of substance P, which modulates pain perception in the spinal cord. *Morphine* also appears to inhibit the release of many excitatory transmitters from nerve terminals carrying nociceptive (painful) stimuli. Some therapeutic uses of *morphine* and other opioids are listed in Figure 14.6.

2. Actions:

a. **Analgesia:** *Morphine* and other opioids cause analgesia (relief of pain without the loss of consciousness) and relieve pain both by raising the pain threshold at the spinal cord level and, more importantly, by altering the brain's perception of pain. Patients treated with opioids are still aware of the presence of pain, but the sensation is not unpleasant. The maximum analgesic efficacy for representative opioid agonists is shown in Figure 14.7.

b. **Euphoria:** *Morphine* produces a powerful sense of contentment and well-being. Euphoria may be caused by disinhibition of the dopamine-containing neurons of the ventral tegmental area.

c. **Respiration:** *Morphine* causes respiratory depression by reduction of the sensitivity of respiratory center neurons to carbon dioxide. This can occur with ordinary doses of *morphine* in patients who are opioid-naïve and can be accentuated as the dose is increased until ultimately respiration ceases. Respiratory depression is the most common cause of death in acute opioid overdoses. Tolerance to this effect does develop quickly with repeated dosing, which allows the safe use of *morphine* for the treatment of pain when the dose is correctly titrated.

d. **Depression of cough reflex:** Both *morphine* and *codeine* have antitussive properties. In general, cough suppression does not correlate closely with the analgesic and respiratory depressant properties of opioid drugs. The receptors involved in the antitussive action appear to be different from those involved in analgesia.

e. **Miosis:** The pinpoint pupil (Figure 14.8) characteristic of *morphine* use results from stimulation of μ and κ receptors. There is little tolerance to the effect, and all *morphine* abusers demonstrate pinpoint pupils. [Note: This is important diagnostically, because many other causes of coma and respiratory depression produce dilation of the pupil.]

f. **Emesis:** *Morphine* directly stimulates the chemoreceptor trigger zone in the area postrema that causes vomiting.

g. **GI tract:** *Morphine* relieves diarrhea by decreasing the motility and increasing the tone of the intestinal circular smooth muscle. *Morphine* also increases the tone of the anal sphincter. Overall, *morphine* and other opioids produce constipation, with little tolerance developing. [Note: A nonprescription laxative combination of the stool softener *docusate* with the stimulant laxative *senna* is useful to treat opioid-induced constipation.] *Morphine* can also increase biliary tract pressure due to contraction of the gallbladder and constriction of the biliary sphincter.

h. **Cardiovascular:** *Morphine* has no major effects on the blood pressure or heart rate at lower dosages. With large doses, hypotension and bradycardia may occur. Because of respiratory depression and carbon dioxide retention, cerebral vessels dilate and increase cerebrospinal fluid pressure. Therefore, *morphine* is usually contraindicated in individuals with head trauma or severe brain injury.

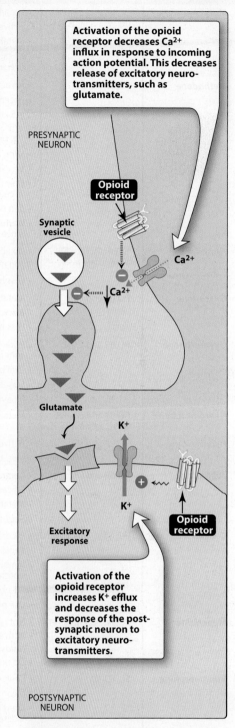

Figure 14.4
Mechanism of action of μ opioid receptor agonists in the spinal cord.

Opioid	Routes of Administration	Comments
Morphine	PO (IR and ER), PR, IM, IV, SC, IA, SL, EA	• For all drugs listed: opioid class side effects (Figure 14.9). • Active metabolites are renally eliminated and accumulate in renal impairment. • Metabolite M3G has no analgesic action, but can be neuroexcitatory. • Metabolite M6G is two to four times more potent than parent drug; accumulation can cause oversedation and respiratory depression.

Methadone	PO, IV, IM, SC	• No active metabolites.
		• Racemic mixture
		  • **S isomer:** NMDA antagonist; aids in preventing opioid tolerance and treatment of neuropathic pain.
		  • **R isomer:** μ agonist in treatment of nociceptive pain.
		• Long and variable half-life increases risks of overdose.
		• Very lipophilic and redistributes to fat stores.
		• Duration of analgesia is much shorter than elimination half-life. Repeated dosing can lead to accumulation.
		• Can prolong QT interval and cause torsades de pointes.
		• Warning: Conversion to and from *methadone* and other opioids should be done with great care, since equianalgesic dosing varies dramatically.

Fentanyl	IV, EA, IA, TD, OTFC, SL, Buccal, Nasal	• No active metabolites; option for patients with renal dysfunction but should be used with caution. • 100 times more potent than *morphine*. • Less histamine release, sedation, and constipation in comparison to *morphine*.
Oxycodone	PO (IR and CR)	• Metabolized by CYP2D6 and CYP3A4. • Black box warning: CYP3A4 drug interactions. • Less histamine release and nausea in comparison to *morphine*.
Oxymorphone	PO (IR and ER), IV	• Immediate release has longer duration of action and elimination half-life (8 hours) compared to other immediate-release opioids. • Oral bioavailability increases with food. • Should be administered 1 to 2 hours after eating. • Bioavailability increased with coadministration of alcohol.
Hydromorphone	PO (IR and ER), PR, IV, SC, EA, IA	• Metabolized via glucuronidation to H6G and H3G which are renally eliminated and can cause CNS side effects in patients with renal insufficiency.
Hydrocodone	PO (IR and ER)	• Active metabolite is *hydromorphone*. • Metabolized by CYP2D6 and CYP3A4.
Tapentadol	PO (IR and ER)	• Centrally acting analgesic; μ agonist activity along with inhibition of norepinephrine reuptake. • Efficacy in treating nociceptive and neuropathic pain. • Metabolized predominately by glucuronidation; no CYP450 interactions. • Seizures and serotonin syndrome can occur in predisposed patients.
Codeine	PO, SC	• Prodrug: Metabolized by CYP2D6 to the active drug *morphine*. • Rapid and poor metabolizers of CYP2D6 can experience toxicity. • Inhibitors of CYP2D6 will prevent conversion of *codeine* to *morphine*, thereby preventing pain control. • Do not use in patients with renal dysfunction. • Use only for mild or moderate pain.
Meperidine	PO, IV, SC, EA, IA	• Not recommended as first-line opioid choice. • Active metabolite normeperidine accumulates with renal dysfunction, leading to toxicity. • *Naloxone* does not antagonize the effects of normeperidine; could worsen seizure activity. • Do not use in elderly, patients with renal dysfunction, or for chronic pain management.
Buprenorphine	SL, TD, IM	• Long duration of action; very lipophilic. • Incompletely reversible by *naloxone*. • Drug interactions: contraindicated with *atazanavir, conivaptan,* MAO inhibitors; also many interactions with CYP450 system, including CYP3A4. • Can prolong QT interval. • Avoid use in patients with hypokalemia, atrial fibrillation, or unstable heart failure, or other predisposing factors increasing QT abnormalities. • Transdermal patch is applied every 7 days.

CR = controlled-release; EA = epidural anesthesia; IA = intrathecal anesthesia; IM = intramuscular; IR = immediate release; IV = intravenous; OTFC = oral transmucosal fentanyl citrate; PO = orally; PR = rectally; SC = subcutaneous; SL = sublingual; TD = transdermal; M3G = morphine-3-glucuronide; M6G = morphine-6-glucuronide; NMDA = N-methyl-D-aspartate; H6G = hydromorphone-6-glucuronide; H3G = hydromorphone-3-glucuronide

Note: There are many different acronyms which may be used to indicate a medication is extended-release. Examples include CR (controlled-release), LA (long-acting), ER (extended-release).

Figure 14.5

Summary of clinically relevant properties for each of the μ receptor agonists.

i. **Histamine release:** *Morphine* releases histamine from mast cells causing urticaria, sweating, and vasodilation. Because it can cause bronchoconstriction, *morphine* should be used with caution in patients with asthma.

j. **Hormonal actions:** *Morphine* increases growth hormone release and enhances prolactin secretion. It increases antidiuretic hormone and leads to urinary retention.

k. **Labor:** *Morphine* may prolong the second stage of labor by transiently decreasing the strength, duration, and frequency of uterine contractions.

3. **Pharmacokinetics:**

a. **Administration:** Because significant first-pass metabolism of *morphine* occurs in the liver, intramuscular, subcutaneous, and IV injections produce the most reliable responses. Absorption of *morphine* from the GI tract after oral absorption is slow and erratic. When used orally, *morphine* is commonly administered in an extended-release form to provide more consistent plasma levels. It is important to note that *morphine* has a linear pharmacokinetic profile that allows dosing to be more predictable and more flexible.

b. **Distribution:** *Morphine* rapidly enters all body tissues, including the fetuses of pregnant women. It should not be used for analgesia during labor. Infants born to addicted mothers show physical dependence on opioids and exhibit withdrawal symptoms if opioids are not administered. Only a small percentage of *morphine* crosses the blood–brain barrier, because *morphine* is the least lipophilic of the common opioids. In contrast, the more lipid-soluble opioids, such as *fentanyl* and *methadone*, readily penetrate into the CNS.

c. **Fate:** *Morphine* is conjugated with glucuronic acid in the liver to two main metabolites. Morphine-6-glucuronide is a very potent analgesic, whereas morphine-3-glucuronide does not have analgesic activity, but is believed to cause the neuroexcitatory effects seen with high doses of *morphine.* The conjugates are excreted primarily in urine, with small quantities appearing in bile. The duration of action of *morphine* is 4 to 5 hours when administered systemically to *morphine*-naïve individuals, but considerably longer when injected epidurally because the low lipophilicity prevents redistribution from the epidural space. [Note: Age can influence the response to *morphine*. Elderly patients are more sensitive to the analgesic effects of the drug, possibly due to decreases in metabolism, lean body mass, or renal function. Lower starting doses should be considered for elderly patients. Neonates should not receive *morphine* because of their low conjugating capacity.]

4. **Adverse effects:** Many adverse effects are common across the entire opioid class (Figure 14.9). With most μ agonists, severe respiratory depression can occur and may result in death from acute opioid overdose. Respiratory drive may be suppressed in patients with emphysema or cor pulmonale. If opioids are used, respiration must

Therapeutic Use	Comments
Analgesia	*Morphine* is the prototype opioid agonist. Opioids are used for pain in trauma, cancer, and other types of severe pain.
Treatment of diarrhea	Opioids decrease the motility and increase the tone of intestinal circular smooth muscle. [Note: Agents commonly used include *diphenoxylate* and *loperamide* (see Chapter 31).]
Relief of cough	*Morphine* does suppress the cough reflex, but *codeine* and *dextromethorphan* are more commonly used.
Treatment of acute pulmonary edema	Intravenous *morphine* dramatically relieves dyspnea caused by pulmonary edema associated with left ventricular failure, possibly via the vasodilatory effect. This, in effect, decreases cardiac preload and afterload, as well as anxiety experienced by the patient.
Anesthesia	Opioids are used as pre-anesthetic medications, for systemic and spinal anesthesia, and for postoperative analgesia.

Figure 14.6
Selected clinical uses of opioids.

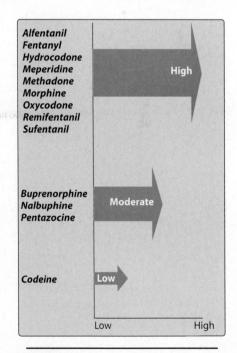

Figure 14.7
A comparison of opioid agonist efficacy.

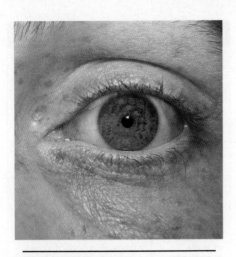

Figure 14.8
Characteristic pinpoint pupil associated with *morphine* use.

be closely monitored. Elevation of intracranial pressure, particularly in head injury, can be serious. *Morphine* should be used with caution in patients with asthma, liver disease, or renal dysfunction.

5. **Tolerance and physical dependence:** Repeated use produces tolerance to the respiratory depressant, analgesic, euphoric, and sedative effects of *morphine*. However, tolerance usually does not develop to the pupil-constricting and constipating effects of the drug. Physical and psychological dependence can occur with *morphine* and with some of the other agonists. Withdrawal produces a series of autonomic, motor, and psychological responses that incapacitate the individual and cause serious symptoms, although it is rare that the effects cause death.

6. **Drug interactions:** Drug interactions with *morphine* are rare, although the depressant actions of *morphine* are enhanced by phenothiazines, monoamine oxidase inhibitors (MAOIs), and tricyclic antidepressants (Figure 14.10).

B. Codeine

Codeine [KOE-deen] is a naturally occurring opioid that is a weak analgesic compared to *morphine*. It should be used only for mild to moderate pain. The analgesic actions of *codeine* are derived from its conversion to *morphine* by the CYP450 2D6 enzyme system (see Chapter 1). CYP450 2D6 activity varies in patients, and ultra-rapid metabolizers may experience higher levels of *morphine*, leading to possible overdose. Drug interactions associated with the CYP450 2D6 enzyme system may alter the efficacy of *codeine* or potentially lead to toxicity. *Codeine* is commonly used in combination with *acetaminophen* for management of pain. *Codeine* exhibits good antitussive activity at doses that do not cause analgesia. [Note: In most nonprescription cough preparations, *codeine* has been replaced by drugs such as *dextromethorphan*, a synthetic cough depressant that has relatively no analgesic action and a relatively low potential for abuse in usual antitussive doses.]

C. Oxycodone and oxymorphone

Oxycodone [ok-see-KOE-done] is a semisynthetic derivative of *morphine*. It is orally active and is sometimes formulated with *aspirin* or *acetaminophen*. Its oral analgesic effect is approximately twice that of *morphine*. *Oxycodone* is metabolized via the CYP450 2D6 and 3A4 enzyme systems and excreted via the kidney. Abuse of the sustained-release preparation (ingestion of crushed tablets) has been implicated in many deaths. It is important that the higher-dosage forms of the latter preparation be used only by patients who are tolerant to opioids. *Oxymorphone* [ox-ee-MOR-fone] is a semisynthetic opioid analgesic. When given parenterally it is approximately ten times more potent than *morphine*. The oral formulation has a lower relative potency and is about three times more potent than oral *morphine*. *Oxymorphone* is available in both immediate-acting and extended-release oral formulations. This agent has no clinically relevant drug–drug interactions associated with the CYP450 enzyme system.

D. Hydromorphone and hydrocodone

Hydromorphone [hye-droe-MORE-fone] and *hydrocodone* [hye-droe-KOE-done] are orally active, semisynthetic analogs of *morphine* and *codeine*, respectively. Oral *hydromorphone* is approximately 8 to 10 times more potent than *morphine*. It is preferred over *morphine* in patients with renal dysfunction due to less accumulation of active metabolites. *Hydrocodone* is the methyl ether of *hydromorphone*, but is a weaker analgesic than *hydromorphone*, with oral analgesic efficacy comparable to that of *morphine*. This agent is often combined with *acetaminophen* or *ibuprofen* to treat moderate to severe pain. It is also used as an antitussive. *Hydrocodone* is metabolized in the liver to several metabolites, one of which is *hydromorphone* via the actions of CYP450 2D6. Metabolism to *hydromorphone* can be affected by drug–drug interactions.

E. Fentanyl

Fentanyl [FEN-ta-nil], a synthetic opioid chemically related to *meperidine*, has 100-fold the analgesic potency of *morphine* and is used for anesthesia. The drug is highly lipophilic and has a rapid onset and short duration of action (15 to 30 minutes). It is usually administered IV, epidurally, or intrathecally. *Fentanyl* is combined with local anesthetics to provide epidural analgesia for labor and postoperative pain. IV *fentanyl* is used in anesthesia for its analgesic and sedative effects. An oral transmucosal preparation and a transdermal patch are also available. The oral transmucosal preparation is used in the treatment of cancer patients with breakthrough pain who are tolerant to opioids. The transdermal patch must be used with caution because death resulting from hypoventilation has been known to occur. Use is contraindicated in opioid-naïve patients, and patches should not be used in managing acute and postoperative pain. [Note: The transdermal patch creates a reservoir of the drug in the skin. Hence, the onset is delayed at least 12 hours, and the offset is prolonged.] *Fentanyl* is metabolized to inactive metabolites by the CYP450 3A4 system, and drugs that inhibit this isoenzyme can potentiate the effect of *fentanyl*. The drug and inactive metabolites are eliminated through the urine.

F. Sufentanil, alfentanil, and remifentanil

Sufentanil [soo-FEN-ta-nil], *alfentanil* [al-FEN-ta-nil], and *remifentanil* [rem-ih-FEN-ta-nil] are three synthetic opioid agonists related to *fentanyl*. They differ in potency and metabolic disposition. *Sufentanil* is even more potent than *fentanyl*, whereas the other two are less potent and shorter acting. These agents are mainly used for their analgesic and sedative properties during surgical procedures requiring anesthesia.

G. Methadone

Methadone [METH-a-done] is a synthetic, orally effective opioid that has variable equianalgesic potency compared to that of *morphine*, and the conversion between the two products is not linear. *Methadone* induces less euphoria and has a longer duration of action.

The actions of *methadone* are mediated by μ receptors. In addition, *methadone* is an antagonist of the *N*-methyl-D-aspartate (NMDA)

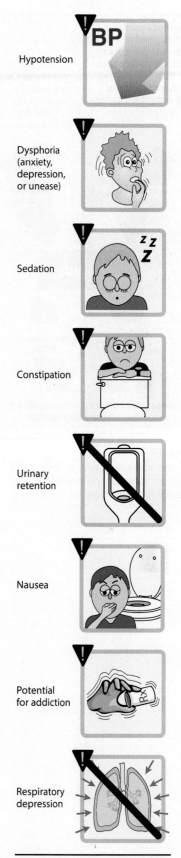

Hypotension

Dysphoria (anxiety, depression, or unease)

Sedation

Constipation

Urinary retention

Nausea

Potential for addiction

Respiratory depression

Figure 14.9
Adverse effects commonly observed in individuals treated with opioids.

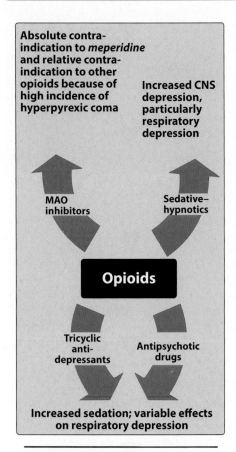

Absolute contra-indication to *meperidine* and relative contra-indication to other opioids because of high incidence of hyperpyrexic coma

Increased CNS depression, particularly respiratory depression

MAO inhibitors

Sedative–hypnotics

Opioids

Tricyclic anti-depressants

Antipsychotic drugs

Increased sedation; variable effects on respiratory depression

Figure 14.10
Drugs interacting with opioids. CNS = central nervous system; MAO = monoamine oxidase.

receptor and a norepinephrine and serotonin reuptake inhibitor. Thus, it has efficacy in the treatment of both nociceptive and neuropathic pain. *Methadone* is also used in the controlled withdrawal of dependent abusers from opioids and *heroin*. Oral *methadone* is administered as a substitute for the opioid of abuse, and the patient is then slowly weaned from *methadone*. The withdrawal syndrome with *methadone* is milder but more protracted (days to weeks) than that with other opioids. Unlike *morphine*, *methadone* is well absorbed after oral administration. It increases biliary pressure and is also constipating, but less so than *morphine*.

An understanding of the pharmacokinetics of *methadone* is important for proper use of this medication. *Methadone* is readily absorbed following oral administration, is biotransformed in the liver, and is excreted almost exclusively in feces. *Methadone* is very lipophilic, leading to accumulation in the fat tissues. The half-life of *methadone* ranges from 12 to 40 hours. It may extend up to 150 hours, although the actual duration of analgesia ranges from 4 to 8 hours. Consequently, the time frame it takes for an individual patient to reach steady state can vary dramatically, from 35 hours to 2 weeks. Upon repeated dosing, *methadone* can accumulate due to the long terminal half-life, thereby leading to toxicity. Overdose is possible when prescribers are unaware of the long half-life of *methadone*, the incomplete cross-tolerance between *methadone* and other opioids, and the proper titration guidelines to avoid its accumulation. The metabolism is variable because it relies on multiple CYP450 isoenzymes, some of which are affected by known genetic polymorphisms and are susceptible to many drug–drug interactions.

Methadone can produce physical dependence like that of *morphine*, but has less neurotoxicity than *morphine* due to the lack of active metabolites. *Methadone* can prolong the QT interval and cause torsades de pointes, possibly by interacting with cardiac potassium channels. It should be used with caution in patients with a family or personal history of QT prolongation or those taking other medications that can prolong the QT interval.

H. Meperidine

Meperidine [me-PER-i-deen] is a lower-potency synthetic opioid structurally unrelated to *morphine*. It is used for acute pain and acts primarily as a κ agonist, with some μ agonist activity also. *Meperidine* is very lipophilic and has anticholinergic effects, resulting in an increased incidence of delirium as compared to other opioids. The duration of action is slightly shorter than that of *morphine* and other opioids. *Meperidine* also has an active metabolite (normeperidine) that is renally excreted. Normeperidine has significant neurotoxic actions that can lead to delirium, hyperreflexia, myoclonus, and possibly seizures. Due to the short duration of action and the potential for toxicity, *meperidine* should only be used for short-term (≤48 hours) management of pain. Other agents are generally preferred. *Meperidine* should not be used in elderly patients or those with renal insufficiency, hepatic insufficiency, preexisting respiratory compromise, or concomitant or recent administration of MAOIs. Serotonin syndrome has also been reported in patients receiving both *meperidine* and selective serotonin reuptake inhibitors (SSRIs).

IV. PARTIAL AGONISTS AND MIXED AGONIST–ANTAGONISTS

Partial agonists bind to the opioid receptor, but have less intrinsic activity than full agonists (see Chapter 2). There is a ceiling to the pharmacologic effects of these agents. Drugs that stimulate one receptor but block another are termed mixed agonist–antagonists. The effects of these drugs depend on previous exposure to opioids. In individuals who have not received opioids (naïve patients), mixed agonist–antagonists show agonist activity and are used to relieve pain. In the patient with opioid dependence, the agonist–antagonist drugs may show primarily blocking effects (that is, produce withdrawal symptoms).

A. Buprenorphine

Buprenorphine [byoo-pre-NOR-feen] is classified as a partial agonist, acting at the µ receptor. It acts like *morphine* in naïve patients, but it can also precipitate withdrawal in users of *morphine* or other full opioid agonists. A major use is in opioid detoxification, because it has shorter and less severe withdrawal symptoms compared to *methadone* (Figure 14.11). It causes little sedation, respiratory depression, or hypotension, even at high doses. In contrast to *methadone*, which is available only at specialized clinics when used for detoxification or maintenance, *buprenorphine* is approved for office-based detoxification or maintenance. *Buprenorphine* is administered sublingually, parenterally, or transdermally and has a long duration of action because of its tight binding to the µ receptor. *Buprenorphine* tablets are indicated for the treatment of opioid dependence and are also available in a combination product containing *buprenorphine* and *naloxone*. *Naloxone* was added to prevent the abuse of *buprenorphine* via IV administration. The injectable form and the once-weekly transdermal patch are indicated for the relief of moderate to severe pain. *Buprenorphine* is metabolized by the liver and excreted in bile and urine. Adverse effects include respiratory depression that cannot easily be reversed by *naloxone* and decreased (or, rarely, increased) blood pressure, nausea, and dizziness.

B. Pentazocine

Pentazocine [pen-TAZ-oh-seen] acts as an agonist on κ receptors and is a weak antagonist at µ and δ receptors. *Pentazocine* promotes analgesia by activating receptors in the spinal cord, and it is used to relieve moderate pain. It may be administered either orally or parenterally. *Pentazocine* produces less euphoria compared to *morphine*. In higher doses, the drug causes respiratory depression and decreases the activity of the GI tract. High doses increase blood pressure and can cause hallucinations, nightmares, dysphoria, tachycardia, and dizziness. The latter properties have led to its decreased use. Despite its antagonist action, *pentazocine* does not antagonize the respiratory depression of *morphine*, but it can precipitate a withdrawal syndrome in a *morphine* abuser. Tolerance and dependence develop with repeated use. *Pentazocine* should be used with caution in patients with angina or coronary artery disease, since it can increase systemic and pulmonary arterial pressure and, thus, increase the work of the heart.

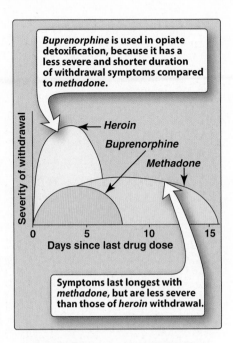

Buprenorphine is used in opiate detoxification, because it has a less severe and shorter duration of withdrawal symptoms compared to *methadone*.

Severity of withdrawal

Heroin
Buprenorphine
Methadone

Days since last drug dose

Symptoms last longest with *methadone*, but are less severe than those of *heroin* withdrawal.

Figure 14.11
Severity of opioid withdrawal symptoms after abrupt withdrawal of equivalent doses of *heroin*, *buprenorphine*, and *methadone*.

C. Nalbuphine and butorphanol

Nalbuphine [NAL-byoo-feen] and *butorphanol* [byoo-TOR-fa-nole] are mixed opioid agonist–antagonists. Like *pentazocine*, they play a limited role in the treatment of chronic pain. *Butorphanol* is available in a nasal formulation that has been used for severe headaches, but has also been associated with abuse. Neither agent is available for oral use. Their propensity to cause psychotomimetic effects (actions mimicking the symptoms of psychosis) is less than that of *pentazocine*. *Nalbuphine* does not affect the heart or increase blood pressure, in contrast to *pentazocine* and *butorphanol*. A benefit of all three medications is that they exhibit a ceiling effect for respiratory depression.

V. OTHER ANALGESICS

A. Tapentadol

Tapentadol [ta-PEN-ta-dol], a centrally acting analgesic, is an agonist at the μ opioid receptor and an inhibitor of norepinephrine reuptake. It has been used to manage moderate to severe pain, both chronic and acute. *Tapentadol* is mainly metabolized to inactive metabolites via glucuronidation, and it does not inhibit or induce the CYP450 enzyme system. Because *tapentadol* does not produce active metabolites, dosing adjustment is not necessary in mild to moderate renal impairment. *Tapentadol* should be avoided in patients who have received MAOIs within the last 14 days. It is available in an immediate-release and extended-release formulation.

B. Tramadol

Tramadol [TRA-ma-dole] is a centrally acting analgesic that binds to the μ opioid receptor. The drug undergoes extensive metabolism via CYP450 2D6, leading to an active metabolite with a much higher affinity for the μ receptor than the parent compound. In addition, it weakly inhibits reuptake of norepinephrine and serotonin. It is used to manage moderate to moderately severe pain. Its respiratory-depressant activity is less than that of *morphine*. *Naloxone* can only partially reverse the analgesia produced by *tramadol* or its active metabolite. Anaphylactoid reactions have been reported. Overdose or drug–drug interactions with medications, such as SSRIs, MAOIs, and tricyclic antidepressants, can lead to toxicity manifested by CNS excitation and seizures. As with other agents that bind the μ opioid receptor, *tramadol* has been associated with misuse and abuse.

VI. ANTAGONISTS

The opioid antagonists bind with high affinity to opioid receptors, but fail to activate the receptor-mediated response. Administration of opioid antagonists produces no profound effects in normal individuals. However, in patients dependent on opioids, antagonists rapidly reverse the effect of agonists, such as *morphine* or any full μ agonist, and precipitate the symptoms of opioid withdrawal. Figure 14.12 summarizes some of the signs and symptoms of opioid withdrawal.

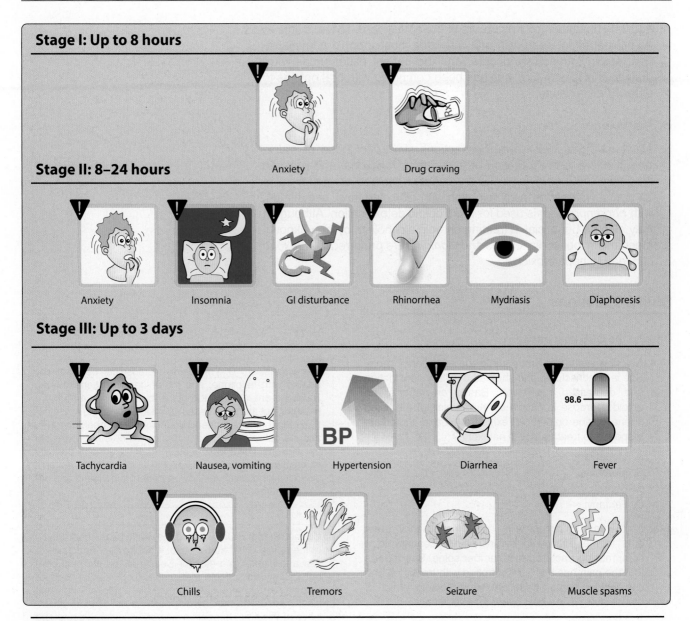

Stage I: Up to 8 hours

Anxiety

Drug craving

Stage II: 8–24 hours

Anxiety

Insomnia

GI disturbance

Rhinorrhea

Mydriasis

Diaphoresis

Stage III: Up to 3 days

Tachycardia

Nausea, vomiting

Hypertension

Diarrhea

Fever

Chills

Tremors

Seizure

Muscle spasms

Figure 14.12
Opiate withdrawal syndrome. GI = gastrointestinal.

A. Naloxone

Naloxone [nal-OX-own] is used to reverse the coma and respiratory depression of opioid overdose. It rapidly displaces all receptor-bound opioid molecules and, therefore, is able to reverse the effect of a *morphine* overdose. Within 30 seconds of IV injection of *naloxone*, the respiratory depression and coma characteristic of high doses of *morphine* are reversed, causing the patient to be revived and alert. *Naloxone* has a half-life of 30 to 81 minutes; therefore, a patient who has been treated and recovered may lapse back into respiratory depression. *Naloxone* is a competitive antagonist at μ, κ, and δ receptors, with a 10-fold higher affinity for μ than for κ receptors. This may explain why *naloxone* readily reverses respiratory depression with only minimal reversal of the analgesia that results from agonist stimulation of κ receptors in the spinal cord. There is little to no clinical effect seen with oral *naloxone*, but, upon IV administration, opioid antagonism occurs, and the patient experiences withdrawal. This is why *naloxone* has been combined with oral opioids to deter IV drug abuse.

B. Naltrexone

Naltrexone [nal-TREX-own] has actions similar to those of *naloxone*. It has a longer duration of action than *naloxone*, and a single oral dose of *naltrexone* blocks the effect of injected *heroin* for up to 24 hours. *Naltrexone* in combination with *clonidine* (and, sometimes, with *buprenorphine*) is used for rapid opioid detoxification. Although it may also be beneficial in treating chronic alcoholism by an unknown mechanism, benzodiazepines and *clonidine* are preferred. *Naltrexone* can lead to hepatotoxicity.

Study Questions

Choose the ONE best answer.

14.1 A young woman is brought into the emergency room. She is unconscious, and she has pupillary constriction and depressed respiration. Based on reports, an opioid overdose is almost certain. Which of the listed phenanthrene opioids will exhibit a full and immediate response to treatment with naloxone?

  A. Meperidine.
  B. Morphine.
  C. Buprenorphine.
  D. Fentanyl.

> Correct answer = B. A morphine overdose can be effectively treated with naloxone, and morphine is a phenanthrene. Naloxone antagonizes the opioid by displacing it from the receptor, but there are cases in which naloxone is not effective. Meperidine is a phenylpiperidine, not a phenanthrene, and the active metabolite, normeperidine, is not reversible by naloxone. The effects of buprenorphine are only partially reversible by naloxone. Naloxone is effective for fentanyl overdoses; however, fentanyl is a phenylpiperidine, and not a phenanthrene.

14.2 A 76-year-old female with renal insufficiency presents to the clinic with severe pain secondary to a compression fracture in the lumbar spine. She reports that the pain has been uncontrolled with tramadol, and it is decided to start treatment with an opioid. Which of the following is the best opioid for this patient?

  A. Meperidine.
  B. Fentanyl transdermal patch.
  C. Hydrocodone.
  D. Morphine.

> Correct answer = C. Hydrocodone would be the best choice of the opioid given in this case. It will be very important to use a low dose and monitor closely for proper pain control and any side effects. Meperidine should not be used for chronic pain, nor should it be used in a patient with renal insufficiency. The transdermal patch is not a good option, since at this time, her pain would be considered acute and she is opioid naïve. Morphine also is not the best choice in this case due to the active metabolites that can accumulate in renal insufficiency.

14.3 Which of the following statements about fentanyl is correct?

  A. Fentanyl is 100 times more potent than morphine.
  B. Its withdrawal symptoms can be relieved by naloxone.
  C. The active metabolites of fentanyl can cause seizures.
  D. It is most effective by oral administration.

> Correct answer = A. Fentanyl is very selective for the μ receptor and is a very potent opioid. Naloxone is an opioid antagonist and can precipitate withdrawal symptoms in patients currently taking opioids. Meperidine is the opioid whose active metabolite, normeperidine, can cause seizures. Fentanyl undergoes hepatic first-pass metabolism and is not effective via oral administration. Due to high lipid solubility, fentanyl has been developed for many routes of administration such as buccal, transmucosal, and transdermal.

14.4 A 56-year-old patient who has suffered with severe chronic pain with radiculopathy secondary to spinal stenosis for years presents to the clinic for pain management. Over the years, this patient has failed to receive relief from the neuropathic pain from the radiculopathy with traditional agents such as tricyclics or anticonvulsants. Based on the mechanism of action, which opioid might be beneficial in this patient to treat both nociceptive and neuropathic pain?

A. Meperidine.
B. Oxymorphone.
C. Morphine.
D. Methadone.

Correct answer = D. Methadone has a unique mechanism of action in comparison to the other choices given. Methadone is a μ agonist, but it also exhibits NMDA receptor antagonism that is thought to aid in the treatment of neuropathic pain and could also aid in prevention of opioid tolerance. All other μ agonists could help manage neuropathic pain, but in some situations, higher doses of opioids are needed to achieve efficacy. It is much better to consider adjuvants such as tricyclics or certain anticonvulsants in the treatment of neuropathic pain.

14.5 Which of the following statements regarding methadone is correct?

A. Methadone is an excellent choice for analgesia in most patients since there are limited drug–drug interactions.
B. The equianalgesic potency of methadone is similar to that of morphine.
C. The duration of analgesia for methadone is much shorter than the elimination half-life.
D. The active metabolites of methadone accumulate in patients with renal dysfunction.

Correct Answer = C. The duration of analgesia is much shorter than the elimination half-life, leading to dangers of accumulation and increased potential for respiratory depression and death. Methadone's equianalgesic potency is extremely variable based on many factors, and it is highly recommended that only prescribers very familiar with methadone should prescribe this agent. The drug interactions associated with methadone are numerous due to the multiple enzymes in the liver that metabolize this drug. Methadone does not have active metabolites, which does make it an option in patients with renal dysfunction.

14.6 Which of the following opioids is the LEAST lipophilic?

A. Fentanyl.
B. Methadone.
C. Meperidine.
D. Morphine.

Correct answer = D. Morphine is the least lipophilic of the opioids listed. Fentanyl, methadone, and meperidine are all very lipophilic opioids.

14.7 A 64-year-old male is preparing for a total knee replacement. He is taking many medications that are metabolized by the CYP450 enzyme system and is worried about drug interactions with the pain medication that will be used following his surgery. Which of the following opioids would have the lowest chance of interacting with his medications that are metabolized by the CYP450 enzyme system?

A. Methadone.
B. Oxymorphone.
C. Oxycodone.
D. Hydrocodone.

Correct answer = B. Oxymorphone is metabolized via glucuronidation and has not been shown to have any drug interactions associated with the CYP enzyme family. All other opioids listed are metabolized by one or more CYP enzymes and increase the risk of drug interactions.

14.8 Which of the following opioids is the best choice for treating pain associated with diabetic peripheral neuropathy?

A. Morphine.
B. Tapentadol.
C. Codeine.
D. Buprenorphine.

Correct answer = B. Tapentadol has a dual mechanism of action (μ agonist and norepinephrine reuptake inhibition) that has demonstrated effectiveness in treating neuropathic pain. Morphine and buprenorphine could decrease some of the pain associated with neuropathic pain, but are not the best choices. Codeine should not be used in chronic pain management.

14.9 KM is a 64-year-old male who has been hospitalized following a car accident in which he sustained a broken leg and broken arm. He has been converted to oral morphine in anticipation of his discharge. What other medication should he receive with his morphine upon discharge?

A. Diphenhydramine.
B. Methylphenidate.
C. Docusate sodium with senna.
D. Docusate sodium.

Correct answer = C. A bowel regimen should be prescribed with the initiation of the opioid. Docusate and senna include both a stool softener and a stimulant, which is recommended for opioid-induced constipation. Treatment with docusate sodium only is ineffective. Constipation is very common with all opioids, and tolerance does not occur. Diphenhydramine can be used for urticaria that might occur with the initiation of an opioid, but this is not reported in this case. Methylphenidate has been used for opioid-induced sedation in certain situations, but is not an issue in this case.

14.10 AN is a 57-year-old male who has been treated with oxycodone for chronic nonmalignant pain for over 2 years. He is now reporting increased pain in the afternoon while at work. Which of the following opioids is a short-acting opioid and is the best choice for this patient's breakthrough pain?

A. Methadone.
B. Pentazocine.
C. Hydrocodone.
D. Nalbuphine.

Correct answer = C. Hydrocodone is a commonly used short-acting agent that is commercially available in combination form with either acetaminophen or ibuprofen. Methadone should not routinely be used for breakthrough pain due to the unique pharmacokinetics and should be reserved for practitioners who have experience with this agent and understand the variables associated with this drug. Pentazocine and nalbuphine are mixed agonist/antagonist analgesics that could precipitate withdrawal in patients who are currently taking a full μ agonist such as oxycodone.

Drugs of Abuse

15

Carol Motycka and Joseph Spillane

I. OVERVIEW

A boy inhales paint fumes to momentarily escape his surroundings of poverty; a new gang member smokes crack with his friends to feel like he belongs; a curious girl swallows a "Molly" to see what it is like; a prescription drug abuser injects heroin to substitute for the pain pills that are more difficult to obtain; and a lonely widower drinks another shot of bourbon to help remember the past and forget the present. In each of these cases, chemicals are being used for nontherapeutic effects on the body or mind. Excessive use or misuse of drugs or alcohol for intoxicating or mind altering effects is considered substance abuse. Figure 15.1 provides a list of commonly abused substances.

Substance abuse in all its many forms has exerted its effects throughout the history of the world, and the lure of addictive substances continues to impact people today. In 2012, approximately 24 million persons in the United States, or about 9% of the population aged 12 years and older, were current users of some form of illicit substance (Figure 15.2). Abused substances have become progressively more potent, and their routes of administration have become increasingly effective, resulting in greater risks of addiction and toxicity (Figure 15.3). Some examples of the methods, mechanisms, and clinical manifestations of toxicity of commonly abused substances are discussed in this chapter.

II. SYMPATHOMIMETICS

Sympathomimetics are stimulants that mimic the sympathetic nervous system, producing "fight-or-flight" responses. Sympathomimetics usually produce a relative increase of adrenergic neurotransmitters at their sites of action (Figure 15.4), thereby causing tachycardia, hypertension, hyperthermia, and tachypnea. These agents come from natural sources, such as plants, or are synthesized in legitimate or clandestine laboratories. Aside from their stimulant effect, many of these have a remarkable

STIMULANTS
Amphetamines
Cocaine
Methylenedioxymethamphetamine (MDMA)
Cocaine
Synthetic cathinones ("bath salts")
HALLUCINOGENS
Lysergic acid diethylamide (LSD)
Marijuana
Synthetic cannabinoids
OTHER DRUGS OF ABUSE
Ethanol
Prescription drugs (particularly opioids)

Figure 15.1
Summary of commonly abused substances.

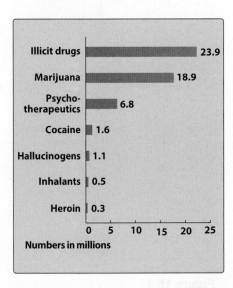

Figure 15.2
Past month illicit drug use among persons aged 12 or older. Ilicit drugs include marijuana/hashish, cocaine (including crack), heroin, hallucinogens, inhalants, or prescription type psychotherapeutics used nonmedically.

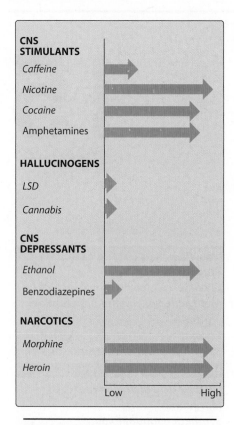

Figure 15.3
Relative potential for physical dependence of commonly abused substances.

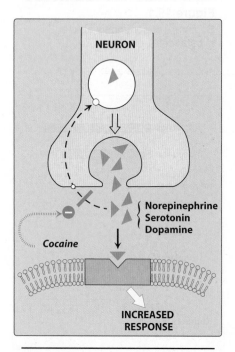

Figure 15.4
Mechanism of action of *cocaine*.

ability to produce pleasure. Consequently, their addictive potential and monetary value on the illicit market offer a huge profit motive.

A. Cocaine

Cocaine is derived from the erythroxylon coca shrub that grows in the foothills of the Andes Mountains in South America. It causes central nervous system (CNS) stimulation by inhibiting the reuptake of norepinephrine into the adrenergic neuron, thus increasing the amount of catecholamines available at the synapse. The profound ability of *cocaine* to stimulate the pleasure center of the human brain is thought to result from inhibition of reuptake of dopamine and serotonin. *Cocaine* has minimal bioavailability when taken by the oral route. Instead, the *cocaine* hydrochloride powder is snorted, or solubilized and injected. The *cocaine* powder cannot be effectively smoked, as it is destroyed upon heating. However, crack *cocaine*, an alkaloidal form, can be smoked. Smoking is an extremely effective route of administration, as the lungs are richly perfused with blood and carry the drug within seconds to its site of action, the brain. This causes an intense euphoria or "rush" that is followed rapidly by an intense dysphoria or "crash." It is this immediate positive reinforcement, followed rapidly by the negative reinforcement, that makes the drug, particularly in this form, so addictive. Like most drugs of abuse, street *cocaine* powder and crack are usually adulterated to increase the bulk, mimic the action, and thereby increase the profitability.

The clinical manifestations of *cocaine* toxicity are not just a function of its inherent toxicity, but also of its adulterants. An example of a common adulterant that has been found in street samples of *cocaine* is *levamisole*, an anthelmintic used to deworm cattle and pigs. *Levamisole* has the ability to cause agranulocytosis, a profound decrease in neutrophils, leaving a weakened immune system prone to opportunistic infections, which have been described among *cocaine* users. A few of the more common reasons for *cocaine* users to come to the emergency department include psychiatric complaints (depression precipitated by *cocaine* dysphoria, agitation/paranoia), convulsions, hyperthermia, and chest pain. The hyperthermia is caused by *cocaine*-induced CNS stimulation that generates increased heat production, coupled with vasoconstrictive effects of *cocaine* that minimize the ability to dissipate the heat. *Cocaine*-related chest pain can be chest muscle pain or cardiac in nature, as *cocaine* causes vasoconstriction of the coronary arteries and accelerates the atherosclerotic process. Commonly, *cocaine* is consumed with alcohol, which creates a secondary metabolite called cocaethylene. This metabolite is cardiotoxic and further contributes to the cardiac issues related to *cocaine* consumption. *Cocaine* chest pain can also be due to pulmonary damage caused by inhaling this hot impure substance. *Cocaine* convulsions are a natural extension of the CNS stimulant effect (Figure 15.5). *Cocaine* toxicity is treated by calming and cooling the patient. Benzodiazepines, such as *lorazepam*, help to calm the agitated patient and can both treat and prevent convulsions. In addition, the calming effect helps cool the patient and manage the hyperthermia. This is an important effect, as hyperthermia is one of the major causes of *cocaine* fatalities. The remainder of *cocaine* toxicity is treated with short-acting antihypertensives, anticonvulsants, and symptomatic supportive care.

B. Amphetamines

Amphetamines such as *methamphetamine* are sympathomimetics with clinical effects very similar to those of *cocaine*. In many cases, these effects may last longer and be associated with more stimulation and less euphoria when compared to *cocaine*. Treatment of *amphetamine* toxicity is similar to that of *cocaine* toxicity. Therapeutic uses of amphetamines are presented in Chapter 16.

C. Methylenedioxymethamphetamine

Methylenedioxymethamphetamine (*MDMA*), commonly known as ecstasy or Molly, is a hallucinogenic *amphetamine* with profound serotonin-releasing effects (Figure 15.6). Its use was first popularized among those attending late-night "rave" parties, dance clubs, and concerts. Because of its unique serotonin properties, it is sometimes referred to as an "empathogen," and tactile stimulation is particularly pleasurable to users. Many users describe a sense of well-being and social interactivity, and sexual offenders have also taken advantage of this. The Internet is replete with warnings to drink plenty of water while using ecstasy, and, indeed, some of the early deaths associated with *MDMA* toxicity involved dehydration and renal failure. Promoters take advantage of this by selling bottled water at a huge profit, and, in fact, water intoxication and hyponatremia have now been described among ecstasy users. Like many amphetamines, *MDMA* can cause bruxism (teeth grinding) and trismus (jaw clenching), which explain the baby pacifiers and lollipops that have been popularized among "ravers." Among the most disturbing properties of *MDMA* abuse is its propensity to cause profound hyperthermia, altered mental status, and movement disorders known as the serotonin syndrome. Treatment for *MDMA* toxicity should be undertaken with the knowledge that like all street drugs, adulterants and coingestants are likely to be involved. Again, benzodiazepines help to calm and cool the patient. Life-threatening hyperthermia has been treated with neuromuscular blockers and endotracheal intubation to control excessive movement and heat generation. *Cyproheptadine* is a serotonin antagonist that has been used to treat serotonin syndrome. However, one of its practical limitations is that it is only available orally.

D. Synthetic Cathinones

Cathinone is the psychoactive component in an evergreen shrub called Khat native to East Africa and the Arabian Peninsula. Synthetic cathinones, also known as "bath salts," have become increasingly popular. These products are packaged and labeled in such a way as to circumvent detection, prosecution, and enforcement. Many of the "bath salts" or "pond water cleaner" packages will read "not for human consumption." These are substances that are sold as something else at large profits with an unstated understanding by seller and buyer that they will produce intoxication. Synthetic cathinones are not easily detected on urine toxicology screens.

Methcathinone, butylone, methylene dioxypyrovalerone, and *naphyrone* are just a few examples of synthetic cathinones. These drugs increase the release and inhibit the reuptake of catecholamines (norepinephrine, epinephrine, and dopamine) in a manner very similar to *cocaine* and amphetamines. A rapid onset of *amphetamine*-like stimulation with psychotomimetic effects of variable duration is common

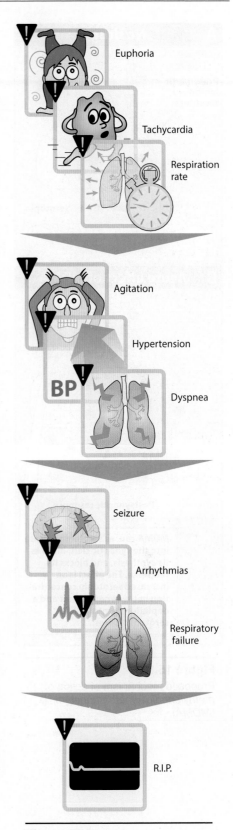

Figure 15.5
Major effects of *cocaine* use.

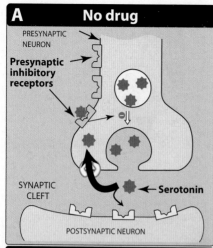

A **No drug**

PRESYNAPTIC
NEURON

**Presynaptic
inhibitory
receptors**

SYNAPTIC
CLEFT

◄— **Serotonin**

POSTSYNAPTIC NEURON

B **Acute effect of MDMA**

MDMA ⊖

Postsynaptic response

MDMA causes serotonin release
into the synaptic cleft, inhibits
its synthesis, and blocks its
reuptake. The effect is an
increased serotonin concentration in the synaptic cleft and a
depletion of intracellular
serotonin stores.

Figure 15.6
Proposed mechanism of action of
methylenedioxymethamphetamine
(*MDMA*).

with synthetic cathinones. Bath salts are generally snorted or ingested, but they may also be injected. Treatment is similar to the emergent treatment of amphetamines and *cocaine*.

III. HALLUCINOGENS

Lysergic acid diethylamide (LSD), marijuana, and synthetic cannabinoids are substances that fall into this category.

A. Lysergic acid diethylamide

LSD, lysergic acid diethylamide, is perhaps the most commonly considered drug in the hallucinogen class. *LSD* was first created from ergot in 1938 by Dr. Albert Hoffman. It was later popularized by Dr. Timothy Leary, a Harvard psychologist who encouraged its use among young people. *LSD* produces its psychedelic effects through serving as a potent partial agonist at 5-HT$_{2A}$ receptors. Aside from the very colorful hallucinations, the drug is also responsible for mood alterations, sleep disturbances, and anxiety. Repeated use rapidly produces tolerance through down-regulation of the serotonin receptors.

Although physical side effects are typically minimal, *LSD* may cause tachycardia, increased blood pressure and body temperature, dizziness, decreased appetite, and sweating. Perhaps, the most troubling side effects are the loss of judgment and impaired reasoning associated with use of *LSD*. This can sometimes be an exaggerated effect with extreme panic, which is known by individuals as a "bad trip," and may lead to unforeseen consequences such as suicide. After long-term use, withdrawal from *LSD* is considered more emotional than physical in nature.

B. Marijuana

Cannabis is a plant that is thought to have been used by humans for over 10,000 years. Centuries-old Chinese documents describe using cannabis for clothing production, food, and as an agent to communicate with spirits. Today, marijuana is the most frequently used illicit drug, and the illicit drug that new users are most likely to try (Figure 15.7). Those numbers are expected to grow as legalization is introduced in several states. Certain cannabis plants can be used for making rope or clothing; however, the species Cannabis sativa is the plant most often used for its hallucinogenic properties. The main psychoactive alkaloid contained in marijuana is Δ⁹-*tetrahydrocannabinol* [tet-ra-HY-dro-can-NAB-i-nol] (*THC*). Growing techniques have evolved over the past 50 years, and *THC* concentrations found in the plant have increased as much as 20-fold during that time period.

Specific receptors in the brain, cannabinoid or CB$_1$ receptors, were discovered in the late 1980s and found to be reactive to *THC*. When CB$_1$ receptors are activated by marijuana, the effects produced include physical relaxation, hyperphagia (increased appetite), increased heart rate, decreased muscle coordination, conjunctivitis, and minor pain control (Figure 15.8). Depending on the social situation, *THC* can produce euphoria, followed by drowsiness and relaxation. Although hallucinations are typically not as robust as those observed with *LSD* use, marijuana is often used for the hallucinogenic effects that it produces. Marijuana stimulates the amygdala, causing the user to have a sense of novelty to anything the user encounters through an enhancement of sensory activity. For this same reason, heavy users have a down-regulation in their CB_1 receptors, leaving them with a feeling of boredom when not taking the drug. The effects of marijuana on γ-aminobutyric acid (GABA) in the hippocampus diminish the capacity for short-term memory in users, and this affect seems to be more pronounced in adolescents. In addition to adversely affecting short-term memory and mental activity, *THC* decreases muscle strength and impairs highly skilled motor activity such as that required to drive a car. The effects of *THC* appear immediately after the drug is smoked, but maximum effects take about 20 minutes. By 3 hours, the effects largely disappear.

Long-term effects of use may include chronic bronchitis, chronic obstructive pulmonary disease, increased progression of HIV and breast cancer, and exacerbation of mental illness. Tolerance develops rapidly in users, and withdrawal has been observed. Marijuana may be found in the body up to 3 months after last usage in heavy chronic users. For this reason, withdrawal occurs much later in individuals who previously used marijuana heavily. Withdrawal may include depression, pain, and irritability.

Although not well studied for medicinal use, marijuana has been used to help in the treatment of chemotherapy-induced nausea and vomiting, cachexia secondary to cancer and AIDS, epilepsy, chronic pain, multiple sclerosis, glaucoma, and anxiety. *THC* is available as the prescription product *dronabinol* [droe-NAB-i-nol]. This product is prescribed to treat emesis and to stimulate the appetite.

C. Synthetic Cannabinoids

Synthetic cannabinoids are sold over the Internet or in head shops (retail outlets specializing in tobacco paraphernalia often used for consumption of marijuana or related substances) and are often known under the names of "Spice" or "K2." The synthetic *THC*-containing compounds were originally created in Germany in 2008 in the hopes that they could be used for medicinal purposes. Since the molecular structure of synthetic cannabinoids is much different from the cannabinoids found in marijuana plants, users do not test positive for *THC* with traditional drug tests. The effects of these designer agents may be up to 800 times greater than the effects observed with cannabis. Sympathomimetic effects may also be seen in users, including tachycardia and hypertension. Possibly the greatest danger includes extreme hallucinations that have been reported with the use of these agents.

IV. ETHANOL

Ethanol (*EtOH*) is a clear colorless hydroxylated hydrocarbon that is the product of fermentation of fruits, grains, or vegetables. It is a major cause of fatal automobile accidents, drownings, and fatal falls and is a related factor in many hospital admissions. Alcohol is the most commonly abused substance in modern society. Alcoholism decreases

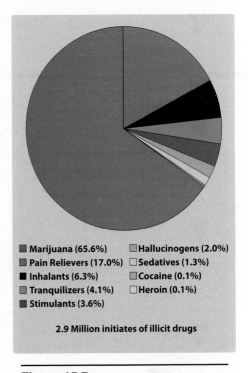

Marijuana (65.6%) Hallucinogens (2.0%)
Pain Relievers (17.0%) Sedatives (1.3%)
Inhalants (6.3%) Cocaine (0.1%)
Tranquilizers (4.1%) Heroin (0.1%)
Stimulants (3.6%)

2.9 Million initiates of illicit drugs

Figure 15.7
First specific drug associated with initiation of illicit drug use among past year illicit drug initiates aged 12 or older.

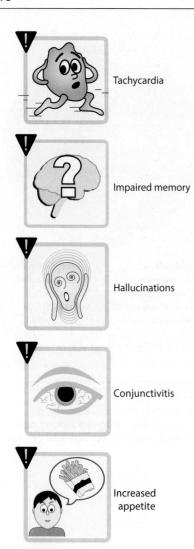

Figure 15.8
Effects of
tetrahydrocannabinol.

Tachycardia

Impaired memory

Hallucinations

Conjunctivitis

Increased
appetite

Impaired
coordination

life expectancy by 10 to 15 years and impacts one in three families. It is thought that *ethanol* exerts its desired and toxic effects through several mechanisms, including enhancing the effects of the inhibitory neurotransmitter GABA, inducing the release of endogenous opioids, and altering levels of serotonin and dopamine. *Ethanol* is a selective CNS depressant at low doses, resulting in decreased inhibitions and the characteristic loquaciousness or drunken behavior. At high doses, it is a general CNS depressant, which can result in coma and respiratory depression.

Drinking *ethanol* traditionally has been the most common route of administration, although recently the inhalation of aerosolized *ethanol* has gained popularity. *Ethanol* is absorbed from the stomach and duodenum, and food slows and decreases absorption. Peak *ethanol* levels are generally achieved in 20 minutes to 1 hour of ingestion. There is a greater subjective feeling of intoxication while levels are ascending (absorption), as compared to when levels are descending. *Ethanol* is metabolized by alcohol dehydrogenase to acetaldehyde and then by aldehyde dehydrogenase to acetate in the liver (Figure 15.9). It is metabolized by zero-order elimination at approximately 15 to 40 mg/dL/h. Since there is a constant blood-to-breath ratio of 2100:1, a breath sample can be used to determine blood alcohol levels. Medical management of acute *ethanol* toxicity includes symptomatic supportive care and the administration of *thiamine* and *folic acid* to prevent/treat Wernicke encephalopathy and macrocytic anemia. Extremely high levels can be dialyzed, although that is rarely necessary, and could precipitate withdrawal in an alcoholic.

Chronic *ethanol* abuse can cause profound hepatic, cardiovascular, pulmonary, hematologic, endocrine, metabolic, and CNS damage (Figure 15.10). Sudden cessation of *ethanol* ingestion in a heavy drinker can precipitate withdrawal manifested by tachycardia, sweating, tremor, anxiety, agitation, hallucinations, and convulsions. Alcohol withdrawal is a life-threatening situation that should be medically managed with symptomatic/supportive care, benzodiazepines, and long-term addiction treatment. The following are drugs used in the treatment of alcohol dependence:

A. Disulfiram

Disulfiram [dye-SUL-fi-ram] blocks the oxidation of acetaldehyde to acetic acid by inhibiting aldehyde dehydrogenase (Figure 15.11). This results in the accumulation of acetaldehyde in the blood, causing flushing, tachycardia, hyperventilation, and nausea. *Disulfiram* has found some use in the patient seriously desiring to stop alcohol ingestion. A conditioned avoidance response is induced so that the patient abstains from alcohol to prevent the unpleasant effects of *disulfiram*-induced acetaldehyde accumulation.

B. Naltrexone

Naltrexone [nal-TREX-own] is a long-acting opioid antagonist that should be used in conjunction with supportive psychotherapy. *Naltrexone* is better tolerated than *disulfiram* and does not produce the aversive reaction that *disulfiram* does.

C. Acamprosate

Acamprosate [a-kam-PROE-sate] is an agent used in alcohol dependence treatment programs with an as-yet poorly understood mechanism of action. This agent should also be used in conjunction with supportive psychotherapy.

V. PRESCRIPTION DRUG ABUSE

This chapter has discussed many of the illicit substances that are abused by individuals. It is important to also mention that parts of the world, including the United States and portions of Europe, are currently experiencing an epidemic of prescription drug abuse. Some commonly abused prescription drugs include opioids, benzodiazepines, and barbiturates, with opioids outpacing the other prescription drugs by a large margin. In the United States, between 1997 and 2007, there was a 600% increase in the prescribing of opioids, and by 2010, enough opioid prescription pain relievers were sold in the United States to medicate every American adult with 5 mg of hydrocodone every 4 hours for 1 month. With the increase in prescribing, has come a commensurate increase in consequences. Visits to the emergency department related to misuse of pharmaceuticals now exceed those related to illicit drug use, and prescription pain relievers

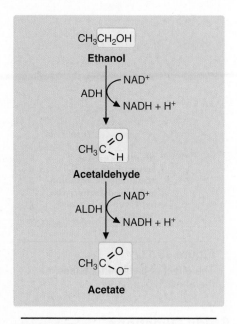

Figure 15.9
The pathway of ethanol metabolism.
ADH = alcohol dehydrogenase;
ALDH = acetaldehyde dehydrogenase.

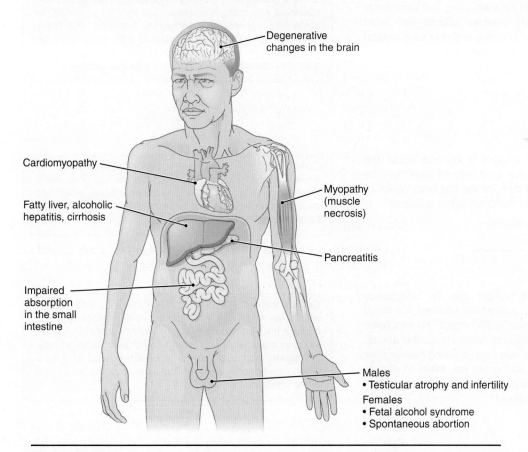

Figure 15.10
The effects of chronic alcohol abuse.

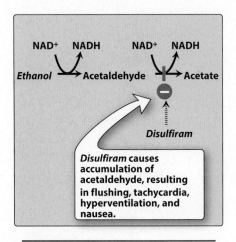

Figure 15.11
The effect of disulfiram on the metabolism of ethanol.

also now account for more deaths than heroin and *cocaine* combined. An increased emphasis on treating pain as the "fifth vital sign," coupled with an exaggerated belief in the beneficial capacity of these medications and a minimization of their inherent toxicity among the lay public and health professionals, is among the many possible explanations for this current epidemic. Medications for the treatment of opioid toxicity and dependence are reviewed in Chapter 14.

Study Questions

Choose the ONE best answer.

15.1 A 22-year-old HIV patient has been told that marijuana may benefit him should he start using the substance. Which of the following adverse effects has been associated with marijuana usage and may be a reason for this patient to avoid use of marijuana?

A. Hyperphagia.
B. Hyperthermia.
C. Hepatitis.
D. Progression of HIV.
E. Hyponatremia.

> Correct answer = D. Although hyperphagia is a side effect observed with marijuana usage, this may be of benefit for some HIV patients. Hyperthermia, hepatitis, and hyponatremia have not been associated with marijuana use. Progression of HIV has been linked to marijuana use and is a serious consideration for anyone with this disease.

15.2 A 21-year-old college student is curious about the effects of LSD. She asks what type of risks may be involved with using the drug for the first time. Which of the following is a correct response to her question?

A. Exaggerated hallucinations.
B. Cardiomyopathy.
C. Hyperphagia.
D. Bronchitis.

> Correct answer = A. Exaggerated hallucinations, sometimes known as "bad trips," may occur, even in first-time users. These hallucinations can lead to extreme panic, which has caused individuals to react in a manner very uncharacteristic of their typical behavior.

15.3 A 58-year-old male is brought into the emergency department following an automobile accident. His blood alcohol level on admission is 280 mg/dL. He has been treated in the past for seizures related to alcohol abuse, and he confirms that he has been drinking heavily over the past month since losing his job. What treatment should be given to this patient if he begins to go into withdrawal while hospitalized?

A. None.
B. Lorazepam.
C. Acamprosate.
D. Naltrexone.
E. Disulfiram.

> Correct answer = B. Should this patient go into alcohol withdrawal, he will likely also have seizures associated with it, given his past history. Benzodiazepines are used to treat seizures associated with alcohol withdrawal. Acamprosate, naltrexone, and disulfiram may be considered at a later time to treat the dependence, but would not be useful in the acute withdrawal setting.

15.4 A 35-year-old man has been abusing cocaine and is agitated, tachycardic, hypertensive, and hyperthermic. Which of the following is correct regarding treatment in this situation?

A. This patient should undergo gastric lavage; that is, he should have his stomach pumped immediately.

B. Cocaine toxicity commonly involves CNS depression that can be reversed with IV atropine.

C. Benzodiazepines would be a good choice, as they should help calm the patient down, decrease heart rate, decrease blood pressure, and decrease body temperature.

D. Phenobarbital should be the first choice as an anticonvulsant.

Correct answer = C. Benzodiazepines such as lorazepam have anxiolytic properties and can calm a cocaine toxic patient down, thereby decreasing heart rate and blood pressure. As the patient becomes less agitated, he/she decreases movement and his or her body temperature drops. In addition, the use of benzodiazepines decreases the chance of the patient experiencing a convulsion and would be the first choice to treat cocaine-induced convulsions.

15.5 A 22-year-old man with a history of substance abuse arrives in the emergency department hypertensive, hyperthermic, and tachycardic, with altered mental status and hyperreflexia. His friends say he has been snorting "bath salts." Which of the following is correct regarding this patient?

A. This patient's clinical presentation is consistent with opioid toxicity and he should receive an opioid antagonist such as naloxone immediately.

B. "Bath salts" are often labeled as "not for human consumption" and sold with an unstated understanding that they contain synthetic cathinones, which are amphetamine-like compounds.

C. Treatment with a serotonin agonist might be beneficial.

D. Along with cooling measures, antihypertensives, β-blockers, and monoamine oxidase inhibitors would be reasonable options for the treatment.

Correct answer = B: "Bath salts" often contain synthetic cathinones and are labeled, marketed, and sold as something "not for human consumption" to avoid law enforcement and prosecution. In addition, they are usually not detected on urine toxicology screening. These products can cause an amphetamine-like sympathomimetic toxidrome, as well as serotonin syndrome, which would be treated with symptomatic/supportive care and possibly a serotonin antagonist (not a serotonin agonist) such as cyproheptadine. The combination of an amphetamine or amphetamine-like substance and a monoamine oxidase inhibitor (MAO inhibitor) can precipitate serotonin syndrome and should be avoided in a hyperdynamic patient such as this.

CNS Stimulants

16

Jose A. Rey

I. OVERVIEW

Psychomotor stimulants and hallucinogens are two groups of drugs that act primarily to stimulate the central nervous system (CNS). The psychomotor stimulants cause excitement and euphoria, decrease feelings of fatigue, and increase motor activity. The hallucinogens produce profound changes in thought patterns and mood, with little effect on the brainstem and spinal cord. As a group, the CNS stimulants have diverse clinical uses and are important as drugs of abuse, as are the CNS depressants (Chapter 9) and the opioids (Chapter 14). Figure 16.1 summarizes the CNS stimulants.

PSYCHOMOTOR STIMULANTS
Amphetamine ADDERALL
Armodafinil NUVIGIL
Atomoxetine STRATTERA
Caffeine CAFCIT, NO DOZ, VIVARIN
Cocaine
Dexmethylphenidate FOCALIN
Dextroamphetamine DEXEDRINE, DEXTROSTAT
Lisdexamfetamine VYVANSE
Methamphetamine DESOXYN
Methylphenidate RITALIN, CONCERTA, DAYTRANA
Modafinil PROVIGIL
Nicotine NICODERM CQ, NICORETTE, NICOTROL
Theophylline ELIXOPHYLLIN, THEO-24, THEOCHRON, UNIPHYL
Varenicline CHANTIX

Figure 16.1
Summary of central nervous system (CNS) stimulants.

II. PSYCHOMOTOR STIMULANTS

A. Methylxanthines

The methylxanthines include *theophylline* [thee-OFF-i-lin], which is found in tea; *theobromine* [thee-oh-BROE-meen], found in cocoa; and *caffeine* [kaf-EEN]. *Caffeine,* the most widely consumed stimulant in the world, is found in highest concentration in certain coffee products (for example, espresso), but it is also present in tea, cola drinks, energy drinks, chocolate candy, and cocoa.

1. **Mechanism of action:** Several mechanisms have been proposed for the actions of methylxanthines, including translocation of extracellular calcium, increase in cyclic adenosine monophosphate and cyclic guanosine monophosphate caused by inhibition of phosphodiesterase, and blockade of adenosine receptors. The latter most likely accounts for the actions achieved by the usual consumption of *caffeine*-containing beverages.

2. **Actions:**

   a. **CNS:** The *caffeine* contained in one to two cups of coffee (100 to 200 mg) causes a decrease in fatigue and increased mental alertness as a result of stimulating the cortex and other areas of the brain. Consumption of 1.5 g of *caffeine* (12 to 15 cups of coffee) produces anxiety and tremors. The spinal cord is stimulated only by very high doses (2 to 5 g) of *caffeine.* Tolerance can rapidly develop to the stimulating properties of *caffeine,* and withdrawal consists of feelings of fatigue and sedation.

b. **Cardiovascular system:** A high dose of *caffeine* has positive inotropic and chronotropic effects on the heart. [Note: Increased contractility can be harmful to patients with angina pectoris. In others, an accelerated heart rate can trigger premature ventricular contractions.]

c. **Diuretic action:** *Caffeine* has a mild diuretic action that increases urinary output of sodium, chloride, and potassium.

d. **Gastric mucosa:** Because methylxanthines stimulate secretion of gastric acid, individuals with peptic ulcers should avoid foods and beverages containing methylxanthines.

3. **Therapeutic uses:** *Caffeine* and its derivatives relax the smooth muscles of the bronchioles. [Note: Previously the mainstay of asthma therapy, *theophylline* has been largely replaced by other agents, such as β_2 agonists and corticosteroids (see Chapter 29).] *Caffeine* is also used in combination with the analgesics *acetaminophen* and *aspirin* for the management of headaches in both prescription and over-the-counter products.

4. **Pharmacokinetics:** The methylxanthines are well absorbed orally. *Caffeine* distributes throughout the body, including the brain. These drugs cross the placenta to the fetus and are secreted into the breast milk. All methylxanthines are metabolized in the liver, generally by the CYP1A2 pathway, and the metabolites are excreted in the urine.

5. **Adverse effects:** Moderate doses of *caffeine* cause insomnia, anxiety, and agitation. A high dosage is required for toxicity, which is manifested by emesis and convulsions. The lethal dose is 10 g of *caffeine* (about 100 cups of coffee), which induces cardiac arrhythmias. Death from *caffeine* is, therefore, highly unlikely. Lethargy, irritability, and headache occur in users who routinely consume more than 600 mg of *caffeine* per day (roughly six cups of coffee per day) and then suddenly stop.

B. Nicotine

Nicotine [NIK-o-teen] is the active ingredient in tobacco. Although this drug is not currently used therapeutically (except in smoking cessation therapy), *nicotine* remains important because it is second only to *caffeine* as the most widely used CNS stimulant, and it is second only to alcohol as the most abused drug. In combination with the tars and carbon monoxide found in cigarette smoke, *nicotine* represents a serious risk factor for lung and cardiovascular disease, various cancers, and other illnesses. Dependency on the drug is not easily overcome.

1. **Mechanism of action:** In low doses, *nicotine* causes ganglionic stimulation by depolarization. At high doses, *nicotine* causes ganglionic blockade. *Nicotine* receptors exist at a number of sites in the CNS, which participate in the stimulant attributes of the drug.

2. Actions:

a. CNS:
Nicotine is highly lipid soluble and readily crosses the blood–brain barrier. Cigarette smoking or administration of low doses of *nicotine* produces some degree of euphoria and arousal, as well as relaxation. It improves attention, learning, problem solving, and reaction time. High doses of *nicotine* result in central respiratory paralysis and severe hypotension caused by medullary paralysis (Figure 16.2). *Nicotine* is also an appetite suppressant.

b. Peripheral effects:
The peripheral effects of *nicotine* are complex. Stimulation of sympathetic ganglia as well as of the adrenal medulla increases blood pressure and heart rate. Thus, use of tobacco is particularly harmful in hypertensive patients. Many patients with peripheral vascular disease experience an exacerbation of symptoms with smoking. In addition, *nicotine*-induced vasoconstriction can decrease coronary blood flow, adversely affecting a patient with angina. Stimulation of parasympathetic ganglia also increases motor activity of the bowel. At higher doses, blood pressure falls and activity ceases in both the gastrointestinal (GI) tract and bladder musculature as a result of a *nicotine*-induced block of parasympathetic ganglia.

3. Pharmacokinetics:
Because *nicotine* is highly lipid soluble, absorption readily occurs via the oral mucosa, lungs, GI mucosa, and skin. *Nicotine* crosses the placental membrane and is secreted in the breast milk. By inhaling tobacco smoke, the average smoker takes in 1 to 2 mg of *nicotine* per cigarette. The acute lethal dose is 60 mg. More than 90% of the *nicotine* inhaled in smoke is absorbed. Clearance of *nicotine* involves metabolism in the lung and the liver and urinary excretion. Tolerance to the toxic effects of *nicotine* develops rapidly, often within days.

4. Adverse effects:
The CNS effects of *nicotine* include irritability and tremors. *Nicotine* may also cause intestinal cramps, diarrhea, and increased heart rate and blood pressure. In addition, cigarette smoking increases the rate of metabolism for a number of drugs.

5. Withdrawal syndrome:
As with the other drugs in this class, *nicotine* is an addictive substance, and physical dependence develops rapidly and can be severe (Figure 16.3). Withdrawal is characterized by irritability, anxiety, restlessness, difficulty concentrating, headaches, and insomnia. Appetite is affected, and GI upset often occurs. [Note: Smoking cessation programs that combine pharmacologic and behavioral therapy are the most successful in helping individuals to stop smoking.] The transdermal patch and chewing gum containing *nicotine* have been shown to reduce *nicotine* withdrawal symptoms and to help smokers stop smoking. For example, the blood concentration of *nicotine* obtained from *nicotine* chewing gum is typically about one-half the peak level observed with

Low doses of *nicotine*

Arousal and relaxation

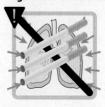

High doses of *nicotine*

Respiratory paralysis

Figure 16.2
Actions of *nicotine* on the CNS.

Potential for addiction

Nicotine

Figure 16.3
Nicotine has potential for addiction.

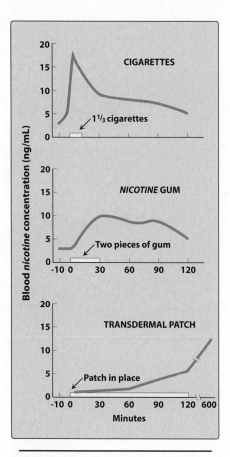

Figure 16.4
Blood concentrations of *nicotine* in individuals who smoked cigarettes, chewed *nicotine* gum, or received *nicotine* by transdermal patch.

Potential for addiction

Cocaine amphetamine

Figure 16.5
Cocaine and *amphetamine* have potential for addiction.

smoking (Figure 16.4). Other forms of *nicotine* replacement used for smoking cessation include the inhaler, nasal spray, and lozenges. *Bupropion,* an antidepressant (Chapter 10), can reduce the craving for cigarettes.

C. Varenicline

Varenicline [ver-EN-ih-kleen] is a partial agonist at neuronal nicotinic acetylcholine receptors in the CNS. Because *varenicline* is only a partial agonist at these receptors, it produces less euphoric effects than *nicotine* (*nicotine* is a full agonist at these receptors). Thus, it is useful as an adjunct in the management of smoking cessation in patients with *nicotine* withdrawal symptoms. Additionally, *varenicline* tends to attenuate the rewarding effects of *nicotine* if a person relapses and uses tobacco. Patients taking *varenicline* should be monitored for suicidal thoughts, vivid nightmares, and mood changes.

D. Cocaine

Cocaine [koe-KANE] is a widely available and highly addictive drug. Because of its abuse potential, *cocaine* is classified as a Schedule II drug by the U.S. Drug Enforcement Agency. The primary mechanism of action underlying the effects of *cocaine* is blockade of reuptake of the monoamines (norepinephrine, serotonin, and dopamine) into the presynaptic terminals. This potentiates and prolongs the CNS and peripheral actions of these monoamines. In particular, the prolongation of dopaminergic effects in the brain's pleasure system (limbic system) produces the intense euphoria that *cocaine* initially causes. Chronic intake of *cocaine* depletes dopamine. This depletion triggers the vicious cycle of craving for *cocaine* that temporarily relieves severe depression (Figure 16.5). A full description of *cocaine* and its effects is provided in Chapter 15.

E. Amphetamine

Amphetamine [am-FET-a-meen] is a sympathetic amine that shows neurologic and clinical effects quite similar to those of *cocaine.* *Dextroamphetamine* [dex-troe-am-FET-a-meen] is the major member of this class of compounds. *Methamphetamine* [meth-am-FET-a-meen] (also known as "speed") is a derivative of *amphetamine* available for prescription use. It can also be smoked and is preferred by many abusers. *3,4-Methylenedioxymethamphetamine* (also known as MDMA, or Ecstasy) is a synthetic derivative of *methamphetamine* with both stimulant and hallucinogenic properties (see Chapter 15).

1. **Mechanism of action:** As with *cocaine,* the effects of *amphetamine* on the CNS and peripheral nervous system are indirect. That is, both depend upon an elevation of the level of catecholamine neurotransmitters in synaptic spaces. *Amphetamine,* however, achieves this effect by releasing intracellular stores of catecholamines (Figure 16.6). Because *amphetamine* also inhibits monoamine oxidase (MAO) and is a weak reuptake transport inhibitor, high levels of catecholamines are readily released into synaptic spaces. Despite different mechanisms of action, the behavioral effects of *amphetamine* and its derivatives are similar to those of *cocaine.*

2. **Actions:**

   a. **CNS:** The major behavioral effects of *amphetamine* result from a combination of its dopamine and norepinephrine release-enhancing properties. *Amphetamine* stimulates the entire cerebrospinal axis, cortex, brainstem, and medulla. This leads to increased alertness, decreased fatigue, depressed appetite, and insomnia. The CNS stimulant effects of *amphetamine* and its derivatives have led to their use in therapy for hyperactivity in children, for narcolepsy, and for appetite control. At high doses, psychosis and convulsions can ensue.

   b. **Sympathetic nervous system:** In addition to its marked action on the CNS, *amphetamine* acts on the adrenergic system, indirectly stimulating the receptors through norepinephrine release.

3. **Therapeutic uses:** Factors that limit the therapeutic usefulness of *amphetamine* include psychological and physiologic dependence similar to those with *cocaine* and, with chronic use, the development of tolerance to the euphoric and anorectic effects.

   a. **Attention deficit hyperactivity disorder (ADHD):** Some young children are hyperkinetic and lack the ability to be involved in any one activity for longer than a few minutes. *Dextroamphetamine*, *methamphetamine*, the *mixed amphetamine salts,* and *methylphenidate* [meth-ill-FEN-ih-date] can help improve attention span and alleviate many of the behavioral problems associated with this syndrome, in addition to reducing hyperkinesia. *Lisdexamfetamine* [lis-dex-am-FET-a-meen] is a prodrug that is converted to the active component *dextroamphetamine* after GI absorption and metabolism. *Atomoxetine* [AT-oh-MOX-ih-teen] is a nonstimulant drug approved for ADHD in children and adults. [Note: This drug should not be taken by individuals on MAO inhibitors and by patients with angle-closure glaucoma.] Unlike *methylphenidate,* which blocks dopamine reuptake more than norepinephrine reuptake, *atomoxetine* is more selective for inhibition of norepinephrine reuptake. Therefore, it is not considered habit forming and is not a controlled substance.

   b. **Narcolepsy:** Narcolepsy is a relatively rare sleep disorder that is characterized by uncontrollable bouts of sleepiness during the day. It is sometimes accompanied by catalepsy, a loss in muscle control, and even paralysis brought on by strong emotions such as laughter. The sleepiness can be treated with drugs, such as the *mixed amphetamine salts* or *methylphenidate. Modafinil* [moe-DA-fi-nil] and its R-enantiomer derivative, *armodafinil* [ar-moe-DA-fi-nil], are considered first-line agents for the treatment of narcolepsy. *Modafinil* promotes wakefulness, but it produces fewer psychoactive and euphoric effects and fewer alterations in mood, perception, thinking, and feelings typical of other CNS stimulants. The mechanism of action remains unclear, but may involve the adrenergic and dopaminergic systems. *Modafinil* is effective orally. It is well distributed

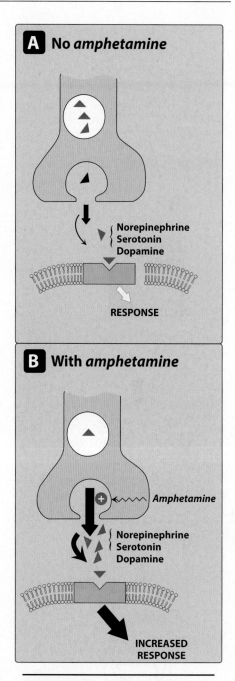

A No *amphetamine*

Norepinephrine
Serotonin
Dopamine

RESPONSE

B With *amphetamine*

Amphetamine

Norepinephrine
Serotonin
Dopamine

INCREASED
RESPONSE

Figure 16.6
Mechanism of action of *amphetamine*.

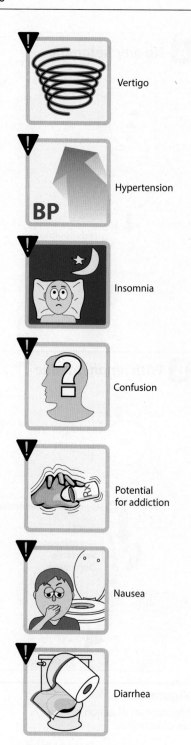

Vertigo

Hypertension

BP

Insomnia

Confusion

Potential for addiction

Nausea

Diarrhea

Figure 16.7
Adverse effects of
amphetamines and
methylphenidate.

throughout the body and undergoes extensive hepatic metabolism. The metabolites are excreted in urine. Headaches, nausea, and nervousness are the primary adverse effects. *Modafinil* and *armodafinil* may have some potential for abuse and physical dependence, and both are classified as controlled substances.

c. **Appetite suppression:** *Phentermine* [FEN-ter-meen] and *diethylpropion* [dye-eth-ill-PROE-pee-on] are sympathomimetic amines that are related structurally to *amphetamine*. These agents are used for their appetite-suppressant effects in the management of obesity (see Chapter 28).

4. **Pharmacokinetics:** *Amphetamine* is completely absorbed from the GI tract, metabolized by the liver, and excreted in the urine. [Note: Administration of urinary alkalinizing agents such as *sodium bicarbonate* will increase the nonionized species of the drug and enhance the reabsorption of *dextroamphetamine* from the renal tubules into the bloodstream.] *Amphetamine* abusers often administer the drugs by IV injection and/or by smoking. The euphoria caused by *amphetamine* lasts 4 to 6 hours, or four- to eightfold longer than the effects of *cocaine.*

5. **Adverse effects:** The *amphetamines* may cause addiction, leading to dependence, tolerance, and drug-seeking behavior. In addition, they have the following undesirable effects.

a. **CNS effects:** Adverse effects of *amphetamine* usage include insomnia, irritability, weakness, dizziness, tremor, and hyperactive reflexes (Figure 16.7). *Amphetamine* can also cause confusion, delirium, panic states, and suicidal tendencies, especially in mentally ill patients. Benzodiazepines, such as *lorazepam*, are often used in the management of agitation and CNS stimulation secondary to *amphetamine* overdose. Chronic *amphetamine* use produces a state of "*amphetamine* psychosis" that resembles the psychotic episodes associated with schizophrenia. Whereas long-term *amphetamine* use is associated with psychic and physical dependence, tolerance to its effects may occur within a few weeks. The anorectic effect of *amphetamine* is due to its action in the lateral hypothalamic feeding center.

b. **Cardiovascular effects:** In addition to its CNS effects, *amphetamine* causes palpitations, cardiac arrhythmias, hypertension, anginal pain, and circulatory collapse. Headache, chills, and excessive sweating may also occur.

c. **GI system effects:** *Amphetamine* acts on the GI system, causing anorexia, nausea, vomiting, abdominal cramps, and diarrhea.

d. **Contraindications:** Patients with hypertension, cardiovascular disease, hyperthyroidism, glaucoma, or a history of drug abuse or those taking MAO inhibitors should not be treated with *amphetamine.*

F. Methylphenidate

Methylphenidate has CNS-stimulant properties similar to those of *amphetamine* and may also lead to abuse, although its addictive potential is controversial. It is a Schedule II drug. *Methylphenidate* is presently one of the most prescribed medications in children. It is estimated that 4 to 6 million children in the United States take *methylphenidate* daily for ADHD. The pharmacologically active isomer, *dexmethylphenidate,* is also a Schedule II drug used for the treatment of ADHD.

1. **Mechanism of action:** Children with ADHD may produce weak dopamine signals, which suggests that once-interesting activities provide fewer rewards to these children. *Methylphenidate* is a dopamine and norepinephrine transport inhibitor and may act by increasing both dopamine and norepinephrine in the synaptic space. [Note: *Methylphenidate* may have less potential for abuse than *cocaine,* because it enters the brain much more slowly than *cocaine* and, thus, does not increase dopamine levels as rapidly.]

2. **Therapeutic uses:** *Methylphenidate* has been used for several decades in the treatment of ADHD. It is also effective in the treatment of narcolepsy. Unlike *methylphenidate, dexmethylphenidate* is not indicated in the treatment of narcolepsy.

3. **Pharmacokinetics:** Both *methylphenidate* and *dexmethylphenidate* are readily absorbed after oral administration. *Methylphenidate* is available in extended-release oral formulations and as a transdermal patch for once-daily application. The de-esterified product, ritalinic acid, is excreted in urine.

4. **Adverse effects:** GI adverse effects are the most common and include abdominal pain and nausea. Other reactions include anorexia, insomnia, nervousness, and fever. In seizure patients, *methylphenidate* may increase seizure frequency, especially if the patient is taking antidepressants. It is contraindicated in patients with glaucoma. *Methylphenidate* can inhibit the metabolism of *warfarin, phenytoin, phenobarbital, primidone,* and the tricyclic antidepressants.

III. HALLUCINOGENS

A few drugs have, as their primary action, the ability to induce altered perceptual states reminiscent of dreams. Many of these altered states are accompanied by visions of bright, colorful changes in the environment and by a plasticity of constantly changing shapes and color. The individual under the influence of these drugs is incapable of normal decision making because the drug interferes with rational thought. These compounds are known as hallucinogens, and *lysergic acid diethylamide (LSD)* and *tetrahydrocannabinol* (from marijuana) are examples of agents in this class. These agents are discussed in detail in Chapter 15.

Study Questions

Choose the ONE best answer.

16.1 A young male was brought to the emergency room by the police due to severe agitation. Psychiatric examination revealed that he had injected dextroamphetamine several times in the past few days, the last time being 10 hours previously. He was given a drug that sedated him, and he fell asleep. Which of the following drugs was most likely used to counter this patient's apparent symptoms of dextroamphetamine withdrawal?

A. Phenobarbital.

B. Lorazepam.

C. Cocaine.

D. Hydroxyzine.

E. Fluoxetine.

Correct answer = B. The anxiolytic properties of benzodiazepines, such as lorazepam, make them the drugs of choice in treating the anxiety and agitation of amphetamine or cocaine abuse. Lorazepam also has hypnotic properties. Phenobarbital has hypnotic properties, but its anxiolytic properties are inferior to those of the benzodiazepines. Hydroxyzine, an antihistamine, is effective as a hypnotic, and it is sometimes used to deal with anxiety, especially if emesis is a problem. Fluoxetine is an antidepressant with no immediate effects on anxiety or agitation.

16.2 JM is a 10-year-old male who is sent to a pediatric neurologist for an evaluation due to receiving poor grades in class. JM's parents have recently received complaints from his teacher that he is performing poorly in school and he is repeatedly caught not paying attention in class. Several times a day during class, JM is noted to be getting out of his chair and socializing with other students. He has also been getting into fights with some children, as he is being singled out by others and teased. JM is given a diagnosis of ADHD with impulsivity and irritability. Which of the following is the most appropriate recommendation for management of the ADHD?

A. Clonidine.

B. Caffeine.

C. Dextroamphetamine.

D. Haloperidol.

E. Buspirone.

Correct answer = C. Dextroamphetamine is the only stimulant medication in the list that is approved for ADHD. Certain symptoms like fighting may improve with haloperidol and hyperactivity may improve with clonidine, but these agents would not improve the patient's academic performance and the underlying problems.

16.3 JM is a 10-year-old male with ADHD. His symptoms are currently controlled with an oral psychostimulant. However, he and his family wish to avoid having to give a second dose of medication at school. They are looking for an alternative treatment option that could be implemented in the morning and last the entire day. Which treatment option would be best for JM's needs?

A. Mixed amphetamine salts in immediate-release oral tablet formulation.

B. Methylphenidate in a transdermal delivery system.

C. Nicotine in a chewing gum formulation for buccal absorption.

D. Methylphenidate in immediate-release pills.

Correct answer = B. Methylphenidate is also a psychostimulant, and the transdermal (patch) formulation is designed for once-per-day use to avoid middle of the day dosing. Immediate-release formulations require dosing at least twice daily. Nicotine is not indicated for ADHD.

16.4 Which of the following treatments for ADHD is a controlled substance (DEA Schedule II)?

A. Clonidine.

B. Guanfacine.

C. Atomoxetine.

D. Dexmethylphenidate.

E. Desipramine.

Correct answer = D. Dexmethylphenidate is the only controlled substance on the list and is DEA scheduled II. The other agents may assist in the management of ADHD but are not controlled substances.

16.5 Amphetamines are contraindicated in patients with all of the following conditions except:

 A. Cardiovascular disease.
 B. Glaucoma.
 C. Hypertension.
 D. Hyperthyroidism.
 E. Obesity.

Correct answer= E. The use of amphetamines in the management of obesity should be closely monitored. However, this is an older use of these agents, and there are amphetamine analogs that are FDA approved for obesity. The other conditions are contraindications when considering the use of amphetamines, because amphetamines may exacerbate these medical conditions.

16.6 Which of the following agents is considered a first-line treatment for narcolepsy?

 A. Donepezil.
 B. Atomoxetine.
 C. Clonidine.
 D. Temazepam.
 E. Modafinil.

Correct answer = E. Modafinil is the only drug listed that is approved for narcolepsy. Temazepam is indicated for insomnia, donepezil for Alzheimer's disease, clonidine for hypertension, and atomoxetine for ADHD.

16.7 Which of the following is a common adverse effect of amphetamines?

 A. Bradycardia.
 B. Somnolence.
 C. Constipation.
 D. Hypertension.
 E. Fatigue.

Correct answer = D. Hypertension is a possible adverse effect that warrants caution, especially in individuals with risk factors for increased blood pressure. Amphetamines cause tachycardia (not bradycardia), insomnia (not somnolence), diarrhea (not constipation), and alertness (not fatigue).

16.8 Which of the following CNS stimulants occurs naturally and can be found in certain candies?

 A. Amphetamine.
 B. Clonidine.
 C. Modafinil.
 D. Caffeine.
 E. Atomoxetine.

Correct answer = D. Caffeine is a naturally occurring substance found in cocoa, chocolate, and many forms of tea. Overuse of cola beverages and other caffeine-containing products may cause adverse effects, including anxiety and insomnia, and even increase the risk for seizures.

16.9 TT is a 35-year-old male who is interested in quitting smoking. In previous quit attempts, he has tried nicotine gum, the nicotine patch, and the "cold turkey" method. He has been unsuccessful in each of these attempts and usually resumed smoking within 4 to 6 weeks. Which of the following may be useful to assist TT in his attempt to quit smoking?

 A. Varenicline.
 B. Dextroamphetamine.
 C. Lorazepam.
 D. Methylphenidate.

Correct answer = A. Varenicline is FDA approved as an adjunctive treatment option for the management of nicotine dependence. It is believed to attenuate the withdrawal symptoms of smoking cessation, though continued observation is needed to monitor for changes in psychiatric status, including suicidal ideation. The use of dextroamphetamine, lorazepam, and methylphenidate will bring the risk of addiction to another substance with abuse potential.

16.10 All of the following drugs are controlled substances with a risk for drug addiction or dependence except:

 A. Armodafinil.
 B. Lisdexamfetamine.
 C. Dexmethylphenidate.
 D. Atomoxetine.
 E. Methamphetamine.

Correct answer = D. Atomoxetine is the only agent listed that is not a controlled substance. All of the other agents are considered to have a risk for addiction and/or dependence.

Antihypertensives

17

Kyle Melin

I. OVERVIEW

Hypertension is defined as either a sustained systolic blood pressure of greater than 140 mm Hg or a sustained diastolic blood pressure of greater than 90 mm Hg. Hypertension results from increased peripheral vascular arteriolar smooth muscle tone, which leads to increased arteriolar resistance and reduced capacitance of the venous system. In most cases, the cause of the increased vascular tone is unknown. Elevated blood pressure is a common disorder, affecting approximately 30% of adults in the United States. Although many patients have no symptoms, chronic hypertension can lead to heart disease and stroke, the top two causes of death in the world. Hypertension is also an important risk factor in the development of chronic kidney disease and heart failure. The incidence of morbidity and mortality significantly decreases when hypertension is diagnosed early and is properly treated. The drugs used in the treatment of hypertension are shown in Figure 17.1. In recognition of the

ANGIOTENSIN II RECEPTOR BLOCKERS
Azilsartan medoxomil EDARBI
Candesartan ATACAND
Eprosartan TEVETEN
Irbesartan AVAPRO
Losartan COZAAR
Olmesartan BENICAR
Telmisartan MICARDIS
Valsartan DIOVAN

RENIN INHIBITORS
Aliskiren TEKTURNA

ACE INHIBITORS
Benazepril LOTENSIN
Captopril CAPOTEN
Enalapril VASOTEC
Fosinopril MONOPRIL
Lisinopril PRINIVIL, ZESTRIL
Moexipril UNIVASC
Quinapril ACCUPRIL
Perindopril ACEON
Ramipril ALTACE
Trandolapril MAVIK

DIURETICS
Amiloride MIDAMOR
Bumetanide BUMEX
Chlorthalidone HYGROTON
Eplerenone INSPRA
Ethacrynic acid EDECRIN
Furosemide LASIX
Hydrochlorothiazide MICROZIDE
Indapamide LOZOL
Metolazone MYKROX, ZAROXOLYN
Spironolactone ALDACTONE
Triamterene DYRENIUM
Torsemide DEMADEX

β-BLOCKERS
Acebutolol SECTRAL
Atenolol TENORMIN
Betaxolol KERLONE
Bisoprolol ZEBETA
Carvedilol COREG, COREG CR
Esmolol BREVIBLOC
Labetalol TRANDATE
Metoprolol LOPRESSOR, TOPROL-XL
Nadolol CORGARD
Nebivolol BYSTOLIC
Penbutolol LEVATOL
Pindolol VISKEN
Propranolol INDERAL LA, INNOPRAN XL
Timolol BLOCADREN

Figure 17.1
Summary of antihypertensive drugs. ACE = angiotensin-converting enzyme.
(Figure continues on next page.)

CALCIUM CHANNEL BLOCKERS

Amlodipine NORVASC
Clevidipine CLEVIPREX
Diltiazem CARDIZEM, CARTIA, DILACOR
Felodipine PLENDIL
Isradipine DYNACIRC CR
Nicardipine CARDENE
Nifedipine ADALAT, NIFEDIAC, PROCARDIA
Nisoldipine SULAR
Verapamil CALAN, ISOPTIN, VERELAN

α-BLOCKERS

Doxazosin CARDURA
Prazosin MINIPRESS
Terazosin HYTRIN

OTHERS

Clonidine CATAPRES, DURACLON
Fenoldopam CORLOPAM
Hydralazine APRESOLINE
Methyldopa ALDOMET
Minoxidil LONITEN
Nitroprusside NITROPRESS

Figure 17.1 (Continued)
Summary of antihypertensive drugs.

	Systolic mm Hg		Diastolic mm Hg
Normal	<120	and	<80
Prehyper-tension	120–139	or	80–89
Stage I	140–159	or	90–99
Stage II	≥160	or	≥100

Figure 17.2
Classification of blood pressure.

progressive nature of hypertension, hypertension is classified into four categories for the purpose of treatment management (Figure 17.2).

II. ETIOLOGY OF HYPERTENSION

Although hypertension may occur secondary to other disease processes, more than 90% of patients have essential hypertension (hypertension with no identifiable cause). A family history of hypertension increases the likelihood that an individual will develop hypertension. The prevalence of hypertension increases with age, but decreases with education and income level. Non-Hispanic blacks have a higher incidence of hypertension than do both non-Hispanic whites and Hispanic whites. Persons with diabetes, obesity, or disability status are all more likely to have hypertension than those without. In addition, environmental factors, such as a stressful lifestyle, high dietary intake of sodium, and smoking, may further predispose an individual to hypertension.

III. MECHANISMS FOR CONTROLLING BLOOD PRESSURE

Arterial blood pressure is regulated within a narrow range to provide adequate perfusion of the tissues without causing damage to the vascular system, particularly the arterial intima (endothelium). Arterial blood pressure is directly proportional to cardiac output and peripheral vascular resistance (Figure 17.3). Cardiac output and peripheral resistance, in turn, are controlled mainly by two overlapping control mechanisms: the baroreflexes and the renin–angiotensin–aldosterone system (Figure 17.4). Most antihypertensive drugs lower blood pressure by reducing cardiac output and/or decreasing peripheral resistance.

A. Baroreceptors and the sympathetic nervous system

Baroreflexes act by changing the activity of the sympathetic nervous system. Therefore, they are responsible for the rapid, moment-to-moment regulation of blood pressure. A fall in blood pressure causes pressure-sensitive neurons (baroreceptors in the aortic arch and carotid sinuses) to send fewer impulses to cardiovascular centers in the spinal cord. This prompts a reflex response of increased sympathetic and decreased parasympathetic output to the heart and vasculature, resulting in vasoconstriction and increased cardiac output. These changes result in a compensatory rise in blood pressure (Figure 17.4).

B. Renin–angiotensin–aldosterone system

The kidney provides long-term control of blood pressure by altering the blood volume. Baroreceptors in the kidney respond to reduced arterial pressure (and to sympathetic stimulation of β_1-adrenoceptors) by releasing the enzyme renin (Figure 17.4). Low sodium intake and greater sodium loss also increase renin release. Renin converts angiotensinogen to angiotensin I, which is converted in turn to angiotensin II, in the presence of angiotensin-converting enzyme (ACE). Angiotensin II is a potent circulating vasoconstrictor, constricting both arterioles and veins, resulting in an increase in blood pressure. Angiotensin II exerts a preferential vasoconstrictor action on the efferent arterioles of the renal glomerulus, increasing glomerular filtration. Furthermore, angiotensin II stimulates aldosterone secretion, leading to increased renal sodium reabsorption and increased blood volume, which contribute to a further increase in blood pressure. These effects of angiotensin II are mediated by stimulation of angiotensin II type 1 (AT$_1$) receptors.

IV. TREATMENT STRATEGIES

The goal of antihypertensive therapy is to reduce cardiovascular and renal morbidity and mortality. The relationship between blood pressure and the risk of cardiovascular events is continuous, and, thus, lowering of even moderately elevated blood pressure significantly reduces cardiovascular disease. The classification of "prehypertension" recognizes this relationship and emphasizes the need for decreasing blood pressure in the general population by education and the adoption of blood pressure–lowering behaviors. For most patients, the blood pressure goal when treating hypertension is a systolic blood pressure of less than 140 mm Hg and a diastolic blood pressure of less than 90 mm Hg. Mild hypertension can sometimes be controlled with monotherapy, but most patients require more than one drug to achieve blood pressure control. Current recommendations are to initiate therapy with a thiazide diuretic, ACE inhibitor, angiotensin receptor blocker (ARB), or

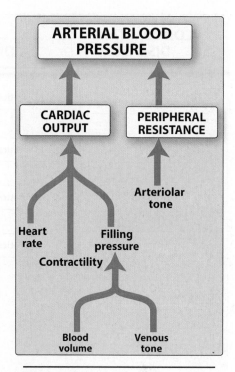

Figure 17.3
Major factors influencing blood pressure.

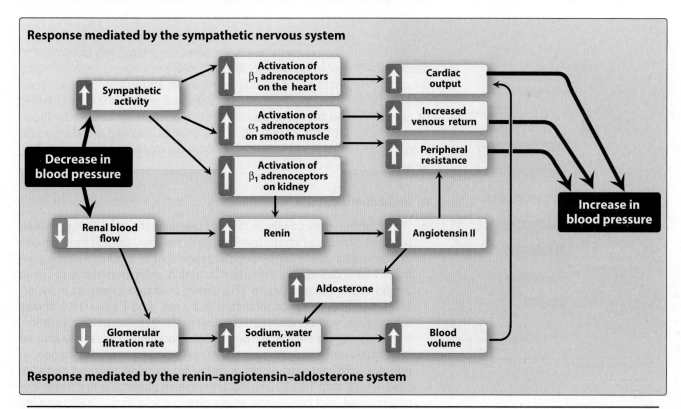

Figure 17.4
Response of the autonomic nervous system and the renin–angiotensin–aldosterone system to a decrease in blood pressure.

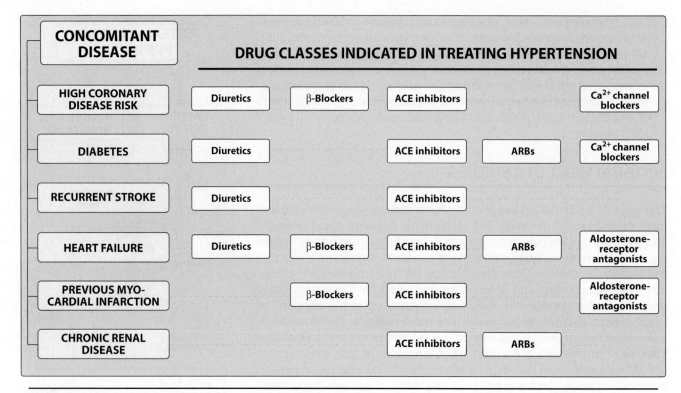

Figure 17.5
Treatment of hypertension in patients with concomitant diseases. [Note: Angiotensin receptor blockers (ARBs) are an alternative to angiotensin-converting enzyme (ACE) inhibitors.]

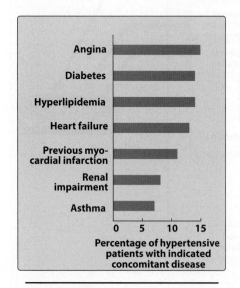

Figure 17.6
Frequency of occurrence of concomitant disease among the hypertensive patient population.

calcium channel blocker. If blood pressure is inadequately controlled, a second drug should be added, with the selection based on minimizing the adverse effects of the combined regimen and achieving goal blood pressure. Patients with systolic blood pressure greater than 160 mm Hg or diastolic blood pressure greater than 100 mm Hg (or systolic blood pressure greater than 20 mm Hg above goal or diastolic blood pressure more than 10 mm Hg above goal) should be started on two antihypertensives simultaneously.

A. Individualized care

Hypertension may coexist with other diseases that can be aggravated by some of the antihypertensive drugs or that may benefit from the use of some antihypertensive drugs independent of blood pressure control. In such cases, it is important to match antihypertensive drugs to the particular patient. Figure 17.5 shows preferred therapies in hypertensive patients with concomitant diseases, and Figure 17.6 shows the frequency of concomitant disease in the hypertensive population. In addition to the choice of therapy, blood pressure goals may also be individualized based on concurrent disease states. For instance, in patients with diabetes, some experts recommend a blood pressure goal of less than 140/80 mm Hg. Likewise, in patients with chronic kidney disease and proteinuria, lower goals of less than 130/80 mm Hg may be considered. Elderly patients may have less stringent goals (for example, less than 150/90 mm Hg).

B. Patient compliance in antihypertensive therapy

Lack of patient compliance is the most common reason for failure of antihypertensive therapy. The hypertensive patient is usually asymptomatic and is diagnosed by routine screening before the occurrence of overt end-organ damage. Thus, therapy is generally directed at preventing future disease sequelae rather than relieving current discomfort. The adverse effects associated with the hypertensive therapy may influence the patient more than the future benefits. For example, β-blockers can cause sexual dysfunction in males, which may prompt discontinuation of therapy. Thus, it is important to enhance compliance by selecting a drug regimen that reduces adverse effects and also minimizes the number of doses required daily. Combining two drug classes in a single pill, at a fixed-dose combination, has been shown to improve patient compliance and the number of patients achieving goal blood pressure.

V. DIURETICS

Thiazide diuretics can be used as initial drug therapy for hypertension unless there are compelling reasons to choose another agent. Regardless of class, the initial mechanism of action of diuretics is based upon decreasing blood volume, which ultimately leads to decreased blood pressure. Low-dose diuretic therapy is safe, inexpensive, and effective in preventing stroke, myocardial infarction, and heart failure. Routine serum electrolyte monitoring should be done for all patients receiving diuretics. A complete discussion of the actions, therapeutic uses, pharmacokinetics, and adverse effects of diuretics can be found in Chapter 18.

A. Thiazide diuretics

Thiazide diuretics, such as *hydrochlorothiazide* [hye-droe-klor-oh-THYE-a-zide] and *chlorthalidone* [klor-THAL-ih-done], lower blood pressure initially by increasing sodium and water excretion. This causes a decrease in extracellular volume, resulting in a decrease in cardiac output and renal blood flow (Figure 17.7). With long-term treatment, plasma volume approaches a normal value, but a hypotensive effect persists that is related to a decrease in peripheral resistance. Thiazides are useful in combination therapy with a variety of other antihypertensive agents, including β-blockers, ACE inhibitors, ARBs, and potassium-sparing diuretics. With the exception of *metolazone* [me-TOL-ah-zone], thiazide diuretics are not effective in patients with inadequate kidney function (estimated glomerular filtration rate less than 30 mL/min/m²). Loop diuretics may be required in these patients. Thiazide diuretics can induce hypokalemia, hyperuricemia and, to a lesser extent, hyperglycemia in some patients.

B. Loop diuretics

The loop diuretics (*furosemide, torsemide, bumetanide,* and *ethacrynic acid*) act promptly by blocking sodium and chloride reabsorption in the kidneys, even in patients with poor renal function or those who have not responded to thiazide diuretics. Loop diuretics cause decreased renal vascular resistance and increased renal blood flow.

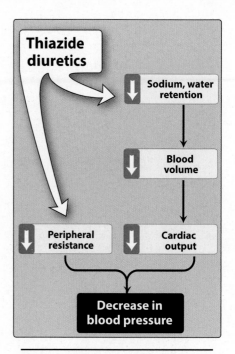

Figure 17.7
Actions of thiazide diuretics.

Like thiazides, they can cause hypokalemia. However, unlike thiazides, loop diuretics increase the Ca^{2+} content of urine, whereas thiazide diuretics decrease it. These agents are rarely used alone to treat hypertension, but they are commonly used to manage symptoms of heart failure and edema.

C. Potassium-sparing diuretics

Amiloride [a-MIL-oh-ride] and *triamterene* [tri-AM-ter-een] (inhibitors of epithelial sodium transport at the late distal and collecting ducts) as well as *spironolactone* [speer-on-oh-LAK-tone] and *eplerenone* [eh-PLEH-reh-none] (aldosterone receptor antagonists) reduce potassium loss in the urine. Aldosterone antagonists have the additional benefit of diminishing the cardiac remodeling that occurs in heart failure (see Chapter 19). Potassium-sparing diuretics are sometimes used in combination with loop diuretics and thiazides to reduce the amount of potassium loss induced by these diuretics.

VI. β-ADRENOCEPTOR–BLOCKING AGENTS

β-Blockers are a treatment option for hypertensive patients with concomitant heart disease or heart failure (Figure 17.5).

A. Actions

The β-blockers reduce blood pressure primarily by decreasing cardiac output (Figure 17.8). They may also decrease sympathetic outflow from the central nervous system (CNS) and inhibit the release of renin from the kidneys, thus decreasing the formation of angiotensin II and the secretion of aldosterone. The prototype β-blocker is *propranolol* [proe PRAN-oh-lol], which acts at both β_1 and β_2 receptors. Selective blockers of β_1 receptors, such as *metoprolol* [met-OH-pro-lol] and *atenolol* [ah-TEN-oh-lol], are among the most commonly prescribed β-blockers. *Nebivolol* is a selective blocker of β_1 receptors, which also increases the production of nitric oxide, leading to vasodilation. The

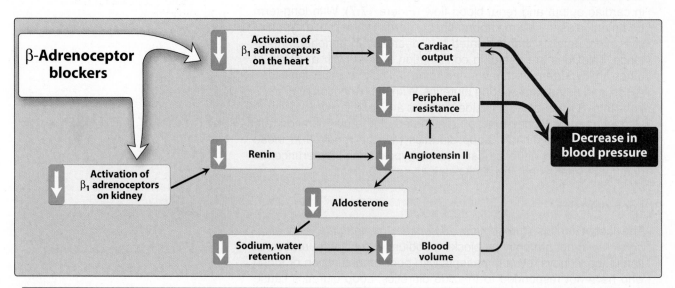

Figure 17.8
Actions of β-adrenoceptor–blocking agents.

selective β-blockers may be administered cautiously to hypertensive patients who also have asthma. The nonselective β-blockers, such as *propranolol* and *nadolol*, are contraindicated in patients with asthma due to their blockade of β_2-mediated bronchodilation. (See Chapter 7 for an in-depth discussion of β-blockers.) β-Blockers should be used cautiously in the treatment of patients with acute heart failure or peripheral vascular disease.

B. Therapeutic uses

The primary therapeutic benefits of β-blockers are seen in hypertensive patients with concomitant heart disease, such as supraventricular tachyarrhythmia (for example, atrial fibrillation), previous myocardial infarction, angina pectoris, and chronic heart failure. Conditions that discourage the use of β-blockers include reversible bronchospastic disease such as asthma, second- and third-degree heart block, and severe peripheral vascular disease.

C. Pharmacokinetics

The β-blockers are orally active for the treatment of hypertension. *Propranolol* undergoes extensive and highly variable first-pass metabolism. Oral β-blockers may take several weeks to develop their full effects. *Esmolol*, *metoprolol*, and *propranolol* are available in intravenous formulations.

D. Adverse effects

1. **Common effects:** The β-blockers may cause bradycardia, hypotension, and CNS side effects such as fatigue, lethargy, and insomnia (Figure 17.9). The β-blockers may decrease libido and cause erectile dysfunction, which can severely reduce patient compliance.

2. **Alterations in serum lipid patterns:** Noncardioselective β-blockers may disturb lipid metabolism, decreasing high-density lipoprotein cholesterol and increasing triglycerides.

3. **Drug withdrawal:** Abrupt withdrawal may induce angina, myocardial infarction, and even sudden death in patients with ischemic heart disease. Therefore, these drugs must be tapered over a few weeks in patients with hypertension and ischemic heart disease.

VII. ACE INHIBITORS

The ACE inhibitors, such as *enalapril* [e-NAL-ah-pril] and *lisinopril* [lye-SIN-oh-pril], are recommended as first-line treatment of hypertension in patients with a variety of compelling indications, including high coronary disease risk or history of diabetes, stroke, heart failure, myocardial infarction, or chronic kidney disease (Figure 17.5).

A. Actions

The ACE inhibitors lower blood pressure by reducing peripheral vascular resistance without reflexively increasing cardiac output, heart rate, or contractility. These drugs block the enzyme ACE which

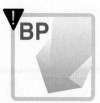
Hypotension

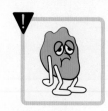
Bradycardia

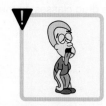
Fatigue

Insomnia

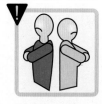
Sexual dysfunction

Figure 17.9
Some adverse effects of β-blockers.

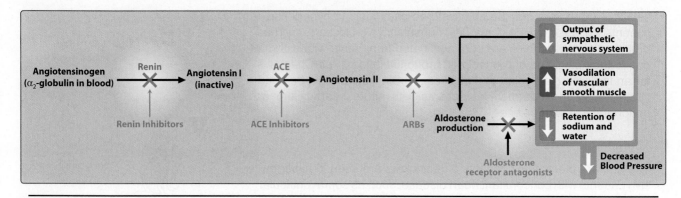

Figure 17.10
Effects of various drug classes on the renin–angiotensin–aldosterone system. Blue = drug target enzymes; red = drug class.

cleaves angiotensin I to form the potent vasoconstrictor angiotensin II (Figure 17.10). ACE is also responsible for the breakdown of bradykinin, a peptide that increases the production of nitric oxide and prostacyclin by the blood vessels. Both nitric oxide and prostacyclin are potent vasodilators. ACE inhibitors decrease angiotensin II and increase bradykinin levels. Vasodilation of both arterioles and veins occurs as a result of decreased vasoconstriction (from diminished levels of angiotensin II) and enhanced vasodilation (from increased bradykinin). By reducing circulating angiotensin II levels, ACE inhibitors also decrease the secretion of aldosterone, resulting in decreased sodium and water retention. ACE inhibitors reduce both cardiac preload and afterload, thereby decreasing cardiac work.

B. Therapeutic uses

Like the ARBs, ACE inhibitors slow the progression of diabetic nephropathy and decrease albuminuria and, thus, have a compelling indication for use in patients with diabetic nephropathy. Beneficial effects on renal function may result from decreasing intraglomerular pressures, due to efferent arteriolar vasodilation. ACE inhibitors are a standard in the care of a patient following a myocardial infarction and first-line agents in the treatment of patients with systolic dysfunction. Chronic treatment with ACE inhibitors achieves sustained blood pressure reduction, regression of left ventricular hypertrophy, and prevention of ventricular remodeling after a myocardial infarction. ACE inhibitors are first-line drugs for treating heart failure, hypertensive patients with chronic kidney disease, and patients at increased risk of coronary artery disease. All of the ACE inhibitors are equally effective in the treatment of hypertension at equivalent doses.

C. Pharmacokinetics

All of the ACE inhibitors are orally bioavailable as a drug or prodrug. All but *captopril* [KAP-toe-pril] and *lisinopril* undergo hepatic conversion to active metabolites, so these agents may be preferred in patients with severe hepatic impairment. *Fosinopril* [foe-SIN-oh-pril] is the only ACE inhibitor that is not eliminated primarily by the kidneys and does not require dose adjustment in patients with renal impairment. *Enalaprilat* [en-AL-a-pril-AT] is the only drug in this class available intravenously.

D. Adverse effects

Common side effects include dry cough, rash, fever, altered taste, hypotension (in hypovolemic states), and hyperkalemia (Figure 17.11). The dry cough, which occurs in up to 10% of patients, is thought to be due to increased levels of bradykinin and substance P in the pulmonary tree and resolves within a few days of discontinuation. The cough occurs more frequently in women. Angioedema is a rare but potentially life-threatening reaction that may also be due to increased levels of bradykinin. Potassium levels must be monitored while on ACE inhibitors, and potassium supplements and potassium-sparing diuretics should be used with caution due to the risk of hyperkalemia. Serum creatinine levels should also be monitored, particularly in patients with underlying renal disease. However, an increase in serum creatinine of up to 30% above baseline is acceptable and by itself does not warrant discontinuation of treatment. ACE inhibitors can induce fetal malformations and should not be used by pregnant women.

VIII. ANGIOTENSIN II RECEPTOR BLOCKERS

The ARBs, such as *losartan* [LOW-sar-tan] and *irbesartan* [ir-be-SAR-tan], are alternatives to the ACE inhibitors. These drugs block the AT_1 receptors, decreasing the activation of AT_1 receptors by angiotensin II. Their pharmacologic effects are similar to those of ACE inhibitors in that they produce arteriolar and venous dilation and block aldosterone secretion, thus lowering blood pressure and decreasing salt and water retention (Figure 17.10). ARBs do not increase bradykinin levels. They may be used as first-line agents for the treatment of hypertension, especially in patients with a compelling indication of diabetes, heart failure, or chronic kidney disease (Figure 17.5). Adverse effects are similar to those of ACE inhibitors, although the risks of cough and angioedema are significantly decreased. ARBs should not be combined with an ACE inhibitor for the treatment of hypertension due to similar mechanisms and adverse effects. These agents are also teratogenic and should not be used by pregnant women. [Note: The ARBs are discussed more fully in Chapter 19.]

IX. RENIN INHIBITOR

A selective renin inhibitor, *aliskiren* [a-LIS-ke-rin], is available for the treatment of hypertension. *Aliskiren* directly inhibits renin and, thus, acts earlier in the renin–angiotensin–aldosterone system than ACE inhibitors or ARBs (Figure 17.10). It lowers blood pressure about as effectively as ARBs, ACE inhibitors, and thiazides. *Aliskiren* should not be routinely combined with an ACE inhibitor or ARB. *Aliskiren* can cause diarrhea, especially at higher doses, and can also cause cough and angioedema, but probably less often than ACE inhibitors. As with ACE inhibitors and ARBs, *aliskiren* is contraindicated during pregnancy. *Aliskiren* is metabolized by CYP 3A4 and is subject to many drug interactions.

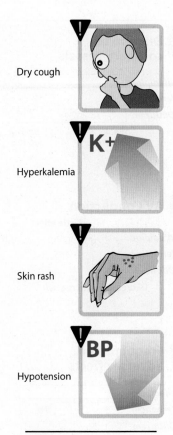

Dry cough

Hyperkalemia

Skin rash

Hypotension

Figure 17.11
Some common adverse effects of the ACE inhibitors.

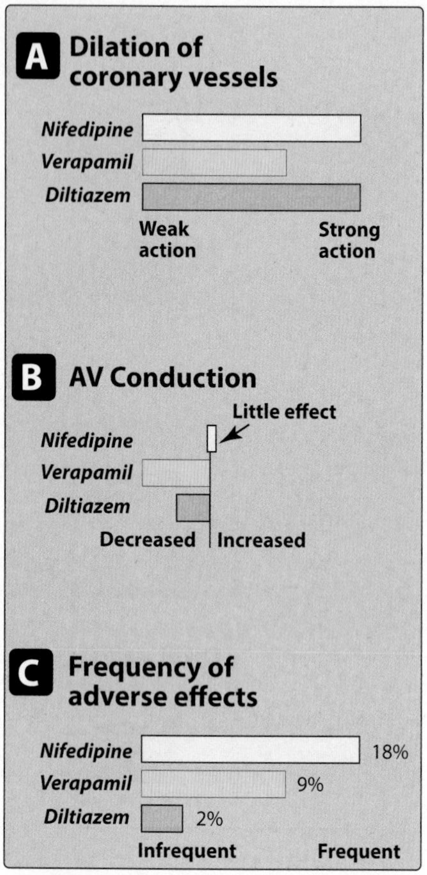

Figure 17.12

Actions of calcium channel blockers. AV = atrioventricular.

X. CALCIUM CHANNEL BLOCKERS

Calcium channel blockers are a recommended treatment option in hypertensive patients with diabetes or angina. High doses of short-acting calcium channel blockers should be avoided because of increased risk of myocardial infarction due to excessive vasodilation and marked reflex cardiac stimulation.

A. Classes of calcium channel blockers

The calcium channel blockers are divided into three chemical classes, each with different pharmacokinetic properties and clinical indications (Figure 17.12).

1. **Diphenylalkylamines:** *Verapamil* [ver-AP-a-mil] is the only member of this class that is available in the United States. *Verapamil* is the least selective of any calcium channel blocker and has significant effects on both cardiac and vascular smooth muscle cells. It is also used to treat angina and supraventricular tachyarrhythmias and to prevent migraine and cluster headaches.

2. **Benzothiazepines:** *Diltiazem* [dil-TYE-a-zem] is the only member of this class that is currently approved in the United States. Like *verapamil*, *diltiazem* affects both cardiac and vascular smooth muscle cells, but it has a less pronounced negative inotropic effect on the heart compared to that of *verapamil. Diltiazem* has a favorable side effect profile.

3. **Dihydropyridines:** This class of calcium channel blockers includes *nifedipine* [nye-FED-i-peen] (the prototype), *amlodipine* [am-LOE-di-peen], *felodipine* [fe-LOE-di-peen], *isradipine* [is-RAD-i-peen], *nicardipine* [nye-KAR-di-peen], and *nisoldipine* [nye-ZOL-di-peen]. These agents differ in pharmacokinetics, approved uses, and drug interactions. All dihydropyridines have a much greater affinity for vascular calcium channels than for calcium channels in the heart. They are, therefore, particularly beneficial in treating hypertension. The dihydropyridines have the advantage in that they show little interaction with other cardiovascular drugs, such as *digoxin* or *warfarin*, which are often used concomitantly with calcium channel blockers.

B. Actions

The intracellular concentration of calcium plays an important role in maintaining the tone of smooth muscle and in the contraction of the myocardium. Calcium enters muscle cells through special voltage-sensitive calcium channels. This triggers release of calcium from the sarcoplasmic reticulum and mitochondria, which further increases the cytosolic level of calcium. Calcium channel antagonists block the inward movement of calcium by binding to L-type calcium channels in the heart and in smooth muscle of the coronary and peripheral arteriolar vasculature. This causes vascular smooth muscle to relax, dilating mainly arterioles. Calcium channel blockers do not dilate veins.

C. Therapeutic uses

In the management of hypertension, CCBs may be used as an initial therapy or as add-on therapy. They are useful in the treatment of hypertensive patients who also have asthma, diabetes, and/or peripheral vascular disease, because unlike β-blockers, they do not have the potential to adversely affect these conditions. All CCBs are useful in the treatment of angina. In addition, *diltiazem* and *verapamil* are used in the treatment of atrial fibrillation.

D. Pharmacokinetics

Most of these agents have short half-lives (3 to 8 hours) following an oral dose. Sustained-release preparations are available and permit once-daily dosing. *Amlodipine* has a very long half-life and does not require a sustained-release formulation.

E. Adverse effects

First-degree atrioventricular block and constipation are common dose-dependent side effects of *verapamil*. *Verapamil* and *diltiazem* should be avoided in patients with heart failure or with atrioventricular block due to their negative inotropic (force of cardiac muscle contraction) and dromotropic (velocity of conduction) effects. Dizziness, headache, and a feeling of fatigue caused by a decrease in blood pressure are more frequent with dihydropyridines (Figure 17.13). Peripheral edema is another commonly reported side effect of this class. *Nifedipine* and other dihydropyridines may cause gingival hyperplasia.

XI. α-ADRENOCEPTOR–BLOCKING AGENTS

Prazosin [PRA-zoe-sin], *doxazosin* [dox-AH-zoe-sin], and *terazosin* [ter-AH-zoe-sin] produce a competitive block of α_1-adrenoceptors. They decrease peripheral vascular resistance and lower arterial blood pressure by causing relaxation of both arterial and venous smooth muscle. These drugs cause only minimal changes in cardiac output, renal blood flow, and glomerular filtration rate. Therefore, long-term tachycardia does not occur, but salt and water retention does. Reflex tachycardia and postural hypotension often occur at the onset of treatment and with dose increases, requiring slow titration of the drug in divided doses. Due to weaker outcome data and their side effect profile, α-blockers are no longer recommended as initial treatment for hypertension, but may be used for refractory cases. Other α_1-blockers with greater selectivity for prostate muscle are used in the treatment of benign prostatic hyperplasia (see Chapter 32).

XII. α-/β-ADRENOCEPTOR–BLOCKING AGENTS

Labetalol [la-BAY-ta-lol] and *carvedilol* [kar-VE-di-lol] block α_1, β_1, and β_2 receptors. *Carvedilol*, although an effective antihypertensive, is mainly used in the treatment of heart failure. *Carvedilol*, as well as *metoprolol succinate*, and *bisoprolol* have been shown to reduce morbidity and mortality associated with heart failure. *Labetalol* is used in the management of gestational hypertension and hypertensive emergencies.

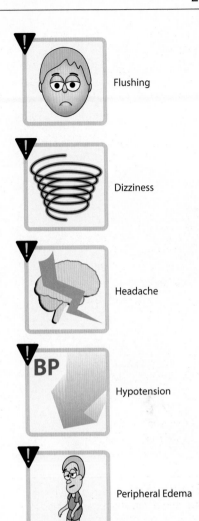

Figure 17.13
Some common adverse effects of the calcium channel blockers.

Flushing

Dizziness

Headache

Hypotension

Peripheral Edema

XIII. CENTRALLY ACTING ADRENERGIC DRUGS

A. Clonidine

Clonidine [KLON-i-deen] acts centrally as an α_2 agonist to produce inhibition of sympathetic vasomotor centers, decreasing sympathetic outflow to the periphery. This leads to reduced total peripheral resistance and decreased blood pressure. *Clonidine* is used primarily for the treatment of hypertension that has not responded adequately to treatment with two or more drugs. *Clonidine* does not decrease renal blood flow or glomerular filtration and, therefore, is useful in the treatment of hypertension complicated by renal disease. *Clonidine* is absorbed well after oral administration and is excreted by the kidney. It is also available in a transdermal patch. Adverse effects include sedation, dry mouth, and constipation. Rebound hypertension occurs following abrupt withdrawal of *clonidine.* The drug should, therefore, be withdrawn slowly if discontinuation is required.

B. Methyldopa

Methyldopa [meth-ill-DOE-pa] is an α_2 agonist that is converted to methylnorepinephrine centrally to diminish adrenergic outflow from the CNS. The most common side effects of *methyldopa* are sedation and drowsiness. Its use is limited due to adverse effects and the need for multiple daily doses. It is mainly used for management of hypertension in pregnancy, where it has a record of safety.

XIV. VASODILATORS

The direct-acting smooth muscle relaxants, such as *hydralazine* [hye-DRAL-a-zeen] and *minoxidil* [min-OX-i-dill], are not used as primary drugs to treat hypertension. These vasodilators act by producing relaxation of vascular smooth muscle, primarily in arteries and arterioles. This results in decreased peripheral resistance and, therefore, blood pressure. Both agents produce reflex stimulation of the heart, resulting in the competing reflexes of increased myocardial contractility, heart rate, and oxygen consumption. These actions may prompt angina pectoris, myocardial infarction, or cardiac failure in predisposed individuals. Vasodilators also increase plasma renin concentration, resulting in sodium and water retention. These undesirable side effects can be blocked by concomitant use of a diuretic and a β-blocker. For example, *hydralazine* is almost always administered in combination with a β-blocker, such as *propranolol, metoprolol,* or *atenolol* (to balance the reflex tachycardia) and a diuretic (to decrease sodium retention). Together, the three drugs decrease cardiac output, plasma volume, and peripheral vascular resistance. *Hydralazine* is an accepted medication for controlling blood pressure in pregnancy-induced hypertension. Adverse effects of *hydralazine* include headache, tachycardia, nausea, sweating, arrhythmia, and precipitation of angina. A lupus-like syndrome can occur with high dosages, but it is reversible upon discontinuation of the drug. *Minoxidil* treatment causes hypertrichosis (the growth of body hair). This drug is used topically to treat male pattern baldness.

XV. HYPERTENSIVE EMERGENCY

Hypertensive emergency is a rare but life-threatening situation characterized by severe elevations in blood pressure (systolic greater than 180 mm Hg or diastolic greater than 120 mm Hg) with evidence of impending or progressive target organ damage (for example, stroke, myocardial infarction). [Note: A severe elevation in blood pressure without evidence of target organ damage is considered a hypertensive urgency.] Hypertensive emergencies require timely blood pressure reduction with treatment administered intravenously to prevent or limit target organ damage. A variety of medications are used, including calcium channel blockers (*nicardipine* and *clevidipine*), nitric oxide vasodilators (*nitroprusside* and *nitroglycerin*), adrenergic receptor antagonists (*phentolamine*, *esmolol*, and *labetalol*), the vasodilator *hydralazine*, and the dopamine agonist *fenoldopam*. Treatment is directed by the type of target organ damage present and/or comorbidities present.

XVI. RESISTANT HYPERTENSION

Resistant hypertension is defined as blood pressure that remains elevated (above goal) despite administration of an optimal three-drug regimen that includes a diuretic. The most common causes of resistant hypertension are poor compliance, excessive ethanol intake, concomitant conditions (diabetes, obesity, sleep apnea, hyperaldosteronism, high salt intake, and/or metabolic syndrome), concomitant medications (sympathomimetics, nonsteroidal anti-inflammatory drugs, or antidepressant medications), insufficient dose and/or drugs, and use of drugs with similar mechanisms of action.

XVII. COMBINATION THERAPY

Combination therapy with separate agents or a fixed-dose combination pill may lower blood pressure more quickly with minimal adverse effects. Initiating therapy with two antihypertensive drugs should be considered in patients with blood pressures that are more than 20/10 mm Hg above the goal. A variety of combination formulations of the various pharmacologic classes are available to increase ease of patient adherence to treatment regimens that require multiple medications to achieve the blood pressure goal.

Study Questions

Choose the ONE best answer.

17.1 A 45-year-old man was just started on therapy for hypertension and developed a persistent, dry cough. Which is most likely responsible for this side effect?

　　A. Enalapril.
　　B. Losartan.
　　C. Nifedipine.
　　D. Prazosin.
　　E. Propranolol.

Correct answer = A. The cough is most likely an adverse effect of the ACE inhibitor enalapril. Losartan is an ARB that has the same beneficial effects as an ACE inhibitor but is less likely to produce a cough. Nifedipine, prazosin, and propranolol do not cause this side effect.

17.2 Which may cause reflex tachycardia and/or postural hypotension on initial administration?

A. Atenolol.

B. Hydrochlorothiazide.

C. Metoprolol.

D. Prazosin.

E. Verapamil.

Correct answer = D. Prazosin produces first-dose hypotension, presumably by blocking α_1 receptors. This effect is minimized by initially giving the drug in small, divided doses. The other agents do not have this adverse effect.

17.3 Which can precipitate a hypertensive crisis following abrupt cessation of therapy?

A. Clonidine.

B. Diltiazem.

C. Enalapril.

D. Losartan.

E. Hydrochlorothiazide.

Correct answer = A. Increased sympathetic nervous system activity occurs if clonidine therapy is abruptly stopped after prolonged administration. Uncontrolled elevation in blood pressure can occur. Patients should be slowly weaned from clonidine while other antihypertensive medications are initiated. The other drugs on the list do not produce this phenomenon.

17.4 A 48-year-old hypertensive patient has been successfully treated with a thiazide diuretic for the last 5 years. Over the last 3 months, his diastolic pressure has steadily increased, and he was started on an additional antihypertensive agent. He complains of several instances of being unable to achieve an erection and not being able to complete three sets of tennis as he once did. Which is the likely second antihypertensive medication?

A. Captopril.

B. Losartan.

C. Metoprolol.

D. Minoxidil.

E. Nifedipine.

Correct answer = C. The side effect profile of β-blockers, such as metoprolol, is characterized by interference with sexual performance and decreased exercise tolerance. None of the other drugs is likely to produce this combination of side effects.

17.5 A 40-year-old male has recently been diagnosed with hypertension due to pressure readings of 163/102 and 165/100 mm Hg. He also has diabetes that is well controlled with oral hypoglycemic medications. Which is the best initial treatment regimen for treatment of hypertension in this patient?

A. Felodipine.

B. Furosemide.

C. Lisinopril.

D. Lisinopril and hydrochlorothiazide.

E. Metoprolol.

Correct answer = D. Because the systolic blood pressure is more than 20 mm Hg above goal (10 mm Hg above goal diastolic), treatment with two different medications is preferred. Because the patient is diabetic, he also has a compelling indication for an ACE inhibitor or ARB.

17.6 A 60-year-old white female has not reached her blood pressure goal after 1 month of treatment with a low dose of lisinopril. All of the following would be appropriate next steps in the treatment of her hypertension except:

A. Increase dose of lisinopril.

B. Add a diuretic medication.

C. Add on a calcium channel blocker medication.

D. Add on an ARB medication.

Correct answer = D. Increasing the dose of lisinopril or adding a second medication from a different class (such as a calcium channel blocker or diuretic) would be appropriate steps to control the blood pressure. Adding an ARB as the second medication is not recommended. ARBs have a similar mechanism of action to ACE inhibitors, and combination therapy may increase the risk of adverse effects.

17.7 A patient returns to her health care provider for routine monitoring 3 months after her hypertension regimen was modified. Labs reveal elevated serum potassium. Which is likely responsible for this hyperkalemia?

A. Chlorthalidone.

B. Clonidine.

C. Furosemide.

D. Losartan.

E. Nifedipine.

Correct answer = D. Losartan, an ARB, can cause an increase in serum potassium similar to ACE inhibitors. Furosemide and chlorthalidone can cause a decrease in serum potassium. Nifedipine and clonidine do not affect potassium levels.

17.8 A 58-year-old female reports that she recently stopped taking her blood pressure medications because of swelling in her feet that began shortly after she started treatment. Which is most likely to cause peripheral edema?

A. Atenolol.

B. Clonidine.

C. Felodipine.

D. Hydralazine.

E. Prazosin.

Correct answer = C. Peripheral edema is one of the most common side effects of calcium channel blockers. None of the other agents commonly cause peripheral edema.

17.9 Which is an appropriate choice for hypertension treatment during pregnancy?

A. Aliskiren.

B. Fosinopril.

C. Hydralazine.

D. Valsartan.

Correct answer = C. Hydralazine is an appropriate choice for a hypertensive pregnant patient. ACE inhibitors, ARBs, and the direct renin inhibitor, aliskiren, are all contraindicated in pregnancy due to their potential for fetal harm.

17.10 DD is a 50-year-old male with newly diagnosed hypertension. His comorbidities include diabetes and chronic hepatitis C infection with moderate liver impairment. He requires two drugs for initial treatment of his hypertension. Which should be prescribed in combination with a thiazide diuretic?

A. Lisinopril.

B. Spironolactone.

C. Fosinopril.

D. Furosemide.

E. Hydralazine.

Correct answer = A. Because DD has diabetes, he has a compelling indication for an ACE inhibitor or ARB for the treatment of his hypertension and prevention of diabetic nephropathy. However, most ACE inhibitors undergo hepatic conversion to active metabolites, so his hepatic impairment is of concern. Because lisinopril is one of the two ACE inhibitors that does not undergo hepatic conversion to active metabolites, it is the best choice. Fosinopril is the only ACE inhibitor that is not eliminated primarily by the kidneys but does undergo hepatic conversion. An additional diuretic like spironolactone or furosemide is not indicated. DD does not have a compelling indication for hydralazine.

Diuretics

Jason Powell

18

I. OVERVIEW

Diuretics are drugs that increase the volume of urine excreted. Most diuretic agents are inhibitors of renal ion transporters that decrease the reabsorption of Na^+ at different sites in the nephron. As a result, Na^+ and other ions, such as Cl^-, enter the urine in greater than normal amounts along with water, which is carried passively to maintain osmotic equilibrium. Diuretics, thus, increase the volume of urine and often change its pH, as well as the ionic composition of the urine and blood. The diuretic effect of the different classes of diuretics varies considerably, with the increase in Na^+ secretion varying from less than 2% for the weak potassium-sparing diuretics to over 20% for the potent loop diuretics. In addition to the ion transport inhibitors, other types of diuretics include osmotic diuretics, aldosterone antagonists, and carbonic anhydrase inhibitors. Diuretics are most commonly used for management of abnormal fluid retention (edema) or treatment of hypertension. In this chapter, the diuretic drugs (Figure 18.1) are discussed according to the frequency of their use.

II. NORMAL REGULATION OF FLUID AND ELECTROLYTES BY THE KIDNEYS

Approximately 16% to 20% of the blood plasma entering the kidneys is filtered from the glomerular capillaries into Bowman's capsule. The filtrate, although normally free of proteins and blood cells, contains most of the low molecular weight plasma components in concentrations similar to that in the plasma. These include glucose, sodium bicarbonate, amino acids, and other organic solutes, as well as electrolytes, such as Na^+, K^+, and Cl^-. The kidney regulates the ionic composition and volume of urine by active reabsorption or secretion of ions and/or passive reabsorption of water at five functional zones along the nephron: 1) the proximal convoluted tubule, 2) the descending loop of Henle, 3) the ascending loop of Henle, 4) the distal convoluted tubule, and 5) the collecting tubule and duct (Figure 18.2).

A. Proximal convoluted tubule

In the proximal convoluted tubule located in the cortex of the kidney, almost all the glucose, bicarbonate, amino acids, and other metabolites are reabsorbed. Approximately two-thirds of the Na^+ is also

---

THIAZIDE DIURETICS

Chlorothiazide DIURIL, SODIUM DIURIL
Chlorthalidone THALITONE
Hydrochlorothiazide (**HCTZ**) MICROZIDE
Indapamide
Metolazone ZAROXOLYN

LOOP DIURETICS

Bumetanide
Ethacrynic acid EDECRIN
Furosemide LASIX
Torsemide DEMADEX

POTASSIUM-SPARING DIURETICS

Amiloride MIDAMOR
Eplerenone INSPRA
Spironolactone ALDACTONE
Triamterene DYRENIUM

CARBONIC ANHYDRASE INHIBITORS

Acetazolamide DIAMOX

OSMOTIC DIURETICS

Mannitol OSMITROL
Urea

Figure 18.1
Summary of diuretic drugs.

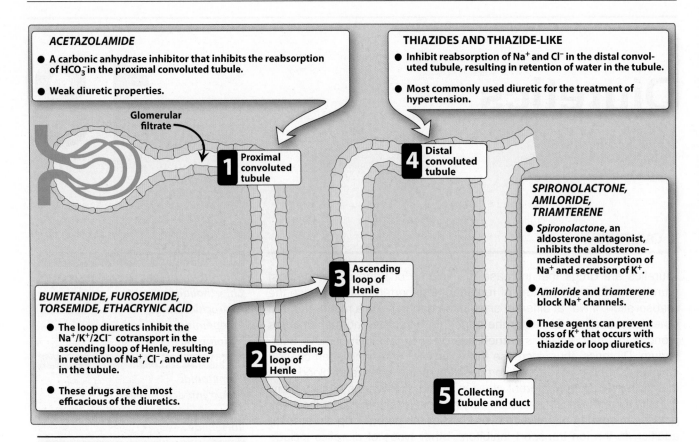

ACETAZOLAMIDE

● A carbonic anhydrase inhibitor that inhibits the reabsorption of HCO_3^- in the proximal convoluted tubule.

● Weak diuretic properties.

THIAZIDES AND THIAZIDE-LIKE

● Inhibit reabsorption of Na^+ and Cl^- in the distal convoluted tubule, resulting in retention of water in the tubule.

● Most commonly used diuretic for the treatment of hypertension.

Glomerular filtrate

1 Proximal convoluted tubule

4 Distal convoluted tubule

SPIRONOLACTONE, AMILORIDE, TRIAMTERENE

● *Spironolactone*, an aldosterone antagonist, inhibits the aldosterone-mediated reabsorption of Na^+ and secretion of K^+.

● *Amiloride* and *triamterene* block Na^+ channels.

● These agents can prevent loss of K^+ that occurs with thiazide or loop diuretics.

3 Ascending loop of Henle

BUMETANIDE, FUROSEMIDE, TORSEMIDE, ETHACRYNIC ACID

● The loop diuretics inhibit the $Na^+/K^+/2Cl^-$ cotransport in the ascending loop of Henle, resulting in retention of Na^+, Cl^-, and water in the tubule.

● These drugs are the most efficacious of the diuretics.

2 Descending loop of Henle

5 Collecting tubule and duct

Figure 18.2
Major locations of ion and water exchange in the nephron, showing sites of action of the diuretic drugs.

reabsorbed. Chloride enters the lumen of the tubule in exchange for an anion, such as oxalate, as well as paracellularly through the lumen. Water follows passively from the lumen to the blood to maintain osmolar equality. If not for the extensive reabsorption of solutes and water in the proximal tubule, the mammalian organism would rapidly become dehydrated and fail to maintain normal osmolarity. The Na^+ that is reabsorbed is pumped into the interstitium by Na^+/K^+-adenosine triphosphatase (ATPase) pump, thereby maintaining normal levels of Na^+ and K^+ in the cell. Carbonic anhydrase in the luminal membrane and cytoplasm of the proximal tubular cells modulates the reabsorption of bicarbonate.

The proximal tubule is the site of the organic acid and base secretory systems (Figure 18.3). The organic acid secretory system, located in the middle-third of the proximal tubule, secretes a variety of organic acids, such as uric acid, some antibiotics, and diuretics, from the bloodstream into the proximal tubular lumen. Most diuretic drugs are delivered to the tubular fluid via this system. The organic acid secretory system is saturable, and diuretic drugs in the bloodstream compete for transfer with endogenous organic acids such as uric acid. A number of other interactions can also occur. For example, *probenecid* interferes with *penicillin* secretion. The organic base secretory system, located in the upper and middle segments of the proximal tubule, is responsible for the secretion of creatinine and choline.

B. Descending loop of Henle

The remaining filtrate, which is isotonic, next enters the descending limb of the loop of Henle and passes into the medulla of the kidney. The osmolarity increases along the descending portion of the loop of Henle because of the countercurrent mechanism that is responsible for water reabsorption. This results in a tubular fluid with a threefold increase in salt concentration. Osmotic diuretics exert part of their action in this region.

C. Ascending loop of Henle

The cells of the ascending tubular epithelium are unique in being impermeable to water. Active reabsorption of Na^+, K^+, and Cl^- is mediated by a $Na^+/K^+/2Cl^-$ cotransporter. Both Mg^{2+} and Ca^{2+} enter the interstitial fluid via the paracellular pathway. The ascending loop is, thus, a diluting region of the nephron. Approximately 25% to 30% of the tubular sodium chloride returns to the interstitial fluid, thereby helping to maintain high osmolarity. Because the ascending loop of Henle is a major site for salt reabsorption, drugs affecting this site, such as loop diuretics (Figure 18.2), have the greatest diuretic effect.

D. Distal convoluted tubule

The cells of the distal convoluted tubule are also impermeable to water. About 10% of the filtered sodium chloride is reabsorbed via a Na^+/Cl^- transporter that is sensitive to thiazide diuretics. Calcium reabsorption is mediated by passage through a channel and then transported by a Na^+/Ca^{2+}-exchanger into the interstitial fluid. The mechanism, thus, differs from that in the loop of Henle. Additionally, Ca^{2+} excretion is regulated by parathyroid hormone in this portion of the tubule.

E. Collecting tubule and duct

The principal cells of the collecting tubule and duct are responsible for Na^+, K^+, and water transport, whereas the intercalated cells affect H^+ secretion. Sodium enters the principal cells through channels (epithelial sodium channels) that are inhibited by *amiloride* and *triamterene*. Once inside the cell, Na^+ reabsorption relies on a Na^+/K^+-ATPase pump to be transported into the blood. Aldosterone receptors in the principal cells influence Na^+ reabsorption and K^+ secretion. Aldosterone increases the synthesis of Na^+ channels and of the Na^+/K^+-ATPase pump, which when combined increase Na^+ reabsorption. Antidiuretic hormone (ADH; vasopressin) receptors promote the reabsorption of water from the collecting tubules and ducts (Figure 18.3).

III. THIAZIDES AND RELATED AGENTS

The thiazides are the most widely used diuretics. They are sulfonamide derivatives. All thiazides affect the distal convoluted tubule, and all have equal maximum diuretic effects, differing only in potency. Thiazides are sometimes called "low ceiling diuretics," because increasing the dose above normal therapeutic doses does not promote further diuretic response.

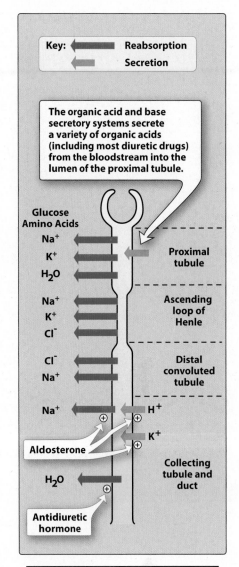

Figure 18.3
Sites of transport of solutes and water along the nephron.

A. Thiazides

Chlorothiazide [klor-oh-THYE-ah-zide] was the first orally active diuretic that was capable of affecting the severe edema often seen in hepatic cirrhosis and heart failure with minimal side effects. Its properties are representative of the thiazide group, although *hydrochlorothiazide* [hi-dro-klor-oh-THYE-ah-zide] and *chlorthalidone* are now used more commonly. *Hydrochlorothiazide* is more potent, so the required dose is considerably lower than that of *chlorothiazide*, but the efficacy is comparable to that of the parent drug. In all other aspects, *hydrochlorothiazide* resembles *chlorothiazide*. [Note: *Chlorthalidone*, *indapamide*, and *metolazone* are referred to as thiazide-like diuretics, because they contain the sulfonamide residue in their chemical structures, and their mechanism of action is similar. However, they are not truly thiazides.]

1. **Mechanism of action:** The thiazide and thiazide-like diuretics act mainly in the cortical region of the ascending loop of Henle and the distal convoluted tubule to decrease the reabsorption of Na^+, apparently by inhibition of a Na^+/Cl^- cotransporter on the luminal membrane of the tubules (Figure 18.2). They have a lesser effect in the proximal tubule. As a result, these drugs increase the concentration of Na^+ and Cl^- in the tubular fluid. [Note: Because the site of action of the thiazide derivatives is on the luminal membrane, these drugs must be excreted into the tubular lumen to be effective. Therefore, with decreased renal function, thiazide diuretics lose efficacy.] The efficacy of these agents may be diminished with concomitant use of NSAIDs, such as *indomethacin*, which inhibit production of renal prostaglandins, thereby reducing renal blood flow.

2. **Actions:**

   a. **Increased excretion of Na^+ and Cl^-:** Thiazide and thiazide-like diuretics cause diuresis with increased Na^+ and Cl^- excretion, which can result in the excretion of very hyperosmolar (concentrated) urine. This latter effect is unique, as the other diuretic classes are unlikely to produce a hyperosmolar urine. The diuretic action is not affected by the acid–base status of the body, and *hydrochlorothiazide* does not change the acid–base status of the blood. Figure 18.4 outlines relative changes in the ionic composition of the urine with thiazide and thiazide-like diuretics.

   b. **Loss of K^+:** Because thiazides increase Na^+ in the filtrate arriving at the distal tubule, more K^+ is also exchanged for Na^+, resulting in a continual loss of K^+ from the body with prolonged use of these drugs. Thus, serum K^+ should be measured periodically (more frequently at the beginning of therapy) to monitor for the development of hypokalemia.

   c. **Loss of Mg^{2+}:** Magnesium deficiency requiring supplementation can occur with chronic use of thiazide diuretics, particularly in elderly patients. The mechanism for the magnesuria is not understood.

   d. **Decreased urinary calcium excretion:** Thiazide and thiazide-like diuretics decrease the Ca^{2+} content of urine by promoting

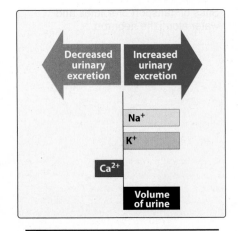

Figure 18.4
Relative changes in the composition of urine induced by thiazides and thiazide-like diuretics.

the reabsorption of Ca^{2+} in the distal convoluted tubule where parathyroid hormone regulates reabsorption. This effect contrasts with the loop diuretics, which increase the Ca^{2+} concentration in the urine. [Note: Epidemiologic evidence suggests that use of thiazides preserves bone mineral density at the hip and spine and may reduce the risk of fractures.]

e. **Reduced peripheral vascular resistance:** An initial reduction in blood pressure results from a decrease in blood volume and, therefore, a decrease in cardiac output. With continued therapy, volume recovery occurs. However, there are continued antihypertensive effects, resulting from reduced peripheral vascular resistance caused by relaxation of arteriolar smooth muscle. How these agents induce vasodilation is unknown.

3. **Therapeutic uses:**

a. **Hypertension:** Clinically, the thiazides are a mainstay of antihypertensive medication, because they are inexpensive, convenient to administer, and well tolerated. They are effective in reducing blood pressure in the majority of patients with mild to moderate essential hypertension. Blood pressure can be maintained with a daily dose of thiazide, which causes lower peripheral resistance without having a major diuretic effect. Some patients can be continued for years on thiazides alone; however, many patients require additional medication for blood pressure control (see Chapter 17), such as adrenergic blockers, angiotensin-converting enzyme inhibitors, or angiotensin receptor blockers. [Note: The antihypertensive actions of angiotensin-converting enzyme inhibitors are enhanced when given in combination with the thiazides.]

b. **Heart failure:** Loop diuretics (not thiazides) are the diuretics of choice in reducing extracellular volume in heart failure. However, thiazide diuretics may be added if additional diuresis is needed. When given in combination, thiazides should be administered 30 minutes prior to loop diuretics in order to allow the thiazide time to reach the site of action and produce effect.

c. **Hypercalciuria:** The thiazides can be useful in treating idiopathic hypercalciuria, because they inhibit urinary Ca^{2+} excretion. This is particularly beneficial for patients with calcium oxalate stones in the urinary tract.

d. **Diabetes insipidus:** Thiazides have the unique ability to produce a hyperosmolar urine. Thiazides can substitute for ADH in the treatment of nephrogenic diabetes insipidus. The urine volume of such individuals may drop from 11 L/d to about 3 L/d when treated with the drug.

4. **Pharmacokinetics:** The drugs are effective orally. Most thiazides take 1 to 3 weeks to produce a stable reduction in blood pressure, and they exhibit a prolonged half-life. All thiazides are secreted by the organic acid secretory system of the kidney (Figure 18.3).

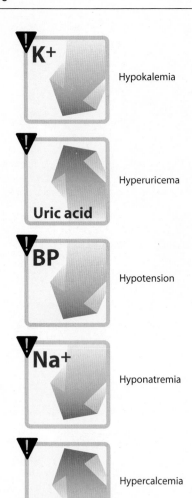

Figure 18.5
Summary of some adverse
effects commonly observed
with thiazides and thiazide-like
diuretics. BP = blood pressure.

5. **Adverse effects:** These mainly involve problems in fluid and electrolyte balance.

   a. **Potassium depletion:** Hypokalemia is the most frequent problem with the thiazide diuretics, and it can predispose patients who are taking *digoxin* to ventricular arrhythmias (Figure 18.5). Often, K$^+$ can be supplemented by dietary measures such as increasing the consumption of citrus fruits, bananas, and prunes. In some cases, K$^+$ supplementation may be necessary. Thiazides decrease the intravascular volume, resulting in activation of the renin–angiotensin–aldosterone system. Increased aldosterone contributes significantly to urinary K$^+$ losses. Under these circumstances, the K$^+$ deficiency can be overcome by *spironolactone*, which interferes with aldosterone action, or by administering *triamterene* or *amiloride*, which act to retain K$^+$. Low-sodium diets blunt the potassium depletion caused by thiazide diuretics.

   b. **Hyponatremia:** Hyponatremia may develop due to elevation of ADH as a result of hypovolemia, as well as diminished diluting capacity of the kidney and increased thirst. Limiting water intake and lowering the diuretic dose can prevent hyponatremia.

   c. **Hyperuricemia:** Thiazides increase serum uric acid by decreasing the amount of acid excreted by the organic acid secretory system. Being insoluble, uric acid deposits in the joints and may precipitate a gouty attack in predisposed individuals. Therefore, thiazides should be used with caution in patients with gout or high levels of uric acid.

   d. **Volume depletion:** This can cause orthostatic hypotension or light-headedness.

   e. **Hypercalcemia:** The thiazides inhibit the secretion of Ca^{2+}, sometimes leading to hypercalcemia (elevated levels of Ca^{2+} in the blood).

   f. **Hyperglycemia:** Therapy with thiazides can lead to glucose intolerance, possibly due to impaired release of insulin and tissue uptake of glucose. New-onset diabetes has been reported more often with thiazides than with other antihypertensive agents. Patients with diabetes who are taking thiazides should monitor glucose to assess the need for an adjustment in diabetes therapy.

B. **Thiazide-like diuretics**

These compounds lack the thiazide structure, but, like the thiazides, they have the unsubstituted sulfonamide group and, therefore, share their mechanism of action. The therapeutic uses and adverse effect profiles are similar to those of the thiazides.

1. **Chlorthalidone:** *Chlorthalidone* [klor-THAL-i-done] is a nonthiazide derivative that behaves pharmacologically like *hydrochlorothiazide*. It has a long duration of action and, therefore, is often used once daily to treat hypertension.

2. **Metolazone:** *Metolazone* [me-TOL-ah-zone] is more potent than the thiazides and, unlike the thiazides, causes Na⁺ excretion even in advanced renal failure.

3. **Indapamide:** *Indapamide* [in-DAP-a-mide] is a lipid-soluble, nonthiazide diuretic that has a long duration of action. At low doses, it shows significant antihypertensive action with minimal diuretic effects. *Indapamide* is metabolized and excreted by the gastrointestinal tract and the kidneys. Thus, it is less likely to accumulate in patients with renal failure and may be useful in their treatment.

IV. LOOP OR HIGH-CEILING DIURETICS

Bumetanide [byoo-MET-ah-nide], *furosemide* [fur-OH-se-mide], *torsemide* [TOR-se-mide], and *ethacrynic* [eth-a-KRIN-ik] *acid* have their major diuretic action on the ascending limb of the loop of Henle (Figure 18.2). Of all the diuretics, these drugs have the highest efficacy in mobilizing Na⁺ and Cl⁻ from the body. They produce copious amounts of urine. *Furosemide* is the most commonly used of these drugs. *Bumetanide* and *torsemide* are much more potent than *furosemide*, and the use of these agents is increasing. *Ethacrynic acid* is used infrequently due to its adverse effect profile.

A. Bumetanide, furosemide, torsemide, and ethacrynic acid

1. **Mechanism of action:** Loop diuretics inhibit the cotransport of Na⁺/K⁺/2Cl⁻ in the luminal membrane in the ascending limb of the loop of Henle. Therefore, reabsorption of these ions is decreased. These agents have the greatest diuretic effect of all the diuretic drugs, since the ascending limb accounts for reabsorption of 25% to 30% of filtered NaCl, and downstream sites are unable to compensate for the increased Na⁺ load.

2. **Actions:** Loop diuretics act promptly, even in patients with poor renal function or lack of response to other diuretics. Changes in the composition of the urine induced by loop diuretics are shown in Figure 18.6. [Note: Unlike thiazides, loop diuretics increase the Ca²⁺ content of urine. In patients with normal serum Ca²⁺ concentrations, hypocalcemia does not result, because Ca²⁺ is reabsorbed in the distal convoluted tubule.] The loop diuretics may increase renal blood flow, possibly by enhancing prostaglandin synthesis. NSAIDs inhibit renal prostaglandin synthesis and can reduce the diuretic action of loop diuretics.

3. **Therapeutic uses:** The loop diuretics are the drugs of choice for reducing acute pulmonary edema and acute/chronic peripheral edema caused from heart failure or renal impairment. Because of their rapid onset of action, particularly when given intravenously, the drugs are useful in emergency situations such as acute pulmonary edema. Loop diuretics (along with hydration) are also useful in treating hypercalcemia, because they stimulate tubular Ca²⁺ excretion. They also are useful in the treatment of hyperkalemia.

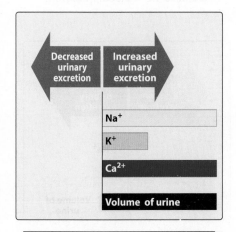

Figure 18.6
Relative changes in the composition of urine induced by loop diuretics.

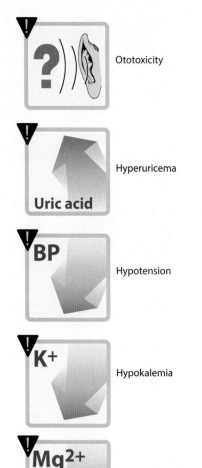

Figure 18.7
Summary of some adverse effects commonly observed with loop diuretics. BP = blood pressure.

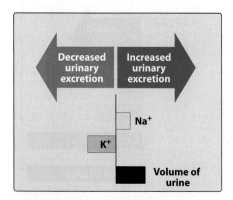

Figure 18.8
Relative changes in the composition of urine induced by potassium-sparing diuretics.

4. **Pharmacokinetics:** Loop diuretics are administered orally or parenterally. Their duration of action is relatively brief (2 to 4 hours), allowing patients to predict the window of diuresis. They are secreted into urine.

5. **Adverse effects:** Figure 18.7 summarizes the adverse effects of the loop diuretics.

   a. **Ototoxicity:** Reversible or permanent hearing loss may occur with loop diuretics, particularly when used in conjunction with other ototoxic drugs (for example, aminoglycoside antibiotics). *Ethacrynic acid* is the most likely to cause deafness. Although less common, vestibular function may also be affected, inducing vertigo.

   b. **Hyperuricemia:** *Furosemide* and *ethacrynic acid* compete with uric acid for the renal secretory systems, thus blocking its secretion and, in turn, causing or exacerbating gouty attacks.

   c. **Acute hypovolemia:** Loop diuretics can cause a severe and rapid reduction in blood volume, with the possibility of hypotension, shock, and cardiac arrhythmias.

   d. **Potassium depletion:** The heavy load of Na^+ presented to the collecting tubule results in increased exchange of tubular Na^+ for K^+, leading to the possibility of hypokalemia. The loss of K^+ from cells in exchange for H^+ leads to hypokalemic alkalosis. Use of potassium-sparing diuretics or supplementation with K^+ can prevent the development of hypokalemia.

   e. **Hypomagnesemia:** Chronic use of loop diuretics combined with low dietary intake of Mg^{2+} can lead to hypomagnesemia, particularly in the elderly. This can be corrected by oral supplementation.

V. POTASSIUM-SPARING DIURETICS

Potassium-sparing diuretics act in the collecting tubule to inhibit Na^+ reabsorption and K^+ excretion (Figure 18.8). The major use of potassium-sparing agents is in the treatment of hypertension (most often in combination with a thiazide) and in heart failure (aldosterone antagonists). It is extremely important that potassium levels are closely monitored in patients treated with potassium-sparing diuretics. These drugs should be avoided in patients with renal dysfunction because of the increased risk of hyperkalemia. Within this class, there are drugs with two distinct mechanisms of action: aldosterone antagonists and sodium channel blockers.

A. Aldosterone antagonists: spironolactone and eplerenone

1. **Mechanism of action:** *Spironolactone* [spear-oh-no-LAK-tone] is a synthetic steroid that antagonizes aldosterone at intracellular cytoplasmic receptor sites rendering the spironolactone–receptor complex inactive. It prevents translocation of the receptor complex into the nucleus of the target cell, ultimately resulting in a failure to produce mediator proteins that normally stimulate the

Na+/K+-exchange sites of the collecting tubule. Thus, a lack of mediator proteins prevents Na+ reabsorption and, therefore, K+ and H+ secretion. *Eplerenone* [eh-PLEH-reh-none] is another aldosterone receptor antagonist, which has actions comparable to those of *spironolactone*, although it may have less endocrine effects than *spironolactone*.

2. **Actions:** In most edematous states, blood levels of aldosterone are high, causing retention of Na+. *Spironolactone* antagonizes the activity of aldosterone, resulting in retention of K+ and excretion of Na+ (Figure 18.8). Similar to thiazides and loop diuretics, the effect of these agents may be diminished by administration of NSAIDs.

3. **Therapeutic uses:**

   a. **Diuretic:** Although the aldosterone antagonists have a low efficacy in mobilizing Na+ from the body in comparison with the other diuretics, they have the useful property of causing the retention of K+. These agents are often given in conjunction with thiazide or loop diuretics to prevent K+ excretion that would otherwise occur with these drugs. Since these drugs work by a mechanism in the later parts of the kidney, these agents can potentiate the effects of more proximally acting agents. *Spironolactone* is the diuretic of choice in patients with hepatic cirrhosis, as edema in these patients is caused by secondary hyperaldosteronism.

   b. **Secondary hyperaldosteronism:** *Spironolactone* is particularly effective in clinical situations associated with secondary hyperaldosteronism, such as hepatic cirrhosis and nephrotic syndrome. In contrast, in patients who have no significant circulating levels of aldosterone, such as in Addison disease (primary adrenal insufficiency), there is no diuretic effect with the use of this drug.

   c. **Heart failure:** Aldosterone antagonists prevent remodeling that occurs as compensation for the progressive failure of the heart. Use of these agents has been shown to decrease mortality associated with heart failure, particularly in those with reduced ejection fraction.

   d. **Resistant hypertension:** Resistant hypertension, defined by the use of three or more medications without reaching the blood pressure goal, often responds well to aldosterone antagonists. This effect can be seen in those with or without elevated aldosterone levels.

   e. **Ascites:** Accumulation of fluid in the abdominal cavity (ascites) is a common complication of hepatic cirrhosis. *Spironolactone* is effective in this condition.

   f. **Polycystic ovary syndrome:** *Spironolactone* is often used off-label for the treatment of polycystic ovary syndrome. It blocks androgen receptors and inhibits steroid synthesis at high doses, thereby helping to offset increased androgen levels seen in this disorder.

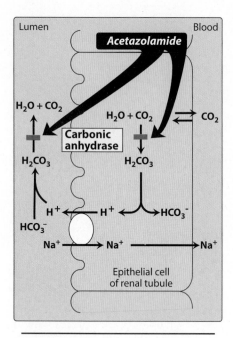

Figure 18.9
Role of carbonic anhydrase in sodium retention by epithelial cells of the renal tubule.

4. **Pharmacokinetics:** Both *spironolactone* and *eplerenone* are absorbed after oral administration and are significantly bound to plasma proteins. S*pironolactone* is extensively metabolized and converted to several active metabolites. The metabolites, along with the parent drug, are thought to be responsible for the therapeutic effects. *Spironolactone* is a potent inhibitor of P-glycoprotein, and *eplerenone* is metabolized by cytochrome P450 3A4.

5. **Adverse effects:** *Spironolactone* can cause gastric upset. Because it chemically resembles some of the sex steroids, *spironolactone* may induce gynecomastia in male patients and menstrual irregularities in female patients. Hyperkalemia, nausea, lethargy, and mental confusion can occur. At low doses, *spironolactone* can be used chronically with few side effects. Potassium-sparing diuretics should be used with caution with other medications that can induce hyperkalemia, such as angiotensin-converting enzyme inhibitors and potassium supplements.

B. Triamterene and amiloride

Triamterene [trye-AM-ter-een] and *amiloride* [a-MIL-oh-ride] block Na^+ transport channels, resulting in a decrease in Na^+/K^+ exchange. Although they have a K^+-sparing diuretic action similar to that of the aldosterone antagonists, their ability to block the Na^+/K^+-exchange site in the collecting tubule does not depend on the presence of aldosterone. Like the aldosterone antagonists, these agents are not very efficacious diuretics. Both *triamterene* and *amiloride* are commonly used in combination with other diuretics, usually for their potassium-sparing properties. Much like the aldosterone antagonists, they prevent the loss of K^+ that occurs with thiazide and loop diuretics. The side effects of *triamterene* include increased uric acid, renal stones, and K^+ retention.

VI. CARBONIC ANHYDRASE INHIBITOR

Acetazolamide [ah-set-a-ZOLE-a-mide] and other carbonic anhydrase inhibitors are more often used for their other pharmacologic actions than for their diuretic effect, because they are much less efficacious than the thiazide or loop diuretics.

A. Acetazolamide

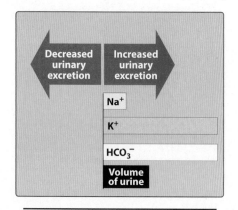

Figure 18.10
Relative changes in the composition of urine induced by *acetazolamide*.

1. **Mechanism of action:** *Acetazolamide* inhibits carbonic anhydrase located intracellularly (cytoplasm) and on the apical membrane of the proximal tubular epithelium (Figure 18.9). [Note: Carbonic anhydrase catalyzes the reaction of CO_2 and H_2O, leading to H_2CO_3, which spontaneously ionizes to H^+ and HCO_3^- (bicarbonate).] The decreased ability to exchange Na^+ for H^+ in the presence of *acetazolamide* results in a mild diuresis. Additionally, HCO_3^- is retained in the lumen, with marked elevation in urinary pH. The loss of HCO_3^- causes a hyperchloremic metabolic acidosis and decreased diuretic efficacy following several days of therapy. Changes in the composition

of urinary electrolytes induced by *acetazolamide* are summarized in Figure 18.10. Phosphate excretion is increased by an unknown mechanism.

2. Therapeutic uses:

a. Glaucoma: *Acetazolamide* decreases the production of aqueous humor and reduces intraocular pressure in patients with chronic open-angle glaucoma, probably by blocking carbonic anhydrase in the ciliary body of the eye. Topical carbonic anhydrase inhibitors, such as *dorzolamide* and *brinzolamide*, have the advantage of not causing systemic effects.

b. Mountain sickness: *Acetazolamide* can be used in the prophylaxis of acute mountain sickness. *Acetazolamide* prevents weakness, breathlessness, dizziness, nausea, and cerebral as well as pulmonary edema characteristic of the syndrome.

3. Pharmacokinetics:
Acetazolamide can be administered orally or intravenously. It is approximately 90% protein bound and eliminated renally by both active tubular secretion and passive reabsorption.

4. Adverse effects:
Metabolic acidosis (mild), potassium depletion, renal stone formation, drowsiness, and paresthesia may occur. The drug should be avoided in patients with hepatic cirrhosis, because it could lead to a decreased excretion of NH_4^+.

VII. OSMOTIC DIURETICS

A number of simple, hydrophilic chemical substances that are filtered through the glomerulus, such as *mannitol* [MAN-i-tol] and *urea* [yu-REE-ah], result in some degree of diuresis. Filtered substances that undergo little or no reabsorption will cause an increase in urinary output. The presence of these substances results in a higher osmolarity of the tubular fluid and prevents further water reabsorption, resulting in osmotic diuresis. Only a small amount of additional salt may also be excreted. Because osmotic diuretics are used to increase water excretion rather than Na^+ excretion, they are not useful for treating conditions in which Na^+ retention occurs. They are used to maintain urine flow following acute toxic ingestion of substances capable of producing acute renal failure. Osmotic diuretics are a mainstay of treatment for patients with increased intracranial pressure or acute renal failure due to shock, drug toxicities, and trauma. Maintaining urine flow preserves long-term kidney function and may save the patient from dialysis. [Note: *Mannitol* is not absorbed when given orally and should be given intravenously.] Adverse effects include extracellular water expansion and dehydration, as well as hypo- or hypernatremia. The expansion of extracellular water results because the presence of *mannitol* in the extracellular fluid extracts water from the cells and causes hyponatremia until diuresis occurs.

Figure 18.11 summarizes the relative changes in urinary composition induced by diuretic drugs.

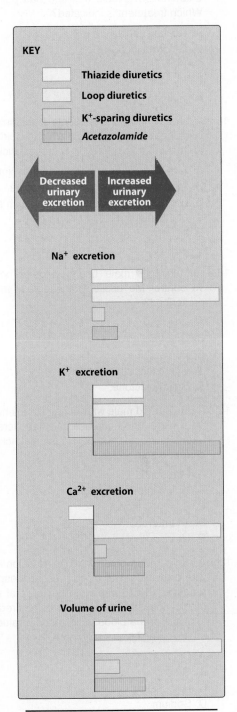

Figure 18.11
Summary of relative changes in urinary composition induced by diuretic drugs.

Study Questions

Choose the ONE best answer.

18.1 An elderly patient with a history of heart disease is brought to the emergency room with difficulty breathing. Examination reveals that she has pulmonary edema. Which treatment is indicated?

A. Acetazolamide.
B. Chlorthalidone.
C. Furosemide.
D. Hydrochlorothiazide.
E. Spironolactone.

Correct answer = C. This is a potentially fatal situation. It is important to administer a diuretic that will reduce fluid accumulation in the lungs and, thus, improve oxygenation and heart function. The loop diuretics are most effective in removing large fluid volumes from the body and are the treatment of choice in this situation. In this situation, furosemide should be administered intravenously. The other choices are inappropriate.

18.2 A group of college students is planning a mountain climbing trip to the Andes. Which would be appropriate for them to take to prevent mountain sickness?

A. A thiazide diuretic such as hydrochlorothiazide.
B. An anticholinergic such as atropine.
C. A carbonic anhydrase inhibitor such as acetazolamide.
D. A loop diuretic such as furosemide.
E. A β-blocker such as metoprolol.

Correct answer = C. Acetazolamide is used prophylactically for several days before an ascent above 10,000 feet. This treatment prevents the cerebral and pulmonary problems associated with the syndrome as well as other difficulties, such as nausea.

18.3 An alcoholic male has developed hepatic cirrhosis. To control the ascites and edema, which should be prescribed?

A. Acetazolamide.
B. Chlorthalidone.
C. Furosemide.
D. Hydrochlorothiazide.
E. Spironolactone.

Correct answer = E. Spironolactone is very effective in the treatment of hepatic edema. These patients are frequently resistant to the diuretic action of loop diuretics, although a combination with spironolactone may be beneficial. The other agents are not indicated.

18.4 A 55-year-old male with kidney stones has been placed on a diuretic to decrease calcium excretion. However, after a few weeks, he develops an attack of gout. Which diuretic was he taking?

A. Furosemide.
B. Hydrochlorothiazide.
C. Spironolactone.
D. Triamterene.
E. Urea.

Correct answer = B. Hydrochlorothiazide is effective in increasing calcium reabsorption, thus decreasing the amount of calcium excreted, and decreasing the formation of kidney stones that contain calcium phosphate or calcium oxalate. However, hydrochlorothiazide can also inhibit the excretion of uric acid and cause its accumulation, leading to an attack of gout in some individuals. Furosemide increases the excretion of calcium, whereas the K+-sparing osmotic diuretics, spironolactone and triamterene, and urea do not have an effect.

18.5 A 75-year-old woman with hypertension is being treated with a thiazide. Her blood pressure responds well and reads at 120/76 mm Hg. After several months on the medication, she complains of being tired and weak. An analysis of the blood indicates low values for which of the following?

A. Calcium.
B. Glucose.
C. Potassium.
D. Sodium.
E. Uric acid.

Correct answer = C. Hypokalemia is a common adverse effect of the thiazides and causes fatigue and lethargy in the patient. Supplementation with potassium chloride or foods high in K+ corrects the problem. Alternatively, a potassium-sparing diuretic, such as spironolactone, may be added. Calcium, uric acid, and glucose are usually elevated by thiazide diuretics. Sodium loss would not weaken the patient.

18.6 Which is contraindicated in a patient with hyperkalemia?

A. Acetazolamide.

B. Chlorthalidone.

C. Chlorothiazide.

D. Ethacrynic acid.

E. Spironolactone.

Correct answer = E. Spironolactone acts in the collecting tubule to inhibit Na^+ reabsorption and K^+ excretion. It is extremely important that patients who are treated with any potassium-sparing diuretic be closely monitored for potassium levels. Exogenous potassium supplementation is usually discontinued when potassium-sparing diuretic therapy is instituted and spironolactone is contraindicated in patients with hyperkalemia. The other drugs promote the excretion of potassium.

18.7 Which of the following should be avoided in a patient with a history of severe anaphylactic reaction to sulfa medications?

A. Amiloride.

B. Hydrochlorothiazide.

C. Mannitol.

D. Spironolactone.

E. Triamterene.

Correct answer = B. Hydrochlorothiazide, like many thiazide and thiazide-like diuretics, contains a sulfa moiety within its chemical structure. It is important to avoid use in those individuals with severe hypersensitivity to sulfa medications. It may be used with caution, however, in those with only minor reaction to sulfa medications.

18.8 A male patient is placed on a new medication and notes that his breasts have become enlarged and tender to the touch. Which medication is he most likely taking?

A. Chlorthalidone.

B. Furosemide.

C. Hydrochlorothiazide.

D. Spironolactone.

E. Triamterene.

Correct answer = D. An adverse drug reaction to spironolactone is gynecomastia due to its effects on androgens and progesterone in the body. Eplerenone may be a suitable alternative if the patient is in need of an aldosterone antagonist but has a history of gynecomastia.

18.9 A patient presents to the emergency department with an extreme headache. After a thorough workup, the attending physician concludes that the pain is due to increased intracranial pressure. Which diuretic would work best to reduce this pressure?

A. Acetazolamide.

B. Indapamide.

C. Furosemide.

D. Hydrochlorothiazide.

E. Mannitol.

Correct answer = E. Osmotic diuretics, such as mannitol, are a mainstay of treatment for patients with increased intracranial pressure or acute renal failure due to shock, drug toxicities, and trauma.

18.10 Which diuretic has been shown to improve blood pressure in resistant hypertension or those already treated with three blood pressure medications including a thiazide or thiazide-like diuretic?

A. Chlorthalidone.

B. Indapamide.

C. Furosemide.

D. Mannitol.

E. Spironolactone.

Correct answer = E. Resistant hypertension, defined by the use of three or more medications without reaching the blood pressure goal, often responds well to aldosterone antagonists. This effect can be seen in those with or without elevated aldosterone levels.

Heart Failure

19

Shawn Anderson and Katherine Vogel Anderson

I. OVERVIEW

Heart failure (HF) is a complex, progressive disorder in which the heart is unable to pump sufficient blood to meet the needs of the body. Its cardinal symptoms are dyspnea, fatigue, and fluid retention. HF is due to an impaired ability of the heart to adequately fill with and/or eject blood. It is often accompanied by abnormal increases in blood volume and interstitial fluid. Underlying causes of HF include arteriosclerotic heart disease, myocardial infarction, hypertensive heart disease, valvular heart disease, dilated cardiomyopathy, and congenital heart disease.

A. Role of physiologic compensatory mechanisms in the progression of HF

Chronic activation of the sympathetic nervous system and the renin–angiotensin–aldosterone system is associated with remodeling of cardiac tissue, loss of myocytes, hypertrophy, and fibrosis. This prompts additional neurohormonal activation, creating a vicious cycle that, if left untreated, leads to death.

B. Goals of pharmacologic intervention in HF

Goals of treatment are to alleviate symptoms, slow disease progression, and improve survival. Accordingly, seven classes of drugs have been shown to be effective: 1) angiotensin-converting enzyme inhibitors, 2) angiotensin-receptor blockers, 3) aldosterone antagonists, 4) β-blockers, 5) diuretics, 6) direct vaso- and venodilators, and 7) inotropic agents (Figure 19.1). Depending on the severity of HF and individual patient factors, one or more of these classes of drugs are administered. Pharmacologic intervention provides the following benefits in HF: reduced myocardial work load, decreased extracellular fluid volume, improved cardiac contractility, and a reduced rate of cardiac remodeling. Knowledge of the physiology of cardiac muscle contraction is essential for understanding the compensatory responses evoked by the failing heart, as well as the actions of drugs used to treat HF.

II. PHYSIOLOGY OF MUSCLE CONTRACTION

The myocardium, like smooth and skeletal muscle, responds to stimulation by depolarization of the membrane, which is followed by shortening of the contractile proteins and ends with relaxation and return to the

ACE INHIBITORS
Captopril CAPOTEN
Enalapril VASOTEC
Fosinopril MONOPRIL
Lisinopril PRINIVIL, ZESTRIL
Quinapril ACCUPRIL
Ramipril ALTACE

ANGIOTENSIN RECEPTOR BLOCKERS
Candesartan ATACAND
Losartan COZAAR
Telmisartan MICARDIS
Valsartan DIOVAN

ALDOSTERONE ANTAGONISTS
Eplerenone INSPRA
Spironolactone ALDACTONE

β–ADRENORECEPTOR BLOCKERS
Bisoprolol ZEBETA
Carvedilol COREG, COREG CR
Metoprolol succinate TOPROL XL
Metoprolol tartrate LOPRESSOR

DIURETICS
Bumetanide BUMEX
Furosemide LASIX
Metolazone ZAROXOLYN
Torsemide DEMADEX

DIRECT VASO - AND VENODILATORS
Hydralazine APRESOLINE
Isosorbide dinitrate DILATRATE-SR, ISORDIL
FDC Hydralazine/Isosorbide dinitrate BIDIL

INOTROPIC AGENTS
Digoxin LANOXIN
Dobutamine DOBUTREX
Milrinone PRIMACOR

Figure 19.1
Summary of drugs used to treat HF.
ACE = angiotensin-converting enzyme;
FDC = fixed dose combination.

resting state (repolarization). Cardiac myocytes are interconnected in groups that respond to stimuli as a unit, contracting together whenever a single cell is stimulated.

A. Action potential

Cardiac myocytes are electrically excitable and have a spontaneous, intrinsic rhythm generated by specialized "pacemaker" cells located in the sinoatrial and atrioventricular (AV) nodes. Cardiac myocytes also have an unusually long action potential, which can be divided into five phases (0 to 4). Figure 19.2 illustrates the major ions contributing to depolarization and repolarization of cardiac myocytes.

B. Cardiac contraction

The force of contraction of the cardiac muscle is directly related to the concentration of free (unbound) cytosolic calcium. Therefore, agents that increase intracellular calcium levels (or that increase the sensitivity of the contractile machinery to calcium) increase the force of contraction (inotropic effect). [Note: The inotropic agents increase the contractility of the heart by directly or indirectly altering the mechanisms that control the concentration of intracellular calcium.] Calcium handling by cardiac myocytes is illustrated in Figure 19.3.

C. Compensatory physiological responses in HF

The failing heart evokes three major compensatory mechanisms to enhance cardiac output (Figure 19.4). Although initially beneficial, these alterations ultimately result in further deterioration of cardiac function.

1. **Increased sympathetic activity:** Baroreceptors sense a decrease in blood pressure and activate the sympathetic nervous system. In an attempt to sustain tissue perfusion, this stimulation of β-adrenergic receptors results in an increased heart rate and a greater force of contraction of the heart muscle. In addition, vasoconstriction enhances venous return and increases cardiac preload. An increase in preload (stretch on the heart) increases stroke volume, which, in turn, increases cardiac output. These compensatory responses increase the work of the heart, which, in the long term, contributes to further decline in cardiac function.

2. **Activation of the renin–angiotensin–aldosterone system:** A fall in cardiac output decreases blood flow to the kidney, prompting the release of renin, and resulting in increased formation of angiotensin II and release of aldosterone. This results in increased peripheral resistance (afterload) and retention of sodium and water. Blood volume increases, and more blood is returned to the heart. If the heart is unable to pump this extra volume, venous pressure increases and peripheral and pulmonary edema occur. Again, these compensatory responses increase the work of the heart, contributing to further decline in cardiac function.

3. **Myocardial hypertrophy:** The heart increases in size, and the chambers dilate and become more globular. Initially, stretching of the heart muscle leads to a stronger contraction of the heart.

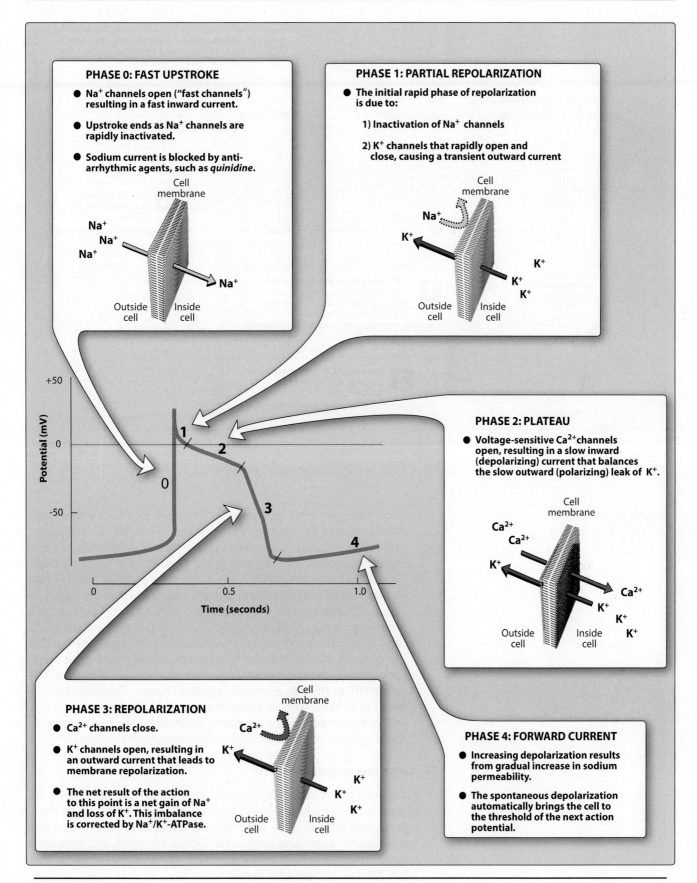

PHASE 0: FAST UPSTROKE

- Na⁺ channels open ("fast channels") resulting in a fast inward current.
- Upstroke ends as Na⁺ channels are rapidly inactivated.
- Sodium current is blocked by anti-arrhythmic agents, such as *quinidine*.

Cell membrane

Na⁺
Na⁺
Na⁺
Na⁺

Outside cell   Inside cell

PHASE 1: PARTIAL REPOLARIZATION

- The initial rapid phase of repolarization is due to:

  1) Inactivation of Na⁺ channels

  2) K⁺ channels that rapidly open and close, causing a transient outward current

Cell membrane

Na⁺

K⁺   K⁺
K⁺
K⁺

Outside cell   Inside cell

PHASE 2: PLATEAU

- Voltage-sensitive Ca²⁺ channels open, resulting in a slow inward (depolarizing) current that balances the slow outward (polarizing) leak of K⁺.

Cell membrane

Ca²⁺
Ca²⁺

K⁺   Ca²⁺
K⁺
K⁺

Outside cell   Inside cell

PHASE 3: REPOLARIZATION

- Ca²⁺ channels close.
- K⁺ channels open, resulting in an outward current that leads to membrane repolarization.
- The net result of the action to this point is a net gain of Na⁺ and loss of K⁺. This imbalance is corrected by Na⁺/K⁺-ATPase.

Cell membrane

Ca²⁺

K⁺

K⁺
K⁺

Outside cell   Inside cell

PHASE 4: FORWARD CURRENT

- Increasing depolarization results from gradual increase in sodium permeability.
- The spontaneous depolarization automatically brings the cell to the threshold of the next action potential.

Potential (mV): +50, 0, -50
Time (seconds): 0, 0.5, 1.0

Figure 19.2

Action potential of a Purkinje fiber. ATPase = adenosine triphosphatase.

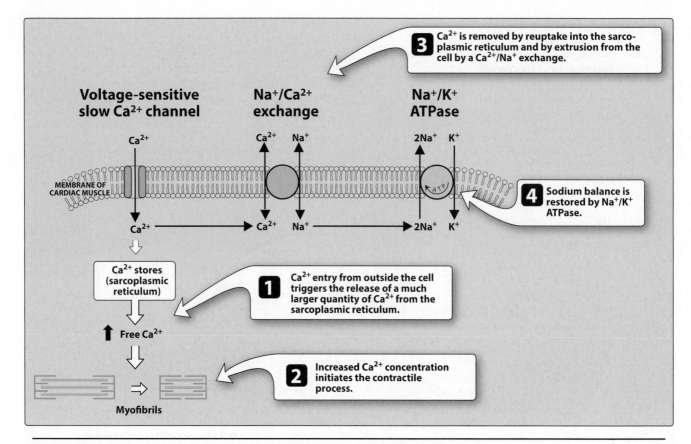

Voltage-sensitive slow Ca²⁺ channel

Na⁺/Ca²⁺ exchange

Na⁺/K⁺ ATPase

3 Ca²⁺ is removed by reuptake into the sarcoplasmic reticulum and by extrusion from the cell by a Ca²⁺/Na⁺ exchange.

MEMBRANE OF CARDIAC MUSCLE

Ca²⁺

Ca²⁺   Na⁺

2Na⁺   K⁺

Ca²⁺

Ca²⁺   Na⁺

2Na⁺   K⁺

4 Sodium balance is restored by Na⁺/K⁺ ATPase.

Ca²⁺ stores (sarcoplasmic reticulum)

1 Ca²⁺ entry from outside the cell triggers the release of a much larger quantity of Ca²⁺ from the sarcoplasmic reticulum.

↑ Free Ca²⁺

2 Increased Ca²⁺ concentration initiates the contractile process.

Myofibrils

Figure 19.3
Ion movements during the contraction of cardiac muscle. ATPase = adenosine triphosphatase.

However, excessive elongation of the fibers results in weaker contractions, and the geometry diminishes the ability to eject blood. This type of failure is termed "systolic failure" or HF with reduced ejection fraction (HFrEF) and is the result of the ventricle being unable to pump effectively. Less commonly, patients with HF may have "diastolic dysfunction," a term applied when the ability of the ventricles to relax and accept blood is impaired by structural changes such as hypertrophy. The thickening of the ventricular wall and subsequent decrease in ventricular volume decrease the ability of heart muscle to relax. In this case, the ventricle does not fill adequately, and the inadequacy of cardiac output is termed "diastolic HF" or HF with preserved ejection fraction. Diastolic dysfunction, in its pure form, is characterized by signs and symptoms of HF in the presence of a normal functioning left ventricle. However, both systolic and diastolic dysfunction commonly coexist in HF.

D. Acute (decompensated) HF

If the adaptive mechanisms adequately restore cardiac output, HF is said to be compensated. If the adaptive mechanisms fail to maintain cardiac output, HF is decompensated and the patient develops worsening HF signs and symptoms. Typical HF signs and symptoms include dyspnea on exertion, orthopnea, paroxysmal nocturnal dyspnea, fatigue, and peripheral edema.

E. Therapeutic strategies in HF

Chronic HF is typically managed by fluid limitations (less than 1.5 to 2 L daily); low dietary intake of sodium (less than 2000 mg/d); treatment of comorbid conditions; and judicious use of diuretics, inhibitors of the renin–angiotensin–aldosterone system, and inhibitors of the sympathetic nervous system. Inotropic agents are reserved for acute HF signs and symptoms in mostly the inpatient setting. Drugs that may precipitate or exacerbate HF, such as nonsteroidal anti-inflammatory drugs (NSAIDs), alcohol, nondihydropyridine calcium channel blockers, and some antiarrhythmic drugs, should be avoided if possible.

III. INHIBITORS OF THE RENIN–ANGIOTENSIN– ALDOSTERONE SYSTEM

HF leads to activation of the renin–angiotensin–aldosterone system via two mechanisms: 1) increased renin release by juxtaglomerular cells in renal afferent arterioles due to diminished renal perfusion pressure produced by the failing heart and 2) renin release by juxtaglomerular cells promoted by sympathetic stimulation and activation of β receptors. The production of angiotensin II, a potent vasoconstrictor, and the subsequent stimulation of aldosterone release that causes salt and water retention lead to increases in both preload and afterload that are characteristic of the failing heart. In addition, high levels of angiotensin II and of aldosterone have direct detrimental effects on the cardiac muscle, favoring remodeling, fibrosis, and inflammatory changes.

A. Angiotensin-converting enzyme inhibitors

Angiotensin-converting enzyme (ACE) inhibitors are a part of standard pharmacotherapy in HFrEF. These drugs block the enzyme that cleaves angiotensin I to form the potent vasoconstrictor angiotensin II. They also diminish the inactivation of bradykinin (Figure 19.5). Vasodilation occurs as a result of decreased levels of the vasoconstrictor angiotensin II and increased levels of bradykinin (a potent vasodilator). By reducing angiotensin II levels, ACE inhibitors also decrease the secretion of aldosterone.

1. **Actions on the heart:** ACE inhibitors decrease vascular resistance (afterload) and venous tone (preload), resulting in increased cardiac output. ACE inhibitors also blunt the usual angiotensin II–mediated increase in epinephrine and aldosterone seen in HF. ACE inhibitors improve clinical signs and symptoms of HF and have been shown to significantly improve patient survival in HF (Figure 19.6).

2. **Indications:** ACE inhibitors may be considered for patients with asymptomatic and symptomatic HFrEF. Importantly, ACE inhibitors are indicated for patients with all stages of left ventricular failure. Patients with the lowest ejection fraction show the greatest benefit from use of ACE inhibitors. Depending on the severity of HF, ACE inhibitors may be used in combination with diuretics, β-blockers, *digoxin*, aldosterone antagonists, and *hydralazine/isosorbide dinitrate* fixed-dose combination. Patients who have had a recent

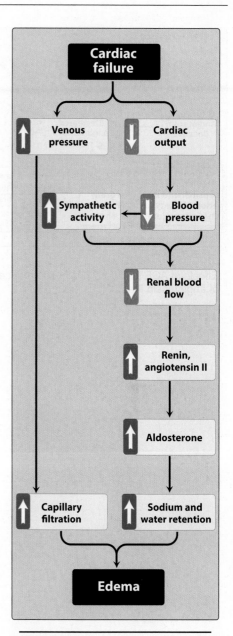

Figure 19.4
Cardiovascular consequences of HF.

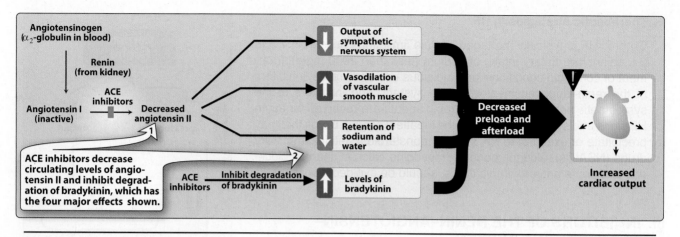

Figure 19.5

Effects of ACE inhibitors. [Note: The reduced retention of sodium and water results from two causes: decreased production of angiotensin II and aldosterone.]

myocardial infarction or are at high risk for a cardiovascular event also benefit from long-term ACE inhibitor therapy. ACE inhibitors are also used for the treatment of hypertension (see Chapter 17).

3. **Pharmacokinetics:** ACE inhibitors are adequately absorbed following oral administration. Food may decrease the absorption of *captopril* [CAP-toe-pril], so it should be taken on an empty stomach. Except for *captopril*, ACE inhibitors are prodrugs that require activation by hydrolysis via hepatic enzymes. Renal elimination of the active moiety is important for most ACE inhibitors except *fosinopril* [foe-SIH-no-pril]. Plasma half-lives of active compounds vary from 2 to 12 hours, although the inhibition of ACE may be much longer.

4. **Adverse effects:** These include postural hypotension, renal insufficiency, hyperkalemia, a persistent dry cough, and angioedema (rare). Potassium levels must be monitored, particularly with concurrent use of potassium supplements, potassium-sparing diuretics, or aldosterone antagonists due to risk of hyperkalemia. Serum creatinine levels should also be monitored, particularly in patients with underlying renal disease. The potential for symptomatic hypotension with ACE inhibitors is much more common if used concomitantly with a diuretic. ACE inhibitors are teratogenic and should not be used in pregnant women. Please see Chapter 17 for a full discussion of ACE inhibitors.

B. Angiotensin receptor blockers

Angiotensin receptor blockers (ARBs) are orally active compounds that are competitive antagonists of the angiotensin II type 1 receptor. ARBs have the advantage of more complete blockade of angiotensin II action, because ACE inhibitors inhibit only one enzyme responsible for the production of angiotensin II. Further, ARBs do not affect bradykinin levels. Although ARBs have actions similar to those of ACE inhibitors, they are not therapeutically identical. Even so, ARBs are a substitute for ACE inhibitors in those patients who cannot tolerate the latter.

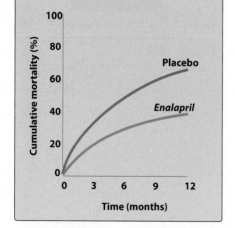

Figure 19.6

Effect of *enalapril* on the mortality of patients with symptomatic heart failure with reduced ejection fraction.

1. **Actions on the cardiovascular system:** Although ARBs have a different mechanism of action than ACE inhibitors, their actions on preload and afterload are similar. Their use in HF is mainly as a substitute for ACE inhibitors in those patients with severe cough or angioedema, which are thought to be mediated by elevated brady-kinin levels. ARBs are also used in the treatment of hypertension (see Chapter 17).

2. **Pharmacokinetics:** All the drugs are orally active and are dosed once-daily, with the exception of *valsartan* [val-SAR-tan] which is twice a day. They are highly plasma protein bound and, except for *candesartan* [kan-de-SAR-tan], have large volumes of distribution. *Losartan* [loe-SAR-tan], the prototype of the class, differs in that it undergoes extensive first-pass hepatic metabolism, including conversion to its active metabolite. The other drugs have inactive metabolites. Elimination of metabolites and parent compounds occurs in urine and feces.

3. **Adverse effects:** ARBs have an adverse effect and drug interaction profile similar to that of ACE inhibitors. However, the ARBs have a lower incidence of cough and angioedema. Like ACE inhibitors, ARBs are contraindicated in pregnancy.

C. Aldosterone antagonists

Patients with advanced heart disease have elevated levels of aldosterone due to angiotensin II stimulation and reduced hepatic clearance of the hormone. *Spironolactone* [spy-ro-no-LAC-tone] is a direct antagonist of aldosterone, thereby preventing salt retention, myocardial hypertrophy, and hypokalemia. *Eplerenone* [eh-PLEH-reh-none] is a competitive antagonist of aldosterone at mineralocorticoid receptors. Although similar in action to *spironolactone* at the mineralocorticoid receptor, *eplerenone* has a lower incidence of endocrine-related side effects due to its reduced affinity for glucocorticoid, androgen, and progesterone receptors. Aldosterone antagonists are indicated in patients with more severe stages of HFrEF or HFrEF and recent myocardial infarction. Please see Chapter 18 for a full discussion of aldosterone receptor antagonists.

IV. β-BLOCKERS

Although it may seem counterintuitive to administer drugs with negative inotropic activity in HF, evidence clearly demonstrates improved systolic functioning and reverse cardiac remodeling in patients receiving β-blockers. These benefits arise in spite of an occasional, initial exacerbation of symptoms. The benefit of β-blockers is attributed, in part, to their ability to prevent the changes that occur because of chronic activation of the sympathetic nervous system. These agents decrease heart rate and inhibit release of renin in the kidneys. In addition, β-blockers prevent the deleterious effects of norepinephrine on the cardiac muscle fibers, decreasing remodeling, hypertrophy, and cell death. Three β-blockers have shown benefit in HF: *bisoprolol* [bis-oh-PROE-lol], *carvedilol* [KAR-ve-dil-ol], and long-acting *metoprolol succinate* [me-TOE-proe-lol SUK-si-nate] (Figure 19.7). *Carvedilol* is a nonselective β-adrenoreceptor

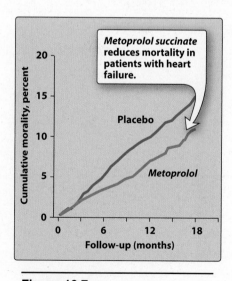

Figure 19.7
Cumulative mortality in patients with HF treated using placebo or *metoprolol succinate*.

antagonist that also blocks α-adrenoreceptors, whereas *bisoprolol* and *metoprolol succinate* are β₁-selective antagonists. [Note: The pharmacology of β-blockers is described in detail in Chapter 7.] β-Blockade is recommended for all patients with chronic, stable HF. *Bisoprolol*, *carvedilol*, and *metoprolol succinate* reduce morbidity and mortality associated with HFrEF. Treatment should be started at low doses and gradually titrated to target doses based on patient tolerance and vital signs. Both *carvedilol* and *metoprolol* are metabolized by the cytochrome P450 2D6 isoenzyme, and inhibitors of this metabolic pathway may increase levels of these drugs and increase the risk of adverse effects. In addition, *carvedilol* is a substrate of P-glycoprotein (P-gp). Increased effects of *carvedilol* may occur if it is coadministered with P-gp inhibitors. β-Blockers should also be used with caution with other drugs that slow AV conduction, such as *amiodarone*, *verapamil*, and *diltiazem*.

V. DIURETICS

Diuretics relieve pulmonary congestion and peripheral edema. These agents are also useful in reducing the symptoms of volume overload, including orthopnea and paroxysmal nocturnal dyspnea. Diuretics decrease plasma volume and, subsequently, decrease venous return to the heart (preload). This decreases cardiac workload and oxygen demand. Diuretics may also decrease afterload by reducing plasma volume, thereby decreasing blood pressure. Loop diuretics are the most commonly used diuretics in HF. These agents are used for patients who require extensive diuresis and those with renal insufficiency. [Note: Overdoses of loop diuretics can lead to profound hypovolemia.] As diuretics have not been shown to improve survival in HF, they should only be used to treat signs and symptoms of volume excess. Please see Chapter 18 for a full discussion of diuretics.

VI. VASO- AND VENODILATORS

Dilation of venous blood vessels leads to a decrease in cardiac preload by increasing venous capacitance. Nitrates are commonly used venous dilators to reduce preload for patients with chronic HF. Arterial dilators, such as *hydralazine* [hye-DRAL-a-zeen] reduce systemic arteriolar resistance and decrease afterload. If the patient is intolerant of ACE inhibitors or β-blockers, or if additional vasodilator response is required, a combination of *hydralazine* and *isosorbide dinitrate* [eye-soe-SOR-bide dye-NYE-trate] may be used. A fixed-dose combination of these agents has been shown to improve symptoms and survival in black patients with HFrEF on standard HF treatment (β-blocker plus ACE inhibitor or ARB). Headache, hypotension, and tachycardia are common adverse effects with this combination. Rarely, *hydralazine* has been associated with drug-induced lupus.

VII. INOTROPIC DRUGS

Positive inotropic agents enhance cardiac contractility and, thus, increase cardiac output. Although these drugs act by different mechanisms, the inotropic action is the result of an increased cytoplasmic calcium concentration that enhances the contractility of cardiac muscle. All positive inotropes in HFrEF that increase intracellular calcium concentration have been associated with reduced survival, especially in patients with HFrEF due to coronary artery disease. For this reason, these agents, with the exception of *digoxin*, are only used for a short period mainly in the inpatient setting.

A. Digitalis glycosides

The cardiac glycosides are often called digitalis or digitalis glycosides, because most of the drugs come from the digitalis (foxglove) plant. They are a group of chemically similar compounds that can increase the contractility of the heart muscle and, therefore, are used in treating HF. The digitalis glycosides have a low therapeutic index, with only a small difference between a therapeutic dose and doses that are toxic or even fatal. The most widely used agent is *digoxin* [di-JOX-in]. *Digitoxin* [dij-i-TOK-sin] is seldom used due to its considerable duration of action.

1. Mechanism of action:

a. **Regulation of cytosolic calcium concentration:** By inhibiting the Na^+/K^+-adenosine triphosphatase (ATPase) enzyme, *digoxin* reduces the ability of the myocyte to actively pump Na^+ from the cell (Figure 19.8). This decreases the Na^+ concentration gradient and, consequently, the ability of the Na^+/Ca^{2+}-exchanger to move calcium out of the cell. Further, the higher cellular Na^+ is exchanged for extracellular Ca^{2+} by the Na^+/Ca^{2+}-exchanger, increasing intracellular Ca^{2+}. A small but physiologically important increase occurs in free Ca^{2+} that is available at the next contraction cycle of the cardiac muscle, thereby increasing cardiac contractility. When Na^+/K^+-ATPase is markedly inhibited by *digoxin*, the resting membrane potential may increase (-70 mV instead of -90 mV), which makes the

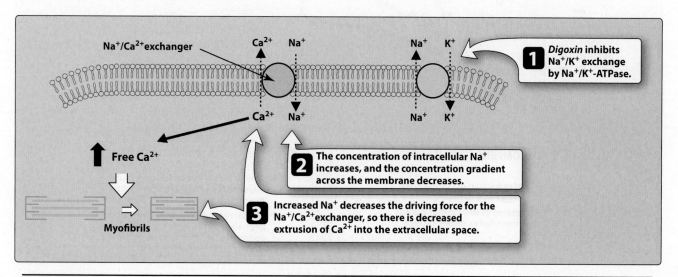

Figure 19.8
Mechanism of action of *digoxin*. ATPase = adenosine triphosphatase.

membrane more excitable, increasing the risk of arrhythmias (toxicity).

b. Increased contractility of the cardiac muscle: *Digoxin* increases the force of cardiac contraction, causing cardiac output to more closely resemble that of the normal heart (Figure 19.9). Vagal tone is also enhanced, so both heart rate and myocardial oxygen demand decrease. *Digoxin* slows conduction velocity through the AV node, making it useful for atrial fibrillation. [Note: In the normal heart, the positive inotropic effect of digitalis glycosides is counteracted by compensatory autonomic reflexes.]

c. Neurohormonal inhibition: Although the exact mechanism of this effect has not been elucidated, low-dose *digoxin* inhibits sympathetic activation with minimal effects on contractility. This effect is the reason a lower serum drug concentration is targeted in HFrEF.

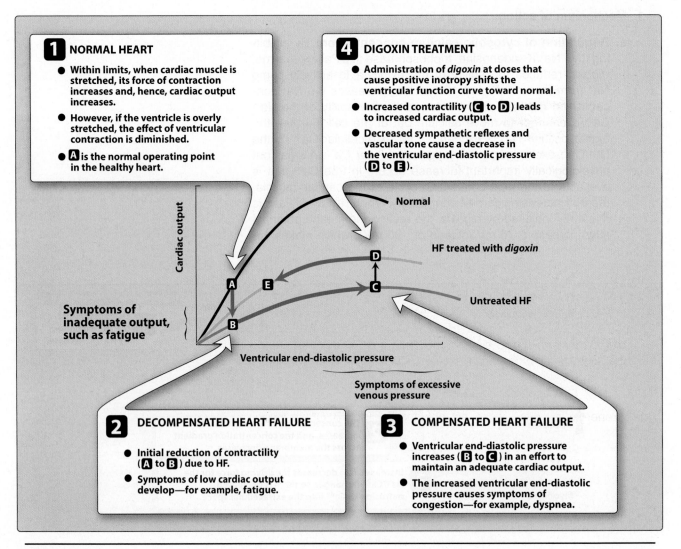

Figure 19.9
Ventricular function curves in the normal heart, in heart failure (HF), and in HF treated with *digoxin*.

2. Therapeutic uses: *Digoxin* therapy is indicated in patients with severe HFrEF after initiation of ACE inhibitor, β-blocker, and diuretic therapy. A low serum drug concentration of *digoxin* (0.5 to 0.8 ng/mL) is beneficial in HFrEF. At this level, patients may see a reduction in HF admissions, along with improved survival. At higher serum drug concentrations, admissions are prevented, but mortality likely increases. *Digoxin* is not indicated in patients with diastolic or right-sided HF unless the patient has concomitant atrial fibrillation or flutter. Patients with mild to moderate HF often respond to treatment with ACE inhibitors, β-blockers, aldosterone antagonists, direct vaso- and venodilators, and diuretics and may not require *digoxin*.

3. Pharmacokinetics: *Digoxin* is available in oral and injectable formulations. It has a large volume of distribution, because it accumulates in muscle. The dosage is based on lean body weight. In acute situations such as symptomatic atrial fibrillation, a loading dose regimen is used. *Digoxin* has a long half-life of 30 to 40 hours. It is mainly eliminated intact by the kidney, requiring dose adjustment in renal dysfunction.

4. Adverse effects: At low serum drug concentrations, *digoxin* is fairly well tolerated. However, it has a very narrow therapeutic index, and *digoxin* toxicity is one of the most common adverse drug reactions leading to hospitalization. Anorexia, nausea, and vomiting may be initial indicators of toxicity. Patients may also experience blurred vision, yellowish vision (xanthopsia), and various cardiac arrhythmias. Toxicity can often be managed by discontinuing *digoxin*, determining serum potassium levels, and, if indicated, replenishing potassium. Decreased levels of serum potassium (hypokalemia) predispose a patient to *digoxin* toxicity, since *digoxin* normally competes with potassium for the same binding site on the Na^+/K^+-ATPase pump. [Note: Patients receiving thiazide or loop diuretics may be prone to hypokalemia.] Severe toxicity resulting in ventricular tachycardia may require administration of antiarrhythmic drugs and the use of antibodies to *digoxin* (*digoxin immune Fab*), which bind and inactivate the drug. With the use of a lower serum drug concentration in HFrEF, toxic levels are infrequent. *Digoxin* is a substrate of P-gp, and inhibitors of P-gp, such as *clarithromycin*, *verapamil*, and *amiodarone*, can significantly increase *digoxin* levels, necessitating a reduced dose of *digoxin*. *Digoxin* should also be used with caution with other drugs that slow AV conduction, such as β-blockers, *verapamil*, and *diltiazem*.

B. β-Adrenergic agonists

β-Adrenergic agonists, such as *dobutamine* [doe-BYOO-ta-meen] and *dopamine* [DOH-puh-meen], improve cardiac performance by causing positive inotropic effects and vasodilation. *Dobutamine* is the most commonly used inotropic agent other than *digoxin*. β-Adrenergic agonists lead to an increase in intracellular cyclic adenosine monophosphate (cAMP), which results in the activation of protein kinase. Protein kinase then phosphorylates slow calcium channels, thereby increasing entry of calcium ions into the myocardial cells and enhancing contraction (Figure 19.10). Both drugs must be given by intravenous infusion and are primarily used in the short-term treatment of acute HF in the hospital setting.

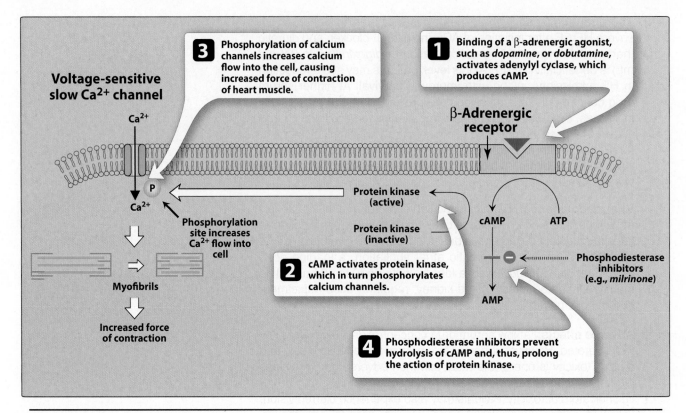

Figure 19.10
Sites of action by β-adrenergic agonists on heart muscle. AMP = adenosine monophosphate; ATP = adenosine triphosphate; cAMP = cyclic adenosine monophosphate; P = phosphate.

C. Phosphodiesterase inhibitors

Milrinone [MIL-rih-nohn] is a phosphodiesterase inhibitor that increases the intracellular concentration of cAMP (Figure 19.10). Like β-adrenergic agonists, this results in an increase of intracellular calcium and, therefore, cardiac contractility. Long-term, *milrinone* therapy may be associated with a substantial increased risk of mortality. However, short-term use of intravenous *milrinone* is not associated with increased mortality in patients without a history of coronary artery disease, and some symptomatic benefit may be obtained in patients with refractory HF.

VIII. ORDER OF THERAPY

Experts have classified HF into four stages, from least severe to most severe. Figure 19.11 shows a treatment strategy using this classification and the drugs described in this chapter. Note that as the disease progresses, polytherapy is initiated. In patients with overt HF, loop diuretics are often introduced first for relief of signs or symptoms of volume overload, such as dyspnea and peripheral edema. ACE inhibitors or ARBs (if ACE inhibitors are not tolerated) are added after the optimization of diuretic therapy. The dosage is gradually titrated to that which is maximally tolerated and/or produces optimal cardiac output. Historically, β-blockers were added after optimization of ACE inhibitor or ARB therapy;

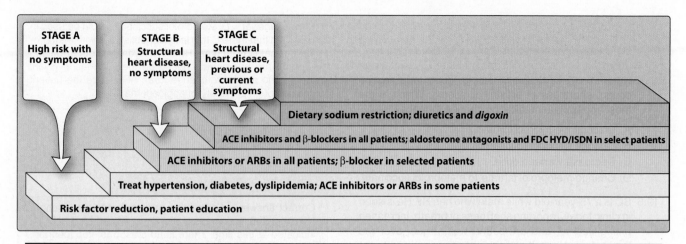

Figure 19.11
Treatment options for various stages of HF. ACE = angiotensin-converting enzyme; ARBs = angiotensin receptor blockers; FDC = fixed dose combination; HYD = hydralazine; ISDN = isosorbide dinitrate. Stage D (refractory symptoms requiring special interventions) is not shown.

however, most patients newly diagnosed with HFrEF are initiated on both low doses of an ACE inhibitor and β-blocker after initial stabilization. These agents are slowly titrated to optimal levels to increase tolerability. *Digoxin*, aldosterone antagonists, and fixed-dose *hydralazine* and *isosorbide dinitrate* are initiated in patients who continue to have HF symptoms despite optimal doses of an ACE inhibitor and β-blocker.

Study Questions

Choose the ONE best answer.

19.1 Which drug may exacerbate HF?

    A. Acetaminophen.

    B. Cetirizine.

    C. Chlorthalidone.

    D. Ibuprofen.

> Correct answer = D. NSAIDs, such as ibuprofen, lead to increased fluid retention and increased blood pressure. If possible, NSAIDs should be avoided in HF patients in order to avoid exacerbations of HF.

19.2 Which best describes the action of ACE inhibitors on the failing heart?

    A. ACE inhibitors increase vascular resistance.

    B. ACE inhibitors decrease cardiac output.

    C. ACE inhibitors reduce preload.

    D. ACE inhibitors increase aldosterone.

> Correct answer = C. ACE inhibitors decrease vascular resistance, decrease preload, decrease afterload, and increase cardiac output. In addition, ACE inhibitors blunt aldosterone release.

19.3 What makes losartan different from other ARBs?

    A. Losartan is renally eliminated.

    B. Losartan has an active metabolite.

    C. Losartan has the shortest half-life.

    D. Losartan has a small volume of distribution.

> Correct answer = B. Losartan is the only ARB that undergoes first-pass metabolism to convert to its active metabolite. Most ARBs have once-daily dosing, and all (except candesartan) have large volumes of distribution.

19.4 How do β-blockers improve cardiac function in HF?

    A. By decreasing cardiac remodeling.

    B. By increasing heart rate.

    C. By increasing renin release.

    D. By activating norepinephrine.

> Correct answer = A. Although it seems counterintuitive to decrease heart rate in HF, β-blockers improve cardiac functioning by slowing heart rate, decreasing renin release, and preventing the direct effects of norepinephrine on cardiac muscle to decrease remodeling.

19.5 BC is a 70-year-old female who is diagnosed with HFrEF. Her past medical history is significant for hypertension and atrial fibrillation. She is taking hydrochlorothiazide, lisinopril, metoprolol tartrate, and warfarin. BC says she is feeling "good" and has no cough, shortness of breath, or edema. Which is the most appropriate medication change to make?

A. Discontinue hydrochlorothiazide.
B. Change lisinopril to losartan.
C. Decrease warfarin dose.
D. Change metoprolol tartrate to metoprolol succinate.

Correct answer = D. Metoprolol succinate should be used in HF, given that there is mortality benefit shown with metoprolol succinate in landmark HF trials. Hydrochlorothiazide and warfarin are appropriate based on the information given; there is no reason to change to an ARB since the patient has no cough or history of angioedema.

19.6 SC is a 75-year-old white male who has HF. He is seen in clinic today, reporting shortness of breath, increased pitting edema, and a 5-pound weight gain over the last 2 days. His current medication regimen includes losartan and metoprolol succinate. SC has no chest pain and is deemed stable for outpatient treatment. Which of the following is the best recommendation?

A. Increase the dose of metoprolol succinate.
B. Start hydrochlorothiazide.
C. Start furosemide.
D. Discontinue losartan.

Correct answer = C. As it is possible that SC is having a HF exacerbation, increasing the dose of the β-blocker is not indicated at this time. There is no reason to stop losartan, based on the information we have. Loop diuretics are preferred over thiazide diuretics when patients require diuresis immediately.

19.7 How is spironolactone beneficial in HF?

A. Promotes potassium secretion.
B. Agonizes aldosterone.
C. Prevents cardiac hypertrophy.
D. Decreases blood glucose.

Correct answer = C. Spironolactone antagonizes aldosterone, which in turn prevents salt/water retention, cardiac hypertrophy, and hypokalemia. Spironolactone has endocrine effects on hormones but not on glucose.

19.8 Which is important to monitor in patients taking digoxin?

A. Chloride.
B. Potassium.
C. Sodium.
D. Zinc.

Correct answer = B. Hypokalemia can lead to life-threatening arrhythmias and increases the potential of cardiac toxicity with digoxin.

19.9 Which describes the mechanism of action of milrinone in HF?

A. Decreases intracellular calcium.
B. Increases cardiac contractility.
C. Decreases cAMP.
D. Activates phosphodiesterase.

Correct answer = B. Milrinone is a phosphodiesterase inhibitor that leads to increased cAMP, increased intracellular calcium, and therefore increased contractility.

19.10 What is the most common adverse effect associated with fixed-dose hydralazine/isosorbide dinitrate?

A. Diarrhea.
B. Drug-induced lupus.
C. Headache.
D. Heartburn.

Correct answer = C. While drug-induced lupus is a possibility with hydralazine, headache is the most common adverse effect.

Antiarrhythmics

Shawn Anderson and Andrew Hendrickson

20

I. OVERVIEW

In contrast to skeletal muscle, which contracts only when it receives a stimulus, the heart contains specialized cells that exhibit automaticity. That is, they intrinsically generate rhythmic action potentials in the absence of external stimuli. These "pacemaker" cells differ from other myocardial cells in showing a slow, spontaneous depolarization during diastole (phase 4), caused by an inward positive current carried by sodium and calcium ions. This depolarization is fastest in the sinoatrial (SA) node (the normal initiation site of the action potential), and it decreases throughout the normal conduction pathway through the atrioventricular (AV) node to the bundle of His and the Purkinje system. Dysfunction of impulse generation or conduction at any of a number of sites in the heart can cause an abnormality in cardiac rhythm. Figure 20.1 summarizes the drugs used to treat cardiac arrhythmias.

II. INTRODUCTION TO THE ARRHYTHMIAS

The arrhythmias are conceptually simple. Dysfunctions cause abnormalities in impulse formation and conduction in the myocardium. However, in the clinical setting, arrhythmias present as a complex family of disorders with a variety of symptoms. To make sense of this large group of disorders, it is useful to organize the arrhythmias into groups according to the anatomic site of the abnormality: the atria, the AV node, or the ventricles. Figure 20.2 summarizes several commonly occurring arrhythmias. Although not shown, each of these abnormalities can be further divided into subgroups depending on the electrocardiogram findings.

A. Causes of arrhythmias

Most arrhythmias arise either from aberrations in impulse generation (abnormal automaticity) or from a defect in impulse conduction.

1. **Abnormal automaticity:** The SA node shows the fastest rate of phase 4 depolarization and, therefore, exhibits a higher rate of discharge than that occurring in other pacemaker cells exhibiting automaticity. Thus, the SA node normally sets the pace of contraction for the myocardium. If cardiac sites other than the SA node show enhanced automaticity, they may generate competing stimuli, and arrhythmias may arise.

CLASS I (Na⁺-channel blockers)
Disopyramide (IA) NORPACE
Flecainide (IC) TAMBOCOR
Lidocaine (IB) XYLOCAINE
Mexiletine (IB) MEXITIL
Procainamide (IA) PRONESTYL
Propafenone (IC) RYTHMOL
Quinidine (IA) QUINIDEX, QUINAGLUTE

CLASS II (ß-adrenoreceptor blockers)
Atenolol TENORMIN
Esmolol BREVIBLOC
Metoprolol LOPRESSOR, TOPROL-XL

CLASS III (K⁺ channel blockers)
Amiodarone CORDARONE, PACERONE
Dofetilide TIKOSYN
Dronedarone MULTAQ
Ibutilide CORVERT
Sotalol BETAPACE, SORINE

CLASS IV (Ca²⁺ channel blockers)
Diltiazem CARDIZEM, CARTIA XT
Verapamil CALAN, ISOPTIN SR, VERELAN

OTHER ANTIARRHYTHMIC DRUGS
Adenosine ADENOCARD
Digoxin LANOXIN
Magnesium sulfate

Figure 20.1
Summary of antiarrhythmic drugs.

269

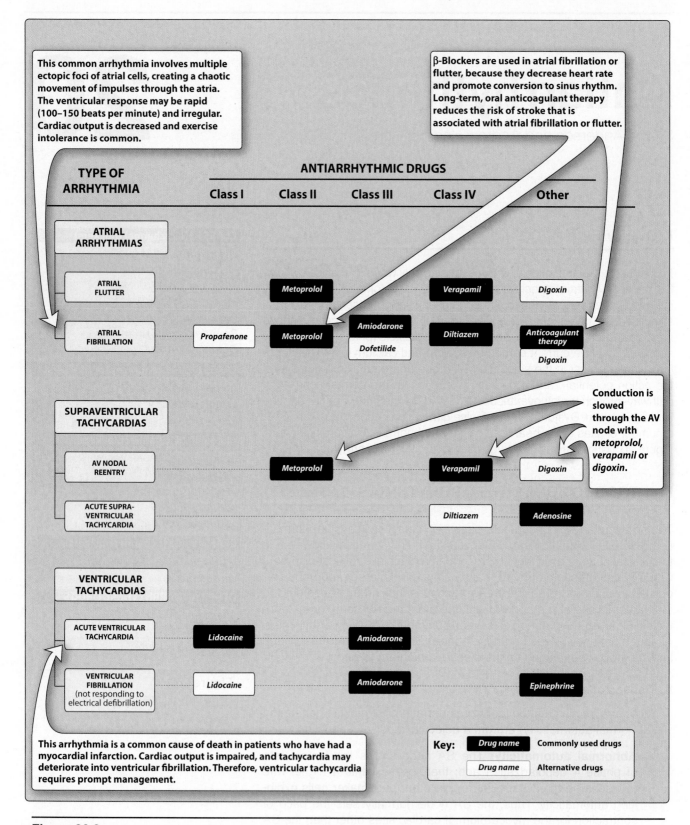

Figure 20.2

Therapeutic indications for some commonly encountered arrhythmias. AV = atrioventricular.

Most of the antiarrhythmic agents suppress automaticity by blocking either Na^+ or Ca^{2+} channels to reduce the ratio of these ions to K^+. This decreases the slope of phase 4 (diastolic) depolarization and/or raises the threshold of discharge to a less negative voltage. Antiarrhythmic drugs cause the frequency of discharge to decrease. This effect is more pronounced in cells with ectopic pacemaker activity than in normal cells.

2. **Abnormalities in impulse conduction:** Impulses from higher pacemaker centers are normally conducted down pathways that bifurcate to activate the entire ventricular surface (Figure 20.3). A phenomenon called reentry can occur if a unidirectional block caused by myocardial injury or a prolonged refractory period results in an abnormal conduction pathway. Reentry is the most common cause of arrhythmias, and it can occur at any level of the cardiac conduction system. This short-circuit pathway results in reexcitation of the ventricular muscle, causing premature contraction or sustained ventricular arrhythmia. Antiarrhythmic agents prevent reentry by slowing conduction (class I drugs) and/or increasing the refractory period (class III drugs), thereby converting a unidirectional block into a bidirectional block.

B. Antiarrhythmic drugs

As noted above, antiarrhythmic drugs can modify impulse generation and conduction to prevent arrhythmias from occurring or to reduce symptoms associated with arrhythmias. Unfortunately, many of the antiarrhythmic agents are known to have dangerous proarrhythmic actions—that is, to cause arrhythmias. Inhibition of potassium (K^+) channels (typically thought of as class III activity) widens the action potential and can, thus, prolong the QT interval. If prolongation is excessive, these drugs increase the risk of developing life-threatening ventricular tachyarrhythmias (torsades de pointes). The most common cause of QT prolongation is drug-induced, although other conditions (for example, ischemia and hypokalemia) and genetic profiles may contribute. QT prolongation is not only seen with class III antiarrhythmics. Drugs such as *cisapride* and *terfenadine* were withdrawn from the market because of severe and fatal arrhythmias. Many drugs are known to prolong the QT interval, such as macrolide antibiotics and antipsychotics. Caution should be employed when combining drugs with additive effects on the QT interval or when giving QT-prolonging antiarrhythmic drugs with drugs known to inhibit their metabolism. As such, the benefit of antiarrhythmic drugs must always be compared to the potential for serious adverse effects or drug interactions. [Note: Implantable cardioverter defibrillators are becoming more widely used to manage ventricular arrhythmias.]

III. CLASS I ANTIARRHYTHMIC DRUGS

Antiarrhythmic drugs can be classified according to their predominant effects on the action potential (Figure 20.4). Although this classification is convenient, it is not entirely clear-cut, because many drugs have actions relating to more than one class or may have active metabolites with a different class of action. Class I antiarrhythmic drugs act by blocking

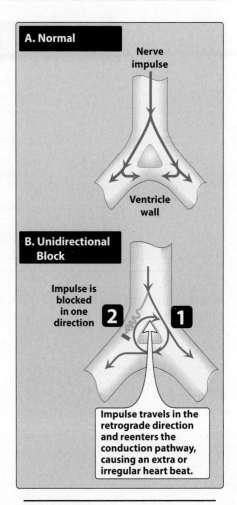

Figure 20.3
Schematic representation of reentry.

CLASSIFICATION OF DRUG	MECHANISM OF ACTION	COMMENT
IA	Na⁺ channel blocker	Slows Phase 0 depolarization in ventricular muscle fibers
IB	Na⁺ channel blocker	Shortens Phase 3 repolarization in ventricular muscle fibers
IC	Na⁺ channel blocker	Markedly slows Phase 0 depolarization in ventricular muscle fibers
II	β-Adrenoreceptor blocker	Inhibits Phase 4 depolarization in SA and AV nodes
III	K⁺ channel blocker	Prolongs Phase 3 repolarization in ventricular muscle fibers
IV	Ca²⁺ channel blocker	Inhibits action potential in SA and AV nodes

Figure 20.4
Actions of antiarrhythmic drugs. SA = sinoatrial; AV = atrioventricular.

voltage-sensitive sodium (Na⁺) channels. The use of sodium channel blockers has declined due to their proarrhythmic effects, particularly in patients with reduced left ventricular function and ischemic heart disease.

A. Use dependence

Class I drugs bind more rapidly to open or inactivated sodium channels than to channels that are fully repolarized following recovery from the previous depolarization cycle. Therefore, these drugs show a greater degree of blockade in tissues that are frequently depolarizing. This property is called use dependence (or state dependence), and it enables these drugs to block cells that are discharging at an abnormally high frequency, without interfering with the normal, low-frequency beating of the heart. The class I drugs have been subdivided into three groups according to their effect on the duration of the ventricular action potential (Figure 20.4).

B. Class IA antiarrhythmic drugs: Quinidine, procainamide, and disopyramide

Quinidine [KWIN-i-deen] is the prototype class IA drug. Other agents in this class include *procainamide* [proe-KANE-a-mide] and *disopyramide* [dye-soe-PEER-a-mide]. Because of their concomitant class III activity, they can precipitate arrhythmias that can progress to ventricular fibrillation.

1. **Mechanism of action:** *Quinidine* binds to open and inactivated sodium channels and prevents sodium influx, thus slowing the rapid upstroke during phase 0 (Figure 20.5). It decreases the slope of phase 4 spontaneous depolarization, inhibits potassium channels, and blocks calcium channels. Because of these actions, it slows conduction velocity and increases refractoriness. *Quinidine* also has mild α-adrenergic blocking and anticholinergic actions. *Procainamide* and *disopyramide* have actions similar to those of *quinidine*. However, there is less anticholinergic activity associated with *procainamide* and more with *disopyramide*. Neither *procainamide* nor *disopyramide* has α-blocking activity.

Disopyramide produces a negative inotropic effect that is greater than the weak effect exerted by *quinidine* and *procainamide*, and unlike the other drugs, it causes peripheral vasoconstriction. The drug may produce a clinically important decrease in myocardial contractility in patients with systolic heart failure.

2. **Therapeutic uses:** *Quinidine* is used in the treatment of a wide variety of arrhythmias, including atrial, AV junctional, and ventricular tachyarrhythmias. *Procainamide* is available in an intravenous formulation only and may be used to treat acute atrial and ventricular arrhythmias. However, electrical cardioversion or defibrillation and *amiodarone* have mostly replaced *procainamide* in clinical use. *Disopyramide* is used in the treatment of ventricular arrhythmias as an alternative to *procainamide* or *quinidine* and may also be used for maintenance of sinus rhythm in atrial fibrillation or flutter.

3. **Pharmacokinetics:** *Quinidine sulfate or gluconate* is rapidly and almost completely absorbed after oral administration. It undergoes extensive metabolism primarily by the hepatic cytochrome P450 3A4 (CYP3A4) isoenzyme, forming active metabolites. *Procainamide* has a relatively short duration of action of 2 to 3 hours. A portion of *procainamide* is acetylated in the liver to *N*-acetylprocainamide (NAPA), which prolongs the duration of the action potential. Thus, NAPA has properties and side effects of a class III drug. NAPA is eliminated via the kidney, and dosages of *procainamide* may need to be adjusted in patients with renal failure. *Disopyramide* is well absorbed after oral administration. It is metabolized in the liver to a less active metabolite and several inactive metabolites. *Disopyramide* is a substrate of CYP3A4. About half of the drug is excreted unchanged by the kidneys.

4. **Adverse effects:** Large doses of *quinidine* may induce the symptoms of cinchonism (for example, blurred vision, tinnitus, headache, disorientation, and psychosis). Drug interactions are common with *quinidine* since it is an inhibitor of both CYP2D6 and P-glycoprotein. Intravenous administration of *procainamide* may cause hypotension. *Disopyramide* has the most anticholinergic adverse effects of the class IA drugs (for example, dry mouth, urinary retention, blurred vision, and constipation). Both *quinidine* and *disopyramide* should be used with caution with potent inhibitors of CYP3A4.

C. Class IB antiarrhythmic drugs: Lidocaine and mexiletine

The class IB agents rapidly associate and dissociate from sodium channels. Thus, the actions of class IB agents are manifested when the cardiac cell is depolarized or firing rapidly. The class IB drugs *lidocaine* [LYE-doe-kane] and *mexiletine* [MEX-i-le-teen] are useful in treating ventricular arrhythmias.

1. **Mechanism of action:** In addition to sodium channel blockade, *lidocaine* and *mexiletine* shorten phase 3 repolarization and decrease the duration of the action potential (Figure 20.6).

2. **Therapeutic uses:** Although *amiodarone* has supplanted *lidocaine* for use in ventricular fibrillation or pulseless ventricular tachycardia (VT), *lidocaine* may be useful as an alternative. *Lidocaine* may also be used in polymorphic VT or in combination

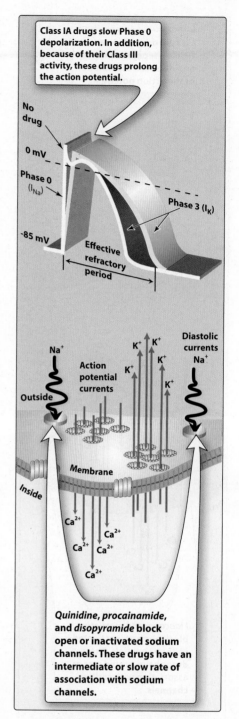

Class IA drugs slow Phase 0 depolarization. In addition, because of their Class III activity, these drugs prolong the action potential.

Quinidine, procainamide, and disopyramide block open or inactivated sodium channels. These drugs have an intermediate or slow rate of association with sodium channels.

Figure 20.5
Schematic diagram of the effects of class IA agents. I_{Na} and I_K are transmembrane currents due to the movement of Na^+ and K^+, respectively.

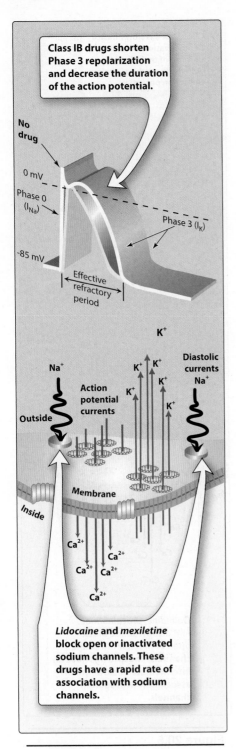

Class IB drugs shorten Phase 3 repolarization and decrease the duration of the action potential.

No drug

0 mV

Phase 0 (I_{Na})

Phase 3 (I_K)

-85 mV

Effective refractory period

K^+

Diastolic currents Na^+

Na^+

K^+ K^+

Action potential currents

K^+

K^+

K^+

Outside

Membrane

Inside

Ca^{2+}

Ca^{2+}

Ca^{2+} Ca^{2+}

Ca^{2+}

Lidocaine and *mexiletine* block open or inactivated sodium channels. These drugs have a rapid rate of association with sodium channels.

Figure 20.6

Schematic diagram of the effects of class IB agents. I_{Na} and I_K are transmembrane currents due to the movement of Na^+ and K^+, respectively.

with *amiodarone* for VT storm. The drug does not markedly slow conduction and, thus, has little effect on atrial or AV junction arrhythmias. *Mexiletine* is used for chronic treatment of ventricular arrhythmias, often in combination with *amiodarone*.

3. **Pharmacokinetics:** *Lidocaine* is given intravenously because of extensive first-pass transformation by the liver, which precludes oral administration. The drug is dealkylated to two less active metabolites, primarily by CYP1A2 with a minor role by CYP3A4. *Lidocaine* should be monitored closely when given in combination with drugs affecting these CYP isoenzymes. As *lidocaine* is a high extraction drug, drugs that lower hepatic blood flow (β-blockers) may require *lidocaine* dose adjustment. *Mexiletine* is well absorbed after oral administration. It is metabolized in the liver primarily by CYP2D6 to inactive metabolites and excreted mainly via the biliary route.

4. **Adverse effects:** *Lidocaine* has a fairly wide therapeutic index. It shows little impairment of left ventricular function and has no negative inotropic effect. Central nervous system (CNS) effects include nystagmus (early indicator of toxicity), drowsiness, slurred speech, paresthesia, agitation, confusion, and convulsions, which often limit the duration of continuous infusions. *Mexiletine* has a narrow therapeutic index and caution should be used when administering the drug with inhibitors of CYP2D6. Nausea, vomiting, and dyspepsia are the most common adverse effects.

D. Class IC antiarrhythmic drugs: Flecainide and propafenone

These drugs slowly dissociate from resting sodium channels and show prominent effects even at normal heart rates. Several studies have cast serious doubts on the safety of the class IC drugs, particularly in patients with structural heart disease.

1. **Mechanism of action:** *Flecainide* [FLEK-a-nide] suppresses phase 0 upstroke in Purkinje and myocardial fibers (Figure 20.7). This causes marked slowing of conduction in all cardiac tissue, with a minor effect on the duration of the action potential and refractoriness. Automaticity is reduced by an increase in the threshold potential, rather than a decrease in slope of phase 4 depolarization. *Flecainide* also blocks potassium channels leading to increased action potential duration, even more so than *propafenone*. *Propafenone* [proe-PA-fen-one], like *flecainide*, slows conduction in all cardiac tissues but does not block potassium channels.

2. **Therapeutic uses:** *Flecainide* is useful in the maintenance of sinus rhythm in atrial flutter or fibrillation in patients without structural heart disease (left ventricular hypertrophy, heart failure, atherosclerotic heart disease) and in treating refractory ventricular arrhythmias. *Flecainide* has a negative inotropic effect and can aggravate chronic heart failure. Use of *propafenone* is restricted mostly to atrial arrhythmias: rhythm control of atrial fibrillation or flutter and paroxysmal supraventricular tachycardia prophylaxis in patients with AV reentrant tachycardias. The latter indication takes advantage of the β-blocking properties of *propafenone*.

3. **Pharmacokinetics:** *Flecainide* is absorbed orally and is metabolized by CYP2D6 to multiple metabolites. The parent drug and metabolites are mostly eliminated renally, and dosage adjustment may be required in renal disease. *Propafenone* is metabolized to active metabolites primarily via CYP2D6, and also by CYP1A2 and CYP3A4. The metabolites are excreted in the urine and the feces.

4. **Adverse effects:** *Flecainide* is generally well tolerated, with blurred vision, dizziness, and nausea occurring most frequently. *Propafenone* has a similar side effect profile, but it may also cause bronchospasm due to its β-blocking effects. It should be avoided in patients with asthma. *Propafenone* is also an inhibitor of P-glycoprotein. Both drugs should be used with caution with potent inhibitors of CYP2D6.

IV. CLASS II ANTIARRHYTHMIC DRUGS

Class II agents are β-adrenergic antagonists, or β-blockers. These drugs diminish phase 4 depolarization and, thus, depress automaticity, prolong AV conduction, and decrease heart rate and contractility. Class II agents are useful in treating tachyarrhythmias caused by increased sympathetic activity. They are also used for atrial flutter and fibrillation and for AV nodal reentrant tachycardia. In addition, β-blockers prevent life-threatening ventricular arrhythmias following a myocardial infarction. [Note: In contrast to the sodium channel blockers, β-blockers and class III compounds, such as *sotalol* and *amiodarone*, are increasing in use.]

Metoprolol [me-TOE-pro-lol] is the β-blocker most widely used in the treatment of cardiac arrhythmias. Compared to nonselective β-blockers, such as *propranolol* [pro-PRAN-oh-lol], it reduces the risk of bronchospasm. It is extensively metabolized in the liver primarily by CYP2D6 and has CNS penetration (less than *propranolol*, but more than *atenolol* [a-TEN-oh-lol]). *Esmolol* [ESS-moe-lol] is a very-short-acting β-blocker used for intravenous administration in acute arrhythmias that occur during surgery or emergency situations. It has a fast onset of action and a short half-life, making it ideal for acute situations and also limiting its adverse effect profile. *Esmolol* is rapidly metabolized by esterases in red blood cells. As such, there are no pharmacokinetic drug interactions.

V. CLASS III ANTIARRHYTHMIC DRUGS

Class III agents block potassium channels and, thus, diminish the outward potassium current during repolarization of cardiac cells. These agents prolong the duration of the action potential without altering phase 0 of depolarization or the resting membrane potential (Figure 20.8). Instead, they prolong the effective refractory period, increasing refractoriness. All class III drugs have the potential to induce arrhythmias.

A. Amiodarone

1. **Mechanism of action:** *Amiodarone* [a-MEE-oh-da-rone] contains iodine and is related structurally to thyroxine. It has complex

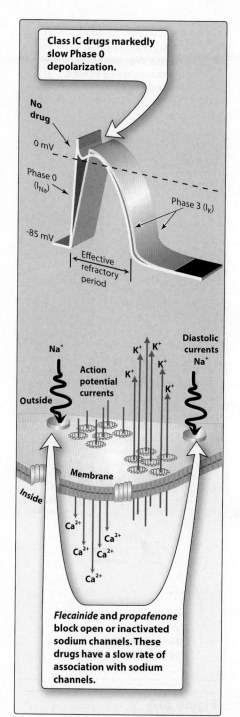

Figure 20.7
Schematic diagram of the effects of class IC agents. I_{Na} and I_K are transmembrane currents due to the movement of Na^+ and K^+, respectively.

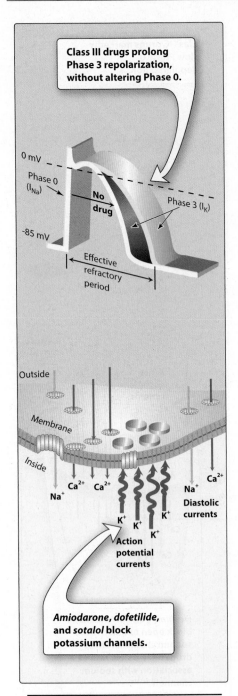

Figure 20.8
Schematic diagram of the effects of class III agents. I_{Na} and I_K are transmembrane currents due to the movement of Na^+ and K^+, respectively.

effects, showing class I, II, III, and IV actions, as well as α-blocking activity. Its dominant effect is prolongation of the action potential duration and the refractory period by blocking K^+ channels.

2. **Therapeutic uses:** *Amiodarone* is effective in the treatment of severe refractory supraventricular and ventricular tachyarrhythmias. *Amiodarone* has been a mainstay of therapy for the rhythm management of atrial fibrillation or flutter. Despite its adverse effect profile, *amiodarone* is the most commonly employed antiarrhythmic and thought to be the least proarrhythmic of the class I and III antiarrhythmic drugs.

3. **Pharmacokinetics:** *Amiodarone* is incompletely absorbed after oral administration. The drug is unusual in having a prolonged half-life of several weeks, and it distributes extensively in adipose tissue. Full clinical effects may not be achieved until months after initiation of treatment, unless loading doses are employed.

4. **Adverse effects:** *Amiodarone* shows a variety of toxic effects, including pulmonary fibrosis, neuropathy, hepatotoxicity, corneal deposits, optic neuritis, blue-gray skin discoloration, and hypo- or hyperthyroidism. However, use of low doses and close monitoring reduce toxicity, while retaining clinical efficacy. *Amiodarone* is subject to numerous drug interactions, since it is metabolized by CYP3A4 and serves as an inhibitor of CYP1A2, CYP2C9, CYP2D6, and P-glycoprotein.

B. Dronedarone

Dronedarone [droe-NE-da-rone] is a benzofuran *amiodarone* derivative, which is less lipophilic, has lower tissue accumulation, and has a shorter serum half-life than *amiodarone*. It does not have the iodine moieties that are responsible for thyroid dysfunction associated with *amiodarone*. Like *amiodarone*, it has class I, II, III, and IV actions. *Dronedarone* has a better adverse effect profile than *amiodarone* but may still cause liver failure. The drug is contraindicated in those with symptomatic heart failure or permanent atrial fibrillation due to an increased risk of death. Currently, *dronedarone* is used to maintain sinus rhythm in atrial fibrillation or flutter, but it is less effective than *amiodarone*.

C. Sotalol

Sotalol [SOE-ta-lol], although a class III antiarrhythmic agent, also has potent nonselective β-blocker activity. The levorotatory isomer (*l-sotalol*) has β-blocking activity, and *d-sotalol* has class III antiarrhythmic action. *Sotalol* blocks a rapid outward potassium current, known as the delayed rectifier. This blockade prolongs both repolarization and duration of the action potential, thus lengthening the effective refractory period. *Sotalol* is used for maintenance of normal sinus rhythm in patients with atrial fibrillation, atrial flutter, or refractory paroxysmal supraventricular tachycardia and in the treatment of ventricular arrhythmias. Since *sotalol* has β-blocking properties, it is commonly used for these indications in patients with left ventricular hypertrophy or atherosclerotic heart disease. This drug can cause the typical adverse effects associated with β-blockers but has a low rate of adverse effects when compared to other antiarrhythmic agents. The dosing interval should be extended in patients with renal disease, since the drug is renally eliminated. To reduce the risk of proarrhythmic effects, *sotalol* is most often initiated in the hospital to monitor QT interval.

D. Dofetilide

Dofetilide [doh-FET-il-ide] is a pure potassium channel blocker. It can be used as a first-line antiarrhythmic agent in patients with persistent atrial fibrillation and heart failure or in those with coronary artery disease. Because of the risk of proarrhythmia, *dofetilide* initiation is limited to the inpatient setting. The half-life of this oral drug is 10 hours. The drug is mainly excreted unchanged in the urine. Drugs that inhibit active tubular secretion are contraindicated.

E. Ibutilide

Ibutilide [eye-BYOO-tih-lide] is a potassium channel blocker that also activates the inward sodium current (mixed class III and IA action). *Ibutilide* is the drug of choice for chemical conversion of atrial flutter, but electrical cardioversion has supplanted its use. *Ibutilide* undergoes extensive first-pass metabolism and is not used orally. Because of the risk of QT prolongation and proarrhythmia, *ibutilide* initiation is limited to the inpatient setting.

VI. CLASS IV ANTIARRHYTHMIC DRUGS

Class IV drugs are the nondihydropyridine calcium channel blockers *verapamil* [ver-AP-a-mil] and *diltiazem* [dil-TYE-a-zem]. Although voltage-sensitive calcium channels occur in many different tissues, the major effect of calcium channel blockers is on vascular smooth muscle and the heart. *Verapamil* shows greater action on the heart than on vascular smooth muscle, and *diltiazem* is intermediate in its actions. In the heart, *verapamil* and *diltiazem* bind only to open depolarized voltage-sensitive channels, thus decreasing the inward current carried by calcium. They prevent repolarization until the drug dissociates from the channel, resulting in a decreased rate of phase 4 spontaneous depolarization. These drugs are therefore use-dependent. They also slow conduction in tissues that are dependent on calcium currents, such as the AV and SA nodes (Figure 20.9). These agents are more effective against atrial than against ventricular arrhythmias. They are useful in treating reentrant supraventricular tachycardia and in reducing the ventricular rate in atrial flutter and fibrillation. Both drugs are metabolized in the liver by CYP3A4. Dosage adjustments may be needed in patients with hepatic dysfunction. Both agents are also inhibitors of CYP3A4, as well as substrates and inhibitors of P-glycoprotein. As such, they are subject to many drug interactions.

VII. OTHER ANTIARRHYTHMIC DRUGS

A. Digoxin

Digoxin [di-JOX-in] inhibits the Na^+/K^+-ATPase pump, ultimately shortening the refractory period in atrial and ventricular myocardial cells while prolonging the effective refractory period and diminishing conduction

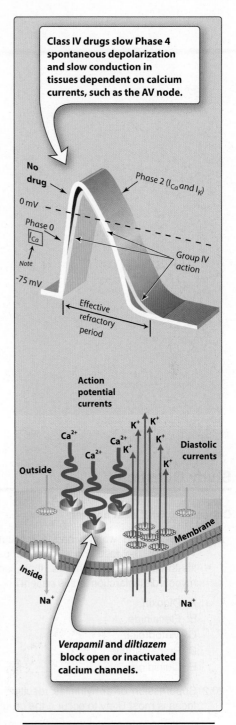

Class IV drugs slow Phase 4 spontaneous depolarization and slow conduction in tissues dependent on calcium currents, such as the AV node.

No drug

Phase 2 (I_{Ca} and I_K)

0 mV

Phase 0

I_{Ca}

Note

−75 mV

Group IV action

Effective refractory period

Action potential currents

Ca^{2+} Ca^{2+} K^+ K^+ K^+ K^+ K^+

Diastolic currents

Outside Ca^{2+}

Membrane

Inside

Na^+ Na^+

Verapamil and diltiazem block open or inactivated calcium channels.

Figure 20.9
Schematic diagram of the effects of class IV agents. I_{Ca} and I_K are transmembrane currents due to the movement of Ca^{2+} and K^+, respectively.

velocity in the AV node. *Digoxin* is used to control ventricular response rate in atrial fibrillation and flutter; however, sympathetic stimulation easily overcomes the inhibitory effects of *digoxin*. At toxic concentrations, *digoxin* causes ectopic ventricular beats that may result in VT and fibrillation. [Note: Serum trough concentrations of 1.0 to 2.0 ng/mL are desirable for atrial fibrillation or flutter, whereas lower concentrations of 0.5 to 0.8 ng/mL are targeted for systolic heart failure.]

B. Adenosine

Adenosine [ah-DEN-oh-zeen] is a naturally occurring nucleoside, but at high doses, the drug decreases conduction velocity, prolongs the refractory period, and decreases automaticity in the AV node. Intravenous *adenosine* is the drug of choice for abolishing acute supraventricular tachycardia. It has low toxicity but causes flushing, chest pain, and hypotension. *Adenosine* has an extremely short duration of action (approximately 10 to 15 seconds) due to rapid uptake by erythrocytes and endothelial cells.

C. Magnesium sulfate

Magnesium is necessary for the transport of sodium, calcium, and potassium across cell membranes. It slows the rate of SA node impulse formation and prolongs conduction time along the myocardial tissue. Intravenous *magnesium sulfate* is the salt used to treat arrhythmias, as oral *magnesium* is not effective in the setting of arrhythmia. Most notably, *magnesium* is the drug of choice for treating the potentially fatal arrhythmia torsades de pointes and *digoxin*-induced arrhythmias.

Study Questions

Choose the ONE best answer.

20.1 A 60-year-old woman had a myocardial infarction. Which of the following should be used to prevent life-threatening arrhythmias that can occur post–myocardial infarction in this patient?

    A. Digoxin.
    B. Flecainide.
    C. Metoprolol.
    D. Procainamide.
    E. Quinidine.

> Correct answer = C. β-Blockers such as metoprolol prevent arrhythmias that occur subsequent to a myocardial infarction. None of the other drugs has been shown to be effective in preventing postinfarct arrhythmias. Flecainide should be avoided in patients with structural heart disease.

20.2 Suppression of arrhythmias resulting from a reentry focus is most likely to occur if the drug:

    A. Has vagomimetic effects on the AV node.
    B. Is a β-blocker.
    C. Converts a unidirectional block to a bidirectional block.
    D. Slows conduction through the atria.
    E. Has atropine-like effects on the AV node.

> Correct answer = C. Current theory holds that a reentrant arrhythmia is caused by damaged heart muscle, so that conduction is slowed through the damaged area in only one direction. A drug that prevents conduction in either direction through the damaged area interrupts the reentrant arrhythmia. Class I antiarrhythmics, such as lidocaine, are capable of producing bidirectional block. The other choices do not have any direct effects on the direction of blockade of conduction through damaged cardiac muscle.

20.3 A 57-year-old man is being treated for an atrial arrhythmia. He complains of dry mouth, blurred vision, and urinary hesitancy. Which antiarrhythmic drug is he mostly like taking?

A. Metoprolol.

B. Disopyramide.

C. Dronedarone.

D. Sotalol.

Correct answer = B. The clustered symptoms of dry mouth, blurred vision, and urinary hesitancy are characteristic of anticholinergic adverse effects which are caused by class IA agents (in this case, disopyramide). The other drugs do not cause anticholinergic effects.

20.4 A 58-year-old woman is being treated for chronic suppression of a ventricular arrhythmia. After 1 week of therapy, she complains about feeling severe upset stomach and heartburn. Which antiarrhythmic drug is the likely cause of these symptoms?

A. Amiodarone.

B. Digoxin.

C. Mexiletine.

D. Propranolol.

E. Quinidine.

Correct answer = C. The patient is exhibiting a classic adverse effect of mexiletine. None of the other agents listed are likely to cause dyspepsia.

20.5 A 78-year-old woman has been newly diagnosed with atrial fibrillation. She is not currently having symptoms of palpitations or fatigue. Which is appropriate to initiate for rate control as an outpatient?

A. Amiodarone.

B. Dronedarone.

C. Esmolol.

D. Flecainide.

E. Metoprolol.

Correct answer = E. Only C and E are options to control rate. The other options are used for rhythm control in patients with atrial fibrillation. Since esmolol is IV only, the only option to start as an outpatient is metoprolol.

20.6 Which of the following is correct regarding digoxin when used for atrial fibrillation?

A. Digoxin works by blocking voltage-sensitive calcium channels.

B. Digoxin is used for rhythm control in patients with atrial fibrillation.

C. Digoxin increases conduction velocity through the AV node.

D. Digoxin levels of 1 to 2 ng/mL are desirable in the treatment of atrial fibrillation.

Correct answer = D. Digoxin works by inhibiting the Na^+/K^+-ATPase pump. It decreases conduction velocity through the AV node and is used for rate control in atrial fibrillation (not rhythm control). Digoxin levels between 1 and 2 ng/mL are more likely to exhibit negative chronotropic effects desired in atrial fibrillation or flutter. A serum drug concentration between 0.5 and 0.8 ng/mL is for symptomatic management of heart failure.

20.7 All of the following are adverse effects of amiodarone except:

A. Cinchonism.

B. Hypothyroidism.

C. Hyperthyroidism.

D. Pulmonary fibrosis.

E. Blue skin discoloration.

Correct answer = A. Cinchonism is a constellation of symptoms (blurred vision, tinnitus, headache, psychosis) that is known to occur with quinidine. All other options are adverse effects with amiodarone that require close monitoring.

20.8 Which arrhythmia can be treated with lidocaine?

A. Paroxysmal supraventricular ventricular tachycardia.

B. Atrial fibrillation.

C. Atrial flutter.

D. Ventricular tachycardia.

Correct answer = D. Lidocaine has little effect on atrial or AV nodal tissue; thus, it used for ventricular arrhythmias such as ventricular tachycardia.

20.9 A clinician would like to initiate a drug for rhythm control of atrial fibrillation. Which of the following coexisting conditions would allow for initiation of flecainide?

   A. Hypertension.
   B. Left ventricular hypertrophy.
   C. Coronary artery disease.
   D. Heart failure.

Correct answer = A. Since flecainide can increase the risk of sudden cardiac death in those with a history of structural heart disease, only A will allow for flecainide initiation. Structural heart disease includes left ventricular hypertrophy, heart failure, and atherosclerotic heart disease.

20.10 Which statement regarding dronedarone is correct?

   A. Dronedarone is more effective than amiodarone.
   B. QT interval prolongation is not a risk with dronedarone.
   C. Dronedarone increases the risk of death in patients with permanent atrial fibrillation or symptomatic heart failure.
   D. There is no need to monitor liver function with dronedarone.

Correct answer = C. Dronedarone is not as effective as amiodarone, QT prolongation is a risk with this drug, and liver function should be monitored when taking dronedarone since it increases the risk of liver failure. The drug is contraindicated in those with symptomatic heart failure or permanent atrial fibrillation due to an increased risk of death.

Antianginal Drugs

21

Kristyn Mulqueen

I. OVERVIEW

Atherosclerotic disease of the coronary arteries, also known as coronary artery disease (CAD) or ischemic heart disease (IHD), is the most common cause of mortality worldwide. Atherosclerotic lesions in coronary arteries can obstruct blood flow, leading to an imbalance in myocardial oxygen supply and demand that presents as stable angina or an acute coronary syndrome (myocardial infarction [MI] or unstable angina). Spasms of vascular smooth muscle may also impede cardiac blood flow, reducing perfusion and causing ischemia and anginal pain.

Typical angina pectoris is a characteristic sudden, severe, crushing chest pain that may radiate to the neck, jaw, back, and arms. Patients may also present with dyspnea or atypical symptoms such as indigestion, nausea, vomiting, or diaphoresis. Transient, self-limited episodes of myocardial ischemia (stable angina) do not result in cellular death; however, acute coronary syndromes and chronic ischemia can lead to deterioration of cardiac function, heart failure, arrhythmias, and sudden death.

All patients with IHD and angina should receive guideline-directed medical therapy with emphasis on lifestyle modifications (smoking cessation, physical activity, weight management) and management of modifiable risk factors (hypertension, diabetes, dyslipidemia) to reduce cardiovascular morbidity and mortality. Medications used for the management of stable angina are summarized in Figure 21.1.

II. TYPES OF ANGINA

Angina pectoris has three patterns: 1) stable, effort-induced, classic, or typical angina; 2) unstable angina; and 3) Prinzmetal, variant, vasospastic, or rest angina. They are caused by varying combinations of increased myocardial demand and decreased myocardial perfusion.

A. Stable angina, effort-induced angina, classic or typical angina

Classic angina is the most common form of angina and, therefore, is also called typical angina pectoris. It is usually characterized by a short-lasting burning, heavy, or squeezing feeling in the chest. Some ischemic episodes may present "atypically"—with extreme fatigue, nausea, or diaphoresis—while others may not be associated with any symptoms (silent angina). Atypical presentations are more common in women, diabetic patients, and the elderly.

ß-BLOCKERS
Atenolol TENORMIN
Bisoprolol ZEBETA
Metoprolol LOPRESSOR, TOPROL XL
Propranolol INDERAL, INDERAL LA

CALCIUM CHANNEL BLOCKERS (DIHYDROPYRIDINES)
Amlodipine NORVASC
Felodipine PLENDIL
Nifedipine PROCARDIA XL

CALCIUM CHANNEL BLOCKERS (NONDIHYDROPYRIDINE)
Diltiazem CARDIZEM
Verapamil CALAN, ISOPTIN

NITRATES
Nitroglycerin NITRO-BID, NITRO-DUR, NITROLINGUAL, NITROSTAT
Isosorbide dinitrate DILATRATE-SR, ISORDIL
Isosorbide mononitrate IMDUR, ISMO

SODIUM CHANNEL BLOCKER
Ranolazine RANEXA

Figure 21.1
Summary of antianginal drugs.

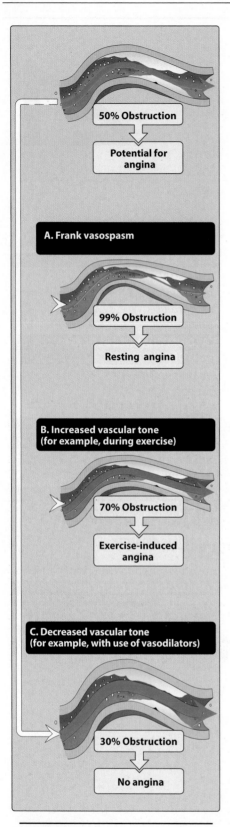

Figure 21.2
Blood flow in a coronary artery partially blocked with atherosclerotic plaques.

Classic angina is caused by the reduction of coronary perfusion due to a fixed obstruction of a coronary artery produced by atherosclerosis. Due to the fixed obstruction, the blood supply cannot increase, and the heart becomes vulnerable to ischemia whenever there is increased demand, such as that produced by physical activity, emotional stress or excitement, or any other cause of increased cardiac workload (Figure 21.2). Typical angina pectoris is promptly relieved by rest or *nitroglycerin* [nye-troe-GLIS-er-in]. When the pattern of the chest pains and the amount of effort needed to trigger the chest pains do not vary over time, the angina is named "stable angina."

B. Unstable angina

Unstable angina is classified between stable angina and MI. In unstable angina, chest pain occurs with increased frequency, duration, and intensity and can be precipitated by progressively less effort. Any episode of rest angina longer than 20 minutes, any new-onset angina, any increasing (crescendo) angina, or even sudden development of shortness of breath is suggestive of unstable angina. The symptoms are not relieved by rest or *nitroglycerin*. Unstable angina is a form of acute coronary syndrome and requires hospital admission and more aggressive therapy to prevent progression to MI and death.

C. Prinzmetal, variant, vasospastic, or rest angina

Prinzmetal angina is an uncommon pattern of episodic angina that occurs at rest and is due to coronary artery spasm. Symptoms are caused by decreased blood flow to the heart muscle from the spasm of the coronary artery. Although individuals with this form of angina may have significant coronary atherosclerosis, the angina attacks are unrelated to physical activity, heart rate, or blood pressure. Prinzmetal angina generally responds promptly to coronary vasodilators, such as *nitroglycerin* and calcium channel blockers.

D. Acute coronary syndrome

Acute coronary syndrome is an emergency that commonly results from rupture of an atherosclerotic plaque and partial or complete thrombosis of a coronary artery. Most cases occur from disruption of an atherosclerotic lesion, followed by platelet activation of the coagulation cascade and vasoconstriction. This process culminates in intraluminal thrombosis and vascular occlusion. If the thrombus occludes most of the blood vessel, and, if the occlusion is untreated, necrosis of the cardiac muscle may ensue. MI (necrosis) is typified by increases in the serum levels of biomarkers such as troponins and creatine kinase. The acute coronary syndrome may present as ST-segment elevation myocardial infarction, non–ST-segment elevation myocardial infarction, or as unstable angina. [Note: In unstable angina, no increases of biomarkers of myocardial necrosis are present.]

III. TREATMENT STRATEGIES

Four types of drugs, used either alone or in combination, are commonly used to manage patients with stable angina: β-blockers, calcium channel blockers, organic nitrates, and the sodium channel–blocking drug, *ranolazine* (Figure 21.1). These agents help to balance the cardiac oxygen supply and demand equation by affecting blood pressure, venous return, heart rate, and contractility. Figure 21.3 summarizes the treatment of angina in patients with concomitant diseases, and Figure 21.4 provides a treatment algorithm for patients with stable angina.

IV. β-ADRENERGIC BLOCKERS

The β-adrenergic blockers decrease the oxygen demands of the myocardium by blocking β_1 receptors, resulting in decreased heart rate, contractility, cardiac output, and blood pressure. These agents reduce myocardial oxygen demand during exertion and at rest. As such, they can reduce both the frequency and severity of angina attacks. β-Blockers can be used to increase exercise duration and tolerance in patients with effort-induced angina. β-Blockers are recommended as initial antianginal therapy in all patients unless contraindicated. [Note: The exception to this rule is vasospastic angina, in which β-blockers are ineffective and may actually worsen symptoms.] β-Blockers reduce the risk of death and MI in patients who have had a prior MI and also improve mortality in patients with hypertension and heart failure with reduced ejection fraction. Agents with intrinsic sympathomimetic activity (ISA) such as *pindolol* should be avoided in patients with angina and those who have had a MI. *Propranolol*

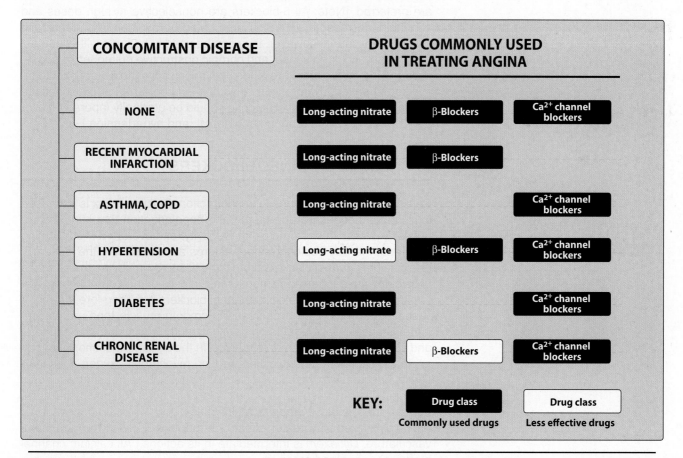

Figure 21.3
Treatment of angina in patients with concomitant diseases.

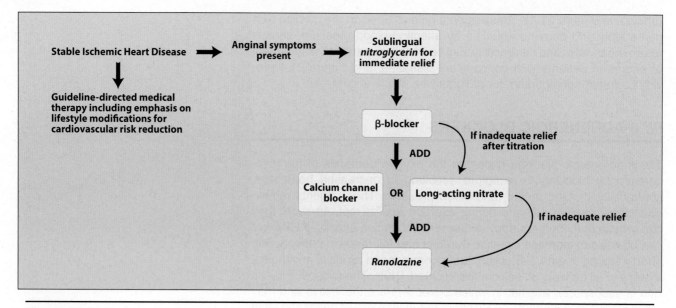

Figure 21.4
Treatment algorithm for improving symptoms in patients with stable angina.

is the prototype for this class of compounds, but it is not cardioselective (see Chapter 7). Thus, other β-blockers, such as *metoprolol* and *atenolol*, are preferred. [Note: All β-blockers are nonselective at high doses and can inhibit β_2 receptors.] β-Blockers should be avoided in patients with severe bradycardia; however, they can be used in patients with diabetes, peripheral vascular disease, and chronic obstructive pulmonary disease, as long as they are monitored closely. Nonselective β-blockers should be avoided in patients with asthma. [Note: It is important not to discontinue β-blocker therapy abruptly. The dose should be gradually tapered off over 2 to 3 weeks to avoid rebound angina, MI, and hypertension.]

V. CALCIUM CHANNEL BLOCKERS

Calcium is essential for muscular contraction. Calcium influx is increased in ischemia because of the membrane depolarization that hypoxia produces. In turn, this promotes the activity of several ATP-consuming enzymes, thereby depleting energy stores and worsening the ischemia. The calcium channel blockers protect the tissue by inhibiting the entrance of calcium into cardiac and smooth muscle cells of the coronary and systemic arterial beds. All calcium channel blockers are, therefore, arteriolar vasodilators that cause a decrease in smooth muscle tone and vascular resistance. These agents primarily affect the resistance of peripheral and coronary arteriolar smooth muscle. In the treatment of effort-induced angina, calcium channel blockers reduce myocardial oxygen consumption by decreasing vascular resistance, thereby decreasing afterload. Their efficacy in vasospastic angina is due to relaxation of the coronary arteries. [Note: *Verapamil* mainly affects the myocardium, whereas *amlodipine* exerts a greater effect on smooth muscle in the peripheral vasculature. *Diltiazem* is intermediate in its actions.] All calcium channel blockers lower blood pressure.

A. Dihydropyridine calcium channel blockers

Amlodipine [am-LOE-di-peen], an oral dihydropyridine, functions mainly as an arteriolar vasodilator. This drug has minimal effect on cardiac conduction. The vasodilatory effect of *amlodipine* is useful in the treatment of variant angina caused by spontaneous coronary spasm. *Nifedipine* [ni-FED-i-pine] is another agent in this class; it is usually administered as an extended-release oral formulation. [Note: Short-acting dihydropyridines should be avoided in CAD because of evidence of increased mortality after an MI and an increase in acute MI in hypertensive patients.]

B. Nondihydropyridine calcium channel blockers

Verapamil [ver-AP-a-mil] slows atrioventricular (AV) conduction directly and decreases heart rate, contractility, blood pressure, and oxygen demand. *Verapamil* has greater negative inotropic effects than *amlodipine*, but it is a weaker vasodilator. *Verapamil* is contraindicated in patients with preexisting depressed cardiac function or AV conduction abnormalities. *Diltiazem* [dil-TYE-a-zem] also slows AV conduction, decreases the rate of firing of the sinus node pacemaker, and is also a coronary artery vasodilator. *Diltiazem* can relieve coronary artery spasm and is particularly useful in patients with variant angina. Nondihydropyridine calcium channel blockers can worsen heart failure due to their negative inotropic effect, and their use should be avoided in this population.

VI. ORGANIC NITRATES

These compounds cause a reduction in myocardial oxygen demand, followed by relief of symptoms. They are effective in stable, unstable, and variant angina.

A. Mechanism of action

Organic nitrates relax vascular smooth muscle by their intracellular conversion to nitrite ions and then to nitric oxide, which activates guanylate cyclase and increases the cells' cyclic guanosine monophosphate (cGMP). Elevated cGMP ultimately leads to dephosphorylation of the myosin light chain, resulting in vascular smooth muscle relaxation (Figure 21.5). Nitrates such as *nitroglycerin* cause dilation of the large veins, which reduces preload (venous return to the heart) and, therefore, reduces the work of the heart. This is believed to be their

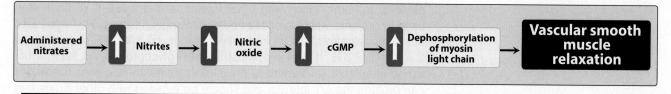

Figure 21.5
Effects of nitrates and nitrites on smooth muscle. cGMP, = cyclic guanosine 3′,5′-monophosphate.

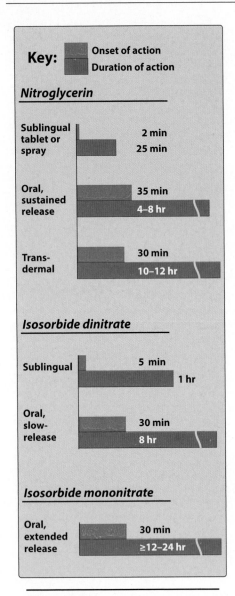

Figure 21.6
Time to peak effect and duration of action for some common organic nitrate preparations.

main mechanism of action in the treatment of angina. Nitrates also dilate the coronary vasculature, providing an increased blood supply to the heart muscle.

B. Pharmacokinetics

Nitrates differ in their onset of action and rate of elimination. The onset of action varies from 1 minute for *nitroglycerin* to 30 minutes for *isosorbide* [eye-soe-SOR-bide] *mononitrate* (Figure 21.6). For prompt relief of an angina attack precipitated by exercise or emotional stress, sublingual (or spray form) *nitroglycerin* is the drug of choice. All patients suffering from angina should have *nitroglycerin* on hand to treat acute angina attacks. Significant first-pass metabolism of *nitroglycerin* occurs in the liver. Therefore, it is commonly administered via the sublingual or transdermal route (patch or ointment), thereby avoiding the hepatic first-pass effect. *Isosorbide mononitrate* owes its improved bioavailability and long duration of action to its stability against hepatic breakdown. Oral *isosorbide dinitrate* undergoes denitration to two mononitrates, both of which possess antianginal activity.

C. Adverse effects

Headache is the most common adverse effect of nitrates. High doses of nitrates can also cause postural hypotension, facial flushing, and tachycardia. Phosphodiesterase type 5 inhibitors such as *sildenafil* potentiate the action of the nitrates. To preclude the dangerous hypotension that may occur, this combination is contraindicated.

Tolerance to the actions of nitrates develops rapidly as the blood vessels become desensitized to vasodilation. Tolerance can be overcome by providing a daily "nitrate-free interval" to restore sensitivity to the drug. This interval of 10 to 12 hours is usually taken at night because demand on the heart is decreased at that time. *Nitroglycerin* patches are worn for 12 hours and then removed for 12 hours. However, variant angina worsens early in the morning, perhaps due to circadian catecholamine surges. Therefore, the nitrate-free interval in these patients should occur in the late afternoon.

VII. SODIUM CHANNEL BLOCKER

Ranolazine inhibits the late phase of the sodium current (late I_{Na}), improving the oxygen supply and demand equation. Inhibition of late I_{Na} reduces intracellular sodium and calcium overload, thereby improving diastolic function. *Ranolazine* has antianginal as well as antiarrhythmic properties. It is indicated for the treatment of chronic angina and may be used alone or in combination with other traditional therapies. It is most often used in patients who have failed other antianginal therapies. *Ranolazine* is extensively metabolized in the liver, mainly by the CYP3A family and also by CYP2D6. It is also a substrate of P-glycoprotein. As such, *ranolazine* is subject to numerous drug interactions. In addition, *ranolazine* can prolong the QT interval and should be avoided with other drugs that cause QT prolongation.

Figure 21.7 provides a summary of characteristics of the antianginal drugs.

DRUG CLASS	COMMON ADVERSE EFFECTS	DRUG INTERACTIONS	NOTES
β-blockers *atenolol* *metoprolol* *propranolol*	Bradycardia, worsening peripheral vascular disease, fatigue, sleep disturbance, depression, blunt hypoglycemia awareness, inhibit β₂-mediated bronchodilation in asthmatics	β₂ agonists (blunted effect); non-dihydropyridine calcium-channel blockers (additive effects)	β₁-selective agents preferred (*atenolol, metoprolol*). Avoid agents with ISA for angina therapy (*pindolol*).
Dihydropyridine calcium-channel blockers *amlodipine* *felodipine* *nifedipine*	Peripheral edema, headache, flushing, rebound tachycardia (immediate release formulations), hypotension	CYP 3A4 substrates (will increase drug concentrations)	Avoid short-acting agents as they can worsen angina (may use extended-release formulations)
Non-dihydropyridine calcium-channel blockers *diltiazem* *verapamil*	Bradycardia, constipation, heart failure exacerbations, gingival hyperplasia (*verapamil*), edema (*diltiazem*)	CYP 3A4 substrates (will increase drug concentrations); increase *digoxin* levels; β-blockers and other drugs affecting AV node conduction (additive effects)	Avoid in patients with heart failure Adjust dose of both agents in patients with hepatic dysfunction
Organic nitrates *isosorbide dinitrate* *isosorbide mononitrate* *nitroglycerin*	Headache, hypotension, flushing, tachycardia	Contraindicated with PDE5 inhibitors (*sildenafil* and others)	Ensure nitrate-free interval to prevent tolerance
Sodium-channel inhibitor *ranolazine*	Constipation, headache, edema, dizziness, QT interval prolongation	Avoid use with CYP 3A4 inducers (*phenytoin, carbamazepine, St. John's wort*) and strong inhibitors (*clarithromycin*, azole antifungals) and agents that prolong QT interval (*citalopram, quetiapine*, others)	No effect on hemodynamic parameters

CYP = cytochrome P450; ISA = intrinsic sympathomimetic activity; PDE5 = phosphodiesterase type 5

Figure 21.7
Summary of characteristics of antianginal drugs.

Study Questions

Choose the ONE best answer.

21.1 What is the clinical term for angina caused by coronary vasospasm?

A. Classic angina.
B. Myocardial infarction.
C. Prinzmetal angina.
D. Unstable angina.

Correct answer = C. Prinzmetal angina is angina caused by vasospasm of the coronary arteries. It is also known as vasospastic or variant angina. The other answers refer to angina (with varying levels of severity) caused by atherosclerosis.

21.2 All of the following medications can be useful for managing stable angina in a patient with coronary artery disease except:

A. Amlodipine.
B. Atenolol.
C. Immediate-release nifedipine.
D. Isosorbide dinitrate.

Correct answer = C. The short-acting dihydropyridine calcium channel blocker nifedipine should be avoided in CAD patients as this can worsen angina; however, the extended-release formulation can be used.

21.3 A 72-year-old male presents to the primary care clinic complaining of chest tightness and pressure that is increasing in severity and frequency. His current medications include atenolol, lisinopril, and nitroglycerin. Which intervention is most appropriate at this time?

    A. Add amlodipine.

    B. Initiate isosorbide mononitrate.

    C. Initiate ranolazine.

    D. Refer the patient to the nearest emergency room for evaluation.

Correct answer = D. Crescendo angina is indicative of unstable angina that requires further workup.

21.4 A 62-year-old patient with a history of asthma and vasospastic angina states that he gets chest pain both with exertion and at rest, about ten times per week. One sublingual nitroglycerin tablet always relieves his symptoms, but this medication gives him an awful headache every time he takes it. Which is the best option for improving his angina?

    A. Change to sublingual nitroglycerin spray.

    B. Add amlodipine.

    C. Add propranolol.

    D. Replace nitroglycerin with ranolazine.

Correct answer = B. Calcium channel blockers are preferred for vasospastic angina. β-Blockers can actually worsen vasospastic angina; furthermore, nonselective β-blockers should be avoided in patients with asthma. The nitroglycerin spray would also be expected to cause headache, so this is not the best choice. Ranolazine is not indicated for immediate relief of an angina attack, nor is it a first-line option.

21.5 Which side effect is associated with amlodipine?

    A. Bradycardia.

    B. Cough.

    C. Edema.

    D. QT prolongation.

Correct answer = C. Edema is the correct answer. The other answers are incorrect.

21.6 Which medication should be prescribed to all anginal patients to treat an acute attack?

    A. Isosorbide dinitrate.

    B. Nitroglycerin patch.

    C. Nitroglycerin sublingual tablet or spray.

    D. Ranolazine.

Correct answer = C. The other options will not provide prompt relief of angina and should not be used to treat an acute attack.

21.7 A 65-year-old male experiences uncontrolled angina attacks that limit his ability to do household chores. He is adherent to a maximized dose of β-blocker with a low heart rate and low blood pressure. He was unable to tolerate an increase in isosorbide mononitrate due to headache. Which is the most appropriate addition to his antianginal therapy?

    A. Amlodipine.

    B. Aspirin.

    C. Ranolazine.

    D. Verapamil.

Correct answer = C. Ranolazine is the best answer. The patient's blood pressure is low, so verapamil and amlodipine may drop blood pressure further. Verapamil may also decrease heart rate. Ranolazine can be used when other agents are maximized, especially when blood pressure is well controlled. The patient will need a baseline ECG and lab work to ensure safe use of this medication.

21.8 A 68-year-old male with a history of angina had a MI last month, and an echocardiogram reveals heart failure with reduced ejection fraction. He was continued on his previous home medications (diltiazem, enalapril, and nitroglycerin), and atenolol was added at discharge. He has only had a few sporadic episodes of stable angina that are relieved with nitroglycerin or rest. What are eventual goals for optimizing this medication regimen?

A. Add isosorbide mononitrate.

B. Increase atenolol.

C. Stop atenolol and increase diltiazem.

D. Stop diltiazem and change atenolol to bisoprolol.

Correct answer = D. Nondihydropyridine calcium channel blockers such as diltiazem should be avoided in patients with heart failure with reduced ejection fraction. Patients should be treated with one of three β-blockers approved for heart failure with reduced ejection fraction (bisoprolol, metoprolol succinate, or carvedilol). It sounds like his angina symptoms are well managed with his current therapy so adding isosorbide mononitrate would not be necessary. These symptoms may become even less frequent as his new β-blocker is titrated.

21.9 Which of the following medications would be safe to use in a patient taking ranolazine?

A. Carbamazepine.

B. Clarithromycin.

C. Enalapril.

D. Quetiapine.

Correct answer = C. All other medications should be avoided due to potential drug–drug interactions.

21.10 A patient whose angina was previously well controlled with once-daily isosorbide mononitrate states that recently he has been taking isosorbide mononitrate twice a day to control angina symptoms that are occurring more frequently during early morning hours. Which of the following is the best option for this patient?

A. Continue once-daily administration of isosorbide mononitrate but advise the patient to take this medication in the evening.

B. Advise continuation of isosorbide mononitrate twice daily for full 24-hour coverage of anginal symptoms.

C. Switch to isosorbide dinitrate, as this has a longer duration of action than the mononitrate.

D. Switch to nitroglycerin patch for consistent drug delivery and advise him to wear the patch around the clock.

Correct answer = A. It is important to maintain a nitrate-free period to prevent the development of tolerance to nitrate therapy. The mononitrate formulation has the longer half-life. The nitroglycerin patch should be taken off for 10 to 12 hours daily to allow for nitrate-free interval.

Anticoagulants and Antiplatelet Agents

Katherine Vogel Anderson and Patrick Cogan

22

I. OVERVIEW

This chapter describes drugs that are useful in treating disorders of hemostasis. Thrombosis, the formation of an unwanted clot within a blood vessel, is the most common abnormality of hemostasis. Thrombotic disorders include acute myocardial infarction (MI), deep vein thrombosis (DVT), pulmonary embolism (PE), and acute ischemic stroke. These conditions are treated with drugs such as anticoagulants and fibrinolytics. Bleeding disorders involving the failure of hemostasis are less common than thromboembolic diseases. These disorders include hemophilia, which is treated with transfusion of recombinant factor VIII, and vitamin K deficiency, which is treated with vitamin K supplementation. Figure 22.1 summarizes the drugs used in treating dysfunctions of hemostasis.

II. THROMBUS VERSUS EMBOLUS

A clot that adheres to a vessel wall is called a "thrombus," whereas an intravascular clot that floats in the blood is termed an "embolus." Thus, a detached thrombus becomes an embolus. Both thrombi and emboli are dangerous, because they may occlude blood vessels and deprive tissues of oxygen and nutrients. Arterial thrombosis most often occurs in medium-sized vessels rendered thrombogenic by atherosclerosis. Arterial thrombosis usually consists of a platelet-rich clot. In contrast, venous thrombosis is triggered by blood stasis or inappropriate activation of the coagulation cascade. Venous thrombosis typically involves a clot that is rich in fibrin, with fewer platelets than are observed with arterial clots.

III. PLATELET RESPONSE TO VASCULAR INJURY

Physical trauma to the vascular system, such as a puncture or a cut, initiates a complex series of interactions between platelets, endothelial cells, and the coagulation cascade. These interactions lead to hemostasis or the cessation of blood loss from a damaged blood vessel. Platelets are central in this process. Initially, there is vasospasm of the damaged blood vessel to prevent further blood loss. The next step involves the formation of a platelet–fibrin plug at the site of the puncture. The creation of an unwanted thrombus involves many of the same steps as normal clot

PLATELET INHIBITORS
Abciximab REOPRO
Aspirin VARIOUS
Cilostazol PLETAL
Clopidogrel PLAVIX
Dipyridamole PERSANTINE
Eptifibatide INTEGRILIN
Prasugrel EFFIENT
Ticagrelor BRILINTA
Ticlopidine TICLID
Tirofiban AGGRASTAT

ANTICOAGULANTS
Apixaban ELIQUIS
Argatroban ARGATROBAN
Bivalirudin ANGIOMAX
Dabigatran PRADAXA
Dalteparin FRAGMIN
Desirudin IPRIVASK
Enoxaparin LOVENOX
Fondaparinux ARIXTRA
Heparin
Rivaroxaban XARELTO
Tinzaparin INNOHEP
Warfarin COUMADIN, JANTOVEN

THROMBOLYTIC AGENTS
Alteplase (tPA) ACTIVASE
Reteplase RETAVASE
Streptokinase
Tenecteplase TNKASE
Urokinase KINLYTIC

TREATMENT OF BLEEDING
Aminocaproic acid AMICAR
Protamine sulfate
Tranexamic acid CYKLOKAPRON, LYSTEDA
Vitamin K₁ (phytonadione) MEPHYTON

Figure 22.1
Summary of drugs used in treating dysfunctions of hemostasis.

formation, except that the triggering stimulus is a pathologic condition in the vascular system, rather than external physical trauma.

A. Resting platelets

Platelets act as vascular sentries, monitoring the integrity of the vascular endothelium. In the absence of injury, resting platelets circulate freely, because the balance of chemical signals indicates that the vascular system is not damaged (Figure 22.2).

1. **Chemical mediators synthesized by endothelial cells:** Chemical mediators, such as prostacyclin and nitric oxide, are synthesized by intact endothelial cells and act as inhibitors of platelet aggregation. Prostacyclin (prostaglandin I_2) acts by binding to platelet membrane receptors that are coupled to the synthesis of cyclic adenosine monophosphate (cAMP), an intracellular messenger (Figure 22.2). Elevated levels of intracellular cAMP are associated with a decrease in intracellular calcium. This prevents platelet activation and the subsequent release of platelet aggregation agents. Damaged endothelial cells synthesize less prostacyclin than healthy cells, resulting in lower prostacyclin levels. Since there is less prostacyclin to bind platelet receptors, less intracellular cAMP is synthesized, which leads to platelet aggregation.

2. **Roles of thrombin, thromboxanes, and collagen:** The platelet membrane also contains receptors that can bind thrombin, thromboxanes, and exposed collagen. In the intact, normal vessel, circulating levels of thrombin and thromboxane are low, and the intact endothelium covers the collagen in the subendothelial layers. The corresponding platelet receptors are, thus, unoccupied, and as a result, platelet activation and aggregation are not

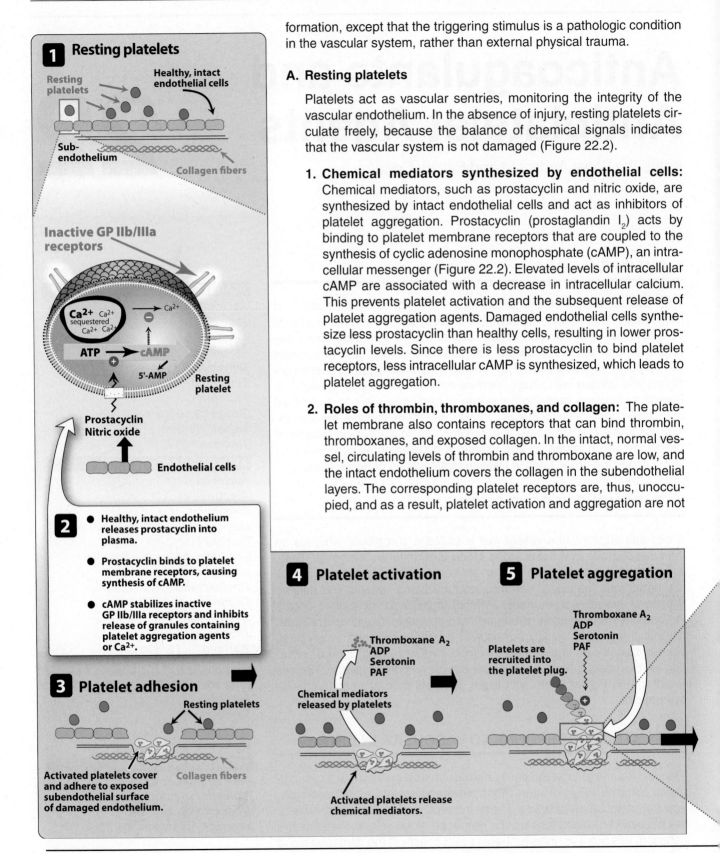

Figure 22.2
Formation of a hemostatic plug. GP = glycoprotein; ATP = adenosine triphosphate; cAMP = cyclic adenosine monophosphate;

initiated. However, when occupied, each of these receptor types triggers a series of reactions leading to the release into the circulation of intracellular granules by the platelets. This ultimately stimulates platelet aggregation.

B. Platelet adhesion

When the endothelium is injured, platelets adhere to and virtually cover the exposed collagen of the subendothelium (Figure 22.2). This triggers a complex series of chemical reactions, resulting in platelet activation.

C. Platelet activation

Receptors on the surface of the adhering platelets are activated by the collagen of the underlying connective tissue. This causes morphologic changes in platelets (Figure 22.3) and the release of platelet granules containing chemical mediators, such as adenosine diphosphate (ADP), thromboxane A$_2$, serotonin, platelet activation factor, and thrombin (Figure 22.2). These signaling molecules bind to receptors in the outer membrane of resting platelets circulating nearby. These receptors function as sensors that are activated by the signals sent from the adhering platelets. The previously dormant platelets become activated and start to aggregate. These actions are mediated by several messenger systems that ultimately result in elevated levels of calcium and a decreased concentration of cAMP within the platelet.

D. Platelet aggregation

The increase in cytosolic calcium accompanying activation is due to a release of sequestered stores within the platelet (Figure 22.2). This leads to 1) the release of platelet granules containing mediators,

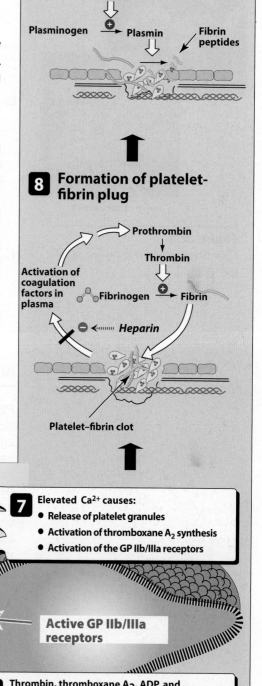

Figure 22.2 (continued)
ADP = adenosine diphosphate; PAF = platelet activation factor.

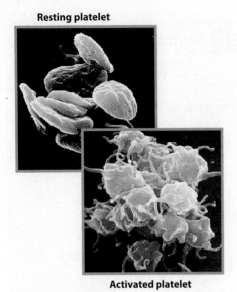

Resting platelet

Activated platelet

Figure 22.3
Scanning electron micrograph of platelets.

such as ADP and serotonin that activate other platelets; 2) activation of thromboxane A$_2$ synthesis; and 3) activation of glycoprotein (GP) IIb/IIIa receptors that bind fibrinogen and, ultimately, regulate platelet–platelet interaction and thrombus formation. Fibrinogen, a soluble plasma GP, simultaneously binds to GP IIb/IIIa receptors on two separate platelets, resulting in platelet cross-linking and platelet aggregation. This leads to an avalanche of platelet aggregation, because each activated platelet can recruit other platelets (Figure 22.4).

E. Formation of a clot

Local stimulation of the coagulation cascade by tissue factors released from the injured tissue and by mediators on the surface of platelets results in the formation of thrombin (factor IIa). In turn, thrombin, a serine protease, catalyzes the hydrolysis of fibrinogen to fibrin, which is incorporated into the clot. Subsequent cross-linking of the fibrin strands stabilizes the clot and forms a hemostatic platelet–fibrin plug (Figure 22.2).

F. Fibrinolysis

During clot formation, the fibrinolytic pathway is locally activated. Plasminogen is enzymatically processed to plasmin (fibrinolysin) by plasminogen activators in the tissue (Figure 22.2). Plasmin limits the growth of the clot and dissolves the fibrin network as wounds heal.

IV. PLATELET AGGREGATION INHIBITORS

Platelet aggregation inhibitors decrease the formation of a platelet-rich clot or decrease the action of chemical signals that promote platelet aggregation (Figure 22.5). The platelet aggregation inhibitors described below inhibit cyclooxygenase-1 (COX-1) or block GP IIb/IIIa or ADP receptors, thereby interfering with the signals that promote platelet aggregation. Because these agents have different mechanisms of actions, synergistic or additive effects may be achieved when agents from different classes are combined. These agents are beneficial in the prevention and treatment of occlusive cardiovascular diseases, in the maintenance of vascular grafts and arterial patency, and as adjuncts to thrombin inhibitors or thrombolytic therapy in MI.

A. Aspirin

1. **Mechanism of action:** Stimulation of platelets by thrombin, collagen, and ADP results in activation of platelet membrane phospholipases that liberate arachidonic acid from membrane phospholipids. Arachidonic acid is first converted to prostaglandin H$_2$ by COX-1 (Figure 22.6). Prostaglandin H$_2$ is further metabolized to thromboxane A$_2$, which is released into plasma. Thromboxane A$_2$ promotes the aggregation process that is essential for the rapid formation of a hemostatic plug. *Aspirin* [AS-pir-in] inhibits thromboxane A$_2$ synthesis by acetylation of a serine residue on the active site of COX-1, thereby irreversibly inactivating the enzyme (Figure 22.7). This shifts the balance of chemical mediators to favor the antiaggregatory effects of prostacyclin, thereby preventing platelet aggregation.

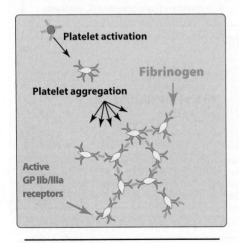

Platelet activation

Fibrinogen

Platelet aggregation

Active GP IIb/IIIa receptors

Figure 22.4
Activation and aggregation of platelets. GP = glycoprotein.

Medication	Adverse Effects	Drug Interactions	Monitoring Parameters
Oral Agents:			
Aspirin	Angioedema Bleeding Bronchospasm GI disturbances Reye syndrome SJS	*ketorolac*—increased bleeding *cidofovir*—nephrotoxicity *probenecid*—decreased uricosuric effects	CBC LFT
Cilostazol	Bleeding GI disturbances Headache Peripheral edema SJS	Food (administer on empty stomach)	CBC
Clopidogrel	Bleeding SJS	Strong CYP2C19 inhibitors reduce antiplatelet effect (e.g., *omeprazole*)	CBC LFT
Dipyridamole	Bleeding Dizziness GI discomfort Rash	Salicylates Thrombolytic agents	None for oral administration
Prasugrel	Angioedema Bleeding Headache Hyperlipidemia Hypertension	Anticoagulants Other antiplatelets	CBC
Ticlopidine	Abnormal LFT Bleeding Dizziness GI disturbances SJS	Antacids—decreases levels *Cimetidine*—reduces clearance	CBC LFT platelet count
Ticagrelor	Bleeding Dyspnea Headache Raised SCr	Strong CYP3A4 inhibitors (e.g., *ketoconazole*) Strong CYP3A4 inducers (e.g., *rifampin*)	CBC LFT
Injectable Agents:			
Abciximab	For all agents:	For all agents:	For all agents:
Eptifibatide	Hypotension Nausea Vomiting Thrombocytopenia	Increased bleeding: *Ginkgo biloba* Antiplatelets Salicylates SSRIs and SNRIs	APTT clotting time H/H platelet count thrombin time
Tirofiban			

APTT=activated partial thromboplastin time, CBC=complete blood count, GI = gastrointestinal, H/H=hemoglobin and hematocrit, LFT=liver function test, SCr=serum creatinine, SJS=Stevens–Johnson Syndrome, SNRI = serotonin–norepinephrine reuptake inhibitor, SSRI = selective serotonin reuptake inhibitor

Figure 22.5
Summary of characteristics of platelet aggregation inhibitors.

The inhibitory effect is rapid, and *aspirin*-induced suppression of thromboxane A$_2$ and the resulting suppression of platelet aggregation last for the life of the platelet, which is approximately 7 to 10 days. Repeated administration of *aspirin* has a cumulative effect on the function of platelets. *Aspirin* is the only antiplatelet agent that irreversibly inhibits platelet function.

2. **Therapeutic use:** *Aspirin* is used in the prophylactic treatment of transient cerebral ischemia, to reduce the incidence of recurrent MI, and to decrease mortality in the setting of primary and secondary prevention of MI. Complete inactivation of platelets occurs with 75 mg of *aspirin* given daily. The recommended dose of *aspirin* ranges from 50 to 325 mg daily.

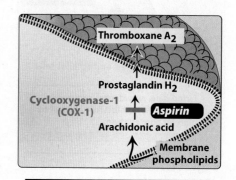

Figure 22.6
Aspirin irreversibly inhibits platelet cyclooxygenase-1.

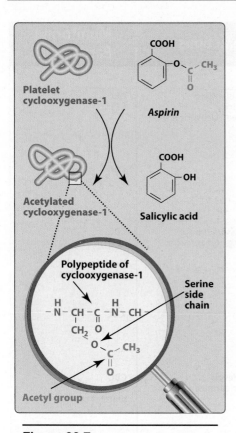

Figure 22.7
Acetylation of cyclooxygenase-1 by
aspirin.

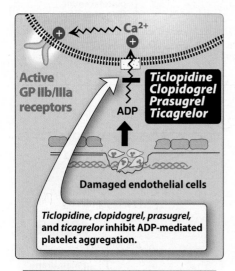

*Ticlopidine, clopidogrel, prasugrel,
and ticagrelor inhibit ADP-mediated
platelet aggregation.*

Figure 22.8
Mechanism of action of *ticlopidine,
clopidogrel prasugrel*, and *ticagrelor*.
GP = glycoprotein.

3. **Pharmacokinetics:** When given orally, *aspirin* is absorbed by passive diffusion and quickly hydrolyzed to salicylic acid in the liver. Salicylic acid is further metabolized in the liver, and some is excreted unchanged in the urine. The half-life of *aspirin* ranges from 15 to 20 minutes and for salicylic acid is 3 to 12 hours.

4. **Adverse effects:** Higher doses of *aspirin* increase drug-related toxicities as well as the probability that *aspirin* may also inhibit prostacyclin production. Bleeding time is prolonged by *aspirin* treatment, causing complications that include an increased incidence of hemorrhagic stroke and gastrointestinal (GI) bleeding, especially at higher doses of the drug. Nonsteroidal anti-inflammatory drugs, such as *ibuprofen*, inhibit COX-1 by transiently competing at the catalytic site. *Ibuprofen*, if taken within the 2 hours prior to *aspirin*, can obstruct the access of *aspirin* to the serine residue and, thereby, antagonize platelet inhibition by *aspirin*. Therefore, immediate release *aspirin* should be taken at least 60 minutes before or at least 8 hours after *ibuprofen*. Although *celecoxib* (a selective COX-2 inhibitor, see Chapter 36) does not interfere with the antiaggregation activity of *aspirin*, there is some evidence that it may contribute to cardiovascular events by shifting the balance of chemical mediators in favor of thromboxane A_2.

B. **Ticlopidine, clopidogrel, prasugrel, and ticagrelor**

Ticlopidine [ti-KLOE-pi-deen], *clopidogrel* [kloh-PID-oh-grel], *prasugrel* [PRA-soo-grel], and *ticagrelor* [tye-KA-grel-or] are $P2Y_{12}$ ADP receptor inhibitors that also block platelet aggregation but by a mechanism different from that of *aspirin*.

1. **Mechanism of action:** These drugs inhibit the binding of ADP to its receptors on platelets and, thereby, inhibit the activation of the GP IIb/IIIa receptors required for platelets to bind to fibrinogen and to each other (Figure 22.8). *Ticagrelor* binds to the $P2Y_{12}$ ADP receptor in a reversible manner. The other agents bind irreversibly. The maximum inhibition of platelet aggregation is achieved in 1 to 3 hours with *ticagrelor*, 2 to 4 hours with *prasugrel*, 3 to 4 days with *ticlopidine*, and 3 to 5 days with *clopidogrel*. When treatment is suspended, the platelet system requires time to recover.

2. **Therapeutic use:** *Clopidogrel* is approved for prevention of atherosclerotic events in patients with a recent MI or stroke and in those with established peripheral arterial disease. It is also approved for prophylaxis of thrombotic events in acute coronary syndromes (unstable angina or non–ST-elevation MI). Additionally, *clopidogrel* is used to prevent thrombotic events associated with percutaneous coronary intervention (PCI) with or without coronary stenting. *Ticlopidine* is similar in structure to *clopidogrel*. It is indicated for the prevention of transient ischemic attacks (TIA) and strokes in patients with a prior cerebral thrombotic event. However, due to life-threatening hematologic adverse reactions, *ticlopidine* is generally reserved for patients who are intolerant to other therapies. *Prasugrel* is approved to decrease thrombotic cardiovascular events in patients with acute coronary syndromes (unstable angina, non–ST-elevation MI, and ST-elevation MI managed with

PCI). *Ticagrelor* is approved for the prevention of arterial thrombo-embolism in patients with unstable angina and acute MI, including those undergoing PCI.

3. **Pharmacokinetics:** These agents require loading doses for quicker antiplatelet effect. Food interferes with the absorption of *ticlopidine* but not with the other agents. After oral ingestion, the drugs are extensively bound to plasma proteins. They undergo hepatic metabolism by the cytochrome P450 (CYP) system to active metabolites. Elimination of the drugs and metabolites occurs by both the renal and fecal routes. *Clopidogrel* is a prodrug, and its therapeutic efficacy relies entirely on its active metabolite, which is produced via metabolism by CYP 2C19. Genetic polymorphism of CYP 2C19 leads to a reduced clinical response in patients who are "poor metabolizers" of *clopidogrel*. Tests are currently available to identify poor metabolizers, and it is recommended that other antiplatelet agents (*prasugrel* or *ticagrelor*) be prescribed for these patients. In addition, other drugs that inhibit CYP 2C19, such as *omeprazole* and *esomeprazole*, should not be administered concurrently with *clopidogrel*.

4. **Adverse effects:** These agents can cause prolonged bleeding for which there is no antidote. *Ticlopidine* is associated with severe hematologic reactions that limit its use, such as agranulocytosis, thrombotic thrombocytopenic purpura (TTP), and aplastic anemia. *Clopidogrel* causes fewer adverse reactions, and the incidence of neutropenia is lower. However, TTP has been reported as an adverse effect for both *clopidogrel* and *prasugrel* (but not for *ticagrelor*). *Prasugrel* is contraindicated in patients with history of TIA or stroke. *Prasugrel* and *ticagrelor* carry black box warnings for bleeding. Additionally, *ticagrelor* carries a black box warning for diminished effectiveness with concomitant use of *aspirin* doses above 100 mg.

C. Abciximab, eptifibatide, and tirofiban

1. **Mechanism of action:** The GP IIb/IIIa receptor plays a key role in stimulating platelet aggregation. A chimeric monoclonal antibody, *abciximab* [ab-SIKS-eh-mab], inhibits the GP IIb/IIIa receptor complex. By binding to GP IIb/IIIa, *abciximab* blocks the binding of fibrinogen and von Willebrand factor and, consequently, aggregation does not occur (Figure 22.9). *Eptifibatide* [ep-ti-FIB-ih-tide] and *tirofiban* [tye-roe-FYE-ban] act similarly to *abciximab*, by blocking the GP IIb/IIIa receptor. *Eptifibatide* is a cyclic peptide that binds to GP IIb/IIIa at the site that interacts with the arginine–glycine–aspartic acid sequence of fibrinogen. *Tirofiban* is not a peptide, but it blocks the same site as *eptifibatide*.

2. **Therapeutic use:** These agents are given intravenously, along with *heparin* and *aspirin*, as an adjunct to PCI for the prevention of cardiac ischemic complications. *Abciximab* is also approved for patients with unstable angina not responding to conventional medical therapy when PCI is planned within 24 hours.

3. **Pharmacokinetics:** *Abciximab* is given by IV bolus, followed by IV infusion, achieving peak platelet inhibition within 30 minutes. The metabolism of *abciximab* is unknown. After cessation of *abciximab* infusion, platelet function gradually returns to normal, with the

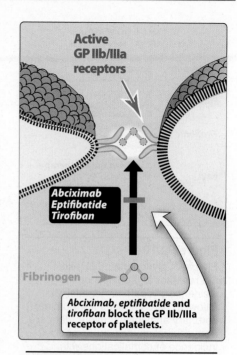

Figure 22.9
Mechanism of action of glycoprotein (GP) IIb/IIIa receptor blockers.

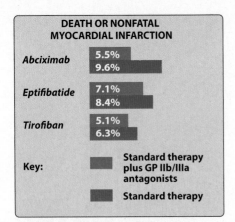

Figure 22.10
Effects of glycoprotein (GP) IIb/
IIIa receptor antagonists on the
incidence of death or nonfatal MI
following percutaneous transluminal
coronary angioplasty. [Note: Data are
from several studies; thus, reported
incidence of complications with
standard therapy, such as *heparin*, is
not the same for each drug.]

antiplatelet effect persisting for 24 to 48 hours. When IV infusion of *eptifibatide* or *tirofiban* is stopped, both agents are rapidly cleared from the plasma. *Eptifibatide* and its metabolites are excreted by the kidney. *Tirofiban* is excreted largely unchanged by the kidney and in the feces.

4. **Adverse effects:** The major adverse effect of these agents is bleeding, especially if used with anticoagulants. Figure 22.10 summarizes the effects of the GP IIb/IIIa receptor antagonists on mortality and MI.

D. Dipyridamole

Dipyridamole [dye-peer-ID-a-mole], a coronary vasodilator, increases intracellular levels of cAMP by inhibiting cyclic nucleotide phosphodiesterase, thereby resulting in decreased thromboxane A_2 synthesis. The drug may potentiate the effect of prostacyclin to antagonize platelet stickiness and, therefore, decrease platelet adhesion to thrombogenic surfaces (Figure 22.2). *Dipyridamole* is used for stroke prevention and is usually given in combination with *aspirin*. *Dipyridamole* has variable bioavailability following oral administration. It is highly protein bound. The drug undergoes hepatic metabolism, as well as glucuronidation, and is excreted mainly in the feces. Patients with unstable angina should not use *dipyridamole* because of its vasodilating properties, which may worsen ischemia (coronary steal phenomenon). *Dipyridamole* commonly causes headache and can lead to orthostatic hypotension (especially if administered IV).

E. Cilostazol

Cilostazol [sill-AH-sta-zole] is an oral antiplatelet agent that also has vasodilating activity. *Cilostazol* and its active metabolites inhibit phosphodiesterase type III, which prevents the degradation of cAMP, thereby increasing levels of cAMP in platelets and vascular tissues. The increase in cAMP levels in platelets and the vasculature prevents platelet aggregation and promotes vasodilation of blood vessels, respectively. *Cilostazol* favorably alters the lipid profile, causing a decrease in plasma triglycerides and an increase in high-density lipoprotein cholesterol. The drug is approved to reduce the symptoms of intermittent claudication. *Cilostazol* is extensively metabolized in the liver by the CYP 3A4, 2C19, and 1A2 isoenzymes. As such, this agent has many drug interactions that require dose modification. The primary route of elimination is via the kidney. Headache and GI side effects (diarrhea, abnormal stools, dyspepsia, and abdominal pain) are the most common adverse effects observed with *cilostazol*. Phosphodiesterase type III inhibitors have been shown to increase mortality in patients with advanced heart failure. As such, *cilostazol* is contraindicated in patients with heart failure.

V. BLOOD COAGULATION

The coagulation process that generates thrombin consists of two interrelated pathways, the extrinsic and the intrinsic systems. The extrinsic system is initiated by the activation of clotting factor VII by tissue factor (also known as thromboplastin). Tissue factor is a membrane protein that is normally separated from the blood by the endothelial cells that line the vasculature. However, in response to vascular injury, tissue factor becomes exposed to blood. There it can bind and activate factor VII, initiating the extrinsic pathway. The intrinsic system is triggered by the activation of clotting factor XII. This occurs when blood comes into contact with the collagen in the damaged wall of a blood vessel.

A. Formation of fibrin

Both the extrinsic and the intrinsic systems involve a cascade of enzyme reactions that sequentially transform various plasma factors (proenzymes) to their active (enzymatic) forms. [Note: The active form of a clotting factor is denoted by the letter "a."] Ultimately, factor Xa is produced, which converts prothrombin (factor II) to thrombin (factor IIa, Figure 22.11). Thrombin plays a key role in coagulation, because it is responsible for generation of fibrin, which forms the mesh-like matrix of the blood clot. If thrombin is not formed or if its function is impeded (for example, by antithrombin III), coagulation is inhibited.

B. Inhibitors of coagulation

It is important that coagulation is restricted to the local site of vascular injury. Endogenously, there are several inhibitors of coagulation factors, including protein C, protein S, antithrombin III, and tissue factor pathway inhibitor. The mechanism of action of several anticoagulant agents, including *heparin* and heparin-related products, involves activation of these endogenous inhibitors (primarily antithrombin III).

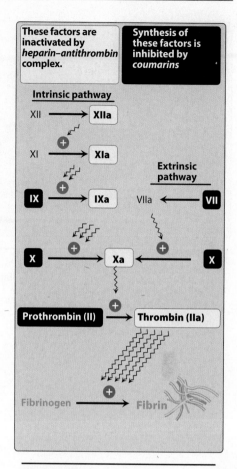

Figure 22.11
Formation of a fibrin clot.

VI. ANTICOAGULANTS

The anticoagulant drugs inhibit either the action of the coagulation factors (for example, *heparin*) or interfere with the synthesis of the coagulation factors (for example, vitamin K antagonists such as *warfarin*).

A. Heparin and low molecular weight heparins

Heparin [HEP-a-rin] is an injectable, rapidly acting anticoagulant that is often used acutely to interfere with the formation of thrombi. *Heparin* occurs naturally as a macromolecule complexed with histamine in mast cells, where its physiologic role is unknown. It is extracted for commercial use from porcine intestinal mucosa. Unfractionated *heparin* is a mixture of straight-chain, anionic glycosaminoglycans with a wide range of molecular weights. It is strongly acidic because of the presence of sulfate and carboxylic acid groups. The realization that low molecular weight forms of *heparin* (*LMWHs*) can also act as anticoagulants led to the isolation of *enoxaparin* [e-NOX-a-par-in], produced by enzymatic depolymerization of unfractionated *heparin*. Other LMWHs include *dalteparin* [DAL-te-PAR-in] and *tinzaparin* [TIN-za-PAR-in]. The *LMWHs* are heterogeneous compounds about one-third the size of unfractionated *heparin*.

1. **Mechanism of action:** *Heparin* acts at a number of molecular targets, but its anticoagulant effect is a consequence of binding to antithrombin III, with the subsequent rapid inactivation of coagulation factors (Figure 22.12). Antithrombin III is an α globulin

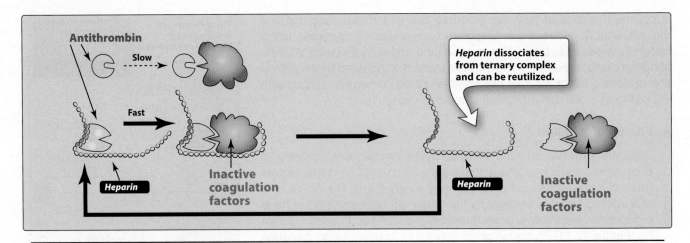

Figure 22.12
Heparin accelerates inactivation of coagulation factors by antithrombin.

that inhibits serine proteases of thrombin (factor IIa) and factor Xa (Figure 22.11). In the absence of *heparin*, antithrombin III interacts very slowly with thrombin and factor Xa. When *heparin* molecules bind to antithrombin III, a conformational change occurs that catalyzes the inhibition of thrombin about 1000-fold (Figure 22.12). *LMWHs* complex with antithrombin III and inactivate factor Xa (including that located on platelet surfaces) but do not bind as avidly to thrombin. A unique pentasaccharide sequence contained in *heparin* and *LMWHs* permits their binding to antithrombin III (Figure 22.13).

2. **Therapeutic use:** *Heparin* and the *LMWHs* limit the expansion of thrombi by preventing fibrin formation. These agents are used for the treatment of acute venous thromboembolism (DVT or PE).

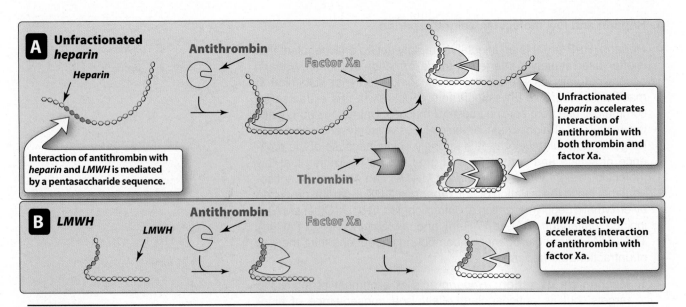

Figure 22.13
Heparin- and *low molecular weight heparin* (*LMWH*)–mediated inactivation of thrombin or factor Xa.

Heparin and *LMWHs* are also used for prophylaxis of postoperative venous thrombosis in patients undergoing surgery (for example, hip replacement) and those with acute MI. These drugs are the anticoagulants of choice for treating pregnant women, because they do not cross the placenta, due to their large size and negative charge. *LMWHs* do not require the same intense monitoring as *heparin*, thereby saving laboratory costs and nursing time. These advantages make *LMWHs* useful for both inpatient and outpatient therapy.

3. **Pharmacokinetics:** *Heparin* must be administered subcutaneously or intravenously, because the drug does not readily cross membranes (Figure 22.14). The *LMWHs* are administered subcutaneously. *Heparin* is often initiated as an intravenous bolus to achieve immediate anticoagulation. This is followed by lower doses or continuous infusion of *heparin*, titrating the dose so that the activated partial thromboplastin time (aPTT) is 1.5- to 2.5-fold that of the normal control. [Note: The aPTT is the standard test used to monitor the extent of anticoagulation with *heparin*.] Whereas the anticoagulant effect with *heparin* occurs within minutes of IV administration (or 1 to 2 hours after subcutaneous injection), the maximum anti–factor Xa activity of the *LMWHs* occurs about 4 hours after subcutaneous injection. It is usually not necessary to monitor coagulation values with *LMWHs* because the plasma levels and pharmacokinetics of these drugs are more predictable. However, in renally impaired, pregnant, and obese patients, monitoring of factor Xa levels is recommended with *LMWHs*.

In the blood, *heparin* binds to many proteins that neutralize its activity, causing unpredictable pharmacokinetics. *Heparin* binding to plasma proteins is variable in patients with thromboembolic diseases. Although generally restricted to the circulation, *heparin* is taken up by the monocyte/macrophage system, and it undergoes depolymerization and desulfation to inactive products. The inactive metabolites, as well as some of the parent *heparin* and *LMWHs*, are excreted into the urine. Renal insufficiency prolongs the half-life of *LMWHs*. Therefore, the dose of *LMWHs* should be reduced in patients with renal impairment. The half-life of *heparin* is approximately 1.5 hours, whereas the half-life of the *LMWHs* is longer than that of heparin, ranging from 3 to 12 hours.

4. **Adverse effects:** The chief complication of *heparin* and *LMWH* therapy is bleeding (Figure 22.15). Careful monitoring of the patient and laboratory parameters is required to minimize bleeding. Excessive bleeding may be managed by discontinuing the drug or by treating with *protamine sulfate*. When infused slowly, the latter combines ionically with *heparin* to form a stable, 1:1 inactive complex. It is very important that the dosage of *protamine sulfate* is carefully titrated (1 mg for every 100 units of *heparin* administered), because *protamine sulfate* is a weak anticoagulant, and excess amounts may trigger bleeding episodes or worsen bleeding potential. *Heparin* preparations are obtained from porcine sources and, therefore, may be antigenic. Possible adverse reactions include chills, fever, urticaria, and anaphylactic shock. *Heparin*-induced thrombocytopenia (HIT) is a serious condition, in which circulating

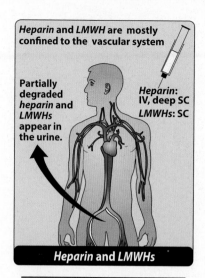

Heparin and *LMWH* are mostly confined to the vascular system

Partially degraded *heparin* and *LMWHs* appear in the urine.

Heparin: IV, deep SC
LMWHs: SC

Heparin and *LMWHs*

Figure 22.14
Administration and fate of *heparin* and *low molecular weight heparins* (*LMWHs*).

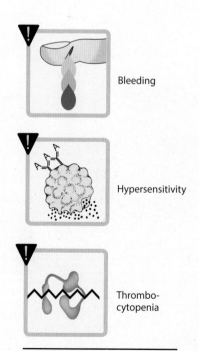

Bleeding

Hypersensitivity

Thrombo-cytopenia

Figure 22.15
Adverse effects of *heparin*.

blood contains an abnormally low number of platelets. This reaction is immune-mediated and carries a risk of venous and arterial embolism. *Heparin* therapy should be discontinued when patients develop HIT or show severe thrombocytopenia. In cases of HIT, *heparin* can be replaced by another anticoagulant, such as *argatroban*. [Note: *LMWHs* can have cross-sensitivity and are not recommended in HIT.] In addition, osteoporosis has been observed in patients on long-term *heparin* therapy. *Heparin* and *LMWHs* are contraindicated in patients who have hypersensitivity to *heparin*, bleeding disorders, alcoholism, or who have had recent surgery of the brain, eye, or spinal cord.

B. Argatroban

Argatroban [ar-GA-troh-ban] is a synthetic parenteral anticoagulant that is derived from L-arginine. It is a direct thrombin inhibitor. *Argatroban* is used for the prophylaxis or treatment of venous thromboembolism in patients with HIT, and it is also approved for use during PCI in patients who have or are at risk for developing HIT. *Argatroban* is metabolized in the liver and has a half-life of about 39 to 51 minutes. Monitoring includes aPTT, hemoglobin, and hematocrit. Because *argatroban* is metabolized in the liver, it may be used in patients with renal dysfunction, but it should be used cautiously in patients with hepatic impairment. As with other anticoagulants, the major side effect is bleeding.

C. Bivalirudin and desirudin

Bivalirudin [bye-VAL-ih-ruh-din] and *desirudin* [deh-SIHR-uh-din] are parenteral anticoagulants that are analogs of hirudin, a thrombin inhibitor derived from medicinal leech saliva. These drugs are selective direct thrombin inhibitors that reversibly inhibit the catalytic site of both free and clot-bound thrombin. *Bivalirudin* is an alternative to *heparin* in patients undergoing PCI who have or are at risk for developing HIT and also in patients with unstable angina undergoing angioplasty. In patients with normal renal function, the half-life of *bivalirudin* is 25 minutes. Dosage adjustments are required in patients with renal impairment. *Desirudin* is indicated for the prevention of DVT in patients undergoing hip replacement surgery. Like the others, bleeding is the major side effect of these agents.

D. Fondaparinux

Fondaparinux [fawn-da-PEAR-eh-nux] is a pentasaccharide anticoagulant that is synthetically derived. This agent selectively inhibits only factor Xa. By selectively binding to antithrombin III, *fondaparinux* potentiates (300- to 1000-fold) the innate neutralization of factor Xa by antithrombin III. *Fondaparinux* is approved for use in the treatment of DVT and PE and for the prophylaxis of venous thromboembolism in the setting of orthopedic and abdominal surgery. The drug is well absorbed from the subcutaneous route with a predictable pharmacokinetic profile and, therefore, requires less monitoring than *heparin*. *Fondaparinux* is eliminated in the urine mainly as unchanged drug with an elimination half-life of 17 to 21 hours. It is contraindicated in patients with severe renal impairment. Bleeding is the major side effect of *fondaparinux*. There is no available agent for the reversal of bleeding associated with *fondaparinux*. HIT is less likely with *fondaparinux* than with *heparin* but is still a possibility. *Fondaparinux* should not be used in the setting of lumbar puncture or spinal cord surgery.

E. Dabigatran etexilate

1. **Mechanism of action:** *Dabigatran etexilate* [da-bi-GAT-ran e-TEX-i-late] is the prodrug of the active moiety *dabigatran*, which is an oral direct thrombin inhibitor. Both clot-bound and free thrombin are inhibited by *dabigatran*.

2. **Therapeutic use:** It is approved for the prevention of stroke and systemic embolism in patients with nonvalvular atrial fibrillation. Because of its efficacy, oral bioavailability, and predictable pharmacokinetic properties, *dabigatran* may be an alternative to *enoxaparin* for thromboprophylaxis in orthopedic surgery.

3. **Pharmacokinetics:** *Dabigatran etexilate* is administered orally. Due to the breakdown of the product and reduction of potency when exposed to moisture, capsules should be stored in the original container and swallowed whole. It is hydrolyzed to the active drug, *dabigatran*, by various plasma esterases. The CYP450 system does not play a role in metabolism of *dabigatran*. Instead, *dabigatran* is a substrate for P-glycoprotein (P-gp) and is eliminated renally.

4. **Adverse effects:** The major adverse effect, like other anticoagulants, is bleeding. *Dabigatran* should be used with caution in renal impairment or in patients over the age of 75, as the risk of bleeding is higher in these groups. There is no approved antidote for reversing bleeding associated with *dabigatran*. *Dabigatran* does not require routine monitoring of the international normalized ratio (INR) and has fewer drug interactions as compared to *warfarin*. [Note: The INR is the standard test used to monitor the anticoagulant activity of *warfarin*.] GI adverse effects are common with this drug and may include dyspepsia, abdominal pain, esophagitis, and GI bleeding. Abrupt discontinuation should be avoided, as patients may be at increased risk for thrombotic events. This drug is contraindicated in patients with mechanical prosthetic heart valves and is not recommended in patients with bioprosthetic heart valves.

F. Rivaroxaban and apixaban

1. **Mechanism of action:** *Rivaroxaban* [RIV-a-ROX-a-ban] and *apixaban* [a-PIX-a-ban] are oral inhibitors of factor Xa. Both agents bind to the active site of factor Xa, thereby preventing its ability to convert prothrombin to thrombin (Figure 22.11).

2. **Therapeutic use:** *Rivaroxaban* is approved for treatment and prevention of DVT and PE and for the prevention of stroke in nonvalvular atrial fibrillation. *Apixaban* is used for stroke prevention in nonvalvular atrial fibrillation.

3. **Pharmacokinetics:** Both drugs are adequately absorbed after oral administration and are highly protein bound. Food may increase the absorption of *rivaroxaban*. *Rivaroxaban* is metabolized

mainly by the CYP 3A4/5 and CYP 2J2 isoenzymes to inactive metabolites. About one-third of the drug is excreted unchanged in the urine, and the inactive metabolites are excreted in the urine and feces. *Apixaban* is primarily metabolized by CYP 3A4, with CYP enzymes 1A2, 2C8, 2C9, 2C19, and 2J2 all sharing minor metabolic roles; approximately 27% is excreted renally. Both *rivaroxaban* and *apixaban* are substrates for P-gp. Compared to *warfarin*, *rivaroxaban* and *apixaban* have fewer drug interactions. There are no laboratory monitoring requirements for either agent.

4. **Adverse effects:** Bleeding is the most serious adverse effect for the factor Xa inhibitors. There is no antidote available to reverse bleeding caused by *rivaroxaban* or *apixaban*. As both drugs are eliminated renally, declining kidney function can prolong the effect of the drugs and, therefore, increase the risk of bleeding. Neither drug should be used in severe renal dysfunction (creatinine clearance less than 15 mL/min). Abrupt discontinuation of these agents should be avoided.

G. Warfarin

The coumarin anticoagulants owe their action to the ability to antagonize the cofactor functions of vitamin K. The only therapeutically relevant coumarin anticoagulant is *warfarin* [WAR-far-in]. Initially used as a rodenticide, *warfarin* is now widely used clinically as an oral anticoagulant. The INR is the standard by which the anticoagulant activity of *warfarin* therapy is monitored. The INR corrects for variations that occur with different thromboplastin reagents used to perform testing at various institutions. The goal of *warfarin* therapy is an INR of 2 to 3 for most indications, with an INR of 2.5 to 3.5 targeted for some mechanical valves and other indications. *Warfarin* has a narrow therapeutic index. Therefore, it is important that the INR is maintained within the optimal range as much as possible, and frequent monitoring may be required.

1. **Mechanism of action:** Factors II, VII, IX, and X (Figure 22.11) require vitamin K as a cofactor for their synthesis by the liver. These factors undergo vitamin K–dependent posttranslational modification, whereby a number of their glutamic acid residues are carboxylated to form γ-carboxyglutamic acid residues (Figure 22.16). The γ-carboxyglutamyl residues bind calcium ions, which are essential for interaction between the coagulation factors and platelet membranes. In the carboxylation reactions, the vitamin K–dependent carboxylase fixes CO_2 to form the new COOH group on glutamic acid. The reduced vitamin K cofactor is converted to vitamin K epoxide during the reaction. Vitamin K is regenerated from the epoxide by vitamin K epoxide reductase, the enzyme that is inhibited by *warfarin*. *Warfarin* treatment results in the production of clotting factors with diminished activity (10% to 40% of normal), due to the lack of sufficient γ-carboxyglutamyl side chains. Unlike *heparin*, the anticoagulant effects of *warfarin* are not observed immediately after drug administration. Instead, peak effects may be delayed for 72 to 96 hours, which is the time required to deplete the pool of circulating clotting factors. The anticoagulant effects of *warfarin* can be overcome by the administration of *vitamin K*. However,

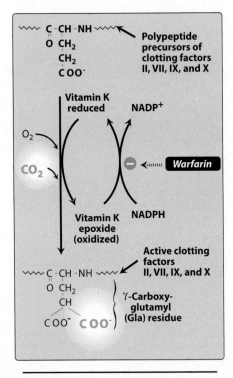

Figure 22.16
Mechanism of action of *warfarin*. NADP+ = oxidized form of nicotinamide adenine dinucleotide phosphate; NADPH = reduced form of nicotinamide adenine dinucleotide phosphate.

reversal following administration of *vitamin K* takes approximately 24 hours (the time necessary for degradation of already synthesized clotting factors).

2. **Therapeutic use:** *Warfarin* is used in the prevention and treatment of DVT and PE, stroke prevention, stroke prevention in the setting of atrial fibrillation and/or prosthetic heart valves, protein C and S deficiency, and antiphospholipid syndrome. It is also used for prevention of venous thromboembolism during orthopedic or gynecologic surgery.

3. **Pharmacokinetics:** *Warfarin* is rapidly absorbed after oral administration (100% bioavailability with little individual patient variation). *Warfarin* is highly bound to plasma albumin, which prevents its diffusion into the cerebrospinal fluid, urine, and breast milk. However, drugs that have a greater affinity for the albumin-binding site, such as sulfonamides, can displace the anticoagulant and lead to a transient, elevated activity. Drugs that affect *warfarin* binding to plasma proteins can lead to variability in the therapeutic response to *warfarin*. *Warfarin* readily crosses the placental barrier. The mean half-life of *warfarin* is approximately 40 hours, but this value is highly variable among individuals. *Warfarin* is metabolized by the CYP450 system (including the 2C9, 2C19, 2C8, 2C18, 1A2, and 3A4 isoenzymes) to inactive components. After conjugation to glucuronic acid, the inactive metabolites are excreted in urine and feces. Agents that affect the metabolism of *warfarin* may alter its therapeutic effects. *Warfarin* has numerous drug interactions that may potentiate or attenuate its anticoagulant effect. The list of interacting drugs is extensive. A summary of some of the important interactions is shown in Figure 22.17.

4. **Adverse effects:** The principal adverse effect of *warfarin* is hemorrhage, and the agent has a black box warning for bleeding risk. Therefore, it is important to frequently monitor the INR and adjust the dose of *warfarin*. Minor bleeding may be treated by withdrawal of the drug or administration of oral *vitamin K_1*, but severe bleeding may require greater doses of *vitamin K* given intravenously. Whole blood, frozen plasma, and plasma concentrates of blood factors may also be used for rapid reversal of *warfarin*. Skin lesions and necrosis are rare complications of *warfarin* therapy. Purple toe syndrome, a rare, painful, blue-tinged discoloration of the toe caused by cholesterol emboli from plaques, has also been observed with *warfarin* therapy. *Warfarin* is teratogenic and should never be used during pregnancy. If anticoagulant therapy is needed during pregnancy, *heparin* or *LMWH* may be administered.

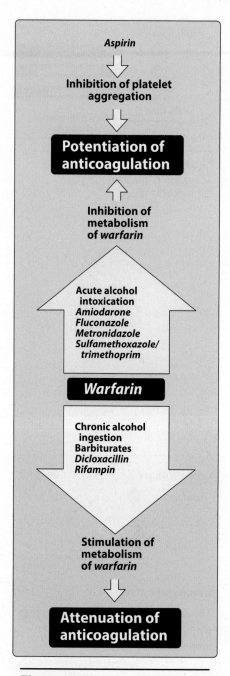

Figure 22.17
Drugs affecting the anticoagulant effect of *warfarin*.

VII. THROMBOLYTIC DRUGS

Acute thromboembolic disease in selected patients may be treated by the administration of agents that activate the conversion of plasminogen to plasmin, a serine protease that hydrolyzes fibrin and, thus, dissolves clots (Figure 22.18). *Streptokinase*, one of the first such agents to be approved, causes a systemic fibrinolytic state that can lead to bleeding problems. *Alteplase* acts more locally on the thrombotic fibrin to

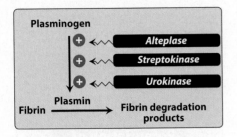

Figure 22.18
Activation of plasminogen by thrombolytic drugs.

produce fibrinolysis. *Urokinase* is produced naturally in human kidneys and directly converts plasminogen into active plasmin. Figure 22.19 compares the thrombolytic agents. Fibrinolytic drugs may lyse both normal and pathologic thrombi.

A. Common characteristics of thrombolytic agents

1. **Mechanism of action:** The thrombolytic agents share some common features. All act either directly or indirectly to convert plasminogen to plasmin, which, in turn, cleaves fibrin, thus lysing thrombi (Figure 22.18). Clot dissolution and reperfusion occur with a higher frequency when therapy is initiated early after clot formation because clots become more resistant to lysis as they age. Unfortunately, increased local thrombi may occur as the clot dissolves, leading to enhanced platelet aggregation and thrombosis. Strategies to prevent this include administration of antiplatelet drugs, such as *aspirin*, or antithrombotics such as *heparin*.

2. **Therapeutic use:** Originally used for the treatment of DVT and serious PE, thrombolytic drugs are now being used less frequently for these conditions. Their tendency to cause bleeding has also blunted their use in treating acute peripheral arterial thrombosis or MI. For MI, intracoronary delivery of the drugs is the most reliable in terms of achieving recanalization. However, cardiac catheterization may not be possible in the 2- to 6-hour "therapeutic window," beyond which significant myocardial salvage becomes less likely. Thus, thrombolytic agents are usually administered intravenously. Thrombolytic agents are helpful in restoring catheter and shunt function, by lysing clots causing occlusions. They are also used to dissolve clots that result in strokes.

3. **Adverse effects:** The thrombolytic agents do not distinguish between the fibrin of an unwanted thrombus and the fibrin of a beneficial hemostatic plug. Thus, hemorrhage is a major side effect. For example, a previously unsuspected lesion, such as a gastric ulcer, may hemorrhage following injection of a thrombolytic agent (Figure 22.20). These drugs are contraindicated in pregnancy, and in patients with healing wounds, a history of cerebrovascular accident, brain tumor, head trauma, intracranial bleeding, and metastatic cancer.

B. Alteplase, reteplase, and tenecteplase

Alteplase [AL-teh-place] (formerly known as *tissue plasminogen activator* or *tPA*) is a serine protease originally derived from cultured human melanoma cells. It is now obtained as a product of recombinant DNA technology. *Reteplase* [RE-teh-place] is a genetically engineered, smaller derivative of recombinant tPA. *Tenecteplase* [ten-EK-te-place] is another recombinant tPA with a longer half-life and greater binding affinity for fibrin than *alteplase*. *Alteplase* has a low affinity for free plasminogen in the plasma, but it rapidly activates plasminogen that is bound to fibrin in a thrombus or a hemostatic plug. Thus, *alteplase* is said to be "fibrin selective" at low doses. *Alteplase* is approved for the treatment of MI, massive PE, and acute ischemic stroke. *Reteplase* and *tenecteplase* are approved only for use in acute MI, although *reteplase* may be used off-label in DVT and massive PE.

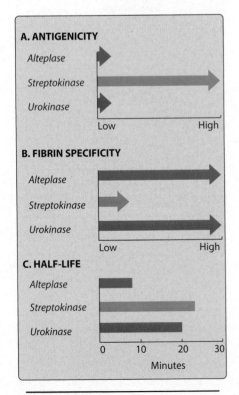

Figure 22.19
A comparison of thrombolytic enzymes.

Alteplase has a very short half-life (5 to 30 minutes), and therefore, 10% of the total dose is injected intravenously as a bolus and the remaining drug is administered over 60 minutes. Both *reteplase* and *tenecteplase* have longer half-lives and, therefore, may be administered as an intravenous bolus. *Alteplase* may cause orolingual angioedema, and there may be an increased risk of this effect when combined with angiotensin-converting enzyme (ACE) inhibitors.

C. Streptokinase

Streptokinase [strep-toe-KYE-nase] is an extracellular protein purified from culture broths of group C β-hemolytic streptococci. It forms an active one-to-one complex with plasminogen. This enzymatically active complex converts uncomplexed plasminogen to the active enzyme plasmin (Figure 22.21). In addition to the hydrolysis of fibrin plugs, the complex also catalyzes the degradation of fibrinogen, as well as clotting factors V and VII (Figure 22.22). With the advent of newer agents, *streptokinase* is rarely used and is no longer available in many markets.

D. Urokinase

Urokinase [URE-oh-KYE-nase] is produced naturally in the body by the kidneys. Therapeutic *urokinase* is isolated from cultures of human kidney cells and has low antigenicity. *Urokinase* directly cleaves the arginine–valine bond of plasminogen to yield active plasmin. It is only approved for lysis of pulmonary emboli. Off-label uses include treatment of acute MI, arterial thromboembolism, coronary artery thrombosis, and DVT. Its use has largely been supplanted by other agents with a more favorable benefit-to-risk ratio.

VIII. DRUGS USED TO TREAT BLEEDING

Bleeding problems may have their origin in naturally occurring pathologic conditions, such as hemophilia, or as a result of fibrinolytic states that may arise after GI surgery or prostatectomy. The use of anticoagulants may also give rise to hemorrhage. Certain natural proteins and *vitamin K*, as well as synthetic antagonists, are effective in controlling this bleeding (Figure 22.23). Concentrated preparations of coagulation factors are available from human donors. However, these preparations carry the risk of transferring viral infections. Blood transfusion is also an option for treating severe hemorrhage.

A. Aminocaproic acid and tranexamic acid

Fibrinolytic states can be controlled by the administration of *aminocaproic* [a-mee-noe-ka-PROE-ic] *acid* or *tranexamic* [tran-ex-AM-ic] *acid*. Both agents are synthetic, orally active, excreted in the urine, and inhibit plasminogen activation. *Tranexamic acid* is 10 times more potent than *aminocaproic acid*. A potential side effect is intravascular thrombosis.

B. Protamine sulfate

Protamine [PROE-ta-meen] *sulfate* antagonizes the anticoagulant effects of *heparin*. This protein is derived from fish sperm or testes and is high in arginine content, which explains its basicity. The positively

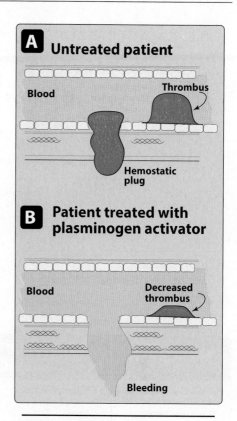

Figure 22.20

Degradation of an unwanted thrombus and a beneficial hemostatic plug by plasminogen activators.

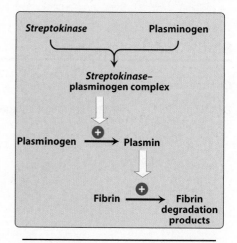

Figure 22.21

Mechanism of action of *streptokinase*.

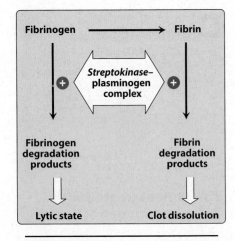

Figure 22.22
Streptokinase degrades both fibrin and fibrinogen.

charged *protamine* interacts with the negatively charged *heparin*, forming a stable complex without anticoagulant activity. Adverse effects of drug administration include hypersensitivity as well as dyspnea, flushing, bradycardia, and hypotension when rapidly injected.

C. Vitamin K

Vitamin K$_1$ (*phytonadione*) administration can stop bleeding problems due to *warfarin* by increasing the supply of active *vitamin K$_1$*, thereby inhibiting the effect of *warfarin*. *Vitamin K$_1$* may be administered via the oral, subcutaneous, or intravenous route. [Note: Intravenous *vitamin K* should be administered by slow IV infusion to minimize the risk of hypersensitivity or anaphylactoid reactions.] For the treatment of bleeding, the subcutaneous route of *vitamin K$_1$* is not preferred, as it is not as effective as oral or IV administration. The response to *vitamin K$_1$* is slow, requiring about 24 hours to reduce INR (time to synthesize new coagulation factors). Thus, if immediate hemostasis is required, fresh frozen plasma should be infused.

Medication	Antidote for Bleeding Caused by	Adverse Effects	Monitoring Parameters
Aminocaproic acid *Tranexamic acid*	**Fibrinolytic state**	**Muscle necrosis Thrombosis CVA Seizure**	**CBC Muscle enzymes Blood pressure**
Protamine sulfate	*Heparin*	**Flushing Nausea/vomiting Dyspnea Bradyarrhythmia Hypotension Anaphylaxis**	**Coagulation monitoring Blood pressure Heart rate**
Vitamin K1	*Warfarin*	**Skin reaction Anaphylaxis**	**PT/INR**

CBC=complete blood count, CVA = cerebrovascular accident, PT=prothrombin time, INR=international normalized ratio

Figure 22.23
Summary of drugs used to treat bleeding.

Study Questions

Choose the ONE best answer.

22.1 Which of the P2Y$_{12}$ ADP receptor antagonists reversibly binds the receptor?

    A. Clopidogrel.
    B. Prasugrel.
    C. Ticagrelor.
    D. Ticlopidine.

Correct answer = C. Of the four P2Y$_{12}$ ADP receptor antagonists, ticagrelor is the only one that reversibly binds the receptor. This is important when it comes to compliance. If a patient is not compliant, then the antiplatelet activity of ticagrelor stops when the drug is missed (since the platelets inhibited are not irreversibly inhibited as they would be with aspirin, clopidogrel, or prasugrel). On the other hand, the waiting period prior to surgery may be shorter in patients taking ticagrelor since it takes less time for the antiplatelet effect to wear off.

22.2 A 70-year-old female is diagnosed with nonvalvular atrial fibrillation. Her past medical history is significant for chronic kidney disease, and her renal function is moderately diminished. All of the following anticoagulants would be expected to require a reduced dosage in this patient except:

A. Apixaban.
B. Dabigatran.
C. Rivaroxaban.
D. Warfarin.

Correct answer = D. Warfarin does not require dosage adjustment in renal dysfunction. The INR is monitored and dosage adjustments are made on the basis of this information. All of the other agents are renally cleared to some extent and require dosage adjustments in renal dysfunction.

22.3 An 80-year-old male is taking warfarin indefinitely for the prevention of deep venous thrombosis. He is a compliant patient with a stable INR and has no issues with bleeding or bruising. He is diagnosed with a urinary tract infection and is prescribed sulfamethoxazole/trimethoprim. What effect will this have on his warfarin therapy?

A. Sulfamethoxazole/trimethoprim will decrease the anticoagulant effect of warfarin.
B. Sulfamethoxazole/trimethoprim will increase the anticoagulant effect of warfarin.
C. Sulfamethoxazole/trimethoprim will activate platelet activity.
D. Sulfamethoxazole/trimethoprim will not change anticoagulation status.

Correct answer = B. Sulfamethoxazole/trimethoprim has a significant drug interaction with warfarin, such that it will inhibit warfarin metabolism. Therefore, sulfamethoxazole/trimethoprim will cause increased anticoagulation, and the patient will need to have his warfarin dose decreased and INR checked frequently while he is on this antibiotic.

22.4 In which disease state is cilostazol contraindicated?

A. Peripheral arterial disease.
B. Gout.
C. Heart failure with reduced ejection fraction.
D. Osteoporosis.

Correct answer = C. Cilostazol is contraindicated in heart failure with reduced ejection fraction because it is a phosphodiesterase inhibitor and acts as a positive inotrope (which can lead to sudden cardiac death).

22.5 Which must heparin bind to in order to exert its anticoagulant effect?

A. GP IIb/IIIa receptor.
B. Thrombin.
C. Antithrombin III.
D. von Willebrand factor.

Correct answer = C. Heparin binds to antithrombin III, causing a conformational change. This heparin/antithrombin III complex then inactivates thrombin and factor Xa.

22.6 Which is considered "fibrin selective" because it rapidly activates plasminogen that is bound to fibrin?

A. Alteplase.
B. Fondaparinux.
C. Streptokinase.
D. Urokinase.

Correct answer = A. Alteplase has a low affinity for free plasminogen in the plasma, but it rapidly activates plasminogen that is bound to fibrin in a thrombus or a hemostatic plug. It has the advantage of lysing only fibrin, without unwanted degradation of other proteins (notably fibrinogen).

22.7 A 56-year-old man presents to the emergency room with complaints of swelling, redness, and pain in his right leg. The patient is diagnosed with acute DVT and requires treatment with an anticoagulant. All of the following are approved for treatment of this patient's DVT except:

A. Rivaroxaban.
B. Dabigatran.
C. Enoxaparin.
D. Heparin.

Correct answer = B. Dabigatran is only approved for the prevention of stroke in nonvalvular atrial fibrillation; it is not approved for the treatment of acute DVT. All of the other options are approved for treatment of acute DVT.

22.8 Which is most appropriate for reversing the anticoagulant effects of heparin?

    A. Aminocaproic acid.
    B. Protamine sulfate.
    C. Vitamin K_1.
    D. Tranexamic acid.

Correct answer = B. Excessive bleeding may be managed by ceasing administration of heparin or by treating with protamine sulfate. Infused slowly, protamine sulfate combines ionically with heparin to form a stable, inactive complex. Aminocaproic acid and tranexamic acid are approved for the treatment of hemorrhage but do not specifically reverse the effects of heparin to stop bleeding. Vitamin K_1 is used to help reverse the effects of warfarin-induced bleeding.

22.9 A 62-year-old male taking warfarin for stroke prevention in atrial fibrillation presents to his primary care physician with an elevated INR of 10.5 without bleeding. He is instructed to hold his warfarin dose and given 2.5 mg of oral vitamin K_1. When would the effects of vitamin K on the INR most likely be noted in this patient?

    A. 1 hour.
    B. 6 hours.
    C. 24 hours.
    D. 72 hours.

Correct answer = C. Vitamin K_1 takes about 24 hours to see a reduction in the INR. This is due to the time required for the body to synthesize new coagulation factors.

22.10 A 58-year-old man receives intravenous alteplase treatment for acute stroke. Five minutes following completion of alteplase infusion, he develops orolingual angioedema. Which of the following drugs may have increased the risk of developing orolingual angioedema in this patient?

    A. ACE inhibitor.
    B. GP IIb/IIIa receptor antagonist.
    C. Phosphodiesterase inhibitor.
    D. Thiazide diuretic.

Correct answer = A. ACE inhibitors, aspirin, and prasugrel all have possible adverse effects including orolingual angioedema. In the setting of alteplase administration, ACE inhibitors have been associated with an increased risk of developing orolingual angioedema with concomitant use.

Drugs for Hyperlipidemia

23

Karen Sando

I. OVERVIEW

Coronary heart disease (CHD) is the leading cause of death worldwide. CHD is correlated with elevated levels of low-density lipoprotein cholesterol (LDL-C; "bad" cholesterol) and triglycerides and low levels of high-density lipoprotein cholesterol (HDL-C; "good cholesterol"). Other risk factors for CHD include cigarette smoking, hypertension, obesity, and diabetes. Cholesterol levels may be elevated due to lifestyle factors (for example, lack of exercise or diet containing excess saturated fats). Hyperlipidemias can also result from an inherited defect in lipoprotein metabolism or, more commonly, from a combination of genetic and lifestyle factors. Appropriate lifestyle changes, along with drug therapy, can lead to a 30% to 40% reduction in CHD mortality. Antihyperlipidemic drugs (Figure 23.1) are often taken indefinitely to control plasma lipid levels. Figure 23.2 illustrates the normal metabolism of serum lipoproteins and the characteristics of the major genetic hyperlipidemias.

II. TREATMENT GOALS

Plasma lipids consist mostly of lipoproteins, which are spherical complexes of lipids and specific proteins (apolipoproteins). The clinically important lipoproteins, listed in decreasing order of atherogenicity, are LDL, very–low-density lipoprotein (VLDL) and chylomicrons, and HDL. The occurrence of CHD is positively associated with high total cholesterol and more strongly with elevated LDL-C. [Note: Total cholesterol is the sum of LDL-C, VLDL-C, and HDL-C.] In contrast to LDL-C, high levels of HDL-C have been associated with a decreased risk for heart disease (Figure 23.3). Reduction of LDL-C is the primary goal of cholesterol-lowering therapy. Previously, cholesterol guidelines recommended treating to specific targets for LDL-C. Recent cholesterol guidelines do not recommend targets but instead emphasize high-intensity or moderate-intensity statin therapy in defined populations with risk for atherosclerotic cardiovascular disease (ASCVD). Higher-intensity therapy is recommended in those with established ASCVD or in those with a higher overall risk of heart disease (Figure 23.4).

A. Treatment options for hypercholesterolemia

Lifestyle changes, such as diet, exercise, and weight reduction, can lead to modest decreases in LDL-C and increases in HDL-C. However,

HMG CoA REDUCTASE INHIBITORS (STATINS)	
Atorvastatin LIPITOR	
Fluvastatin LESCOL	
Lovastatin MEVACOR	
Pitavastatin LIVALO	
Pravastatin PRAVACHOL	
Rosuvastatin CRESTOR	
Simvastatin ZOCOR	
NIACIN	
Niacin NIASPAN, SLO-NIACIN	
FIBRATES	
Gemfibrozil LOPID	
Fenofibrate TRICOR, LOFIBRA, TRIGLIDE	
BILE ACID SEQUESTRANTS	
Colesevelam WELCHOL	
Colestipol COLESTID	
Cholestyramine QUESTRAN, PREVALITE	
CHOLESTEROL ABSORPTION INHIBITOR	
Ezetimibe ZETIA	
OMEGA-3 FATTY ACIDS	
Docosahexaenoic and *eicosapentaenoic acids* LOVAZA, various OTC preparations	
Icosapent ethyl VASCEPA	

Figure 23.1
Summary of antihyperlipidemic drugs. HMG CoA = 3-hydroxy-3-methylglutaryl coenzyme A; OTC = over-the-counter.

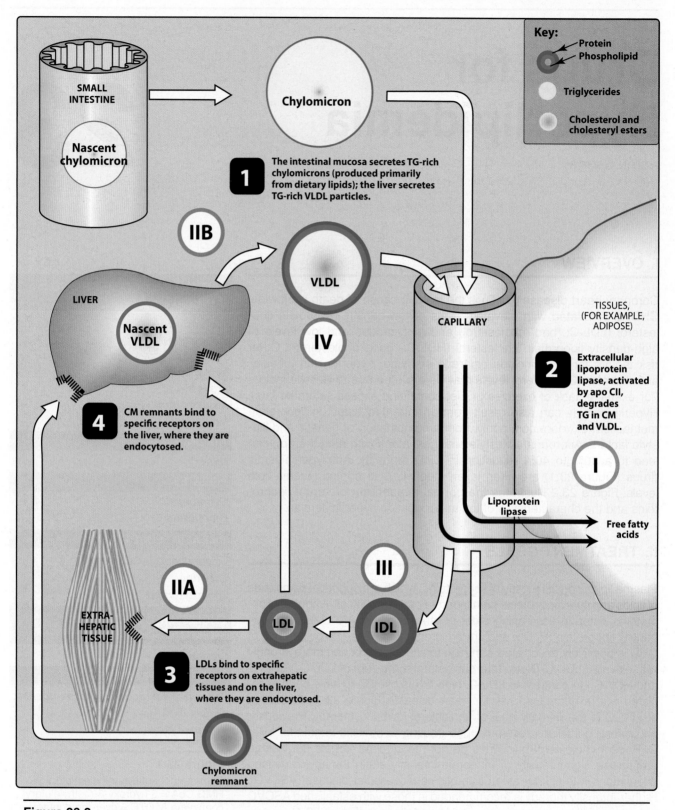

Figure 23.2
Metabolism of plasma lipoproteins and related genetic diseases. Roman numerals in the *white circles* refer to specific genetic types of hyperlipidemias summarized on the facing page. CM = chylomicron; TG = triglyceride; VLDL = very–low-density lipoprotein; LDL = low-density lipoprotein; IDL = intermediate-density lipoprotein; apo CII = apolipoprotein CII found in chylomicrons and VLDL. (Figure continues on next page.)

Type I (FAMILIAL HYPERCHYLOMICRONEMIA)

- Massive fasting hyperchylomicronemia, even following normal dietary fat intake, resulting in greatly elevated serum TG levels.
- Deficiency of lipoprotein lipase or deficiency of normal apolipoprotein CII (rare).
- Type I is not associated with an increase in coronary heart disease.
- Treatment: Low-fat diet. No drug therapy is effective for Type I hyperlipidemia.

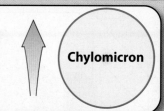

Type IIA (FAMILIAL HYPERCHOLESTEROLEMIA)

- Elevated LDL with normal VLDL levels due to a block in LDL degradation. This results in increased serum cholesterol but normal TG levels.
- Caused by defects in the synthesis or processing of LDL receptors.
- Ischemic heart disease is greatly accelerated.
- Treatment: Diet. Heterozygotes: *Cholestyramine* and *niacin*, or a statin.

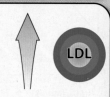

Type IIB (FAMILIAL COMBINED [MIXED] HYPERLIPIDEMIA)

- Similar to Type IIA except that VLDL is also increased, resulting in elevated serum TG as well as cholesterol levels.
- Caused by overproduction of VLDL by the liver.
- Relatively common.
- Treatment: Diet. Drug therapy is similar to that for Type IIA .

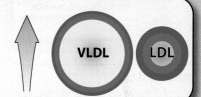

Type III (FAMILIAL DYSBETALIPOPROTEINEMIA)

- Serum concentrations of IDL are increased, resulting in increased TG and cholesterol levels.
- Cause is either overproduction or underutilization of IDL due to mutant apolipoprotein E.
- Xanthomas and accelerated vascular disease develop in patients by middle age.
- Treatment: Diet. Drug therapy includes *niacin* and *fenofibrate*, or a statin.

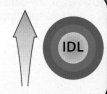

Type IV (FAMILIAL HYPERTRIGLYCERIDEMIA)

- VLDL levels are increased, whereas LDL levels are normal or decreased, resulting in normal to elevated cholesterol, and greatly elevated circulating TG levels.
- Cause is overproduction and/or decreased removal of VLDL and TG in serum.
- This is a relatively common disease. It has few clinical manifestations other than accelerated ischemic heart disease. Patients with this disorder are frequently obese, diabetic, and hyperuricemic.
- Treatment: Diet. If necessary, drug therapy includes *niacin* and/or *fenofibrate*.

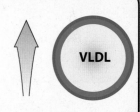

Type V (FAMILIAL MIXED HYPERTRIGLYCERIDEMIA)

- Serum VLDL and chylomicrons are elevated. LDL is normal or decreased. This results in elevated cholesterol and greatly elevated TG levels.
- Cause is either increased production or decreased clearance of VLDL and chylomicrons. Usually, it is a genetic defect.
- Occurs most commonly in adults who are obese and/or diabetic.
- Treatment: Diet. If necessary, drug therapy includes *niacin*, and/or *fenofibrate*, or a statin.

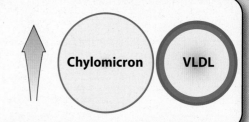

Figure 23.2 (Continued)

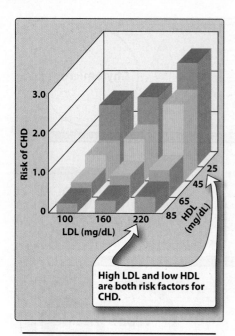

Figure 23.3
Effect of circulating LDL and HDL on the risk of coronary heart disease (CHD). LDL = low-density lipoprotein; HDL = high-density lipoprotein.

most patients are unable to achieve significant LDL-C reductions with lifestyle modifications alone, and drug therapy may be required. Treatment with HMG CoA reductase inhibitors (statins) is the primary treatment option for hypercholesterolemia. Statin therapy is recommended for four major groups as outlined in Figure 23.4.

B. Treatment options for hypertriglyceridemia

Elevated triglycerides are independently associated with increased risk of CHD. Diet and exercise are the primary modes of treating hypertriglyceridemia. If indicated, *niacin* and fibric acid derivatives are the most efficacious in lowering triglycerides. Omega-3 fatty acids (fish oil) in adequate doses may also be beneficial. Triglyceride reduction is a secondary benefit of the statins, with the primary benefit being reduction of LDL-C.

III. DRUGS FOR HYPERLIPIDEMIA

Antihyperlipidemic drugs include the statins, *niacin*, fibrates, bile acid–binding resins, a cholesterol absorption inhibitor, and omega-3 fatty acids. These agents may be used alone or in combination. However, drug therapy should always be accompanied by lifestyle modifications, such as exercise and a diet low in saturated fats.

A. HMG CoA reductase inhibitors

3-Hydroxy-3-methylglutaryl coenzyme A (HMG CoA) reductase inhibitors (commonly known as statins) lower elevated LDL-C, resulting in a substantial reduction in coronary events and death from CHD. They are considered first-line treatment for patients with elevated risk of ASCVD. Therapeutic benefits include plaque stabilization, improvement of coronary endothelial function, inhibition of platelet thrombus formation, and anti-inflammatory activity. The value of lowering LDL-C with statins has been demonstrated in patients with and without established CHD.

1. **Mechanism of action:** *Lovastatin* [LOE-vah-stat-in], *simvastatin* [sim-vah-STAT-in], *pravastatin* [PRAH-vah-stat-in], *atorvastatin* [a-TOR-vah-stat-in], *fluvastatin* [FLOO-vah-stat-in], *pitavastatin* [pit-AV-a-STAT-in], and *rosuvastatin* [roe-SOO-va-stat-in] are competitive inhibitors of HMG CoA reductase, the rate-limiting step in cholesterol synthesis. By inhibiting de novo cholesterol synthesis, they deplete the intracellular supply of cholesterol (Figure 23.5). Depletion of intracellular cholesterol causes the cell to increase the number of cell surface LDL receptors that can bind and internalize circulating LDLs. Thus, plasma cholesterol is reduced, by both decreased cholesterol synthesis and increased LDL catabolism. *Pitavastatin, rosuvastatin*, and *atorvastatin* are the most potent LDL cholesterol–lowering statins, followed by *simvastatin, pravastatin*, and then *lovastatin* and *fluvastatin*. [Note: Because these agents undergo a marked first-pass extraction by the liver, their dominant effect is on that organ.] The HMG CoA reductase inhibitors also decrease triglyceride levels and may increase HDL cholesterol levels in some patients.

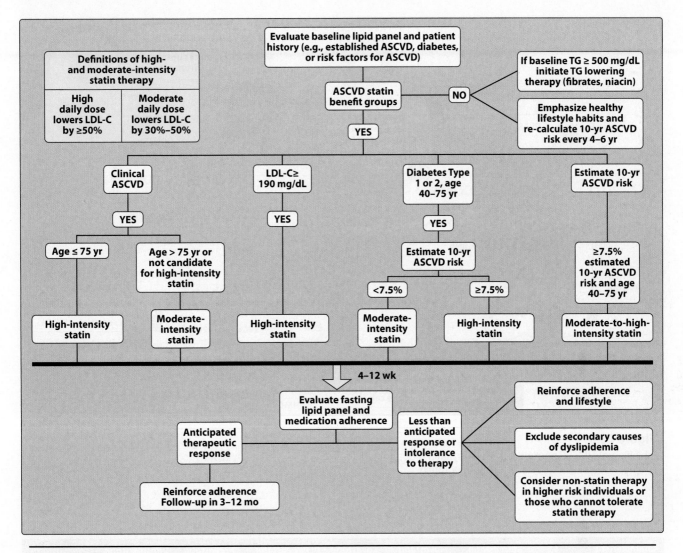

Figure 23.4
Treatment guidelines for hyperlipidemia. ASCVD = atherosclerotic cardiovascular disease; LDL-C = low-density lipoprotein cholesterol; TG = triglycerides.

2. **Therapeutic uses:** These drugs are effective in lowering plasma cholesterol levels in all types of hyperlipidemias. However, patients who are homozygous for familial hypercholesterolemia lack LDL receptors and, therefore, benefit much less from treatment with these drugs.

3. **Pharmacokinetics:** *Lovastatin* and *simvastatin* are lactones that are hydrolyzed to the active drug. The remaining statins are all administered in their active form. Absorption of the statins is variable (30% to 85%) following oral administration. All statins are metabolized in the liver, with some metabolites retaining activity. Excretion takes place principally through bile and feces, but some urinary elimination also occurs. Their half-lives are variable. Some characteristics of the statins are summarized in Figure 23.6.

4. **Adverse effects:** Elevated liver enzymes may occur with statin therapy. Therefore, liver function should be evaluated prior to

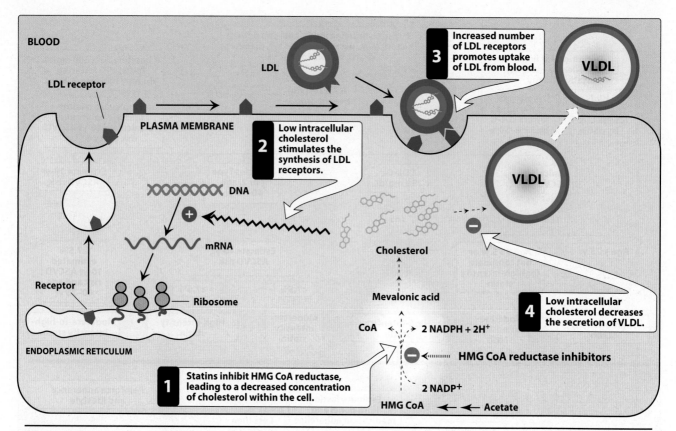

Figure 23.5
Inhibition of HMG CoA reductase by the statin drugs. HMG CoA = 3-hydroxy-3-methylglutaryl coenzyme A; LDL = low-density lipoprotein; VLDL = very–low-density lipoprotein.

Characteristic	Atorvastatin	Fluvastatin	Lovastatin	Pitavastatin	Pravastatin	Rosuvastatin	Simvastatin
Serum LDL cholesterol reduction produced (%)	55	24	34	43	34	60	41
Serum triglyceride reduction produced (%)	29	10	16	18	24	18	18
Serum HDL cholesterol increase produced (%)	6	8	9	8	12	8	12
Plasma half-life (h)	14	1–2	2	12	1–2	19	1–2
Penetration of central nervous system	No	No	Yes	Yes	No	No	Yes
Renal excretion of absorbed dose (%)	2	<6	10	15	20	10	13

Figure 23.6
Summary of 3-hydroxy-3-methylglutaryl coenzyme A (HMG CoA) reductase inhibitors. LDL = low-density lipoprotein; HDL = high-density lipoprotein.

starting therapy and if a patient has symptoms consistent with liver dysfunction. [Note: Hepatic insufficiency can cause drug accumulation.] Myopathy and rhabdomyolysis (disintegration of skeletal muscle; rare) have been reported (Figure 23.7). In most of these cases, patients usually had renal insufficiency or were taking drugs such as *erythromycin*, *gemfibrozil*, or *niacin*. *Simvastatin* is metabolized by cytochrome P450 3A4, and inhibitors of this enzyme may increase the risk of rhabdomyolysis. Plasma creatine kinase levels should be determined in patients with muscle complaints. The HMG CoA reductase inhibitors may also increase the effect of *warfarin*. Thus, it is important to evaluate international normalized ratio (INR) frequently. These drugs are contraindicated during pregnancy and lactation.

B. Niacin (nicotinic acid)

Niacin [NYE-uh-sin] can reduce LDL-C by 10% to 20% and is the most effective agent for increasing HDL-C. It also lowers triglycerides by 20% to 35% at typical doses of 1.5 to 3 grams/day. *Niacin* can be used in combination with statins, and a fixed-dose combination of *lovastatin* and long-acting *niacin* is available.

1. **Mechanism of action:** At gram doses, *niacin* strongly inhibits lipolysis in adipose tissue, thereby reducing production of free fatty acids (Figure 23.8). The liver normally uses circulating free fatty acids as a major precursor for triglyceride synthesis. Reduced liver triglyceride levels decrease hepatic VLDL production, which in turn reduces LDL-C plasma concentrations.

2. **Therapeutic uses:** Since *niacin* lowers plasma levels of both cholesterol and triglycerides, it is useful in the treatment of familial hyperlipidemias. It is also used to treat other severe hypercholesterolemias, often in combination with other agents.

3. **Pharmacokinetics:** *Niacin* is administered orally. It is converted in the body to nicotinamide, which is incorporated into the cofactor nicotinamide adenine dinucleotide (NAD$^+$). *Niacin*, its nicotinamide derivative, and other metabolites are excreted in the urine. [Note: Nicotinamide alone does not decrease plasma lipid levels.]

4. **Adverse effects:** The most common side effects of *niacin* are an intense cutaneous flush (accompanied by an uncomfortable feeling of warmth) and pruritus. Administration of *aspirin* prior to taking *niacin* decreases the flush, which is prostaglandin mediated. Some patients also experience nausea and abdominal pain. Slow titration of the dosage or usage of the sustained-release formulation of *niacin* reduces bothersome initial adverse effects. *Niacin* inhibits tubular secretion of uric acid and, thus, predisposes to hyperuricemia and gout. Impaired glucose tolerance and hepatotoxicity have also been reported. The drug should be avoided in hepatic disease.

C. Fibrates

Fenofibrate [fen-oh-FIH-brate] and *gemfibrozil* [jem-FI-broh-zill] are derivatives of fibric acid that lower serum triglycerides and increase HDL levels.

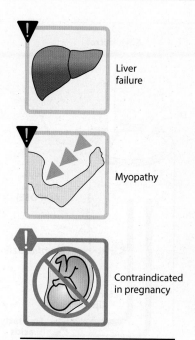

Figure 23.7
Some adverse effects and precautions associated with 3-hydroxy-3-methylglutaryl coenzyme A (HMG CoA) reductase inhibitors.

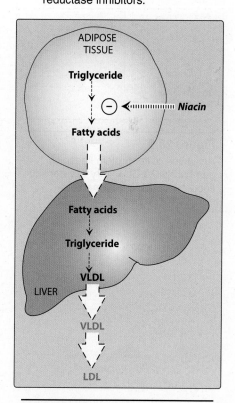

Figure 23.8
Niacin inhibits lipolysis in adipose tissue, resulting in decreased hepatic VLDL synthesis and production of LDLs in the plasma. VLDL= very-low-density lipoprotein; LDL = low-density lipoprotein.

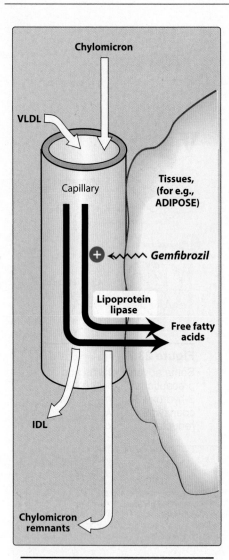

Figure 23.9
Activation of lipoprotein lipase by
gemfibrozil. VLDL = very-low-density
lipoprotein; IDL = intermediate-
density lipoprotein.

1. **Mechanism of action:** The peroxisome proliferator–activated receptors (PPARs) are members of the nuclear receptor family that regulates lipid metabolism. PPARs function as ligand-activated transcription factors. Upon binding to their natural ligands (fatty acids or eicosanoids) or antihyperlipidemic drugs, PPARs are activated. They then bind to peroxisome proliferator response elements, which ultimately leads to decreased triglyceride concentrations through increased expression of lipoprotein lipase (Figure 23.9) and decreasing apolipoprotein (apo) CII concentration. *Fenofibrate* is more effective than *gemfibrozil* in lowering triglyceride levels. Fibrates also increase the level of HDL cholesterol by increasing the expression of apo AI and apo AII.

2. **Therapeutic uses:** The fibrates are used in the treatment of hypertriglyceridemias. They are particularly useful in treating type III hyperlipidemia (dysbetalipoproteinemia), in which intermediate-density lipoprotein particles accumulate.

3. **Pharmacokinetics:** *Gemfibrozil* and *fenofibrate* are completely absorbed after oral administration and distribute widely, bound to albumin. *Fenofibrate* is a prodrug, which is converted to the active moiety fenofibric acid. Both drugs undergo extensive biotransformation and are excreted in the urine as glucuronide conjugates.

4. **Adverse effects:** The most common adverse effects are mild gastrointestinal (GI) disturbances. These lessen as the therapy progresses. Because these drugs increase biliary cholesterol excretion, there is a predisposition to form gallstones. Myositis (inflammation of a voluntary muscle) can occur, and muscle weakness or tenderness should be evaluated. Patients with renal insufficiency may be at risk. Myopathy and rhabdomyolysis have been reported in patients taking *gemfibrozil* and statins together. The use of *gemfibrozil* is contraindicated with *simvastatin*. Both fibrates may increase the effects of *warfarin*. INR should, therefore, be monitored more frequently when a patient is taking both drugs. Fibrates should not be used in patients with severe hepatic or renal dysfunction or in patients with preexisting gallbladder disease.

D. Bile acid–binding resins

Bile acid sequestrants (resins) have significant LDL cholesterol–lowering effects, although the benefits are less than those observed with statins.

1. **Mechanism of action:** *Cholestyramine* [koe-LES-tir-a-meen], *colestipol* [koe-LES-tih-pole], and *colesevelam* [koh-le-SEV-e-lam] are anion-exchange resins that bind negatively charged bile acids and bile salts in the small intestine (Figure 23.10). The resin/bile acid complex is excreted in the feces, thus lowering the bile acid concentration. This causes hepatocytes to increase conversion of cholesterol to bile acids, which are essential components of the bile. Consequently, intracellular cholesterol concentrations decrease, which activates an increased hepatic uptake of cholesterol-containing LDL particles, leading to a fall in plasma LDL-C. [Note: This increased uptake is mediated by an up-regulation of cell surface LDL receptors.]

2. **Therapeutic uses:** The bile acid–binding resins are useful (often in combination with diet or *niacin*) for treating type IIA and type IIB hyperlipidemias. [Note: In those rare individuals who are homozygous for type IIA and functional LDL receptors are totally lacking, these drugs have little effect on plasma LDL levels.] *Cholestyramine* can also relieve pruritus caused by accumulation of bile acids in patients with biliary stasis. *Colesevelam* is also indicated for type 2 diabetes due to its glucose-lowering effects.

3. **Pharmacokinetics:** Bile acid sequestrants are insoluble in water and have large molecular weights. After oral administration, they are neither absorbed nor metabolically altered by the intestine. Instead, they are totally excreted in feces.

4. **Adverse effects:** The most common side effects are GI disturbances, such as constipation, nausea, and flatulence. *Colesevelam* has fewer GI side effects than other bile acid sequestrants. These agents may impair the absorption of the fat-soluble vitamins (A, D, E, and K), and they interfere with the absorption of many drugs (for example, *digoxin*, *warfarin*, and thyroid hormone). Therefore, other drugs should be taken at least 1 to 2 hours before, or 4 to 6 hours after, the bile acid–binding resins. These agents may raise triglyceride levels and are contraindicated in patients with significant hypertriglyceridemia (≥400 mg/dL).

E. Cholesterol absorption inhibitor

Ezetimibe [eh-ZEH-teh-mib] selectively inhibits absorption of dietary and biliary cholesterol in the small intestine, leading to a decrease in the delivery of intestinal cholesterol to the liver. This causes a reduction of hepatic cholesterol stores and an increase in clearance of cholesterol from the blood. *Ezetimibe* lowers LDL cholesterol by approximately 17%. Due its modest LDL-lowering effects, *ezetimibe* is often used as an adjunct to statin therapy or in statin-intolerant patients. *Ezetimibe* is primarily metabolized in the small intestine and liver via glucuronide conjugation, with subsequent biliary and renal excretion. Patients with moderate to severe hepatic insufficiency should not be treated with *ezetimibe*. Adverse effects are uncommon with use of *ezetimibe*.

F. Omega-3 fatty acids

Omega-3 polyunsaturated fatty acids (PUFAs) are essential fatty acids that are predominately used for triglyceride lowering. Essential fatty acids inhibit VLDL and triglyceride synthesis in the liver. The omega-3 PUFAs eicosapentaenoic acid (EPA) and docosahexaenoic acid (DHA) are found in marine sources such as tuna, halibut, and salmon. Approximately 4 g of marine-derived omega-3 PUFAs daily decreases serum triglyceride concentrations by 25% to 30%, with small increases in LDL-C and HDL-C. Over-the-counter or prescription fish oil capsules (EPA/DHA) can be used for supplementation, as it is difficult to consume enough omega-3 PUFAs from dietary sources alone. *Icosapent* [eye-KOE-sa-pent] *ethyl* is a prescription product that contains only EPA and, unlike other fish oil supplements, does not significantly raise LDL-C. Omega-3 PUFAs can be considered as an adjunct to other

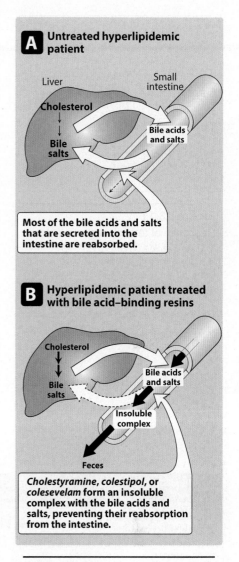

A Untreated hyperlipidemic patient

Liver — Small intestine

Cholesterol ↓ Bile salts

Bile acids and salts

Most of the bile acids and salts that are secreted into the intestine are reabsorbed.

B Hyperlipidemic patient treated with bile acid–binding resins

Cholesterol ↓ Bile salts

Bile acids and salts

Insoluble complex

Feces

Cholestyramine, colestipol, or *colesevelam* form an insoluble complex with the bile acids and salts, preventing their reabsorption from the intestine.

Figure 23.10
Mechanism of bile acid–binding resins.

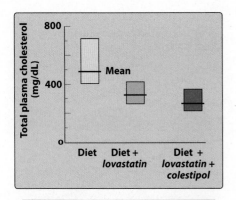

Figure 23.11
Response of total plasma cholesterol in patients with heterozygous familial hypercholesterolemia to a diet (low in cholesterol, low in saturated fat) and antihyperlipidemic drugs.

lipid-lowering therapies for individuals with significantly elevated triglycerides (≥500 mg/dL). Although effective for triglyceride lowering, omega-3 PUFA supplementation has not been shown to reduce cardiovascular morbidity and mortality. The most common side effects of omega-3 PUFAs include GI effects (abdominal pain, nausea, diarrhea) and a fishy aftertaste. Bleeding risk can be increased in those who are concomitantly taking anticoagulants or antiplatelets.

G. Combination drug therapy

It is often necessary to use two antihyperlipidemic drugs to achieve treatment goals in plasma lipid levels. The combination of an HMG CoA reductase inhibitor with a bile acid–binding agent has been shown to be very useful in lowering LDL-C levels (Figure 23.11). *Simvastatin* and *ezetimibe*, as well as *simvastatin* and *niacin*, are currently available combined in one pill to treat elevated LDL cholesterol. However, more clinical information is needed to determine whether combination therapy produces better long-term benefits than the use of a high-dose statin. Until this uncertainty is resolved, many experts recommend maximizing statin dosages and adding *niacin* or fibrates only in those with persistently elevated triglycerides (greater than 500 mg/dL) or those with low HDL cholesterol levels (less than 40 mg/dL). Combination drug therapy is not without risks. Liver and muscle toxicity occurs more frequently with lipid-lowering drug combinations. Figure 23.12 summarizes some actions of the antihyperlipidemic drugs.

TYPE OF DRUG	EFFECT ON LDL	EFFECT ON HDL	EFFECT ON TRIGLYCERIDES
HMG CoA reductase inhibitors (statins)	↓↓↓↓	↑↑	↓↓
Fibrates	↓	↑↑↑	↓↓↓↓
Niacin	↓↓	↑↑↑↑	↓↓↓
Bile acid sequestrants	↓↓↓	↑	↑
Cholesterol absorption inhibitor	↓	↑	↓

Figure 23.12
Characteristics of antihyperlipidemic drug families. HDL = high-density lipoprotein; HMG CoA = 3-hydroxy-3-methylglutaryl coenzyme A; LDL = low-density lipoprotein.

Study Questions

Choose the ONE best answer.

23.1 Which one of the following is the most common side effect of antihyperlipidemic drug therapy?

A. Elevated blood pressure.
B. Gastrointestinal disturbance.
C. Neurologic problems.
D. Heart palpitations.
E. Migraine headaches.

> Correct answer = B. Gastrointestinal disturbances frequently occur as a side effect of antihyperlipidemic drug therapy. The other choices are not seen as commonly.

23.2 Which one of the following hyperlipidemias is characterized by elevated plasma levels of chylomicrons and has no drug therapy available to lower the plasma lipoprotein levels?

A. Type I.
B. Type II.
C. Type III.
D. Type IV.
E. Type V.

> Correct answer = A. Type I hyperlipidemia (hyperchylomicronemia) is treated with a low-fat diet. No drug therapy is effective for this disorder.

23.3 Which one of the following drugs decreases cholesterol synthesis by inhibiting the enzyme 3-hydroxy-3-methylglutaryl coenzyme A reductase?

A. Fenofibrate.
B. Niacin.
C. Cholestyramine.
D. Lovastatin.
E. Gemfibrozil.

> Correct answer = D. Lovastatin decreases cholesterol synthesis by inhibiting HMG CoA reductase. Fenofibrate and gemfibrozil increase the activity of lipoprotein lipase, thereby increasing the removal of VLDL from plasma. Niacin inhibits lipolysis in adipose tissue, thus eliminating the building blocks needed by the liver to produce triglycerides and, therefore, VLDL. Cholestyramine lowers the amount of bile acids returning to the liver via the enterohepatic circulation.

23.4 Which one of the following drugs causes a decrease in liver triglyceride synthesis by limiting available free fatty acids needed as building blocks for this pathway?

A. Niacin.
B. Fenofibrate.
C. Cholestyramine.
D. Gemfibrozil.
E. Lovastatin.

> Correct answer = A. At gram doses, niacin strongly inhibits lipolysis in adipose tissue—the primary producer of circulating free fatty acids. The liver normally utilizes these circulating fatty acids as a major precursor for triglyceride synthesis. Thus, niacin causes a decrease in liver triglyceride synthesis, which is required for VLDL production. The other choices do not inhibit lipolysis in adipose tissue.

23.5 Which one of the following drugs binds bile acids in the intestine, thus preventing their return to the liver via the enterohepatic circulation?

A. Niacin.
B. Fenofibrate.
C. Cholestyramine.
D. Fluvastatin.
E. Lovastatin.

> Correct answer = C. Cholestyramine is an anion-exchange resin that binds negatively charged bile acids and bile salts in the small intestine. The resin/bile acid complex is excreted in the feces, thus preventing the bile acids from returning to the liver by the enterohepatic circulation. The other choices do not bind intestinal bile acids.

23.6 JS is a 65-year-old man who presents to his physician for management of hyperlipidemia. His most recent lipid panel reveals an LDL cholesterol level of 165 mg/dL. His physician wishes to begin treatment to lower his LDL cholesterol levels. Which of the following therapies is the best option to lower JS's LDL cholesterol levels?

A. Fenofibrate.

B. Colesevelam.

C. Niacin.

D. Simvastatin.

E. Ezetimibe.

Correct answer = D. Simvastatin, an HMG CoA reductase inhibitor (statin), is the most effective option for lowering LDL cholesterol, achieving reductions of 30% to 41% from baseline levels. Fenofibrate and niacin are more effective at lowering triglyceride levels or raising HDL levels (niacin). Colesevelam can reduce LDL levels but not as effectively as statins. Ezetimibe lowers LDL levels modestly compared to the LDL reduction achieved by statins.

23.7 WW is a 62-year-old female with hyperlipidemia and hypothyroidism. Her current medications include cholestyramine and levothyroxine (thyroid hormone). What advice would you give to WW to avoid a drug interaction between her cholestyramine and levothyroxine?

A. Stop taking the levothyroxine as it can interact with cholestyramine.

B. Take levothyroxine 1 hour before cholestyramine on an empty stomach.

C. Switch cholestyramine to colesevelam as this will eliminate the interaction.

D. Switch cholestyramine to colestipol as this will eliminate the interaction.

E. Take levothyroxine and cholestyramine at the same time to minimize the interaction.

Correct answer = B. Cholestyramine and the bile acid resins can bind several medications causing decreased absorption. Cholestyramine can decrease absorption of medications such as levothyroxine. Taking levothyroxine 1 hour before or 4 to 6 hours after cholestyramine can help to avoid this interaction. Choices C and D are incorrect, as all bile acid resins cause this interaction. Choice A is incorrect, as this patient should not stop her thyroid medication. Choice E will worsen this drug interaction.

23.8 AJ is a 42-year-old man who was started on niacin sustained-release tablets 2 weeks ago for elevated triglycerides and low HDL levels. He is complaining of an uncomfortable flushing and itchy feeling that he thinks is related to the niacin. Which of the following options can help AJ manage this adverse effect of niacin therapy?

A. Administer aspirin 30 minutes prior to taking niacin.

B. Administer aspirin 30 minutes after taking niacin.

C. Increase the dose of niacin SR to 1000 mg.

D. Continue the current dose of niacin.

E. Change the sustained-release niacin to immediate-release niacin.

Correct answer = A. Flushing associated with niacin is prostaglandin mediated; therefore, use of aspirin (a prostaglandin inhibitor) can help to minimize this adverse effect. It must be administered 30 minutes prior to the dose of the niacin; therefore, choice B is incorrect. Increasing the dose of niacin is likely to increase these complaints; therefore, choice C is incorrect. Continuing the current dose is unlikely to relieve these complaints, which are bothersome to AJ. The sustained-release formulation of niacin has less incidence of flushing versus that of the immediate release; therefore, choice E is incorrect.

23.9 CN is a 72-year-old male who is treated for hyperlipidemia with high-dose atorvastatin for the past 6 months. He also has a history of renal insufficiency. His most recent lipid panel shows an LDL cholesterol level of 131 mg/dL, triglycerides of 510 mg/dL, and HDL cholesterol of 32 mg/dL. His physician wishes to add an additional agent for his hyperlipidemia. Which of the following choices is the best option to address CN's dyslipidemia?

A. Fenofibrate.

B. Niacin.

C. Colesevelam.

D. Gemfibrozil.

E. Ezetimibe.

Correct answer = B. This patient has significantly elevated triglycerides and low HDL. Niacin can lower triglycerides by 35% to 50% and also raise HDL levels. The fibrates (fenofibrate and gemfibrozil) should not be used due to CN's history of renal insufficiency. Use of colesevelam is contraindicated because triglycerides are greater than 400 mg/dL. Ezetimibe can further lower LDL cholesterol but has modest effects on triglycerides versus niacin.

23.10 Which of the following patient populations is more likely to experience myalgia (muscle pain) or myopathy with use of HMG CoA reductase inhibitors?

A. Patients with diabetes mellitus.

B. Patients with renal insufficiency.

C. Patients with gout.

D. Patients with hypertriglyceridemia.

E. Patients taking warfarin (blood thinner).

Correct answer = B. Patients with a history of renal insufficiency have a higher incidence of developing myalgias, myopathy, and rhabdomyolysis with use of HMG CoA reductase inhibitors (statins), especially with those that are renally eliminated as drug accumulation can occur. The other populations have not been reported to have a higher incidence of this adverse effect with HMG CoA reductase inhibitors.

Pituitary and Thyroid

Karen Whalen

24

I. OVERVIEW

The neuroendocrine system, which is controlled by the pituitary and hypothalamus, coordinates body functions by transmitting messages between individual cells and tissues. This contrasts with the nervous system, which communicates locally through electrical impulses and neurotransmitters directed through neurons to other neurons or to specific target organs, such as muscle or glands. Nerve impulses generally act within milliseconds. The endocrine system releases hormones into the bloodstream, which carries chemical messengers to target cells throughout the body. Hormones have a much broader range of response time than do nerve impulses, requiring from seconds to days, or longer, to cause a response that may last for weeks or months. The two regulatory systems are closely interrelated. For example, in several instances, the release of hormones is stimulated or inhibited by the nervous system, and some hormones can stimulate or inhibit nerve impulses. Chapters 25 to 27 focus on drugs that affect the synthesis and/or secretion of specific hormones and their actions. In this chapter, the central role of the hypothalamic and pituitary hormones in regulating body functions is briefly presented. In addition, drugs affecting thyroid hormone synthesis and/or secretion are discussed (Figure 24.1).

II. HYPOTHALAMIC AND ANTERIOR PITUITARY HORMONES

The hormones secreted by the hypothalamus and the pituitary are all peptides or low molecular weight proteins that act by binding to specific receptor sites on their target tissues. The hormones of the anterior

Figure 24.1
Some of the hormones and drugs affecting the hypothalamus, pituitary, and thyroid.

HYPOTHALAMIC AND ANTERIOR PITUITARY HORMONES

Choriogonadotropin alfa OVIDREL
Corticotropin H.P. ACTHAR
Cosyntropin CORTROSYN
Follitropin alfa GONAL-F
Follitropin beta FOLLISTIM
Goserelin ZOLADEX
Histrelin VANTAS
Human chorionic gonadotropin
PREGNYL
Lanreotide SOMATULINE
Leuprolide LUPRON
Menotropins MENOPUR, REPRONEX
Nafarelin SYNAREL
Octreotide SANDOSTATIN
Pegvisomant SOMAVERT
Somatropin HUMATROPE
Urofollitropin BRAVELLE

HORMONES OF THE POSTERIOR PITUITARY

Desmopressin DDAVP
Oxytocin PITOCIN
Vasopressin **(ADH)** PITRESSIN

DRUGS AFFECTING THE THYROID

Iodine and potassium iodide LUGOL'S SOLUTION
Liothyronine CYTOMEL
Levothyroxine LEVOXYL, SYNTHROID
Methimazole TAPAZOLE
Propylthiouracil **(PTU)**
Liotrix THYROLAR

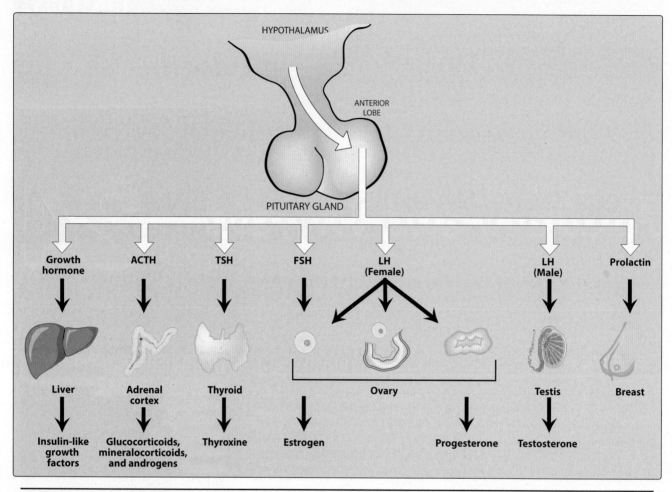

Figure 24.2
Anterior pituitary hormones. ACTH = adrenocorticotropic hormone; TSH = thyroid-stimulating hormone; FSH = follicle-stimulating hormone; LH = luteinizing hormone.

pituitary are regulated by neuropeptides that are called either "releasing" or "inhibiting" factors or hormones. These are produced in the hypothalamus, and they reach the pituitary by the hypophyseal portal system (Figure 24.2). The interaction of the releasing hormones with their receptors results in the activation of genes that promote the synthesis of protein precursors. The protein precursors then undergo posttranslational modification to produce hormones, which are released into the circulation. Each hypothalamic regulatory hormone controls the release of a specific hormone from the anterior pituitary. Although a number of pituitary hormone preparations are currently used therapeutically for specific hormonal deficiencies, most of these agents have limited therapeutic applications. Hormones of the anterior and posterior pituitary are administered intramuscularly (IM), subcutaneously, or intranasally because their peptidyl nature makes them susceptible to destruction by the proteolytic enzymes of the digestive tract.

A. Adrenocorticotropic hormone (corticotropin)

Corticotropin-releasing hormone (CRH) is responsible for the synthesis and release of the peptide pro-opiomelanocortin by the pituitary

(Figure 24.3). *Adrenocorticotropic hormone* (ACTH) or *corticotropin* [kor-ti-koe-TROE-pin] is a product of the posttranslational processing of this precursor polypeptide. [Note: CRH is used diagnostically to differentiate between Cushing syndrome and ectopic ACTH-producing cells.] Normally, ACTH is released from the pituitary in pulses with an overriding diurnal rhythm, with the highest concentration occurring in the early morning and the lowest in the late evening. Stress stimulates its secretion, whereas cortisol acting via negative feedback suppresses its release.

1. **Mechanism of action:** ACTH binds to receptors on the surface of the adrenal cortex, thereby activating G protein–coupled processes that ultimately stimulate the rate-limiting step in the adrenocorticosteroid synthetic pathway (cholesterol to pregnenolone; Figure 24.3).This pathway ends with the synthesis and release of the adrenocorticosteroids and the adrenal androgens.

2. **Therapeutic uses:** The availability of synthetic adrenocorticosteroids with specific properties has limited the use of *corticotropin* mainly to serving as a diagnostic tool for differentiating between primary adrenal insufficiency (Addison disease, associated with adrenal atrophy) and secondary adrenal insufficiency (caused by the inadequate secretion of ACTH by the pituitary).Therapeutic *corticotropin* preparations are extracts from the anterior pituitaries of domestic animals or synthetic human ACTH.The latter, *cosyntropin* [ko-sin-TROE-pin], is preferred for the diagnosis of adrenal insufficiency. ACTH is also used in the treatment of infantile spasm (West syndrome).

3. **Adverse effects:** Short-term use of ACTH for diagnostic purposes is usually well tolerated.With longer use, toxicities are similar to those of glucocorticoids and include hypertension, peripheral edema, hypokalemia, emotional disturbances, and increased risk of infection.

B. Growth hormone (somatotropin)

Somatotropin is a large polypeptide that is released by the anterior pituitary in response to growth hormone (GH)-releasing hormone produced by the hypothalamus (Figure 24.4). Secretion of GH is inhibited by another hypothalamic hormone, somatostatin (see below). GH is released in a pulsatile manner, with the highest levels occurring during sleep. With increasing age, GH secretion decreases, accompanied by a decrease in lean muscle mass. Somatotropin influences a wide variety of biochemical processes (for example, cell proliferation and bone growth are promoted). Synthetic human GH (*somatropin* [soe-mah-TROE pin]) is produced using recombinant DNA technology.

1. **Mechanism of action:** Although many physiologic effects of GH are exerted directly at its targets, others are mediated through the somatomedins—insulin-like growth factors 1 and 2 (IGF-1 and IGF-2). [Note: In acromegaly (a syndrome of excess GH due to hormone-secreting tumors), IGF-1 levels are consistently high, reflecting elevated GH.]

2. **Therapeutic uses:** *Somatropin* is used in the treatment of GH deficiency or growth failure in children. *Somatropin* is also indicated for growth failure due to Prader-Willi syndrome, management of AIDS

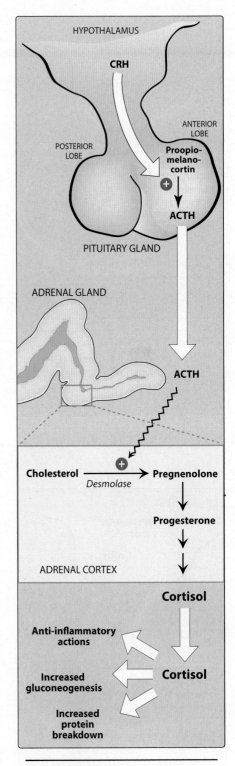

Figure 24.3
Secretion and actions of adrenocorticotropic hormone (ACTH). CRH = corticotropin-releasing hormone.

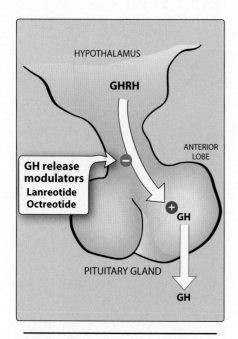

Figure 24.4
Secretion of growth hormone (GH).
GHRH = growth hormone-releasing
hormone.

wasting syndrome, and GH replacement in adults with confirmed GH deficiency. [Note: GH administered to adults increases lean body mass, bone density, and skin thickness, whereas adipose tissue is decreased. Many consider GH an "antiaging" hormone. This has led to off-label use of GH by older individuals and by athletes seeking to enhance performance.] *Somatropin* is administered by subcutaneous or IM injection. Although the half-life of GH is short (approximately 25 minutes), it induces the release of IGF-1 from the liver, which is responsible for subsequent GH-like actions.

3. **Adverse effects:** Adverse effects of *somatropin* include pain at the injection site, edema, arthralgias, myalgias, flu-like symptoms, and an increased risk of diabetes. *Somatropin* should not be used in pediatric patients with closed epiphyses, patients with diabetic retinopathy, or obese patients with Prader-Willi syndrome.

C. Somatostatin (Growth hormone-inhibiting hormone)

In the pituitary, somatostatin binds to receptors that suppress GH and thyroid-stimulating hormone release. Originally isolated from the hypothalamus, somatostatin is a small polypeptide that is also found in neurons throughout the body as well as in the intestine, stomach, and pancreas. Somatostatin not only inhibits the release of GH but also that of insulin, glucagon, and gastrin. *Octreotide* [ok-TREE-oh-tide] and *lanreotide* [lan-REE-oh-tide] are synthetic analogs of somatostatin. Their half-lives are longer than that of the natural compound, and depot formulations are available, allowing for administration once every 4 weeks. They have found use in the treatment of acromegaly and in diarrhea and flushing associated with carcinoid tumors. An intravenous infusion of *octreotide* is also used for the treatment of bleeding esophageal varices. Adverse effects of *octreotide* include diarrhea, abdominal pain, flatulence, nausea, and steatorrhea. Gallbladder emptying is delayed, and asymptomatic cholesterol gallstones can occur with long-term treatment. [Note: Acromegaly that is refractory to other modes of therapy may be treated with *pegvisomant* (peg-VIH-soe-mant), a GH receptor antagonist.]

D. Gonadotropin-releasing hormone

Pulsatile secretion of gonadotropin-releasing hormone (GnRH) from the hypothalamus is essential for the release of the gonadotropins follicle-stimulating hormone (FSH) and luteinizing hormone (LH) from the anterior pituitary. However, continuous administration of GnRH inhibits gonadotropin release through down-regulation of the GnRH receptors on the pituitary. Continuous administration of synthetic GnRH analogs, such as *leuprolide* [loo-PROE-lide], *goserelin* [GOE-se-rel-in], *nafarelin* [NAFF-a-rel-in], and *histrelin* [his-TREL-in], is effective in suppressing production of the gonadotropins (Figure 24.5). [Note: Several of these agents are available as implantable formulations that provide convenient continuous delivery of the drug.] Suppression of gonadotropins, in turn, leads to reduced production of gonadal steroid hormones (androgens and estrogens). Thus, these agents are effective in the treatment of prostate cancer, endometriosis, and precocious puberty. In women, the GnRH analogs may cause hot flushes and sweating, as well as diminished libido, depression, and ovarian cysts. They are

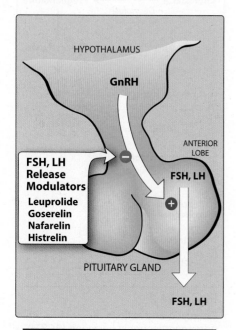

Figure 24.5
Secretion of follicle-stimulating
hormone (FSH) and luteinizing
hormone (LH). GnRH = gonadotropin-
releasing hormone.

contraindicated in pregnancy and breast-feeding. In men, they initially cause a rise in testosterone that can result in bone pain. Hot flushes, edema, gynecomastia, and diminished libido may also occur.

E. Gonadotropins

The gonadotropins (FSH and LH) are glycoproteins that are produced in the anterior pituitary. The regulation of gonadal steroid hormones depends on these agents. They find use in the treatment of infertility. *Menotropins* [men-oh-TROE-pinz] (also known as *human menopausal gonadotropins* or *hMG*) are obtained from the urine of postmenopausal women and contain both FSH and LH. *Urofollitropin* [yoor-oh-fol-li-TROE-pin] is FSH obtained from postmenopausal women and is devoid of LH. *Follitropin* [fol-ih-TROE-pin] *alfa* and *follitropin beta* are human FSH products manufactured using recombinant DNA technology. *Human chorionic gonadotropin* (*hCG*) is a placental hormone that is excreted in the urine of pregnant women. The effects of *hCG* and *choriogonadotropin* [kore-ee-oh-goe-NAD-oh-troe-pin] *alfa* (made using recombinant DNA technology) are essentially identical to those of LH. All of these hormones are injected via the IM or subcutaneous route. Injection of *hMG* or FSH products over a period of 5 to 12 days causes ovarian follicular growth and maturation, and with subsequent injection of *hCG*, ovulation occurs. Adverse effects include ovarian enlargement and possible ovarian hyperstimulation syndrome, which may be life threatening. Multiple births are not uncommon.

F. Prolactin

Prolactin is a peptide hormone that is also secreted by the anterior pituitary. Its primary function is to stimulate and maintain lactation. In addition, it decreases sexual drive and reproductive function. Its secretion is inhibited by dopamine acting at D_2 receptors. [Note: Drugs that act as dopamine antagonists (for example, *metoclopramide* and antipsychotics such as *risperidone*) can increase the secretion of prolactin.] Hyperprolactinemia, which is associated with galactorrhea and hypogonadism, is treated with D_2 receptor agonists, such as *bromocriptine* and *cabergoline*. Both of these agents also find use in the treatment of pituitary microadenomas. *Bromocriptine* is also indicated for the treatment of type 2 diabetes. Among their adverse effects are nausea, headache and, sometimes, psychiatric problems.

III. HORMONES OF THE POSTERIOR PITUITARY

In contrast to the hormones of the anterior lobe of the pituitary, those of the posterior lobe, *vasopressin* and *oxytocin*, are not regulated by releasing hormones. Instead, they are synthesized in the hypothalamus, transported to the posterior pituitary, and released in response to specific physiologic signals, such as high plasma osmolarity or parturition. Both hormones are administered intravenously and have very short half-lives. Their actions are summarized in Figure 24.6.

A. Oxytocin

Oxytocin [ok-se-TOE-sin] is used in obstetrics to stimulate uterine contraction and induce labor. *Oxytocin* also causes milk ejection by contracting the myoepithelial cells around the mammary alveoli. Although toxicities are uncommon when the drug is used properly, hypertension, uterine rupture, water retention, and fetal death have been reported. Its antidiuretic and pressor activities are much less pronounced than those of *vasopressin*.

B. Vasopressin

Vasopressin [vas-oh-PRESS-in] (antidiuretic hormone) is structurally related to *oxytocin*. *Vasopressin* has both antidiuretic and vasopressor effects (Figure 24.6). In the kidney, it binds to the V_2 receptor to increase water permeability and reabsorption in the collecting tubules. Thus, the major use of *vasopressin* is to treat diabetes insipidus. It also finds use in the management of cardiac arrest and in controlling bleeding due to esophageal varices. Other effects of *vasopressin* are mediated by the V_1 receptor, which is found in liver, vascular smooth muscle (where it causes constriction), and other tissues. The major toxicities of *vasopressin* are water intoxication and hyponatremia. Abdominal pain, tremor, and vertigo can also occur. *Desmopressin* [des-moe-PRESS-in], an analog of *vasopressin*, has minimal activity at the V_1 receptor, making it largely free of pressor effects. This analog is longer acting than *vasopressin* and is preferred for the treatment of diabetes insipidus and nocturnal enuresis. For these indications, *desmopressin* may be administered intranasally or orally. [Note: The nasal spray should not be used for enuresis due to reports of seizures in children using this formulation.] Local irritation may occur with the nasal spray.

IV. THYROID HORMONES

The thyroid gland facilitates normal growth and maturation by maintaining a level of metabolism in the tissues that is optimal for their normal function. The two major thyroid hormones are triiodothyronine (T_3; the most active form) and thyroxine (T_4). Inadequate secretion of thyroid hormone (hypothyroidism) results in bradycardia, poor resistance to cold, and mental and physical slowing. In children, this can cause mental retardation and dwarfism. In contrast, excess secretion of thyroid hormones (hyperthyroidism) can cause tachycardia and cardiac arrhythmias, body wasting, nervousness, tremor, and heat intolerance.

A. Thyroid hormone synthesis and secretion

The thyroid gland is made up of multiple follicles that consist of a single layer of epithelial cells surrounding a lumen filled with thyroglobulin, which is the storage form of thyroid hormone. A summary of the steps in thyroid hormone synthesis and secretion is shown in Figure 24.7. Thyroid function is controlled by thyroid-stimulating hormone (TSH; thyrotropin), which is synthesized by the anterior pituitary (Figure 24.2). [Note: TSH generation is governed by the hypothalamic thyrotropin-releasing hormone (TRH).] TSH action is mediated by cAMP and leads to stimulation of iodide (I⁻) uptake by the thyroid gland. Oxidation to iodine (I_2) by a peroxidase is followed by iodination of tyrosines on thyroglobulin. [Note: Antibodies to thyroid peroxidase are diagnostic for Hashimoto thyroiditis, a common cause of hypothyroidism.] Condensation of two diiodotyrosine residues gives rise to T_4,

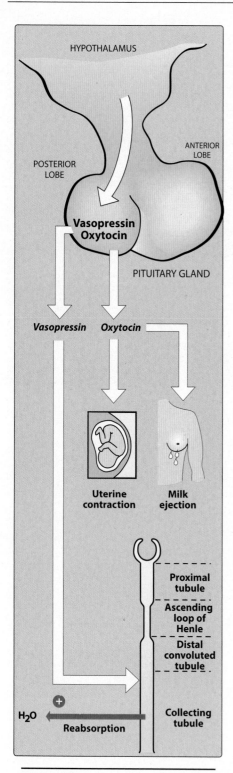

Figure 24.6
Actions of *oxytocin* and *vasopressin*.

HYPOTHALAMUS

POSTERIOR LOBE

ANTERIOR LOBE

Vasopressin
Oxytocin

PITUITARY GLAND

Vasopressin   *Oxytocin*

Uterine contraction   Milk ejection

Proximal tubule

Ascending loop of Henle

Distal convoluted tubule

Collecting tubule

H₂O   Reabsorption

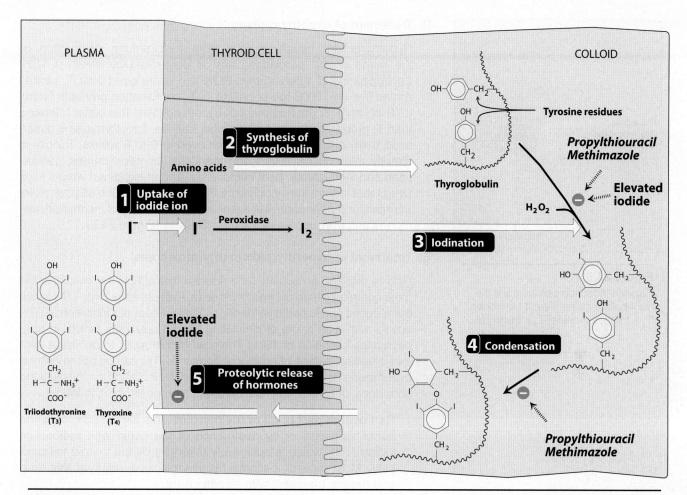

Figure 24.7
Biosynthesis of thyroid hormones.

whereas condensation of a monoiodotyrosine residue with a diiodo-tyrosine residue generates T_3. The hormones are released following proteolytic cleavage of the thyroglobulin.

B. Mechanism of action

Most of the hormone (T_3 and T_4) is bound to thyroxine-binding globulin in the plasma. The hormones must dissociate from thyroxine-binding globulin prior to entry into cells. In the cell, T_4 is enzymatically deiodinated to T_3, which enters the nucleus and attaches to specific receptors. The activation of these receptors promotes the formation of RNA and subsequent protein synthesis, which is responsible for the effects of T_4.

C. Pharmacokinetics

Both T_4 and T_3 are absorbed after oral administration. Food, calcium preparations, and aluminum-containing antacids can decrease the absorption of T_4. Deiodination is the major route of metabolism of T_4. T_3 also undergoes sequential deiodination. The hormones are also metabolized via conjugation with glucuronides and sulfates and excreted into the bile.

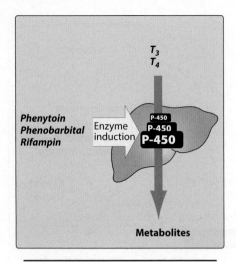

Figure 24.8
Enzyme induction can increase the metabolism of the thyroid hormones. T_3 = triiodothyronine; T_4 = thyroxine.

D. Treatment of hypothyroidism

Hypothyroidism usually results from autoimmune destruction of the gland or the peroxidase and is diagnosed by elevated TSH. *Levothyroxine* (T_4) [leh-vo-thye-ROK-sin] is preferred over T_3 (*liothyronine* [lye-oh-THYE-roe-neen]) or T_3/T_4 combination products (*liotrix* [LYE-oh-trix]) for the treatment of hypothyroidism. It is better tolerated than T_3 preparations and has a longer half-life. *Levothyroxine* is dosed once daily, and steady state is achieved in 6 to 8 weeks. Toxicity is directly related to T_4 levels and manifests as nervousness, palpitations and tachycardia, heat intolerance, and unexplained weight loss. Drugs that induce the cytochrome P450 enzymes, such as *phenytoin, rifampin*, and *phenobarbital*, accelerate metabolism of the thyroid hormones and may decrease the effectiveness (Figure 24.8).

E. Treatment of hyperthyroidism (thyrotoxicosis)

Graves disease, an autoimmune disease that affects the thyroid, is the most common cause of hyperthyroidism. In these situations, TSH levels are reduced due to negative feedback. [Note: Feedback inhibition of TRH occurs with high levels of circulating thyroid hormone, which, in turn, decreases secretion of TSH.] The goal of therapy is to decrease synthesis and/or release of additional hormone. This can be accomplished by removing part or all of the thyroid gland, by inhibiting synthesis of the hormones, or by blocking release of the hormones from the follicle.

1. **Removal of part or all of the thyroid:** This can be accomplished either surgically or by destruction of the gland with radioactive iodine (^{131}I), which is selectively taken up by the thyroid follicular cells. Most patients become hypothyroid as a result of this drug and require treatment with *levothyroxine.*

2. **Inhibition of thyroid hormone synthesis:** The thioamides, *propylthiouracil* [proe-pil-thye-oh-YOOR-ah-sil] (*PTU*) and *methimazole* [me-THIM-ah-zole], are concentrated in the thyroid, where they inhibit both the oxidative processes required for iodination of tyrosyl groups and the condensation (coupling) of iodotyrosines to form T_3 and T_4 (Figure 24.7). *PTU* also blocks the peripheral conversion of T_4 to T_3. [Note: These drugs have no effect on thyroglobulin already stored in the gland. Therefore, clinical effects of these drugs may be delayed until thyroglobulin stores are depleted (Figure 24.9).] *Methimazole* is preferred over *PTU* because it has a longer half-life, allowing for once-daily dosing, and a lower incidence of adverse effects. However, *PTU* is recommended during the first trimester of pregnancy due to a greater risk of teratogenic effects with *methimazole*. *PTU* has been associated with hepatotoxicity and, rarely, agranulocytosis.

3. **Blockade of hormone release:** A pharmacologic dose of *iodide* inhibits the iodination of tyrosines ("Wolff-Chaikoff effect"), but this effect lasts only a few days. More importantly, *iodide* inhibits the release of thyroid hormones from thyroglobulin by mechanisms not yet understood. *Iodide* is employed to treat thyroid storm or prior to surgery, because it decreases the vascularity of the thyroid gland. *Iodide* is not useful for long-term therapy, because the thyroid ceases to respond to the drug after a few weeks. *Iodide* is administered orally. Adverse effects include sore mouth and throat,

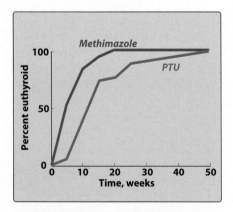

Figure 24.9
Time required for patients with Graves hyperthyroidism to become euthyroid with normal serum T_4 and T_3 concentrations.

swelling of the tongue or larynx, rashes, ulcerations of mucous membranes, and a metallic taste in the mouth.

4. **Thyroid storm:** Thyroid storm presents with extreme symptoms of hyperthyroidism. The treatment of thyroid storm is the same as that for hyperthyroidism, except that the drugs are given in higher doses and more frequently. β-blockers, such as *metoprolol* or *propranolol*, are effective in blunting the widespread sympathetic stimulation that occurs in hyperthyroidism.

Study Questions

Choose the ONE best answer.

24.1 All of the following drugs may be beneficial in the treatment of patients with acromegaly except:

A. Lanreotide.
B. Octreotide.
C. Pegvisomant.
D. Somatropin.

Correct answer = D. Acromegaly is characterized by an excess of GH. Somatropin is synthetic human GH, so it would not be beneficial in this setting. Lanreotide and octreotide are synthetic analogs of somatostatin, which inhibits GH. Pegvisomant is an antagonist at GH receptors and is used to treat acromegaly.

24.2 A 40-year-old female is undergoing infertility treatments. Which of the following drugs might be included in her treatment regimen?

A. Cabergoline.
B. Follitropin.
C. Methimazole.
D. Vasopressin.

Correct answer = B. Follitropin is a recombinant version of FSH that causes ovarian follicular growth and maturation. Cabergoline is a dopamine agonist that is used for hyperprolactinemia. Methimazole is the treatment of choice for hyperthyroidism. Vasopressin is an antidiuretic hormone.

24.3 Which of the following is the treatment of choice for hypothyroidism?

A. Iodide.
B. Levothyroxine.
C. Liothyronine.
D. Liotrix.
E. Propylthiouracil.

Correct answer = B. Levothyroxine is preferred due to its long half-life and better tolerability. Liothyronine (T_3) and liotrix (T_3/T_4) are not as well tolerated. Iodide and propylthiouracil are used in the treatment of hyperthyroidism.

24.4 All of the following agents are correctly paired with an appropriate clinical use of the drug except:

A. Desmopressin—treatment of diabetes insipidus.
B. hCG—treatment of infertility.
C. Octreotide—treatment of bleeding esophageal varices.
D. Oxytocin—induction of labor.
E. Goserelin—growth hormone deficiency.

Correct answer = E. Goserelin is a GnRH analog that may be used for the treatment of prostate cancer or endometriosis. The other choices are paired correctly with their respective clinical uses.

Drugs for Diabetes

25

Karen Whalen

I. OVERVIEW

The pancreas produces the peptide hormones *insulin*, glucagon, and somatostatin. The peptide hormones are secreted from cells in the islets of Langerhans (β cells produce *insulin*, α cells produce glucagon, and δ cells produce somatostatin). These hormones play an important role in regulating metabolic activities of the body, particularly glucose homeostasis. A relative or absolute lack of *insulin*, as seen in diabetes mellitus, can cause serious hyperglycemia. Left untreated, retinopathy, nephropathy, neuropathy, and cardiovascular complications may result. Administration of *insulin* preparations or other glucose-lowering agents (Figure 25.1) can reduce morbidity and mortality associated with diabetes.

II. DIABETES MELLITUS

The incidence of diabetes is growing rapidly in the United States and worldwide. An estimated 25.8 million people in the United States and 347 million people worldwide are afflicted with diabetes. Diabetes is not a single disease. Rather, it is a heterogeneous group of syndromes characterized by elevated blood glucose attributed to a relative or absolute deficiency of *insulin.* The American Diabetes Association (ADA) recognizes four clinical classifications of diabetes: type 1 diabetes (formerly insulin-dependent diabetes mellitus), type 2 diabetes (formerly non–insulin-dependent diabetes mellitus), gestational diabetes, and diabetes due to other causes such as genetic defects or medications. Figure 25.2 summarizes the characteristics of type 1 and type 2 diabetes. Gestational diabetes is defined as carbohydrate intolerance with onset or first recognition during pregnancy. Uncontrolled gestational diabetes can lead to fetal macrosomia (abnormally large body) and shoulder dystocia (difficult delivery), as well as neonatal hypoglycemia. Diet, exercise, and/or *insulin* administration are effective in this condition. *Glyburide* and *metformin* may be reasonable alternatives to *insulin* therapy for gestational diabetes.

A. Type 1 diabetes

Type 1 diabetes most commonly afflicts children, adolescents, or young adults, but some latent forms occur later in life. The disease is characterized by an absolute deficiency of *insulin* due to destruction of β cells. Loss of β-cell function results from autoimmune-mediated processes that may be triggered by viruses or other environmental toxins.

INSULIN
Insulin aspart NOVOLOG
Insulin detemir LEVEMIR
Insulin glargine LANTUS
Insulin glulisine APIDRA
Insulin lispro HUMALOG
NPH insulin suspension HUMULIN N, NOVOLIN N
Regular insulin HUMULIN R, NOVOLIN R

AMYLIN ANALOG
Pramlintide SYMLIN

ORAL AGENTS
Acarbose PRECOSE
Alogliptin NESINA
Bromocriptine CYCLOSET
Canagliflozin INVOKANA
Colesevelam WELCHOL
Dapagliflozin FARXIGA
Glimepiride AMARYL
Glipizide GLUCOTROL
Glyburide DIABETA, GLYNASE PRESTAB
Linagliptin TRADJENTA
Metformin FORTAMET, GLUCOPHAGE
Miglitol GLYSET
Nateglinide STARLIX
Pioglitazone ACTOS
Repaglinide PRANDIN
Rosiglitazone AVANDIA
Saxagliptin ONGLYZA
Sitagliptin JANUVIA
Tolbutamide TOLBUTAMIDE

INCRETIN MIMETIC
Exenatide BYETTA, BYDUREON
Liraglutide VICTOZA

Figure 25.1
Summary of drugs used in the treatment of diabetes.

	Type 1	Type 2
Age of onset	Usually during childhood or puberty	Commonly over age 35
Nutritional status at time of onset	Commonly undernourished	Obesity usually present
Prevalence	5% to 10% of diagnosed diabetics	90% to 95% of diagnosed diabetics
Genetic predisposition	Moderate	Very strong
Defect or deficiency	β cells are destroyed, eliminating the production of insulin	Inability of β cells to produce appropriate quantities of insulin; insulin resistance; other defects

Figure 25.2
Comparison of type 1 and type 2 diabetes.

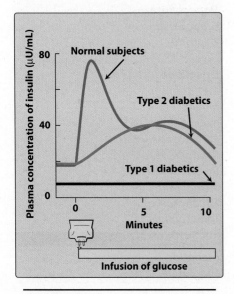

Figure 25.3
Release of *insulin* that occurs in response to an IV glucose load in normal subjects and diabetic patients.

Without functional β cells, the pancreas fails to respond to glucose, and a person with type 1 diabetes shows classic symptoms of *insulin* deficiency (polydipsia, polyphagia, polyuria, and weight loss). Type 1 diabetics require exogenous *insulin* to avoid severe hyperglycemia and the life-threatening catabolic state of ketoacidosis.

1. **Cause of type 1 diabetes:** In a normal postabsorptive period, constant β-cell secretion maintains low basal levels of circulating *insulin*. This suppresses lipolysis, proteolysis, and glycogenolysis. A burst of *insulin* secretion occurs within 2 minutes after ingesting a meal, in response to transient increases in circulating glucose and amino acids. This lasts for up to 15 minutes, followed by the postprandial secretion of *insulin*. However, without functional β cells, those with type 1 diabetes can neither maintain basal secretion of *insulin* nor respond to variations in circulating glucose (Figure 25.3).

2. **Treatment:** A person with type 1 diabetes must rely on exogenous *insulin* to control hyperglycemia, avoid ketoacidosis, and maintain acceptable levels of glycosylated hemoglobin (HbA$_{1c}$). [Note: The rate of formation of HbA$_{1c}$ is proportional to the average blood glucose concentration over the previous 3 months. A higher average glucose results in a higher HbA$_{1c}$.] The goal of *insulin* therapy in type 1 diabetes is to maintain blood glucose as close to normal as possible and to avoid wide swings in glucose. The use of home blood glucose monitors facilitates frequent self-monitoring and treatment with *insulin*.

B. Type 2 diabetes

Type 2 diabetes accounts for greater than 90% of cases. Type 2 diabetes is influenced by genetic factors, aging, obesity, and peripheral *insulin* resistance, rather than autoimmune processes. The metabolic alterations are generally milder than those observed with type 1 (for example, patients with type 2 diabetes typically are not ketotic), but the long-term clinical consequences are similar.

1. **Cause:** Type 2 diabetes is characterized by a lack of sensitivity of target organs to *insulin* (Figure 25.4). In type 2 diabetes, the pancreas retains some β-cell function, but *insulin* secretion is insufficient to maintain glucose homeostasis (Figure 25.3) in the face of increasing peripheral *insulin* resistance. The β-cell mass may gradually decline over time in type 2 diabetes. In contrast to patients with type 1, those with type 2 diabetes are often obese. Obesity contributes to *insulin* resistance, which is considered the major underlying defect of type 2 diabetes.

2. **Treatment:** The goal in treating type 2 diabetes is to maintain blood glucose within normal limits and to prevent the development of long-term complications. Weight reduction, exercise, and dietary modification decrease *insulin* resistance and correct hyperglycemia in some patients with type 2 diabetes. However, most patients require pharmacologic intervention with oral glucose-lowering agents. As the disease progresses, β-cell function declines and *insulin* therapy is often needed to achieve satisfactory glucose levels (Figure 25.5).

III. INSULIN AND INSULIN ANALOGS

Insulin [IN-su-lin] is a polypeptide hormone consisting of two peptide chains that are connected by disulfide bonds. It is synthesized as a precursor (proinsulin) that undergoes proteolytic cleavage to form *insulin* and C-peptide, both of which are secreted by the β cells of the pancreas. [Note: Because *insulin* undergoes significant hepatic and renal extraction, plasma *insulin* levels may not accurately reflect *insulin* production. Thus, measurement of C-peptide provides a better index of *insulin* levels.] *Insulin* secretion is regulated by blood glucose levels, certain amino acids, other hormones, and autonomic mediators. Secretion is most often triggered by increased blood glucose, which is taken up by the glucose transporter into the β cells of the pancreas. There, it is phosphorylated by glucokinase, which acts as a glucose sensor. The products of glucose metabolism enter the mitochondrial respiratory chain and generate adenosine triphosphate (ATP). The rise in ATP levels causes a blockade of K^+ channels, leading to membrane depolarization and an influx of Ca^{2+}. The increase in intracellular Ca^{2+} causes pulsatile *insulin* exocytosis.

A. Mechanism of action

Exogenous *insulin* is administered to replace absent *insulin* secretion in type 1 diabetes or to supplement insufficient *insulin* secretion in type 2 diabetes.

B. Pharmacokinetics and fate

Human *insulin* is produced by recombinant DNA technology using strains of Escherichia coli or yeast that are genetically altered to contain the gene for human *insulin*. Modification of the amino acid sequence of human *insulin* produces insulins with different pharmacokinetic properties. *Insulin* preparations vary primarily in their onset and duration of activity. For example, *insulin lispro, aspart,* and *glulisine* have a faster onset and shorter duration of action than *regular insulin,* because they do not aggregate or form complexes. Dose, injection site, blood supply, temperature, and physical activity can also affect the onset and duration of various *insulin* preparations. Because *insulin* is a polypeptide, it is degraded in the gastrointestinal tract if taken orally. Therefore, it is generally administered by subcutaneous injection. [Note: In a hyperglycemic emergency, *regular insulin* is administered intravenously (IV).] Continuous subcutaneous *insulin* infusion (also called the *insulin* pump) is another method of *insulin* delivery. This method of administration may be more convenient for some patients, eliminating multiple daily injections of *insulin*. The pump is programmed to deliver a basal rate of *insulin*. In addition, it allows the patient to deliver a bolus of *insulin* to cover mealtime carbohydrate intake and compensate for high blood glucose.

C. Adverse reactions to insulin

Hypoglycemia is the most serious and common adverse reaction to *insulin* (Figure 25.6). Other adverse reactions include weight gain, local injection site reactions, and lipodystrophy. Lipodystrophy can be minimized by rotation of injection sites. Diabetics with renal insufficiency may require a decrease in *insulin* dose.

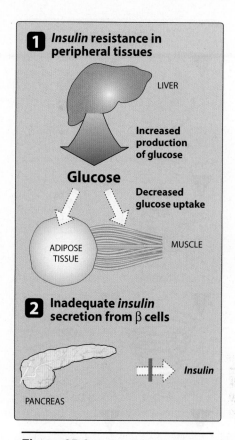

Figure 25.4
Major factors contributing to hyperglycemia observed in type 2 diabetes.

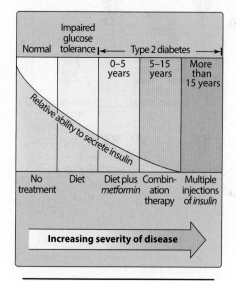

Figure 25.5
Duration of type 2 diabetes mellitus, sufficiency of endogenous *insulin*, and recommended sequence of therapy.

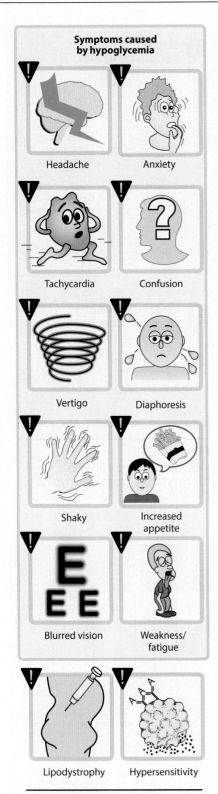

Symptoms caused by hypoglycemia

Headache

Anxiety

Tachycardia

Confusion

Vertigo

Diaphoresis

Shaky

Increased appetite

Blurred vision

Weakness/ fatigue

Lipodystrophy

Hypersensitivity

Figure 25.6
Adverse effects observed with *insulin*. [Note: Lipodystrophy is a local atrophy or hypertrophy of subcutaneous fatty tissue at the site of injections.]

IV. INSULIN PREPARATIONS AND TREATMENT

Insulin preparations are classified as rapid-, short-, intermediate-, or long-acting. Figure 25.7 summarizes onset of action, timing of peak level, and duration of action for the various types of *insulin*. It is important that clinicians exercise caution when adjusting *insulin* treatment, paying strict attention to the dose and type of *insulin*.

A. Rapid-acting and short-acting insulin preparations

Four preparations fall into this category: *regular insulin, insulin lispro* [LIS-proe], *insulin aspart* [AS-part], and *insulin glulisine* [gloo-LYSE-een]. *Regular insulin* is a short-acting, soluble, crystalline zinc *insulin*. *Insulin lispro, aspart,* and *glulisine* are classified as rapid-acting insulins. Modification of the amino acid sequence of *regular insulin* produces analogs that are rapid-acting insulins. For example, *insulin lispro* differs from *regular insulin* in that the lysine and proline at positions 28 and 29 in the B chain are reversed. This modification results in more rapid absorption, a quicker onset, and a shorter duration of action after subcutaneous injection. Peak levels of *insulin lispro* are seen at 30 to 90 minutes, as compared with 50 to 120 minutes for *regular insulin*. *Insulin aspart* and *insulin glulisine* have pharmacokinetic and pharmacodynamic properties similar to those of *insulin lispro*. Rapid- or short-acting insulins are administered to mimic the prandial (mealtime) release of *insulin* and to control postprandial glucose. They may also be used in cases where swift correction of elevated glucose is needed. Rapid- and short-acting insulins are usually used in conjunction with a longer-acting basal *insulin* that provides control of fasting glucose. *Regular insulin* should be injected subcutaneously 30 minutes before a meal, whereas rapid-acting insulins are administered in the 15 minutes proceeding a meal or within 15 to 20 minutes after starting a meal. Rapid-acting insulins are commonly used in external *insulin* pumps, and they are suitable for IV administration, although *regular insulin* is most commonly used when the IV route is needed.

B. Intermediate-acting insulin

Neutral protamine Hagedorn (*NPH*) *insulin* is an intermediate-acting *insulin* formed by the addition of zinc and protamine to *regular insulin*. [Note: Another name for this preparation is *insulin isophane*.] The combination with protamine forms a complex that is less soluble, resulting in delayed absorption and a longer duration of action. *NPH insulin* is used for basal (fasting) control in type 1 or 2 diabetes and is usually given along with rapid- or short-acting *insulin* for mealtime control. *NPH insulin* should be given only subcutaneously (**never IV**), and it should not be used when rapid glucose lowering is needed (for example, diabetic ketoacidosis). Figure 25.8 shows common regimens that use combinations of insulins.

C. Long-acting insulin preparations

The isoelectric point of *insulin glargine* [GLAR-geen] is lower than that of human *insulin,* leading to formation of a precipitate at the injection site that releases *insulin* over an extended period. It has a slower onset than *NPH insulin* and a flat, prolonged hypoglycemic

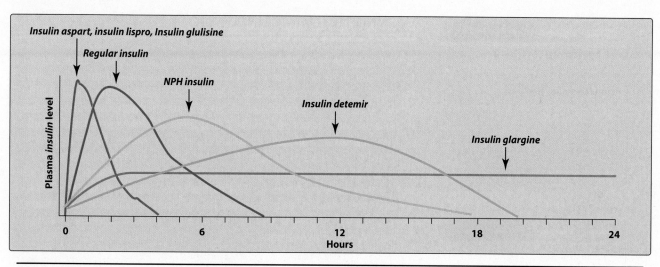

Figure 25.7
Onset and duration of action of human *insulin* and *insulin* analogs. NPH = neutral protamine Hagedorn.

effect with no peak (Figure 25.7). *Insulin detemir* [deh-TEE-meer] has a fatty acid side chain that enhances association to albumin. Slow dissociation from albumin results in long-acting properties similar to those of *insulin glargine.* As with *NPH insulin, insulin glargine* and *insulin detemir* are used for basal control and should only be administered subcutaneously. Neither long-acting *insulin* should be mixed in the same syringe with other insulins, because doing so may alter the pharmacodynamic profile.

D. Insulin combinations

Various premixed combinations of human insulins, such as 70% *NPH insulin* plus 30% *regular insulin* (Figure 25.8), or 50% of each of these are also available. Use of premixed combinations decreases the number of daily injections but makes it more difficult to adjust individual components of the *insulin* regimen.

E. Standard treatment versus intensive treatment

Standard *insulin* therapy involves twice-daily injections. In contrast, intensive treatment utilizes three or more injections daily with frequent monitoring of blood glucose levels. The ADA recommends a target mean blood glucose level of 154 mg/dL or less (HbA$_{1c}$ ≤ 7%), and intensive treatment is more likely to achieve this goal. [Note: Normal mean blood glucose is approximately 115 mg/dL or less (HbA$_{1c}$ < 5.7%).] The frequency of hypoglycemic episodes, coma, and seizures is higher with intensive *insulin* regimens (Figure 25.9A). However, patients on intensive therapy show a significant reduction in microvascular complications of diabetes such as retinopathy, nephropathy, and neuropathy compared to patients receiving standard care (Figure 25.9B). Intensive therapy should not be recommended for patients with long-standing diabetes, significant microvascular complications, advanced age, and those with hypoglycemic unawareness. Intensive therapy has not been shown to significantly reduce macrovascular complications of diabetes.

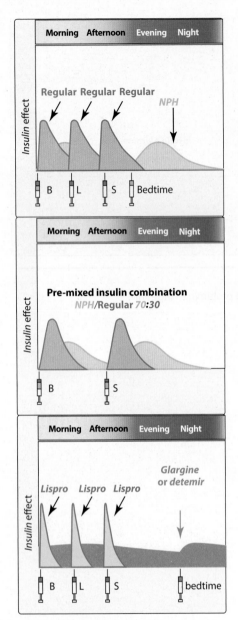

Figure 25.8
Examples of three regimens that provide both prandial and basal *insulin* replacement. B = breakfast; L = lunch; S = supper. NPH = neutral protamine Hagedorn.

V. SYNTHETIC AMYLIN ANALOG

Amylin is a hormone that is cosecreted with *insulin* from β cells following food intake. It delays gastric emptying, decreases postprandial glucagon secretion, and improves satiety. *Pramlintide* [PRAM-lin-tide] is a synthetic amylin analog that is indicated as an adjunct to mealtime *insulin* therapy in patients with type 1 and type 2 diabetes. *Pramlintide* is administered by subcutaneous injection immediately prior to meals. When *pramlintide* is initiated, the dose of mealtime *insulin* should be decreased by 50% to avoid a risk of severe hypoglycemia. Other adverse effects include nausea, anorexia, and vomiting. *Pramlintide* may not be mixed in the same syringe with *insulin*, and it should be avoided in patients with diabetic gastroparesis (delayed stomach emptying), cresol hypersensitivity, or hypoglycemic unawareness.

VI. INCRETIN MIMETICS

Oral glucose results in a higher secretion of *insulin* than occurs when an equal load of glucose is given IV. This effect is referred to as the "incretin effect" and is markedly reduced in type 2 diabetes. The incretin effect occurs because the gut releases incretin hormones, notably glucagon-like peptide-1 (GLP-1) and glucose-dependent insulinotropic polypeptide, in response to a meal. Incretin hormones are responsible for 60% to 70% of postprandial *insulin* secretion. *Exenatide* [EX-e-nah-tide] and *liraglutide* [LIR-a-GLOO-tide] are injectable incretin mimetics used for the treatment of type 2 diabetes.

A. Mechanism of action

The incretin mimetics are analogs of GLP-1 that exert their activity by acting as GLP-1 receptor agonists. These agents improve glucose-dependent *insulin* secretion, slow gastric emptying time, reduce food intake by enhancing satiety (a feeling of fullness), decrease postprandial glucagon secretion, and promote β-cell proliferation. Consequently, weight gain and postprandial hyperglycemia are reduced, and HbA$_{1c}$ levels decline.

B. Pharmacokinetics and fate

Being polypeptides, *exenatide* and *liraglutide* must be administered subcutaneously. *Liraglutide* is highly protein bound and has a long half-life, allowing for once-daily dosing without regard to meals. *Exenatide* is eliminated mainly via glomerular filtration and has a much shorter half-life. Because of the short duration of action, *exenatide* should be injected twice daily within 60 minutes prior to morning and evening meals. A once-weekly extended-release preparation is also available. *Exenatide* should be avoided in patients with severe renal impairment.

C. Adverse effects

The main adverse effects of the incretin mimetics consist of nausea, vomiting, diarrhea, and constipation. *Exenatide* and *liraglutide* have been associated with pancreatitis. Patients should be advised

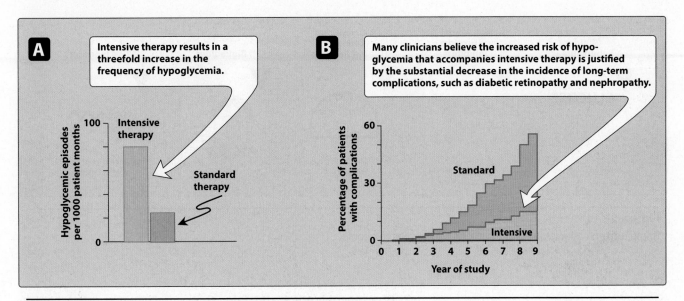

Figure 25.9
A. Effect of tight glucose control on hypoglycemic episodes in a population of patients with type 1 diabetes receiving intensive or standard therapy. **B.** Effect of standard and intensive care on the long-term complications of diabetes.

to discontinue these agents and contact their health care provider immediately if they experience severe abdominal pain. *Liraglutide* causes thyroid C-cell tumors in rodents. However, it is unknown if it causes these tumors or thyroid carcinoma in humans.

VII. ORAL AGENTS

Oral agents are useful in the treatment of patients who have type 2 diabetes that is not controlled with diet. Patients who developed diabetes after age 40 and have had diabetes less than 5 years are most likely to respond well to oral glucose-lowering agents. Patients with long-standing disease may require a combination of oral agents with or without *insulin* to control hyperglycemia. Figure 25.10 summarizes the duration of action of some of the oral glucose-lowering drugs, and Figure 25.11 illustrates some of the common adverse effects.

A. Sulfonylureas

These agents are classified as *insulin* secretagogues, because they promote *insulin* release from the β cells of the pancreas. The sulfonylureas in current use are the second-generation drugs *glyburide* [GLYE-byoor-ide], *glipizide* [GLIP-ih-zide], and *glimepiride* [GLYE-me-pih-ride].

1. **Mechanism of action:** The main mechanism of action includes stimulation of *insulin* release from the β cells of the pancreas. Sulfonylureas block ATP-sensitive K^+ channels, resulting in depolarization, Ca^{2+} influx, and *insulin* exocytosis. In addition, sulfonylureas may reduce hepatic glucose production and increase peripheral *insulin* sensitivity.

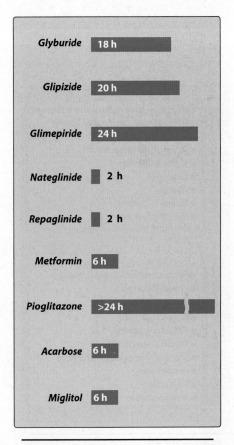

Figure 25.10
Duration of action of some oral hypoglycemic agents.

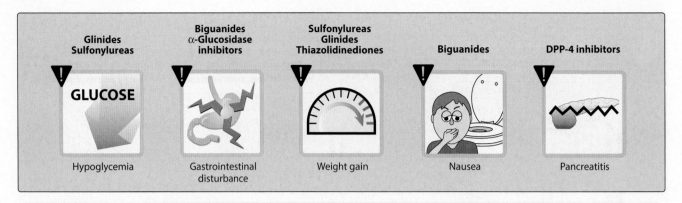

Figure 25.11
Some adverse effects observed with oral hypoglycemic agents.

2. **Pharmacokinetics and fate:** Given orally, these drugs bind to serum proteins, are metabolized by the liver, and are excreted in the urine and feces. The duration of action ranges from 12 to 24 hours.

3. **Adverse effects:** Major adverse effects of the sulfonylureas are weight gain, hyperinsulinemia, and hypoglycemia. They should be used with caution in hepatic or renal insufficiency, since accumulation of sulfonylureas may cause hypoglycemia. Renal impairment is a particular problem for *glyburide*, as it may increase the duration of action and increase the risk of hypoglycemia significantly. *Glipizide* or *glimepiride* are safer options in renal dysfunction and in elderly patients. *Glyburide* has minimal transfer across the placenta and may be an alternative to *insulin* for diabetes in pregnancy. Figure 25.12 summarizes some drug interactions with sulfonylureas.

B. Glinides

This class of agents includes *repaglinide* [re-PAG-lin-ide] and *nateglinide* [nuh-TAY-gli-nide]. Glinides are also considered *insulin* secretagogues.

1. **Mechanism of action:** Like the sulfonylureas, the glinides stimulate *insulin* secretion. They bind to a distinct site on the β cell, closing ATP-sensitive K⁺ channels, and initiating a series of reactions that results in the release of *insulin*. In contrast to the sulfonylureas, the glinides have a rapid onset and a short duration of action. They are particularly effective in the early release of *insulin* that occurs after a meal and are categorized as postprandial glucose regulators. Glinides should not be used in combination with sulfonylureas due to overlapping mechanisms of action. This would increase the risk of serious hypoglycemia.

2. **Pharmacokinetics and fate:** Glinides should be taken prior to a meal and are well absorbed after oral administration. Both glinides are metabolized to inactive products by cytochrome P450 3A4

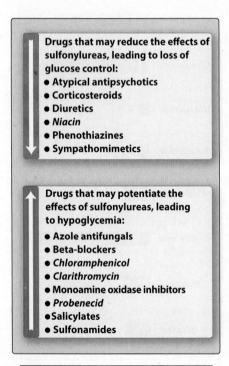

Drugs that may reduce the effects of sulfonylureas, leading to loss of glucose control:
- Atypical antipsychotics
- Corticosteroids
- Diuretics
- *Niacin*
- Phenothiazines
- Sympathomimetics

Drugs that may potentiate the effects of sulfonylureas, leading to hypoglycemia:
- Azole antifungals
- Beta-blockers
- *Chloramphenicol*
- *Clarithromycin*
- Monoamine oxidase inhibitors
- *Probenecid*
- Salicylates
- Sulfonamides

Figure 25.12
Drugs interacting with sulfonylureas.

(CYP3A4; see Chapter 1) in the liver and are excreted through the bile.

3. Adverse effects: Although glinides can cause hypoglycemia and weight gain, the incidence is lower than that with sulfonylureas. [Note: Drugs that inhibit CYP3A4, such as *itraconazole, fluconazole, erythromycin,* and *clarithromycin,* may enhance the glucose-lowering effect of *repaglinide.* Drugs that induce CYP3A4, such as barbiturates, *carbamazepine,* and *rifampin,* may have the opposite effect.] By inhibiting hepatic metabolism, the lipid-lowering drug *gemfibrozil* may significantly increase the effects of *repaglinide,* and concurrent use is contraindicated. These agents should be used with caution in patients with hepatic impairment.

C. Biguanides

Metformin [met-FOR-min], the only biguanide, is classified as an *insulin* sensitizer. It increases glucose uptake and use by target tissues, thereby decreasing *insulin* resistance. Unlike sulfonylureas, *metformin* does not promote *insulin* secretion. Therefore, hyperinsulinemia is not a problem, and the risk of hypoglycemia is far less than that with sulfonylureas.

1. Mechanism of action: The main mechanism of action of *metformin* is reduction of hepatic gluconeogenesis. [Note: Excess glucose produced by the liver is a major source of high blood glucose in type 2 diabetes, accounting for high fasting blood glucose.] *Metformin* also slows intestinal absorption of sugars and improves peripheral glucose uptake and utilization. Weight loss may occur because *metformin* causes loss of appetite. The ADA recommends *metformin* as the initial drug of choice for type 2 diabetes. *Metformin* may be used alone or in combination with other oral agents or *insulin.* Hypoglycemia may occur when *metformin* is taken in combination with *insulin* or *insulin* secretagogues, so adjustment in dosage may be required.

2. Pharmacokinetics and fate: *Metformin* is well absorbed orally, is not bound to serum proteins, and is not metabolized. Excretion is via the urine.

3. Adverse effects: These are largely gastrointestinal. *Metformin* is contraindicated in renal dysfunction due to the risk of lactic acidosis. It should be discontinued in cases of acute myocardial infarction, exacerbation of heart failure, sepsis, or other disorders that can cause acute renal failure. *Metformin* should be used with caution in patients older than 80 years and in those with heart failure or alcohol abuse. It should be temporarily discontinued in patients undergoing procedures requiring IV radiographic contrast. Rarely, potentially fatal lactic acidosis has occurred. Long-term use may interfere with vitamin B_{12} absorption.

4. Other uses: In addition to type 2 diabetes, *metformin* is effective in the treatment of polycystic ovary syndrome. It lowers *insulin* resistance seen in this disorder and can result in ovulation and, therefore, possibly pregnancy.

D. Thiazolidinediones

The thiazolidinediones (TZDs) are also *insulin* sensitizers. The two members of this class are *pioglitazone* [pye-oh-GLI-ta-zone] and *rosiglitazone* [roe-si-GLIH-ta-zone]. Although *insulin* is required for their action, the TZDs do not promote its release from the β cells, so hyperinsulinemia is not a risk.

1. **Mechanism of action:** The TZDs lower *insulin* resistance by acting as agonists for the peroxisome proliferator–activated receptor-γ (PPARγ), a nuclear hormone receptor. Activation of PPARγ regulates the transcription of several *insulin* responsive genes, resulting in increased *insulin* sensitivity in adipose tissue, liver, and skeletal muscle. Effects of these drugs on cholesterol levels are of interest. *Rosiglitazone* increases LDL cholesterol and triglycerides, whereas *pioglitazone* decreases triglycerides. Both drugs increase HDL cholesterol. The TZDs can be used as monotherapy or in combination with other glucose-lowering agents or *insulin.* The dose of *insulin* may have to be lowered when used in combination with these agents. The ADA recommends *pioglitazone* as a second- or third-line agent for type 2 diabetes. *Rosiglitazone* is less utilized due to concerns regarding cardiac adverse effects.

2. **Pharmacokinetics and fate:** *Pioglitazone* and *rosiglitazone* are well absorbed after oral administration and are extensively bound to serum albumin. Both undergo extensive metabolism by different CYP450 isozymes (see Chapter 1). Some metabolites of *pioglitazone* have activity. Renal elimination of *pioglitazone* is negligible, with the majority of active drug and metabolites excreted in the bile and eliminated in the feces. Metabolites of *rosiglitazone* are primarily excreted in the urine. No dosage adjustment is required in renal impairment. These agents should be avoided in nursing mothers.

3. **Adverse effects:** A few cases of liver toxicity have been reported with these drugs, and periodic monitoring of liver function is recommended. Weight gain can occur because TZDs may increase subcutaneous fat and cause fluid retention. [Note: Fluid retention can worsen heart failure. These drugs should be avoided in patients with severe heart failure.] TZDs have been associated with osteopenia and increased fracture risk. *Pioglitazone* may also increase the risk of bladder cancer. Several meta-analyses identified a potential increased risk of myocardial infarction and death from cardiovascular causes with *rosiglitazone.* As a result, use of *rosiglitazone* was limited to patients enrolled in a special restricted access program. After a further review of safety data, the restrictions on *rosiglitazone* use were subsequently lifted.

4. **Other uses:** As with *metformin,* the relief of *insulin* resistance with the TZDs can cause ovulation to resume in premenopausal women with polycystic ovary syndrome.

E. α-Glucosidase inhibitors

Acarbose [AY-car-bose] and *miglitol* [MIG-li-tol] are oral agents used for the treatment of type 2 diabetes.

1. **Mechanism of action:** Located in the intestinal brush border, α-glucosidase enzymes break down carbohydrates into glucose and other simple sugars that can be absorbed. *Acarbose* and *miglitol* reversibly inhibit α-glucosidase enzymes. When taken at the start of a meal, these drugs delay the digestion of carbohydrates, resulting in lower postprandial glucose levels. Since they do not stimulate *insulin* release or increase *insulin* sensitivity, these agents do not cause hypoglycemia when used as monotherapy. However, when used with *insulin* secretagogues or *insulin,* hypoglycemia may develop. [Note: It is important that hypoglycemia in this context be treated with glucose rather than sucrose, because sucrase is also inhibited by these drugs.]

2. **Pharmacokinetics and fate:** *Acarbose* is poorly absorbed. It is metabolized primarily by intestinal bacteria, and some of the metabolites are absorbed and excreted into the urine. *Miglitol* is very well absorbed but has no systemic effects. It is excreted unchanged by the kidney.

3. **Adverse effects:** The major side effects are flatulence, diarrhea, and abdominal cramping. Adverse effects limit the use of these agents in clinical practice. Patients with inflammatory bowel disease, colonic ulceration, or intestinal obstruction should not use these drugs.

F. Dipeptidyl peptidase-4 inhibitors

Alogliptin [al-oh-GLIP-tin], *linagliptin* [lin-a-GLIP-tin], *saxagliptin* [sax-a-GLIP-tin], and *sitagliptin* [si-ta-GLIP-tin] are orally active dipeptidyl peptidase-4 (DPP-4) inhibitors used for the treatment of type 2 diabetes.

1. **Mechanism of action:** These drugs inhibit the enzyme DPP-4, which is responsible for the inactivation of incretin hormones such as GLP-1. Prolonging the activity of incretin hormones increases *insulin* release in response to meals and reduces inappropriate secretion of glucagon. DPP-4 inhibitors may be used as monotherapy or in combination with sulfonylureas, *metformin,* TZDs, or *insulin.* Unlike incretin mimetics, these drugs do not cause satiety, or fullness, and are weight neutral.

2. **Pharmacokinetics and fate:** The DPP-4 inhibitors are well absorbed after oral administration. Food does not affect the extent of absorption. *Alogliptin* and *sitagliptin* are mostly excreted unchanged in the urine. *Saxagliptin* is metabolized via CYP450 3A4/5 to an active metabolite. The primary route of elimination for *saxagliptin* and the metabolite is renal. *Linagliptin* is primarily eliminated via the enterohepatic system. All DPP-4 inhibitors except *linagliptin* require dosage adjustments in renal dysfunction.

3. **Adverse effects:** In general, DPP-4 inhibitors are well tolerated, with the most common adverse effects being nasopharyngitis and headache. Although infrequent, pancreatitis has occurred with use of all DPP-4 inhibitors. Strong inhibitors of CYP450 3A4/5, such

as *ritonavir, atazanavir, itraconazole,* and *clarithromycin,* may increase levels of *saxagliptin.* Therefore, reduced doses of *saxagliptin* should be used.

G. Sodium–glucose cotransporter 2 inhibitors

Canagliflozin [kan-a-gli-FLOE-zin] and *dapagliflozin* [dap-a-gli-FLOE-zin] are the agents in this category of drugs for type 2 diabetes.

1. **Mechanism of action:** The sodium–glucose cotransporter 2 (SGLT2) is responsible for reabsorbing filtered glucose in the tubular lumen of the kidney. By inhibiting SGLT2, these agents decrease reabsorption of glucose, increase urinary glucose excretion, and lower blood glucose. Inhibition of SGLT2 also decreases reabsorption of sodium and causes osmotic diuresis. Therefore, SGLT2 inhibitors may reduce systolic blood pressure. However, they are not indicated for the treatment of hypertension.

2. **Pharmacokinetics and fate:** These agents are given once daily in the morning. *Canagliflozin* should be taken before the first meal of the day. Both drugs are mainly metabolized by glucuronidation to inactive metabolites. While the primary route of excretion for *canagliflozin* is via the feces, about one-third of a dose is renally eliminated. These agents should be avoided in patients with renal dysfunction.

3. **Adverse effects:** The most common adverse effects with SGLT2 inhibitors are female genital mycotic infections (for example, vulvovaginal candidiasis), urinary tract infections, and urinary frequency. Hypotension has also occurred, particularly in the elderly or patients on diuretics. Thus, volume status should be evaluated prior to starting these agents.

H. Other agents

Both the dopamine agonist *bromocriptine* and the bile acid sequestrant *colesevelam* produce modest reductions in HbA_{1c}. The mechanism of action of glucose lowering is unknown for both of these drugs. Although *bromocriptine* and *colesevelam* are indicated for the treatment of type 2 diabetes, their modest efficacy, adverse effects, and pill burden limit their use in clinical practice.

Figure 25.13 provides a summary of the oral antidiabetic agents.

Figure 25.14 shows treatment guidelines for type 2 diabetes.

DRUG CLASS	MECHANISM OF ACTION	EFFECT ON PLASMA INSULIN	RISK OF HYPO-GLYCEMIA	COMMENTS
Sulfonylureas *Glimepiride* *Glipizide* *Glyburide*	Stimulates insulin secretion	⬆	Yes	Well-established history of effectiveness. Weight gain can occur. Hypoglycemia most common with this class of oral agents.
Glinides *Nateglinide* *Repaglinide*	Stimulates insulin secretion	⬆	Yes (rarely)	Taken with meals. Short action with less hypoglycemia. Postprandial effect.
Biguanides *Metformin*	Decreases hepatic production of glucose	⬇	No	Preferred agent for type 2 diabetes. Well-established history of effectiveness. Weight loss may occur. Monitor renal function.
Thiazolidinediones (glitazones) *Pioglitazone* *Rosiglitazone*	Binds to peroxisome proliferator–activated receptor-γ in muscle, fat and liver to decrease insulin resistance	⬇⬇	No	Effective in highly insulin-resistant patients. Once-daily dosing for *pioglitazone*. Check liver function before initiation. Avoid in liver disease or heart failure.
α-Glucosidase inhibitors *Acarbose* *Miglitol*	Decreases glucose absorption	⬄	No	Taken with meals. Adverse gastro-intestinal effects.
DPP-4 inhibitors *Alogliptin* *Linagliptin* *Sitagliptin* *Saxagliptin*	Increases glucose-dependent insulin release; decreases secretion of glucagon	⬆	No	Once-daily dosing. May be taken with or without food. Well tolerated. Risk of pancreatitis.
Incretin mimetics *Exenatide* *Liraglutide*	Increases glucose-dependent insulin release; decreases secretion of glucagon; slows gastric emptying; increases satiety	⬆	No	Injection formulation. *Exenatide* should be injected twice daily within 60 minutes prior to morning and evening meals. Extended-release *exenatide* is given once weekly. *Liraglutide* is dosed once-daily without regard to meals. Weight loss may occur. Risk of pancreatitis.
SGLT2 inhibitors *Canagliflozin* *Dapaglifozin*	Increases urinary glucose excretion	⬄	No	Once-daily dosing in the morning. Risk of hypotension, hyperkalemia. Avoid in severe renal impairment.

Figure 25.13

Summary of oral agents used to treat diabetes. ⇔ = little or no change. DPP-4 = dipeptidyl peptidase-4.

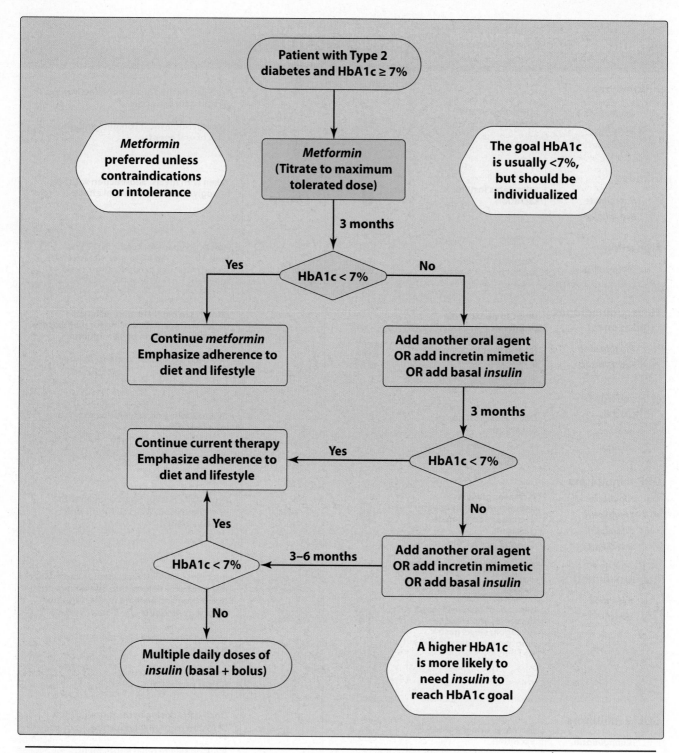

Figure 25.14
Treatment guidelines for type 2 diabetes.

Study Questions

Choose the ONE best answer.

25.1 Which of the following statements is correct regarding insulin glargine?

   A. It is primarily used to control postprandial hyperglycemia.
   B. It is a "peakless" insulin.
   C. The prolonged duration of activity is due to slow dissociation from albumin.
   D. It should not be used in a regimen with insulin lispro or glulisine.
   E. It may be administered intravenously in emergency cases.

Correct answer = B. Insulin glargine has a relatively flat, prolonged hypoglycemic effect. Because of this it is used for basal glucose control, not postprandial. The prolonged duration is due to its low pH, which leads to precipitation at the injection site and resultant extended action. Insulin glargine is often used for basal control in a regimen where insulin lispro, glulisine, or aspart are used for mealtime glucose control. [Note: Glargine should not be combined with other insulins in the same syringe, as it may alter the pharmacodynamic properties of the medication.]

25.2 DW is a patient with type 2 diabetes who has a blood glucose of 400 mg/dL today at his office visit. The physician would like to give some insulin to bring the glucose down before he leaves the office. Which of the following would lower the glucose in the quickest manner in DW?

   A. Insulin aspart.
   B. Insulin glargine.
   C. NPH insulin.
   D. Regular insulin.

Correct answer = A. Insulin aspart is a rapid-acting insulin that has an onset of action within 15 to 20 minutes. Insulin glargine is a long-acting insulin that is used for basal control. NPH insulin is an intermediate-acting insulin that is used for basal control. Although regular insulin can be used to bring the glucose down, its onset is not as quick as insulin aspart. The onset of regular insulin is about 30 to 60 minutes.

25.3 Which of the following classes of oral diabetes drugs is paired most appropriately with its primary mechanism of action?

   A. DPP-4 inhibitor—inhibits breakdown of complex carbohydrates.
   B. Glinide—increases insulin sensitivity.
   C. Sulfonylurea—increases insulin secretion.
   D. Thiazolidinedione—decreases hepatic gluconeogenesis.

Correct answer = C. Sulfonylureas work primarily by increasing insulin secretion through stimulation of the β cells of the pancreas. DPP-4 inhibitors work by inhibiting breakdown of incretins, thereby increasing postprandial insulin secretion, decreasing postprandial glucagon, etc. Glinides work primarily by increasing insulin secretion. TZDs work primarily by increasing insulin sensitivity.

25.4 Which of the following statements is characteristic of metformin?

   A. Metformin is inappropriate for initial management of type 2 diabetes.
   B. Metformin decreases hepatic glucose production.
   C. Metformin undergoes significant metabolism via the cytochrome P450 system.
   D. Metformin should not be combined with sulfonylureas or insulin.
   E. Weight gain is a common adverse effect.

Correct answer = B. Metformin works by inhibiting hepatic gluconeogenesis. It is the preferred initial agent for management of type 2 diabetes. Metformin is not metabolized. It may be combined with sulfonylureas, insulin, or TZDs. Unlike the sulfonylureas and insulin, weight gain is not an adverse effect, and some patients actually lose weight due to GI side effects.

25.5 Which of the following is the most appropriate initial oral agent for management of type 2 diabetes in patients with no other comorbid conditions?

   A. Glipizide.
   B. Insulin.
   C. Metformin.
   D. Pioglitazone.

Correct answer = C. Metformin is the preferred initial agent for management of type 2 diabetes. See Figure 25.14.

25.6 A 64-year-old woman with a history of type 2 diabetes is diagnosed with heart failure. Which of the following medications would be a poor choice for controlling her diabetes?

A. Exenatide.
B. Glyburide.
C. Nateglinide.
D. Pioglitazone.
E. Sitagliptin.

Correct answer = D. The TZDs (pioglitazone and rosiglitazone) can cause fluid retention and lead to a worsening of heart failure. They should be used with caution and dose reduction, if at all, in patients with heart failure. Exenatide, glyburide, nateglinide, and sitagliptin do not have precautions for use in heart failure patients.

25.7 KD is a 69-year-old male with type 2 diabetes and advanced chronic kidney disease. Which of the following diabetes medications is contraindicated in this patient?

A. Glipizide.
B. Insulin lispro.
C. Metformin.
D. Saxagliptin.

Correct answer = C. Metformin should not be used in patients with kidney disease due to the possibility of lactic acidosis. Glipizide can be used safely in patients with CrCl as low as 10 mL/min. Insulin is not contraindicated in renal dysfunction, although the dosage may need to be adjusted. While the dose of the DPP-4 inhibitor saxagliptin may need to be reduced in renal dysfunction, it is not contraindicated.

25.8 Which of the following drugs for diabetes would be LEAST likely to cause weight gain?

A. Glimepiride.
B. Liraglutide.
C. Pioglitazone.
D. Repaglinide.
E. Insulin glulisine.

Correct answer = B. Incretin mimetics are usually associated with weight loss due to their ability to enhance satiety. All of the other agents are associated with weight gain.

25.9 A patient with type 2 diabetes is taking metformin. The fasting glucose levels are in range, but the postprandial glucose is uncontrolled. All of the following drugs would be appropriate to add to metformin to target postprandial glucose except:

A. Acarbose.
B. Exenatide.
C. Insulin aspart.
D. Pramlintide.

The correct answer = D. Although all of these drugs target postprandial glucose, pramlintide should only be used in conjunction with mealtime insulin. Since this patient is not on insulin, pramlintide is not indicated.

25.10 Which of the following diabetes medications is most appropriately paired with an adverse effect associated with its use?

A. Canagliflozin—lactic acidosis.
B. Metformin—urinary tract infections.
C. Nateglinide—heart failure.
D. Liraglutide—pancreatitis.

Correct answer = D. The incretin mimetics are associated with a risk of pancreatitis. Lactic acidosis is a rare but serious side effect of metformin (not canagliflozin). Adverse effects of canagliflozin are genital mycotic infections, urinary tract infections, and urinary frequency. Nateglinide may cause hypoglycemia but has not been associated with heart failure. The TZDs have been associated with heart failure.

Estrogens and Androgens

Karen Whalen

26

I. OVERVIEW

Sex hormones produced by the gonads are necessary for conception, embryonic maturation, and development of primary and secondary sexual characteristics at puberty. The gonadal hormones are used therapeutically in replacement therapy, for contraception, and in management of menopausal symptoms. Several antagonists are effective in cancer chemotherapy. All gonadal hormones are synthesized from the precursor, cholesterol, in a series of steps that includes shortening of the hydrocarbon side chain and hydroxylation of the steroid nucleus. Aromatization is the last step in estrogen synthesis. Figure 26.1 lists the steroid hormones discussed in this chapter.

II. ESTROGENS

Estradiol [ess-tra-DYE-ole], also known as *17β-estradiol*, is the most potent estrogen produced and secreted by the ovary. It is the principal estrogen in premenopausal women. *Estrone* [ESS-trone] is a metabolite of *estradiol* that has approximately one-third the estrogenic potency of *estradiol*. *Estrone* is the primary circulating estrogen after menopause, and it is generated mainly from conversion of androstenedione in peripheral tissues. *Estriol* [ess-TRI-ole], another metabolite of *estradiol*, is significantly less potent than is *estradiol*. It is present in significant amounts during pregnancy, because it is the principal estrogen produced by the placenta. A preparation of conjugated estrogens containing sulfate esters of *estrone* and *equilin* (obtained from urine of pregnant mares) is an oral preparation used for hormone replacement therapy. Plant-derived conjugated estrogen products are also available. Synthetic estrogens, such as *ethinyl estradiol* [ETH-ih-nil ess-tra-DYE-ole], undergo less first-pass metabolism than do naturally occurring steroids and, thus, are effective when administered orally at lower doses. Nonsteroidal compounds that bind to estrogen receptors and exert either estrogenic or antiestrogenic effects on target tissues are called selective estrogen receptor modulators (SERMs). These include *tamoxifen* and *raloxifene*, among others.

A. Mechanism of action

After dissociation from their binding sites on sex hormone–binding globulin or albumin in the plasma, steroid hormones diffuse across the cell membrane and bind with high affinity to specific nuclear

ESTROGENS

Estradiol USED IN MANY COMBINATIONS
Estrone MENEST
Ethinyl estradiol USED IN MANY COMBINATIONS
Mestranol (w/norethindrone) NECON 1/50, NORINYL 1+50

SELECTIVE ESTROGEN-RECEPTOR MODULATORS (SERMs)

Clomiphene CLOMID, SEROPHENE
Ospemifene OSPHENA
Raloxifene EVISTA
Tamoxifen TAMOXIFEN, NOLVADEX
Toremifene FARESTON

PROGESTOGENS

Desogestrel USED IN MANY COMBINATIONS
Dienogest (w/estradiol valerate) NATAZIA
Drospirenone (w/ethinyl estradiol) BEYAZ, YAZ, YASMIN
Etonogestrel (w/ethinyl estradiol) NUVA RING
Etonogestrel (subdermal) IMPLANON, NEXPLANON
Levonorgestrel MIRENA, NEXT CHOICE, PLAN B ONE-STEP
Medroxyprogesterone PROVERA
Norelgestromin (w/ethinyl estradiol) ORTHO EVRA
Norethindrone NOR-QD, ORTHO MICRONOR
Norethindrone acetate AYGESTIN
Norgestimate USED IN MANY COMBINATIONS
Norgestrel (w/ethinyl estradiol) LO/OVRAL
Progesterone USED IN MANY COMBINATIONS

PROGESTERONE AGONIST/ANTAGONIST

Ulipristal acetate ELLA

Figure 26.1

Summary of sex hormones. (Figure continues on next page.)

PROGESTERONE ANTAGONIST

Mifepristone MIFEPREX

ANDROGENS

Danazol DANOCRINE

Fluoxymesterone ANDROXY

Methyltestosterone ANDROID, TESTRED, METHITEST

Oxandrolone OXANDRIN

Oxymetholone ANADROL

Testosterone ANDRODERM, ANDROGEL, AXIRON, FORTESTA, STRIANT, TESTIM, TESTOPEL

Testosterone cypionate DEPO-TESTOSTERONE

Testosterone enanthate DELATESTRYL

ANTIANDROGENS

Bicalutamide CASODEX

Dutasteride AVODART

Enzalutamide XTANDI

Finasteride PROPECIA, PROSCAR

Flutamide EULEXIN

Nilutamide NILANDRON

Figure 26.1 (Continued)
Summary of sex hormones.

receptor proteins (Figure 26.2). The activated steroid–receptor complex interacts with nuclear chromatin to initiate hormone-specific RNA synthesis. This results in the synthesis of specific proteins that mediate a number of physiologic functions. [Note: The steroid hormones may elicit the synthesis of different RNA species in diverse target tissues and, therefore, are both receptor and tissue specific.] Other pathways that require these hormones have been identified that lead to more rapid actions. For example, activation of an estrogen receptor in the membranes of hypothalamic cells has been shown to couple to a G protein, thereby initiating a second-messenger cascade. In addition, estrogen-mediated dilation of coronary arteries occurs by the increased formation and release of nitric oxide and prostacyclin in endothelial cells.

B. Therapeutic uses

Estrogens are most frequently used for contraception and postmenopausal hormone therapy (HT). Estrogens were previously widely used for prevention of osteoporosis, but current guidelines recommend use of other therapies such as *alendronate* (see Chapter 35) over estrogen. Estrogens are also used for replacement therapy in premenopausal patients who are deficient in this hormone. Estrogen deficiency can be due to inadequate functioning of the ovaries (hypogonadism), premature menopause, or surgical menopause.

1. **Postmenopausal HT:** The primary indication for estrogen therapy in postmenopausal women is menopausal symptoms, such as vasomotor instability (for example, "hot flashes" or "hot flushes") and vaginal atrophy (Figure 26.3). For women who have an intact uterus, a progestogen is always included with the estrogen therapy, because the combination reduces the risk of endometrial carcinoma associated with unopposed estrogen. For women who have undergone a hysterectomy, unopposed estrogen therapy

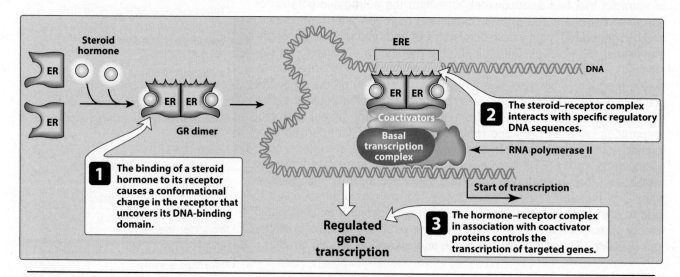

Figure 26.2

Transcriptional regulation by intracellular steroid hormone receptors. ERE = estrogen response element; ER = estrogen receptor.

is recommended because progestins may unfavorably alter the beneficial effects of estrogen on lipid parameters. [Note: The amount of estrogen used in replacement therapy is substantially less than the doses used in oral contraception. Thus, the adverse effects of estrogen replacement therapy are usually less pronounced than those seen in women taking estrogen for contraceptive purposes.] Delivery of *estradiol* by transdermal patch or gel is also effective in treating postmenopausal symptoms. Due to concerns over the risks of HT (increased risk of cardiovascular events and breast cancer), HT should be prescribed at the lowest effective dose for the shortest possible time to relieve menopausal symptoms. Women who only have urogenital symptoms, such as vaginal atrophy, should be treated with vaginal rather than systemic estrogen.

2. **Contraception:** The combination of an estrogen and progestogen provides effective contraception via the oral, transdermal, or vaginal route.

3. **Other uses:** Estrogen therapy mimicking the natural cyclic pattern, and usually in combination with a progestogen, is instituted to stimulate development of secondary sex characteristics in young women with primary hypogonadism. Continued treatment is required after growth is completed. Similarly, estrogen and progestogen replacement therapy is used for women who have premature menopause or premature ovarian failure.

C. Pharmacokinetics

1. **Naturally occurring estrogens:** These agents and their esterified or conjugated derivatives are readily absorbed through the gastrointestinal tract, skin, and mucous membranes. Taken orally, *estradiol* is rapidly metabolized (and partially inactivated) by the microsomal enzymes of the liver. Micronized *estradiol* is available and has better bioavailability. Although there is some first-pass metabolism, it is not sufficient to lessen the effectiveness when taken orally.

2. **Synthetic estrogen analogs:** These compounds, such as *ethinyl estradiol*, *mestranol* [MES-trah-nole], and *estradiol valerate*, are well absorbed after oral administration. *Mestranol* is quickly demethylated to *ethinyl estradiol*, which is metabolized more slowly than the naturally occurring estrogens by the liver and peripheral tissues. *Estradiol valerate* is rapidly cleaved to *estradiol* and valeric acid. Being fat soluble, they are stored in adipose tissue, from which they are slowly released. Therefore, the synthetic estrogen analogs have a prolonged action and a higher potency compared to those of natural estrogens.

3. **Metabolism:** Estrogens are transported in the blood bound to serum albumin or sex hormone–binding globulin. As mentioned above, bioavailability of estrogen taken orally is low due to first-pass metabolism. To reduce first-pass metabolism, the drugs may be administered via the transdermal route (patch, topical gel, topical emulsion, or spray), intravaginally (tablet, cream, or ring), or by injection. They are hydroxylated in the liver to derivatives that

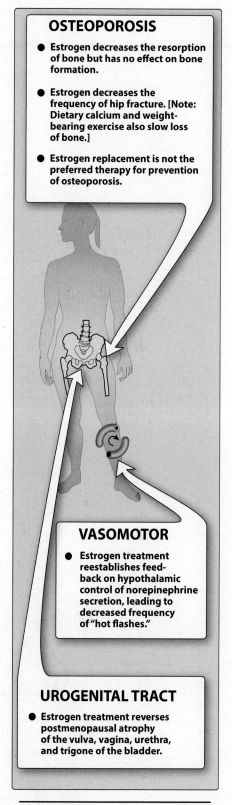

OSTEOPOROSIS

● Estrogen decreases the resorption of bone but has no effect on bone formation.

● Estrogen decreases the frequency of hip fracture. [Note: Dietary calcium and weight-bearing exercise also slow loss of bone.]

● Estrogen replacement is not the preferred therapy for prevention of osteoporosis.

VASOMOTOR

● Estrogen treatment reestablishes feedback on hypothalamic control of norepinephrine secretion, leading to decreased frequency of "hot flashes."

UROGENITAL TRACT

● Estrogen treatment reverses postmenopausal atrophy of the vulva, vagina, urethra, and trigone of the bladder.

Figure 26.3
Benefits associated with postmenopausal estrogen replacement.

are subsequently glucuronidated or sulfated. The parent drugs and their metabolites undergo excretion into bile and are then reabsorbed through the enterohepatic circulation. Inactive products are excreted in urine.

D. Adverse effects

Nausea and breast tenderness are among the most common adverse effects of estrogen therapy. In addition, the risk of thromboembolic events, myocardial infarction, and breast and endometrial cancer is increased with use of estrogen therapy. [Note: The increased risk of endometrial cancer can be offset by including a progestogen along with the estrogen therapy.] Other effects of estrogen therapy are shown in Figure 26.4.

III. SELECTIVE ESTROGEN RECEPTOR MODULATORS

SERMs are a class of estrogen-related compounds that display selective agonism or antagonism for estrogen receptors depending on the tissue type. This category includes *tamoxifen*, *toremifene*, *raloxifene*, *clomiphene*, and *ospemifene*.

A. Mechanism of action

Tamoxifen [tah-MOKS-ih-fen], *toremifene* [tore-EM-i-feen], and *raloxifene* [rah-LOX-ih-feen] compete with estrogen for binding to the estrogen receptor in breast tissue. [Note: Normal breast growth is stimulated by estrogens. Therefore, some breast tumors regress following treatment with these agents.] In addition, *raloxifene* acts as an estrogen agonist in bone, leading to decreased bone resorption, increased bone density, and decreased vertebral fractures (Figure 26.5). Unlike estrogen and *tamoxifen*, *raloxifene* does not have appreciable estrogen receptor agonist activity in the endometrium and, therefore, does not predispose to endometrial cancer. *Raloxifene* also lowers serum total cholesterol and low-density lipoprotein (LDL). *Clomiphene* [KLOE-mi-feen] acts as a partial estrogen agonist and interferes with the negative

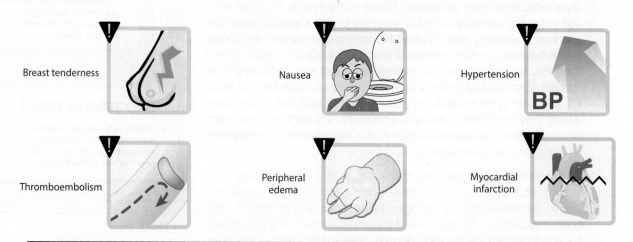

Figure 26.4
Some adverse effects associated with estrogen therapy. BP = blood pressure.

feedback of estrogens on the hypothalamus. This effect increases the secretion of gonadotropin-releasing hormone and gonadotropins, thereby leading to stimulation of ovulation.

B. Therapeutic uses

Tamoxifen is currently used in the treatment of metastatic breast cancer, or as adjuvant therapy following mastectomy or radiation for breast cancer. Both *tamoxifen* and *raloxifene* can be used as prophylactic therapy to reduce the risk of breast cancer in high-risk patients. *Raloxifene* is also approved for the prevention and treatment of osteoporosis in postmenopausal women. *Clomiphene* is useful for the treatment of infertility associated with anovulatory cycles. *Ospemifene* is indicated for the treatment of dyspareunia (painful sexual intercourse) related to menopause.

C. Pharmacokinetics

The SERMs are rapidly absorbed after oral administration. *Tamoxifen* is extensively metabolized by cytochrome P450 isoenzymes, including formation of active metabolites via the CYP3A4/5 and CYP2D6 isoenzymes. [Note: Patients with a genetic polymorphism in CYP2D6 may produce less active metabolite, resulting in diminished activity of *tamoxifen*.] *Raloxifene* is rapidly converted to glucuronide conjugates through first-pass metabolism. These agents undergo enterohepatic cycling, and the primary route of excretion is through the bile into feces.

D. Adverse effects

The most frequent adverse effects of *tamoxifen* and *toremifene* are hot flashes and nausea. Due to its estrogenic activity in the endometrium, endometrial hyperplasia and malignancies have been reported with *tamoxifen* therapy. This has led to recommendations for limiting the length of time on the drug for some indications. Because it is metabolized by various CYP450 isoenzymes, *tamoxifen* is subject to many drug interactions. [Note: *Tamoxifen* is also an inhibitor of CYP3A4 and P-glycoprotein.] Some CYP450 inhibitors may prevent the formation of active metabolites of *tamoxifen* and possibly reduce the efficacy (for example, *amiodarone, haloperidol, risperidone*). Hot flashes and leg cramps are common adverse effects with *raloxifene*. In addition, there is an increased risk of deep vein thrombosis, pulmonary embolism, and retinal vein thrombosis. Women who have a past or active history of venous thromboembolic events should not take the drug. *Cholestyramine* can significantly reduce the absorption of *raloxifene*, and concurrent use should be avoided. Adverse effects of *clomiphene* are dose related and include headache, nausea, vasomotor flushes, visual disturbances, and ovarian enlargement. Use of *clomiphene* increases the risk of multiple births (twins or triplets).

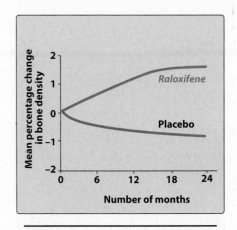

Figure 26.5
Hip bone density increases with *raloxifene* in postmenopausal women.

IV. PROGESTOGENS

Progesterone, the natural progestogen, is produced in response to luteinizing hormone (LH) by both females (secreted by the corpus luteum, primarily during the second half of the menstrual cycle, and by the placenta)

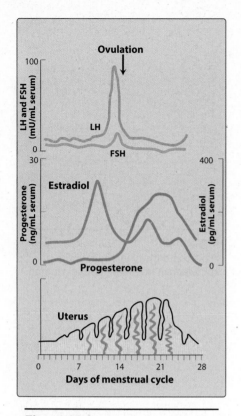

Figure 26.6
The menstrual cycle with plasma
levels of pituitary and ovarian
hormones and a schematic
representation of changes in the
morphology of the uterine lining.
FSH = follicle-stimulating hormone;
LH = luteinizing hormone.

and by males (secreted by the testes). It is also synthesized by the adrenal cortex in both sexes.

A. Mechanism of action

Progestogens exert their mechanism of action in a manner analogous to that of the other steroid hormones. In females, *progesterone* promotes the development of a secretory endometrium that can accommodate implantation of a newly forming embryo. The high levels of *progesterone* that are released during the second half of the menstrual cycle (the luteal phase) inhibit the production of gonadotropin and, therefore, prevent further ovulation. If conception takes place, *progesterone* continues to be secreted, maintaining the endometrium in a favorable state for the continuation of the pregnancy and reducing uterine contractions. If conception does not take place, the release of *progesterone* from the corpus luteum ceases abruptly. This decline stimulates the onset of menstruation. Figure 26.6 summarizes the hormones produced during the menstrual cycle.

B. Therapeutic uses of progestogens

The major clinical uses of progestogens are for contraception or the treatment of hormone deficiency. For contraception, they are often used in combination with estrogens. *Progesterone* by itself is not used widely as a contraceptive therapy because of its rapid metabolism, resulting in low bioavailability. Synthetic progestogens (that is, progestins) used in contraception are more stable to first-pass metabolism, allowing lower doses when administered orally. These agents include *desogestrel* [des-oh-JES-trel], *dienogest* [dye-EN-oh-jest], *drospirenone* [droe-SPY-re-none], *levonorgestrel* [lee-voe-nor-JES-trel], *norethindrone* [nor-ETH-in-drone], *norethindrone acetate*, *norgestimate* [nor-JES-tih-mate], and *norgestrel* [nor-JES-trel]. *Medroxyprogesterone* [me-DROK-see-proe-JES-ter-one] *acetate* is an injectable contraceptive, and the oral form is a common progestin component of postmenopausal HT. Progestins are also used for the control of dysfunctional uterine bleeding, treatment of dysmenorrhea, and management of endometriosis and infertility.

C. Pharmacokinetics

A micronized preparation of *progesterone* is rapidly absorbed after oral administration. It has a short half-life in the plasma and is almost completely metabolized by the liver. The glucuronidated metabolite is excreted primarily by the kidney. Synthetic progestins are less rapidly metabolized. Oral *medroxyprogesterone acetate* has a half-life of 30 days. When injected intramuscularly or subcutaneously, it has a half-life of about 40 to 50 days and provides contraceptive activity for approximately 3 months. The other progestins have half-lives of 1 to 3 days, allowing for once-daily dosing.

D. Adverse effects

The major adverse effects associated with the use of progestins are headache, depression, weight gain, and changes in libido (Figure 26.7). Progestins that are derived from 19-nortestosterone (for example, *norethindrone*, *norethindrone acetate*, *norgestrel*, *levonorgestrel*) possess some androgenic activity because of their structural similarity to *testosterone* and can cause acne and hirsutism. Less androgenic progestins, such as *norgestimate* and *drospirenone*, may be preferred in women with acne. *Drospirenone* may raise serum potassium due to antimineralocorticoid effects, and concurrent use with other drugs that increase potassium (for example, angiotensin-converting enzyme inhibitors) may increase the risk of hyperkalemia.

E. Antiprogestin

Mifepristone [mih-feh-PRIH-stone] (also designated as RU-486) is a progesterone antagonist with partial agonist activity. Administration of this drug to females early in pregnancy usually results in abortion of the fetus due to interference with the *progesterone* needed to maintain pregnancy. *Mifepristone* is often combined with the prostaglandin analog *misoprostol* (administered orally or intravaginally) to induce uterine contractions. The major adverse effects are significant uterine bleeding and the possibility of an incomplete abortion.

V. CONTRACEPTIVES

Currently, interference with ovulation is the most common pharmacologic intervention for prevention of pregnancy. Figure 26.8 outlines the frequency of use for various hormonal and nonhormonal methods of contraception.

A. Major classes of contraceptives

1. **Combination oral contraceptives:** Products containing a combination of an estrogen and a progestin are the most common type of oral contraceptives. Monophasic combination pills contain a constant dose of estrogen and progestin given over 21 to 24 days.

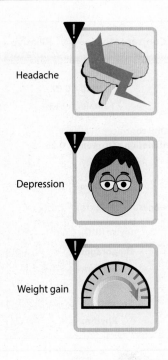

Figure 26.7
Some adverse effects associated with progestin therapy.

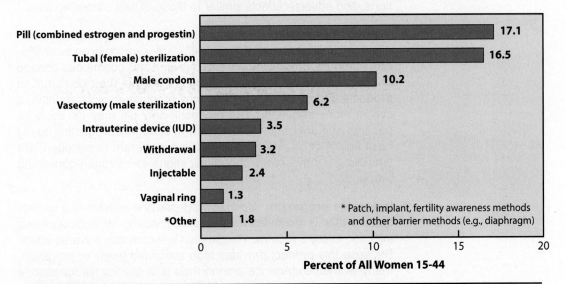

Figure 26.8
Comparison of contraceptive use among U.S. women ages 15 to 44 years.

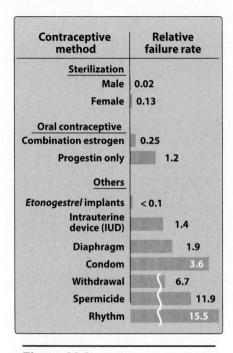

Contraceptive method	Relative failure rate
Sterilization	
Male	0.02
Female	0.13
Oral contraceptive	
Combination estrogen	0.25
Progestin only	1.2
Others	
Etonogestrel implants	< 0.1
Intrauterine device (IUD)	1.4
Diaphragm	1.9
Condom	3.6
Withdrawal	6.7
Spermicide	11.9
Rhythm	15.5

Figure 26.9
Comparison of failure rate for various methods of contraception. *Longer bars* indicate a higher failure rate—that is, more pregnancies.

Triphasic oral contraceptive products attempt to mimic the natural female cycle and most contain a constant dose of estrogen with increasing doses of progestin given over three successive 7-day periods. [Note: The combination of *estradiol valerate* and *dienogest* is available as a four-phasic oral contraceptive.] With most oral contraceptives, active pills are taken for 21 to 24 days, followed by 4 to 7 days of placebo, for a total regimen of 28 days. Withdrawal bleeding occurs during the hormone-free (placebo) interval. [Note: The most common estrogen in the combination pills is *ethinyl estradiol*. The most common progestins are *norethindrone, norethindrone acetate, levonorgestrel, desogestrel, norgestimate,* and *drospirenone*.] These preparations are highly effective in achieving contraception (Figure 26.9). Use of extended-cycle contraception (84 active pills followed by 7 days of placebo) results in less frequent withdrawal bleeding. A continuous oral contraceptive product (active pills taken every day) is also available.

2. **Transdermal patch:** An alternative to combination oral contraceptives is a transdermal patch containing *ethinyl estradiol* and the progestin *norelgestromin*. One contraceptive patch is applied each week for 3 weeks to the abdomen, upper torso, or buttock. No patch is worn during the 4th week, and withdrawal bleeding occurs. The transdermal patch has efficacy comparable to that of the oral contraceptives, but it is less effective in women weighing greater than 90 kg. Contraindications and adverse effects for the patch are similar to those of oral contraceptives. Total estrogen exposure with the transdermal patch may be significantly greater than that seen with oral contraceptives. Increased exposure to estrogen may increase the risk of adverse events such as thromboembolism.

3. **Vaginal ring:** An additional contraceptive option is a vaginal ring containing *ethinyl estradiol* and *etonogestrel*. The ring is inserted into the vagina and is left in place for 3 weeks and then removed. No ring is used during the fourth week, and withdrawal bleeding occurs. The contraceptive vaginal ring has efficacy, contraindications, and adverse effects similar to those of oral contraceptives.

4. **Progestin-only pills:** Products containing a progestin only, usually *norethindrone* (called a "mini-pill"), are taken daily on a continuous schedule. Progestin-only pills deliver a low, continuous dosage of drug. These preparations are less effective than combination products (Figure 26.9), and they may produce irregular menstrual cycles more frequently. The progestin-only pill may be used for patients who are breast-feeding (unlike estrogen, progestins do not have an effect on milk production), are intolerant to estrogen, are smokers, or have other contraindications to estrogen-containing products.

5. **Injectable progestin:** *Medroxyprogesterone acetate* is a contraceptive that is administered via intramuscular or subcutaneous injection every 3 months. Weight gain is a common adverse effect. Because this product provides high sustained levels of progestin, many women experience amenorrhea with *medroxyprogesterone acetate*. In addition, return to fertility may be delayed for several months after discontinuation. *Medroxyprogesterone acetate* may

contribute to bone loss and predispose patients to osteoporosis and/or fractures. Therefore, the drug should not be continued for more than 2 years unless the patient is unable to tolerate other contraceptive options.

6. **Progestin implants:** After subdermal placement, the *etonogestrel* implant offers contraception for approximately 3 years. The implant is nearly as reliable as sterilization, and the effect is totally reversible when surgically removed. Principal side effects of the implant are irregular menstrual bleeding and headaches. The *etonogestrel* implant has not been studied in women who weigh more than 130% of ideal body weight and may be less effective in this population.

7. **Progestin intrauterine device:** A *levonorgestrel*-releasing intrauterine system offers a highly effective method of contraception for 3 to 5 years depending on the system. It is a suitable method of contraception for women who desire long-term contraception and those who have contraindications to estrogen therapy. It should be avoided in patients with pelvic inflammatory disease or a history of ectopic pregnancy.

8. **Postcoital contraception:** Postcoital or emergency contraception reduces the probability of pregnancy after an episode of coitus without effective contraception (Figure 26.10) to between 0.2% and 3%. Emergency contraception uses high doses of *levonorgestrel* (preferred) or high doses of *ethinyl estradiol* plus *levonorgestrel*. For maximum effectiveness, emergency contraception should be taken as soon as possible after unprotected intercourse and preferably within 72 hours. The progestin-only emergency contraceptive regimens are generally better tolerated than the estrogen–progestin combination regimens. An alternative emergency contraceptive is the progesterone agonist/antagonist *ulipristal* [ue-li-PRIS-tal]. It is indicated for emergency contraception within 5 days of unprotected intercourse.

B. Mechanism of action

Estrogen provides a negative feedback on the release of LH and follicle-stimulating hormone (FSH) by the pituitary gland, thus preventing ovulation. Progestin also thickens the cervical mucus, thus hampering the transport of sperm. Withdrawal of the progestin stimulates menstrual bleeding during the placebo week.

C. Adverse effects

The incidence of adverse effects with oral contraceptives is determined by the specific compounds and combinations used. The most common adverse effects with estrogens are breast fullness, fluid retention, headache, and nausea. Increased blood pressure may also occur. Progestins may be associated with depression, changes in libido, hirsutism, and acne. Although rare, thromboembolism, thrombophlebitis, myocardial infarction, and stroke may occur with use of oral contraceptives. These severe adverse effects are most common among women who are over age 35 and smoke. The incidence of cervical cancer may be increased with oral contraceptives, because

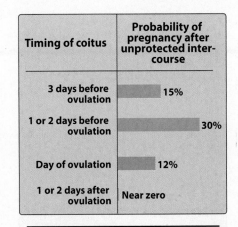

Timing of coitus	Probability of pregnancy after unprotected intercourse
3 days before ovulation	15%
1 or 2 days before ovulation	30%
Day of ovulation	12%
1 or 2 days after ovulation	Near zero

Figure 26.10
Risk of pregnancy after unprotected intercourse in young couples in their mid twenties.

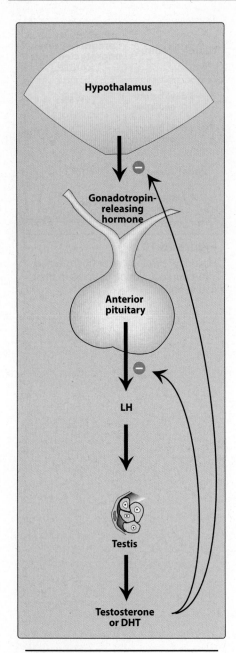

Figure 26.11
Regulation of secretion
of testosterone.
DHT = 5-α-dihydrotestosterone;
LH = luteinizing hormone.

women are less likely to use additional barrier methods of contraception that reduce exposure to human papillomavirus (the primary risk factor for cervical cancer). [Note: Oral contraceptives are associated with a decreased risk of cervical and ovarian cancer.] Oral contraceptives are contraindicated in the presence of cerebrovascular and thromboembolic disease, estrogen-dependent neoplasms, liver disease, and pregnancy. Combination oral contraceptives should not be used in patients over the age of 35 who are heavy smokers. Drugs that induce the CYP3A4 isoenzyme (for example, *rifampin* and *bosentan*) may significantly reduce the efficacy of oral contraceptives. Concurrent use of these agents with oral contraceptives should be avoided, or an alternate barrier method of contraception should be utilized. Antibiotics that alter the normal gastrointestinal flora may reduce enterohepatic recycling of the estrogen component of oral contraceptives, thereby diminishing the effectiveness. Patients should be warned of the possible interaction between antibiotics and oral contraceptives, along with the potential need for an alternate method of contraception during antibiotic therapy.

VI. ANDROGENS

The androgens are a group of steroids that have anabolic and/or masculinizing effects in both males and females. *Testosterone* [tess-TOSS-te-rone], the most important androgen in humans, is synthesized by Leydig cells in the testes and, in smaller amounts, by thecal cells in the ovaries and by the adrenal gland in both sexes. Other androgens secreted by the testes are 5α-dihydrotestosterone (DHT), androstenedione, and dehydroepiandrosterone (DHEA) in small amounts. In adult males, *testosterone* secretion by Leydig cells is controlled by gonadotropin-releasing hormone from the hypothalamus, which stimulates the anterior pituitary gland to secrete FSH and LH. *Testosterone* or its active metabolite, DHT, inhibits production of these specific trophic hormones through a negative feedback loop and, thus, regulates *testosterone* production (Figure 26.11). The androgens are required for 1) normal maturation in the male, 2) sperm production, 3) increased synthesis of muscle proteins and hemoglobin, and 4) decreased bone resorption. Synthetic modifications of the androgen structure modify solubility and susceptibility to enzymatic breakdown (thus prolonging the half-life of the hormone) and separate anabolic and androgenic effects.

A. Mechanism of action

Like the estrogens and progestins, androgens bind to a specific nuclear receptor in a target cell. Although *testosterone* itself is the active ligand in muscle and liver, in other tissues it must be metabolized to derivatives, such as DHT. For example, after diffusing into the cells of the prostate, seminal vesicles, epididymis, and skin, *testosterone* is converted by 5α-reductase to DHT, which binds to the receptor.

B. Therapeutic uses

Androgenic steroids are used for males with primary hypogonadism (caused by testicular dysfunction) or secondary hypogonadism (due to failure of the hypothalamus or pituitary). Anabolic steroids can be used to treat chronic wasting associated with human immunodeficiency virus or cancer. An unapproved use of anabolic steroids is to increase lean body mass, muscle strength, and endurance in athletes and body builders (see below). DHEA (a precursor of *testosterone* and estrogen) has been touted as an antiaging hormone as well as a "performance enhancer." There is no definitive evidence that it slows aging, however, or that it improves performance at normal therapeutic doses. *Danazol* [DAH-nah-zole], a weak androgen, is used in the treatment of endometriosis (ectopic growth of the endometrium) and fibrocystic breast disease. [Note: *Danazol* also possesses antiestrogenic activity.] Weight gain, acne, decreased breast size, deepening voice, increased libido, and increased hair growth are among the adverse effects.

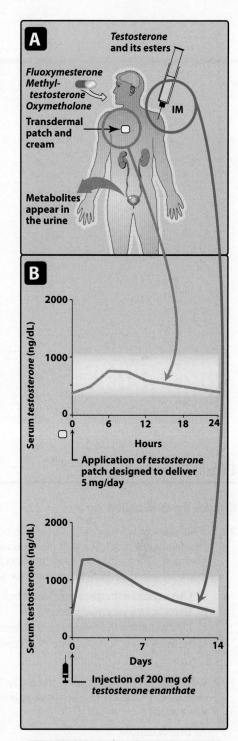

C. Pharmacokinetics

1. **Testosterone:** This agent is ineffective orally because of inactivation by first-pass metabolism. As with the other sex steroids, *testosterone* is rapidly absorbed and is metabolized to relatively or completely inactive compounds that are excreted primarily in the urine. C_{17}-esters of *testosterone* (for example, *testosterone cypionate* or *enanthate*) are administered intramuscularly. [Note: The addition of the esterified lipid makes the hormone more lipid soluble, thereby increasing its duration of action.] Transdermal patches, topical gels, and buccal tablets of *testosterone* are also available. Figure 26.12 shows serum levels of *testosterone* achieved by injection and by a transdermal patch in hypogonadal men. *Testosterone* and its esters demonstrate a 1:1 relative ratio of androgenic to anabolic activity.

2. **Testosterone derivatives:** Alkylation of the 17α position of *testosterone* allows oral administration of the hormone. Agents such as *fluoxymesterone* [floo-ox-ee-MESS-teh-rone] have a longer half-life in the body than that of the naturally occurring androgen. *Fluoxymesterone* is effective when given orally, and it has a 1:2 androgenic-to-anabolic ratio. *Oxandrolone* [ox-AN-droe-lone] is another orally active testosterone derivative with anabolic activity 3 to 13 times that of *testosterone*. Hepatic adverse effects have been associated with the 17α-alkylated androgens.

D. Adverse effects

1. **In females:** Androgens can cause masculinization, acne, growth of facial hair, deepening of the voice, male pattern baldness, and excessive muscle development. Menstrual irregularities may also occur. *Testosterone* should not be used by pregnant women because of possible virilization of the female fetus.

2. **In males:** Excess androgens can cause priapism, impotence, decreased spermatogenesis, and gynecomastia. Cosmetic changes such as those described for females may occur as well. Androgens can also stimulate growth of the prostate.

3. **In children:** Androgens can cause abnormal sexual maturation and growth disturbances resulting from premature closing of the epiphyseal plates.

Figure 26.12
A. Administration and fate of androgens. IM = intramuscularly.
B. Serum testosterone concentrations after administration by injection or transdermal patch to hypogonadal men. The *yellow band* indicates the upper and lower limits of normal.

4. General effects: Androgens can increase serum LDL and lower serum high-density lipoprotein levels. Whether these changes in the lipid profile predispose patients to heart disease is unknown. Androgens can also cause fluid retention, leading to edema.

5. In athletes: Use of anabolic steroids (for example, DHEA) by athletes can cause premature closing of the epiphysis of the long bones, which stunts growth and interrupts development. High doses taken by young athletes may result in reduction of testicular size, hepatic abnormalities, increased aggression ("roid rage"), major mood disorders, and other adverse effects described above.

E. Antiandrogens

Antiandrogens counter male hormonal action by interfering with the synthesis of androgens or by blocking their receptors. *Finasteride* [fin-AS-ter-ide] and *dutasteride* [doo-TAS-ter-ride] inhibit 5α-reductase resulting in decreased formation of dihydrotestosterone. These agents are used for the treatment of benign prostatic hyperplasia (see Chapter 32). Antiandrogens, such as *flutamide* [FLOO-tah-mide], *bicalutamide* [bye-ka-LOO-ta-mide], *enzalutamide* [enz-a-LOO-ta-mide], and *nilutamide* [nye-LOO-ta-mide], act as competitive inhibitors of androgens at the target cell and are effective orally for the treatment of prostate cancer (see Chapter 46).

Study Questions

Choose the ONE best answer.

26.1 A 53-year-old woman has severe vasomotor symptoms (hot flushes) associated with menopause. She has no pertinent past medical or surgical history. Which of the following would be most appropriate for her symptoms?

A. Conjugated estrogens vaginal cream.
B. Estradiol transdermal patch.
C. Oral estradiol and medroxyprogesterone acetate.
D. Injectable medroxyprogesterone acetate.

Correct answer = C. Estrogen vaginal cream only treats vaginal symptoms of menopause such as vaginal atrophy and does not treat hot flushes. Since this patient has an intact uterus, a progestin such as medroxyprogesterone needs to be used along with the estrogen to prevent the development of endometrial hyperplasia. Unopposed estrogen (for example, the estradiol transdermal patch) should not be used. Injectable medroxyprogesterone acetate is used for contraception.

26.2 A 70-year-old woman is being treated with raloxifene for osteoporosis. Which of the following is a concern with this therapy?

A. Breast cancer.
B. Endometrial cancer.
C. Venous thrombosis.
D. Hypercholesterolemia.

Correct answer = C. Raloxifene can increase the risk of venous thromboembolism. Unlike estrogen and tamoxifen, raloxifene does not result in an increased incidence of endometrial cancer. Raloxifene lowers the risk of breast cancer in high-risk women, and it also lowers LDL cholesterol.

26.3 Which of the following is the most appropriate oral contraceptive for a patient with moderate acne?

A. Ethinyl estradiol/levonorgestrel.
B. Ethinyl estradiol/norethindrone acetate.
C. Ethinyl estradiol/norgestimate.
D. Ulipristal.

Correct answer = C. The progestins levonorgestrel and norethindrone acetate may have androgenic activity and contribute to acne. Norgestimate has less androgenic activity and is preferred for this patient. Ulipristal is an emergency contraceptive and should not be used as a regular method of contraception.

26.4 A 26-year-old female is using injectable medroxy-progesterone acetate as a method of contraception. Which of the following adverse effects is a concern if she wishes to use this therapy long-term?

A. Hyperkalemia.
B. Male pattern baldness.
C. Osteoporosis.
D. Weight loss.

Correct answer = C. Medroxyprogesterone acetate may contribute to bone loss and predispose patients to osteoporosis and/or fractures. Therefore, the drug should not be continued for more than 2 years if possible. The drug often causes weight gain, not weight loss. The other adverse effects are not associated with medroxyprogesterone.

Adrenal Hormones

27

Karen Whalen

I. OVERVIEW

The adrenal gland consists of the cortex and the medulla. The medulla secretes catecholamines, whereas the cortex, the subject of this chapter, secretes two types of corticosteroids (glucocorticoids and mineralocorticoids; Figure 27.1) and the adrenal androgens. The adrenal cortex has three zones, and each zone synthesizes a different type of steroid hormone from cholesterol (Figure 27.2). The outer zona glomerulosa produces mineralocorticoids (for example, aldosterone) that are responsible for regulating salt and water metabolism. Production of aldosterone is regulated primarily by the renin–angiotensin system (see Chapter 17). The middle zona fasciculata synthesizes glucocorticoids (for example, cortisol) that are involved with metabolism and response to stress. The inner zona reticularis secretes adrenal androgens (see Chapter 26 for a discussion of androgens). Secretion by the two inner zones and, to a lesser extent, the outer zone is controlled by pituitary adrenocorticotropic hormone (ACTH; also called corticotropin), which is released in response to hypothalamic corticotropin-releasing hormone (CRH). Glucocorticoids serve as feedback inhibitors of ACTH and CRH secretion.

II. CORTICOSTEROIDS

The corticosteroids bind to specific intracellular cytoplasmic receptors in target tissues. Glucocorticoid receptors are widely distributed throughout the body, whereas mineralocorticoid receptors are confined mainly to excretory organs, such as the kidney, colon, salivary glands and sweat glands. Both types of receptors are found in the brain. After dimerizing, the receptor–hormone complex recruits coactivator (or corepressor) proteins and translocates into the nucleus, where it attaches to gene promoter elements. There it acts as a transcription factor to turn genes on (when complexed with coactivators) or off (when complexed with corepressors), depending on the tissue (Figure 27.3). This mechanism requires time to produce an effect. However, other glucocorticoid effects are immediate, such as the interaction with catecholamines to mediate relaxation of bronchial musculature. This section describes normal actions and therapeutic uses of corticosteroids.

A. Glucocorticoids

Cortisol is the principal human glucocorticoid. Normally, its production is diurnal, with a peak early in the morning followed by a decline and

CORTICOSTEROIDS
Betamethasone CELESTONE, DIPROLENE, LUXIQ
Cortisone CORTISONE ACETATE
Dexamethasone DECADRON
Fludrocortisone FLORINEF
Hydrocortisone
Methylprednisolone MEDROL
Prednisolone ORAPRED, PEDIAPRED
Prednisone
Triamcinolone KENALOG, NASACORT, ARISTOSPAN

INHIBITORS OF ADRENOCORTICOID BIOSYNTHESIS OR FUNCTION
Eplerenone INSPRA
Ketoconazole NIZORAL
Spironolactone ALDACTONE

Figure 27.1
Summary of adrenal corticosteroids.

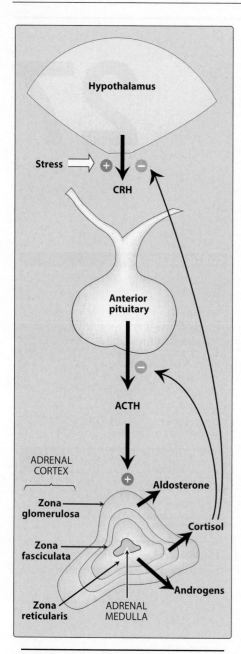

Figure 27.2
Regulation of corticosteroid secretion.
ACTH = adrenocorticotropic hormone;
CRH = corticotropin-releasing hormone.

then a secondary, smaller peak in the late afternoon. Factors such as stress and levels of the circulating steroid influence secretion. The effects of cortisol are many and diverse. In general, all glucocorticoids:

1. **Promote normal intermediary metabolism:** Glucocorticoids favor gluconeogenesis through increasing amino acid uptake by the liver and kidney and elevating activities of gluconeogenic enzymes. They stimulate protein catabolism (except in the liver) and lipolysis, thereby providing the building blocks and energy that are needed for glucose synthesis. [Note: Glucocorticoid insufficiency may result in hypoglycemia (for example, during stressful periods or fasting).]

2. **Increase resistance to stress:** By raising plasma glucose levels, glucocorticoids provide the body with energy to combat stress caused by trauma, fright, infection, bleeding, or debilitating disease.

3. **Alter blood cell levels in plasma:** Glucocorticoids cause a decrease in eosinophils, basophils, monocytes, and lymphocytes by redistributing them from the circulation to lymphoid tissue. Glucocorticoids also increase hemoglobin, erythrocytes, platelets, and polymorphonuclear leukocytes.

4. **Have anti-inflammatory action:** The most important therapeutic properties of the glucocorticoids are their potent anti-inflammatory and immunosuppressive activities. These therapeutic effects of glucocorticoids are the result of a number of actions. The lowering of circulating lymphocytes is known to play a role. In addition, these agents inhibit the ability of leukocytes and macrophages to respond to mitogens and antigens. Glucocorticoids also decrease the production and release of proinflammatory cytokines. They inhibit phospholipase A_2, which blocks the release of arachidonic acid (the precursor of the prostaglandins and leukotrienes) from membrane-bound phospholipid. The decreased production of prostaglandins and leukotrienes is believed to be central to the anti-inflammatory action. Lastly, these agents influence the inflammatory response by stabilizing mast cell and basophil membranes, resulting in decreased histamine release.

5. **Affect other systems:** High levels of glucocorticoids serve as feedback inhibitors of ACTH production and affect the endocrine system by suppressing further synthesis of glucocorticoids and thyroid-stimulating hormone. In addition, adequate cortisol levels are essential for normal glomerular filtration. The effects of corticosteroids on other systems are mostly associated with adverse effects of the hormones (see Adverse Effects below).

B. Mineralocorticoids

Mineralocorticoids help to control fluid status and concentration of electrolytes, especially sodium and potassium. Aldosterone acts on distal tubules and collecting ducts in the kidney, causing reabsorption of sodium, bicarbonate, and water. Conversely, aldosterone decreases reabsorption of potassium, which, with H^+, is then lost in the urine. Enhancement of sodium reabsorption by aldosterone also occurs in gastrointestinal mucosa and in sweat and salivary glands.

[Note: Elevated aldosterone levels may cause alkalosis and hypokalemia, retention of sodium and water, and increased blood volume and blood pressure. Hyperaldosteronism is treated with *spironolactone*.] Target cells for aldosterone contain mineralocorticoid receptors that interact with the hormone in a manner analogous to that of glucocorticoid receptors.

C. Therapeutic uses of the corticosteroids

Several semisynthetic derivatives of corticosteroids are available. These agents vary in anti-inflammatory potency, mineralocorticoid activity, and duration of action (Figure 27.4). Corticosteroids are used in replacement therapy and in the treatment of severe allergic reactions, asthma, rheumatoid arthritis, other inflammatory disorders, and some cancers.

1. **Replacement therapy for primary adrenocortical insufficiency (Addison disease):** Addison disease is caused by adrenal cortex dysfunction (as diagnosed by the lack of response to ACTH administration). *Hydrocortisone* [hye-droe-KOR-tih-sone], which is identical to natural cortisol, is given to correct the deficiency. Failure to do so results in death. The dosage of *hydrocortisone* is divided so that two-thirds of the daily dose is given in the morning and one-third is given in the afternoon. [Note: The goal of this regimen is to mimic the normal diurnal variation in cortisol levels.] Administration of *fludrocortisone* [floo-droe-KOR-tih-sone], a potent synthetic mineralocorticoid with some glucocorticoid activity, may also be necessary to supplement mineralocorticoid deficiency.

2. **Replacement therapy for secondary or tertiary adrenocortical insufficiency:** These disorders are caused by a defect in CRH production by the hypothalamus or in ACTH production by the pituitary. [Note: Under these conditions, the synthesis of mineralocorticoids in the adrenal cortex is less impaired than that of glucocorticoids.] *Hydrocortisone* is used for treatment of these deficiencies.

3. **Diagnosis of Cushing syndrome:** Cushing syndrome is caused by hypersecretion of glucocorticoids (hypercortisolism) that results from excessive release of ACTH by the anterior pituitary or an adrenal tumor. [Note: Chronic treatment with high doses of glucocorticoids is a frequent cause of iatrogenic Cushing syndrome.] Cortisol levels (urine, plasma, and saliva) and the *dexamethasone* [dex-a-METH-a-sone] suppression test are used to diagnose Cushing syndrome. The synthetic glucocorticoid *dexamethasone* suppresses cortisol release in normal individuals, but not those with Cushing syndrome.

4. **Replacement therapy for congenital adrenal hyperplasia (CAH):** CAH is a group of diseases resulting from an enzyme defect in the synthesis of one or more of the adrenal steroid hormones. CAH may lead to virilization in females due to overproduction of adrenal androgens. Treatment of the condition requires administration of sufficient corticosteroids to normalize hormone

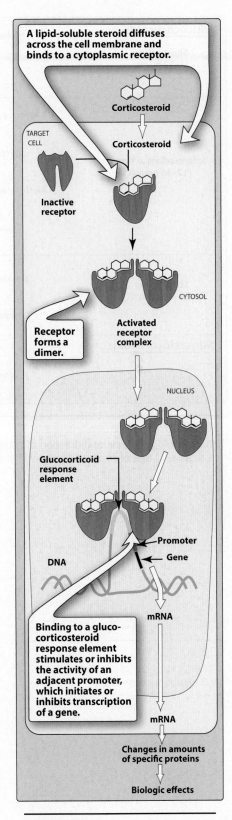

Figure 27.3
Gene regulation by glucocorticoids.

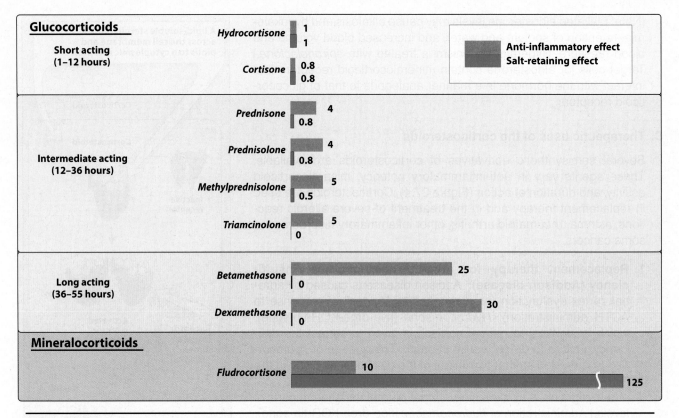

Figure 27.4
Pharmacologic effects and duration of action of some commonly used natural and synthetic corticosteroids. Activities are all relative to that of *hydrocortisone,* which is considered to be 1.

levels by suppressing release of CRH and ACTH. This decreases production of adrenal androgens. The choice of replacement hormone depends on the specific enzyme defect.

5. **Relief of inflammatory symptoms:** Corticosteroids significantly reduce the manifestations of inflammation associated with rheumatoid arthritis and inflammatory skin conditions, including redness, swelling, heat, and tenderness that may be present at the site of inflammation. These agents are also important for maintenance of symptom control in persistent asthma, as well as management of asthma exacerbations and active inflammatory bowel disease. In noninflammatory disorders such as osteoarthritis, intra-articular corticosteroids may be used for treatment of a disease flare. Corticosteroids are not curative in these disorders.

6. **Treatment of allergies:** Corticosteroids are beneficial in the treatment of allergic rhinitis, as well as drug, serum, and transfusion allergic reactions. [Note: In the treatment of allergic rhinitis and asthma, *fluticasone* [floo-TIK-a-sone] and others (see Figure 27.5) are applied topically to the respiratory tract through inhalation from a metered dose dispenser. This minimizes systemic effects and allows the patient to reduce or eliminate the use of oral corticosteroids.]

7. **Acceleration of lung maturation:** Respiratory distress syndrome is a problem in premature infants. Fetal cortisol is a regulator of

lung maturation. Consequently, a regimen of *betamethasone* or *dexamethasone* administered intramuscularly to the mother within the 48 hours proceeding premature delivery can accelerate lung maturation in the fetus.

D. Pharmacokinetics

1. **Absorption and fate:** Orally administered corticosteroid preparations are readily absorbed. Selected compounds can also be administered intravenously, intramuscularly, intra-articularly (for example, into arthritic joints), topically, or via inhalation or intranasal delivery (Figure 27.5). All topical and inhaled glucocorticoids are absorbed to some extent and, therefore, have the potential to cause hypothalamic–pituitary–adrenal (HPA) axis suppression. Greater than 90% of absorbed glucocorticoids are bound to plasma proteins, mostly corticosteroid-binding globulin or albumin. Corticosteroids are metabolized by the liver microsomal oxidizing enzymes. The metabolites are conjugated to glucuronic acid or sulfate, and the products are excreted by the kidney. [Note: The half-life of corticosteroids may increase substantially in hepatic dysfunction.] *Prednisone* [PRED-nih-sone] is preferred in pregnancy because it minimizes steroid effects on the fetus. It is a prodrug that is not converted to the active compound, *prednisolone* [pred-NIH-so-lone], in the fetal liver. Any *prednisolone* formed in the mother is biotransformed to *prednisone* by placental enzymes.

2. **Dosage:** Many factors should be considered in determining the dosage of corticosteroids, including glucocorticoid versus mineralocorticoid activity, duration of action, type of preparation, and time of day when the drug is administered. When large doses of the hormone are required for more than 2 weeks, suppression of the HPA axis occurs. Alternate-day administration of the corticosteroid may prevent this adverse effect by allowing the HPA axis to recover/function on days the hormone is not taken.

E. Adverse effects

Common side effects of long-term corticosteroid therapy are summarized in Figure 27.6. Adverse effects are often dose related. For example, in patients with rheumatoid arthritis, the daily dose of *prednisone* was the strongest predictor of occurrence of adverse effects (Figure 27.7). Osteoporosis is the most common adverse effect due to the ability of glucocorticoids to suppress intestinal Ca^{2+} absorption, inhibit bone formation, and decrease sex hormone synthesis. Patients are advised to take calcium and vitamin D supplements. Bisphosphonates may also be useful in the treatment of glucocorticoid-induced osteoporosis. [Note: Increased appetite is not necessarily an adverse effect. In fact, it is one of the reasons for the use of *prednisone* in cancer chemotherapy.] The classic Cushing-like syndrome (redistribution of body fat, puffy face, hirsutism, and increased appetite) is observed in excess corticosteroid replacement. Cataracts may also occur with long-term corticosteroid therapy. Hyperglycemia may develop and lead to diabetes mellitus. Diabetic patients should monitor blood glucose and adjust medications accordingly if taking corticosteroids. Coadministration of medications that induce or inhibit the hepatic mixed-function oxidases may require adjustment of the

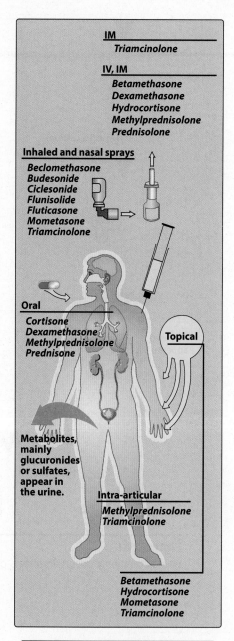

Figure 27.5
Routes of administration and elimination of corticosteroids.

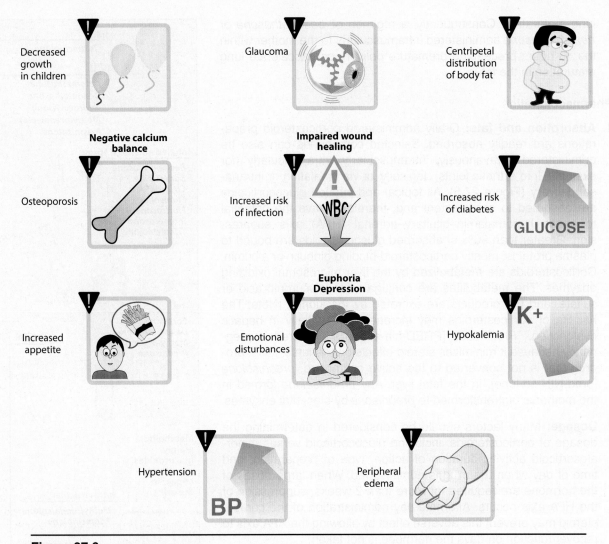

Figure 27.6
Some commonly observed effects of long-term corticosteroid therapy. BP = blood pressure.

glucocorticoid dose. Topical therapy can also cause skin atrophy, ecchymosis, and purple striae.

F. Discontinuation

Sudden discontinuation of these drugs can be a serious problem if the patient has suppression of the HPA axis. In this case, abrupt removal of corticosteroids causes acute adrenal insufficiency that can be fatal. This risk, coupled with the possibility that withdrawal might cause an exacerbation of the disease, means that the dose must be tapered slowly according to individual tolerance. The patient must be monitored carefully.

G. Inhibitors of adrenocorticoid biosynthesis or function

Several substances have proven to be useful as inhibitors of the synthesis or function of adrenal steroids: *ketoconazole, spironolactone,* and *eplerenone.*

1. **Ketoconazole:** *Ketoconazole* [kee-toe-KON-ah-zole] is an anti-fungal agent that strongly inhibits all gonadal and adrenal steroid hormone synthesis. It is used in the treatment of patients with Cushing syndrome.

2. **Spironolactone:** This antihypertensive drug competes for the mineralocorticoid receptor and, thus, inhibits sodium reabsorption in the kidney. It can also antagonize aldosterone and testosterone synthesis. It is effective for hyperaldosteronism and is used along with other standard therapies for the treatment of heart failure with reduced ejection fraction. *Spironolactone* [speer-oh-no-LAK-tone] is also useful in the treatment of hirsutism in women, probably due to interference at the androgen receptor of the hair follicle. Adverse effects include hyperkalemia, gynecomastia, menstrual irregularities, and skin rashes.

3. **Eplerenone:** *Eplerenone* [e-PLER-ih-none] specifically binds to the mineralocorticoid receptor, where it acts as an aldosterone antagonist. This specificity avoids the side effect of gynecomastia that is associated with the use of *spironolactone*. It is approved for the treatment of hypertension and also for heart failure with reduced ejection fraction.

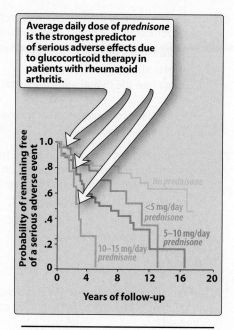

Figure 27.7
Probability of remaining free of a serious adverse event in patients with rheumatoid arthritis treated with no or different doses of *prednisone*.

Study Questions

Choose the ONE best answer.

27.1 Which of the following zones of the adrenal gland is correctly paired with the type of substance it secretes?

A. Adrenal medulla—corticotropin.
B. Zona fasciculata—cortisol.
C. Zona glomerulosa—androgens.
D. Zona reticularis—catecholamines.

Correct answer = B. The adrenal medulla secretes catecholamines. Corticotropin is secreted by the anterior pituitary. The zona glomerulosa secretes aldosterone, and the zona reticularis secretes androgens.

27.2 Corticosteroids are useful in the treatment of all of the following disorders except:

A. Addison disease.
B. Allergic rhinitis.
C. Cushing syndrome.
D. Inflammatory bowel disease.
E. Rheumatoid arthritis.

Correct answer = C. Cushing syndrome is an excess secretion of glucocorticoids. Dexamethasone may be used in the diagnosis of Cushing syndrome, but not its treatment. Treatment of Cushing syndrome usually consists of surgery or suppression of glucocorticoid production with ketoconazole or other agents. Corticosteroids are used frequently in the management of the other disorders listed.

27.3 All of the following adverse effects commonly occur with glucocorticoid therapy except:

A. Glaucoma.
B. Increased risk of infection.
C. Hypotension.
D. Emotional disturbances.
E. Peripheral edema.

Correct answer = C. Glucocorticoid therapy may cause hypertension, not hypotension. All the other adverse effects are associated with the use of glucocorticoids.

27.4 Osteoporosis is a major adverse effect caused by the glucocorticoids. It is due to their ability to:

A. Increase the excretion of calcium.

B. Inhibit absorption of calcium.

C. Stimulate the hypothalamic–pituitary–adrenal axis.

D. Decrease production of prostaglandins.

E. Decrease collagen synthesis.

Correct answer = B. Glucocorticoid-induced osteoporosis is attributed to inhibition of calcium absorption as well as bone formation. Increased intake of calcium plus vitamin D, bisphosphonates, or other drugs that are effective in this condition is indicated. Glucocorticoids suppress rather than stimulate the hypothalamic–pituitary–adrenal axis. The decreased production of prostaglandins does not play a role in bone formation.

27.5 A child with severe asthma is being treated with high doses of inhaled corticosteroids. Which of the following adverse effects is of particular concern?

A. Hypoglycemia.

B. Hirsutism.

C. Growth suppression.

D. Cushing syndrome.

E. Cataract formation.

Correct answer = C. Corticosteroids may retard bone growth. Chronic treatment with the medication therefore may lead to growth suppression, so linear growth should be monitored periodically. Hyperglycemia, not hypoglycemia, is a possible adverse effect. Hirsutism, Cushing syndrome, and cataract formation are unlikely with the dose that the child would receive by inhalation.

27.6 The diagnosis of congenital adrenal hyperplasia (CAH) is confirmed in a child. This condition can be effectively treated by:

A. Administering a glucocorticoid.

B. Administering an androgen antagonist.

C. Administering ketoconazole to decrease cortisol synthesis.

D. Removing the adrenal gland surgically.

E. Administering adrenocorticotropic hormone.

Correct answer = A. Congenital adrenal hyperplasia is seen in infancy and childhood. Because cortisol synthesis is decreased, feedback inhibition of adrenocorticotropic hormone (ACTH) formation and release is also decreased, resulting in enhanced ACTH formation. This in turn leads to increased levels of adrenal androgens and/or mineralocorticoids. The treatment is to administer a glucocorticoid, such as hydrocortisone (in infants) or prednisone, which would restore the feedback inhibition. The other options are inappropriate.

27.7 A patient with Addison disease is being treated with hydrocortisone but is still having problems with dehydration and hyponatremia. Which of the following drugs would be best to add to the patient's therapy?

A. Dexamethasone.

B. Fludrocortisone.

C. Prednisone.

D. Triamcinolone.

Correct answer = B. To combat dehydration and hyponatremia, a corticosteroid with high mineralocorticoid activity is needed. Fludrocortisone has the greatest mineralocorticoid activity of the agents provided. The other drugs have little or no mineralocorticoid activity.

27.8 All of the following are strategies to minimize the development of HPA axis suppression with corticosteroid therapy except:

A. Alternate-day administration of therapy.

B. Administration via topical or inhalation routes when possible.

C. Using the lowest dose of corticosteroid that adequately controls symptoms.

D. Administration of two-thirds of the daily dose in the morning and one-third in the afternoon.

Correct answer = D. Administration of two-thirds of the dose in the morning and one-third in the afternoon is a strategy to mimic the normal diurnal variation of cortisol secretion. However, it is not a strategy to prevent suppression of the HPA axis. All of the other methods will help prevent the likelihood of suppression of the HPA axis.

27.9 Which of the following patients would most likely have suppression of the HPA axis and require a slow taper of corticosteroid therapy?

A. A patient taking 40 mg of prednisone daily for 7 days to treat an asthma exacerbation.

B. A patient taking 10 mg of prednisone daily for 3 months for rheumatoid arthritis.

C. A patient using mometasone nasal spray daily for 6 months for allergic rhinitis.

D. A patient receiving an intra-articular injection of methylprednisolone for osteoarthritis.

Correct answer = B. Suppression of the HPA axis usually occurs with higher doses of corticosteroids when used for a duration of 2 weeks or more. Although the dose of prednisone is higher in the asthma patient, the duration of therapy is short, so the risk of HPA axis suppression is lower. The risk of HPA axis suppression is low with topical therapies like intranasal mometasone and with one-time joint injections.

27.10 Which of the following corticosteroids is most appropriate to administer to a woman in preterm labor to accelerate fetal lung maturation?

    A. Betamethasone.

    B. Fludrocortisone.

    C. Hydrocortisone.

    D. Prednisone.

Correct answer = A. A corticosteroid with high glucocorticoid activity is needed to speed fetal lung maturation prior to delivery. Betamethasone has high glucocorticoid activity and is one of the recommended drugs in this context. Dexamethasone is the other. Fludrocortisone mainly has mineralocorticoid activity and would not be useful in this situation. Hydrocortisone has much lower glucocorticoid activity. Prednisone has a higher glucocorticoid activity than hydrocortisone, but the fetus is not able to convert it to prednisolone, the active form.

Drugs for Obesity

28

Carol Motycka

I. OVERVIEW

The term obesity is given to individuals with a body mass index (BMI) of 30 kg/m² or greater. Obesity is due in part to an energy imbalance. Simply put, calorie consumption exceeds calorie expenditure. However, it is now well understood that genetics, metabolism, behavior, environment, culture, and socioeconomic status play a role in obesity, as well. An individual whose BMI is greater than 30 or greater than 27 with at least two comorbidities (for example, hypertension and diabetes) is considered a potential candidate for pharmacological treatment of obesity. A summary of medications for obesity is provided in Figure 28.1.

The majority of drugs approved to treat obesity have short-term indications for usage. However, some of the newer medications have been approved for long-term weight management. The older medications approved for short-term usage are the anorexiants *phentermine* and *diethylpropion*. There is a much larger list of anorexiants used off-label for weight loss; however, those drugs are not included in this chapter (see Chapter 16). The lipase inhibitor, *orlistat*, has been available for several years, and other lipase inhibitors are being considered for approval. Recently, a serotonin agonist, *lorcaserin*, and a combination drug, *phentermine and topiramate*, were also approved for the treatment of obesity. Drugs for obesity are considered effective if they demonstrate at least a 5% greater reduction in body weight as compared to placebo (no treatment). The medications discussed in this chapter have been shown in clinical trials to help patients lose approximately 5% to 10% of their body weight.

II. ANOREXIANTS (APPETITE SUPPRESSANTS)

Phentermine [FEN-ter-meen] and *diethylpropion* [dye-eth-ill-PROE-pee-on] are considered appetite suppressants.

A. Mechanism of action: *Phentermine* exerts its pharmacologic action by increasing the release of norepinephrine and dopamine from the nerve terminals and by inhibiting reuptake of these neurotransmitters, thereby increasing levels of neurotransmitters in the brain. The increase in norepinephrine signals a "fight-or-flight" response by the body, which, in turn, decreases appetite. *Diethylpropion* has similar

ANOREXIANTS
Diethylpropion TENUATE
Phentermine ADIPEX-P
LIPASE INHIBITORS
Orlistat ALLI, XENICAL
SEROTONIN AGONISTS
Lorcaserin BELVIQ
COMBINATION DRUGS
Phentermine/Topiramate QSYMIA

Figure 28.1
Summary of drugs used in the treatment of obesity.

effects on norepinephrine. Tolerance to the weight loss effect of these agents develops within weeks, and weight loss typically plateaus. An increase in the dosage generally does not result in further weight loss, and discontinuation of the drug is usually recommended once the plateau is reached.

B. Pharmacokinetics: Limited information is available regarding the pharmacokinetics of *phentermine*. The duration of activity is dependent on the formulation, and the primary route of excretion is via the kidneys. *Diethylpropion* is rapidly absorbed and undergoes extensive first-pass metabolism. Many of the metabolites are active. *Diethylpropion* and its metabolites are excreted mainly via the kidneys. The half-life of the metabolites is 4 to 8 hours.

C. Adverse effects: All of the anorexiants are classified as controlled substances due to the potential for dependence or abuse. Dry mouth, headache, insomnia, and constipation are common adverse effects. Heart rate and blood pressure may be increased with these agents. Therefore, these drugs should be avoided in patients with a history of uncontrolled hypertension, cardiovascular disease, arrhythmias, heart failure, or stroke. Concomitant use of anorexiants with monoamine oxidase inhibitors (MAOIs) or other sympathomimetics should be avoided.

III. LIPASE INHIBITORS

Orlistat [OR-lih-stat] is currently the only available agent in a class of antiobesity drugs known as lipase inhibitors. It is indicated for weight loss or weight maintenance. The clinical utility of *orlistat* is limited by gastrointestinal adverse effects.

A. Mechanism of action: *Orlistat* is a pentanoic acid ester that inhibits gastric and pancreatic lipases, thus decreasing the breakdown of dietary fat into smaller molecules that can be absorbed. Administration of *orlistat* decreases fat absorption by about 30%. The loss of calories from decreased absorption of fat is the main cause of weight loss. However, adverse gastrointestinal effects associated with the drug may also contribute to an overall decreased intake of food. Figure 28.2 shows the effects of *orlistat* treatment.

B. Pharmacokinetics: *Orlistat* is administered orally with each meal that contains fat. It has minimal systemic absorption and is mainly excreted in the feces. No dosage adjustments are required in patients with renal or hepatic dysfunction.

C. Adverse effects: The most common adverse effects associated with *orlistat* are gastrointestinal symptoms, such as oily spotting, flatulence with discharge, fecal urgency, and increased defecation. These effects may be minimized through a low-fat diet and the use of concomitant *cholestyramine*. Pancreatitis and liver injury have occurred rarely in people taking *orlistat*. *Orlistat* is contraindicated in pregnancy and in patients with chronic malabsorption syndrome or cholestasis. The drug also interferes with the absorption of fat-soluble vitamins and β-carotene. Thus, patients should be advised to take a multivitamin supplement that contains vitamins A, D, E, and K and also β-carotene. The vitamin supplement should not be taken within 2 hours of *orlistat*.

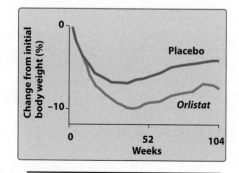

Figure 28.2

Effect of *orlistat* treatment on body weight.

Orlistat can also interfere with the absorption of other medications, such as *amiodarone, cyclosporine,* and *levothyroxine,* and clinical response to these medications should be monitored if *orlistat* is initiated. The dose of *levothyroxine* should be separated from *orlistat* by at least 4 hours.

IV. SEROTONIN AGONISTS

Lorcaserin [lor-KAS-er-in] is a newer serotonin agonist, with selectivity for the 2C serotonin receptor (5-HT$_{2C}$). It is used for chronic weight management. Previous serotonin agonists used for weight loss were pulled from the market following an increase in potentially fatal adverse effects, including valvular heart disease. It is believed that valvulopathy, which may lead to pulmonary hypertension, is linked to 5-HT$_{2B}$ receptors.

A. **Mechanism of action:** *Lorcaserin* selectively activates 5-HT$_{2C}$ receptors, which are almost exclusively found in the central nervous system. This activation, in turn, stimulates pro-opiomelanocortin neurons, which activate melanocortin receptors, thereby causing a decrease in appetite (Figure 28.3). If a patient does not lose at least 5% of their body weight after 12 weeks of use, the drug should be discontinued.

B. **Pharmacokinetics:** *Lorcaserin* is extensively metabolized in the liver to two inactive metabolites that are then eliminated in the urine. *Lorcaserin* has not been studied for use in severe hepatic impairment and is not recommended in severe renal impairment.

C. **Adverse effects:** The most common adverse effects observed with *lorcaserin* are nausea, headache, dry mouth, dizziness, constipation, and lethargy. Although rare, mood changes and suicidal ideation can occur. The development of life-threatening serotonin syndrome or neuroleptic malignant syndrome has been reported with the use of serotonin agonists. Therefore, patients should be monitored for the emergence of these conditions while on *lorcaserin*. Because of the increased risk of serotonin syndrome, concomitant use of *lorcaserin* with selective serotonin reuptake inhibitors, serotonin–norepinephrine reuptake inhibitors, MAOIs, or other serotonergic drugs should be avoided. As mentioned above, valvulopathy has been associated with the use of 5-HT$_{2B}$ receptor agonists. Although the incidence of valvulopathy was not significantly increased in studies of *lorcaserin*, a 5-HT$_{2C}$ receptor agonist, patients should still be monitored for the development of this condition. For that reason, individuals with a history of heart failure should use this agent with caution.

V. COMBINATION DRUGS

The combination of *phentermine* and *topiramate* has been approved for long-term use in the treatment of obesity. In initial studies of the anticonvulsant *topiramate*, it was observed that patients lost weight while taking the medication. This prompted further investigation into the use of *topiramate* for weight loss in obese individuals. Because of the sedating effects of *topiramate*, the stimulant *phentermine* was added to counteract the sedation and promote additional weight loss. The *phentermine/topiramate* combination is dosed in steps, escalating the dose every

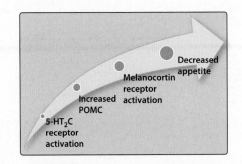

Figure 28.3
Lorcaserin mechanism of action.
POMC = pro-opiomelanocortin.

2 weeks, depending on the response. If a patient does not achieve a 5% weight loss after 12 weeks on the highest dose of this medication, then it should be discontinued. It is also important to note that this medication should not be stopped abruptly as seizures may be precipitated.

Topiramate has been associated with birth defects including cleft palate, and, thus, the combination of *phentermine/topiramate* is contraindicated in pregnancy. Other serious adverse effects with the *topiramate* component include paresthesias, suicidal ideation, and cognitive dysfunction. As discussed previously, potential adverse effects such as increased heart rate may be observed with the *phentermine* component. Several drug interactions may occur with this combination. Concomitant use of MAOIs should be avoided due to the possibility of serotonin syndrome with the *phentermine* component. The use of non–potassium-sparing diuretics with this combination may increase the risk of hypokalemia (low potassium). *Topiramate* is also a weak carbonic anhydrase inhibitor, and use of other carbonic anhydrase inhibitors with this combination increases the risk of kidney stones. *Topiramate* may reduce the efficacy of oral contraceptives, and this is a concern, given the risk of birth defects with this agent.

Study Questions

Choose the ONE best answer.

28.1 A 45-year-old female presents seeking treatment for weight loss. She has tried several fad diets in the past with very little success. She exercises twice weekly at the gym for 30 minutes and tries to watch what she eats. Her BMI is 31 and she has diabetes and uncontrolled hypertension. Which of the following medications would be most appropriate to treat her obesity?

A. Phentermine.
B. Phentermine/topiramate.
C. Orlistat.
D. Diethylpropion.

> Correct answer = C. Orlistat is the only medication of those listed that does not increase heart rate and blood pressure. Since this patient's blood pressure is currently uncontrolled, choosing a drug that does not affect blood pressure would be best at this time.

28.2 Which of the following drugs requires patients to take a multivitamin while on the medication?

A. Phentermine.
B. Phentermine/topiramate.
C. Orlistat.
D. Diethylpropion.
E. Lorcaserin.

> Correct answer = C. Orlistat interferes with the absorption of fat-soluble vitamins and β-carotene. It is important that individuals take the multivitamin 2 hours before or after administration of the orlistat.

28.3 A 38-year-old obese male with depression is considering a weight loss medication following several failed attempts with diet and exercise. Which of the following medications should be avoided in this individual?

A. Phentermine.
B. Phentermine/topiramate.
C. Orlistat.
D. Diethylpropion.
E. Lorcaserin.

> Correct answer = E. Lorcaserin may cause suicidal ideation and would not be advisable for an individual with depression. Also, he is likely on a medication that may increase serotonin levels. The addition of lorcaserin, a serotonin receptor agonist, could lead to serotonin syndrome. Therefore, avoidance of the combination is advisable.

28.4 A 27-year-old recently married female is asking about treatment options for her obesity. She recently stopped taking her birth control medications, as she felt these were contributing to her weight gain. Which of the following medications should be avoided in this patient?

A. Phentermine.
B. Phentermine/topiramate.
C. Orlistat.
D. Diethylpropion.
E. Lorcaserin.

Correct answer = B. The topiramate component of this medication is contraindicated in pregnancy. Since this patient stopped her birth control, she is at risk of becoming pregnant and her fetus is at risk of developing birth defects if she is taking this medication.

28.5 A fellow health care provider is concerned about prescribing orlistat to his adolescent patients. He understands that it is approved for adolescents aged 12 years and older and, therefore, prescribes this medication more often than any other for adolescent obesity. Unfortunately, many of his adolescent patients are stopping the medication during the first month of treatment. Which of the following side effects is the most likely reason these adolescents are stopping the drug?

A. Tachycardia.
B. Valvulopathy.
C. Suicidal ideation.
D. Drowsiness.
E. Flatulence.

Correct answer = E. Flatulence is a very common side effect with orlistat, along with several other GI disturbances. For adolescents, these side effects may be embarrassing and difficult to manage. It is important to counsel patients about these gastrointestinal side effects with orlistat and recommend a low-fat diet as well as cholestyramine to counteract the effects should they become bothersome. The other side effects listed have been seen with other obesity medications, but not with orlistat.

Drugs for Disorders of the Respiratory System

29

Kyle Melin

I. OVERVIEW

Asthma, chronic obstructive pulmonary disease (COPD), and allergic rhinitis are commonly encountered respiratory disorders. Each of these conditions may be associated with a troublesome cough, which may be the only presenting complaint. Asthma is a chronic disease characterized by hyperresponsive airways, affecting over 25 million patients in the United States, and resulting in 2 million emergency room visits and 500,000 hospitalizations annually. More than 12 million Americans have been diagnosed with COPD, and it is currently the fourth leading cause of death in the world. Allergic rhinitis affects approximately 20% of the American population. It is characterized by itchy, watery eyes, runny nose, and a nonproductive cough that can significantly decrease quality of life. Each of these respiratory conditions may be managed with a combination of lifestyle changes and medications. Drugs used to treat respiratory conditions can be delivered topically to the nasal mucosa, inhaled into the lungs, or given orally or parenterally for systemic absorption. Local delivery methods, such as nasal sprays or inhalers, are preferred to target affected tissues while minimizing systemic side effects. Medications used to treat common respiratory disorders are summarized in Figure 29.1.

II. PREFERRED DRUGS USED TO TREAT ASTHMA

Asthma is a chronic inflammatory disease of the airways characterized by episodes of acute bronchoconstriction causing shortness of breath, cough, chest tightness, wheezing, and rapid respiration.

A. Pathophysiology of asthma

Airflow obstruction in asthma is due to bronchoconstriction that results from contraction of bronchial smooth muscle, inflammation of

MEDICATION	INDICATION
SHORT-ACTING β₂ ADRENERGIC AGONISTS	
Albuterol PROAIR, PROVENTIL, VENTOLIN	Asthma, COPD
Levalbuterol XOPENEX	Asthma, COPD
LONG-ACTING β₂ ADRENERGIC AGONISTS	
Arformoterol BROVANA	COPD
Formoterol FORADIL, PERFOROMIST	Asthma, COPD
Indacaterol ARCAPTA	COPD
Salmeterol SEREVENT	Asthma, COPD
INHALED CORTICOSTEROIDS	
Beclomethasone BECONASE AQ, QVAR	Allergic rhinitis, Asthma, COPD
Budesonide PULMICORT, RHINOCORT	Allergic rhinitis, Asthma, COPD
Ciclesonide ALVESCO, OMNARIS, ZETONNA	Allergic rhinitis
Fluticasone FLONASE, FLOVENT	Allergic rhinitis, Asthma, COPD
Mometasone ASMANEX, NASONEX	Allergic rhinitis, Asthma
Triamcinolone NASACORT AQ	Allergic rhinitis
LONG-ACTING β₂ ADRENERGIC AGONIST/CORTICOSTEROID COMBINATION	
Formoterol/budesonide SYMBICORT	Asthma, COPD
Formoterol/mometasone DULERA	Asthma, COPD
Salmeterol/fluticasone ADVAIR	Asthma, COPD
Vilanterol/fluticasone BREO ELLIPTA	COPD
SHORT-ACTING ANTICHOLINERGIC	
Ipratropium ATROVENT	Allergic rhinitis, COPD
LONG-ACTING ANTICHOLINERGIC	
Aclidinium bromide TUDORZA PRESSAIR	COPD
Tiotropium SPIRIVA	COPD
LEUKOTRIENE MODIFIERS	
Montelukast SINGULAIR	Asthma, Allergic rhinitis
Zafirlukast ACCOLATE	Asthma
Zileuton ZYFLO CR	Asthma
ANTIHISTAMINES (H₁-RECEPTOR BLOCKERS)	
Azelastine ASTELIN, ASTEPRO	Allergic rhinitis
Cetirizine ZYRTEC	Allergic rhinitis
Desloratadine CLARINEX	Allergic rhinitis
Fexofenadine ALLEGRA	Allergic rhinitis
Loratadine CLARITIN	Allergic rhinitis
α-ADRENERGIC AGONISTS	
Oxymetazoline AFRIN, DRISTAN	Allergic rhinitis
Phenylephrine NEOSYNEPHRINE, SUDAFED PE	Allergic rhinitis
Pseudoephedrine SUDAFED	Allergic rhinitis
AGENTS FOR COUGH	
Benzonatate TESSALON PERLES	Cough suppressant
Codeine (with guaifenesin) VARIOUS	Cough suppressant/expectorant
Dextromethorphan VARIOUS	Cough suppressant
Dextromethorphan (with guaifenesin) VARIOUS	Cough suppressant/expectorant
Guaifenesin VARIOUS	Expectorant
OTHER AGENTS	
Cromolyn NASALCROM	Asthma, Allergic rhinitis
Omalizumab XOLAIR	Asthma
Roflumilast DALIRESP	COPD
Theophylline ELIXOPHYLLIN, THEO-24, UNIPHYL	Asthma

Figure 29.1

Summary of drugs affecting the respiratory system.

the bronchial wall, and increased secretion of mucus (Figure 29.2). The underlying inflammation of the airways contributes to airway hyperresponsiveness, airflow limitation, respiratory symptoms, and disease chronicity. Asthma attacks may be triggered by exposure to allergens, exercise, stress, and respiratory infections. Unlike COPD, cystic fibrosis, and bronchiectasis, asthma is usually not a progressive disease (that is, it does not inevitably lead to incapacitated airways). However, if untreated, asthma may cause airway remodeling, resulting in increased severity and incidence of asthma exacerbations and/or death.

B. Goals of therapy

The goals of asthma therapy are to decrease the intensity and frequency of asthma symptoms and the degree to which the patient is limited by these symptoms. All patients need to have a "quick-relief" medication to treat acute asthma symptoms. Drug therapy for long-term control of asthma is designed to reverse and prevent airway inflammation. First-line treatment agents based on disease classification are presented in Figure 29.3.

C. β_2-Adrenergic agonists

Inhaled β_2-adrenergic agonists directly relax airway smooth muscle. They are used for the quick relief of asthma symptoms, as well as adjunctive therapy for long-term control of the disease.

1. **Quick relief:** Short-acting β_2 agonists (SABAs) have a rapid onset of action (5 to 30 minutes) and provide relief for 4 to 6 hours. They are used for symptomatic treatment of bronchospasm, providing quick relief of acute bronchoconstriction. All patients with asthma should be prescribed a SABA inhaler. β_2 agonists have no anti-inflammatory effects, and they should never be used as the sole therapeutic agents for patients with persistent asthma. However, monotherapy with SABAs may be appropriate for patients with intermittent asthma or exercise-induced bronchospasm. Direct-acting β_2-selective agonists include *albuterol* [al-BYOO-ter-all] and *levalbuterol* [leh-val-BYOO-ter-all]. These agents provide significant bronchodilation with little of the undesired effect of α or β_1 stimulation (see Chapter 6). Adverse effects, such as tachycardia, hyperglycemia, hypokalemia, and hypomagnesemia, are minimized with inhaled delivery versus systemic administration. These agents can cause β_2-mediated skeletal muscle tremors.

2. **Long-term control:** *Salmeterol* [sal-MEE-ter-all] and *formoterol* [for-MOE-ter-all] are long-acting β_2 agonists (LABAs) and chemical analogs of *albuterol. Salmeterol* and *formoterol* have a long duration of action, providing bronchodilation for at least 12 hours. Neither *salmeterol* nor *formoterol* should be used for quick relief of an acute asthma attack. Use of LABA monotherapy is contraindicated, and LABAs should be used only in combination with an asthma controller medication. Inhaled corticosteroids (ICS) remain the long-term controllers of choice in asthma, and LABAs are considered to be useful adjunctive therapy for attaining asthma control. Some LABAs are available as a combination product with an ICS (Figure 29.1). Adverse effects of LABAs are similar to quick-relief β_2 agonists.

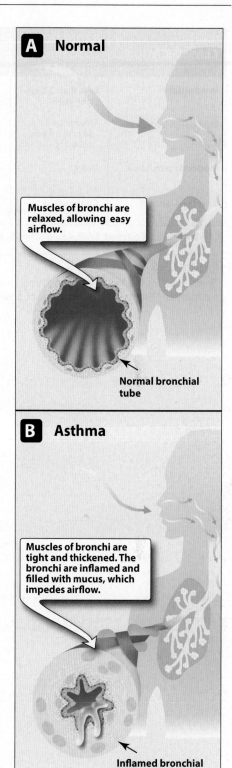

A Normal

Muscles of bronchi are relaxed, allowing easy airflow.

Normal bronchial tube

B Asthma

Muscles of bronchi are tight and thickened. The bronchi are inflamed and filled with mucus, which impedes airflow.

Inflamed bronchial tube

Figure 29.2
Comparison of bronchi of normal and asthmatic individuals.

CLASSIFICATION	BRONCHO-CONSTRICTIVE EPISODES	RESULTS OF PEAK FLOW OR SPIROMETRY	LONG-TERM CONTROL	QUICK RELIEF OF SYMPTOMS
Intermittent	Less than 2 days per week	Near normal*	No daily medication	Short-acting β_2 agonist
Mild persistent	More than 2 days per week, not daily	Near normal*	Low-dose ICS	Short-acting β_2 agonist
Moderate persistent	Daily	60% to 80% of normal	Low-dose ICS + LABA OR Medium-dose ICS	Short-acting β_2 agonist
Severe persistent	Continual	Less than 60% of normal	Medium-dose ICS + LABA OR High-dose ICS + LABA	Short-acting β_2 agonist

ICS = inhaled corticosteroid. LABA = long-acting β_2 agonist.

Figure 29.3
Guidelines for the treatment of asthma. In all asthmatic patients, quick relief is provided by a SABA as needed for symptoms. *Eighty percent or more of predicted function.

D. Corticosteroids

ICS are the drugs of choice for long-term control in patients with any degree of persistent asthma (Figure 29.3). Corticosteroids inhibit the release of arachidonic acid through phospholipase A_2 inhibition, thereby producing direct anti-inflammatory properties in the airways (Figure 29.4). A full discussion of the mechanism of action of corticosteroids is found in Chapter 27. No other medications are as effective as ICS in the long-term control of asthma in children and adults. To be effective in controlling inflammation, glucocorticoids must be used regularly. Severe persistent asthma may require the addition of a short course of oral glucocorticoid treatment.

1. **Actions on lung:** ICS do not directly affect the airway smooth muscle. Instead, ICS therapy directly targets underlying airway inflammation by decreasing the inflammatory cascade (eosinophils, macrophages, and T lymphocytes), reversing mucosal edema, decreasing the permeability of capillaries, and inhibiting the release of leukotrienes. After several months of regular use, ICS reduce the hyperresponsiveness of the airway smooth muscle to a variety of bronchoconstrictor stimuli, such as allergens, irritants, cold air, and exercise.

2. **Routes of administration**

    a. **Inhalation:** The development of ICS has markedly reduced the need for systemic corticosteroid treatment to achieve asthma control. However, as with all inhaled medications, appropriate inhalation technique is critical to the success of therapy (see section on Inhaler Technique).

    b. **Oral/systemic:** Patients with a severe exacerbation of asthma (status asthmaticus) may require intravenous *methylprednisolone* or oral *prednisone* to reduce airway inflammation. In most cases, suppression of the hypothalamic–pituitary–adrenal cortex axis will not occur during the short course of oral *prednisone* "burst" typically prescribed for an asthma exacerbation.

Therefore, prednisone dose taper is unnecessary prior to discontinuation. Due to the increased incidence of adverse effects with oral therapy, chronic maintenance with systemic administration of corticosteroids should be reserved for patients who are not controlled on an ICS.

3. **Adverse effects:** Oral or parenteral glucocorticoids have a variety of potentially serious side effects (see Chapter 27), whereas ICS, particularly if used with a spacer, have few systemic effects. ICS deposition on the oral and laryngeal mucosa can cause adverse effects, such as oropharyngeal candidiasis (due to local immune suppression) and hoarseness. Patients should be instructed to rinse the mouth in a "swish-and-spit" method with water following use of the inhaler to decrease the chance of these adverse events.

III. ALTERNATIVE DRUGS USED TO TREAT ASTHMA

These drugs are useful for treatment of asthma in patients who are poorly controlled by conventional therapy or experience adverse effects secondary to corticosteroid treatment. These drugs should be used in conjunction with ICS therapy for most patients, not as monotherapy.

A. Leukotriene modifiers

Leukotrienes (LT) B_4 and the cysteinyl leukotrienes, LTC_4, LTD_4, and LTE_4, are products of the 5-lipoxygenase pathway of arachidonic acid metabolism and part of the inflammatory cascade. 5-Lipoxygenase is found in cells of myeloid origin, such as mast cells, basophils, eosinophils, and neutrophils. LTB_4 is a potent chemoattractant for neutrophils and eosinophils, whereas the cysteinyl leukotrienes constrict bronchiolar smooth muscle, increase endothelial permeability, and promote mucus secretion. *Zileuton* [zye-LOO-ton] is a selective and specific inhibitor of 5-lipoxygenase, preventing the formation of both LTB_4 and the cysteinyl leukotrienes. Because *zafirlukast* [za-FIR-loo-kast] and *montelukast* [mon-te-LOO-kast] are selective antagonists of the cysteinyl leukotriene-1 receptor, they block the effects of cysteinyl leukotrienes (Figure 29.4). All three drugs are approved for the prevention of asthma symptoms. They should not be used in situations where immediate bronchodilation is required. Leukotriene receptor antagonists have also shown efficacy for the prevention of exercise-induced bronchospasm.

1. **Pharmacokinetics:** All three drugs are orally active and highly protein bound. Food impairs the absorption of *zafirlukast*. The drugs are metabolized extensively by the liver. *Zileuton* and its metabolites are excreted in urine, whereas *zafirlukast*, *montelukast*, and their metabolites undergo biliary excretion.

2. **Adverse effects:** Elevations in serum hepatic enzymes have occurred with all three agents, requiring periodic monitoring and discontinuation when enzymes exceed three to five times the upper limit of normal. Other effects include headache and dyspepsia.

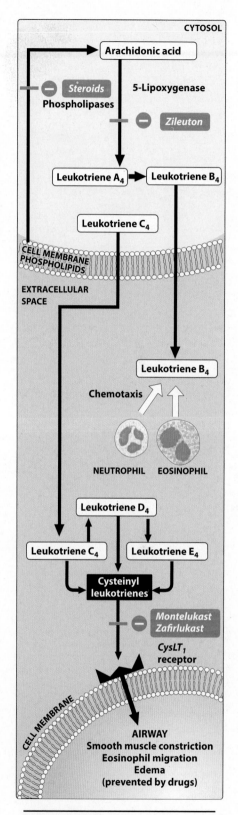

Figure 29.4
Sites of action for various respiratory medications. $CysLT_1$ = cysteinyl leukotriene-1.

Zafirlukast is an inhibitor of cytochrome P450 (CYP) isoenzymes 2C8, 2C9, and 3A4, and *zileuton* inhibits CYP1A2.

B. Cromolyn

Cromolyn [KRO-moe-lin] is a prophylactic anti-inflammatory agent that inhibits mast cell degranulation and release of histamine. It is an alternative therapy for mild persistent asthma. However, it is not useful in managing an acute asthma attack, because it is not a bronchodilator. *Cromolyn* is available as a nebulized solution for use in asthma. Due to its short duration of action, this agent requires dosing three or four times daily, which affects adherence and limits its use. Adverse effects are minor and include cough, irritation, and unpleasant taste.

C. Cholinergic antagonists

The anticholinergic agents block vagally mediated contraction of airway smooth muscle and mucus secretion (see Chapter 5). Inhaled *ipratropium* [IP-ra-TROE-pee-um], a quaternary derivative of *atropine*, is not recommended for the routine treatment of acute bronchospasm in asthma, as its onset is much slower than inhaled SABAs. However, it may be useful in patients who are unable to tolerate a SABA or patients with concomitant COPD. *Ipratropium* also offers additional benefit when used with a SABA for the treatment of acute asthma exacerbations in the emergency department. Adverse effects such as xerostomia and bitter taste are related to local anticholinergic effects.

D. Theophylline

Theophylline [thee-OFF-i-lin] is a bronchodilator that relieves airflow obstruction in chronic asthma and decreases its symptoms. It may also possess anti-inflammatory activity, although the mechanism of action is unclear. Previously, the mainstay of asthma therapy, *theophylline* has been largely replaced with β_2 agonists and corticosteroids due to its narrow therapeutic window, adverse effect profile, and potential for drug interactions. Overdose may cause seizures or potentially fatal arrhythmias. *Theophylline* is metabolized in the liver and is a CYP1A2 and 3A4 substrate. It is subject to numerous drug interactions. Serum concentration monitoring should be performed when *theophylline* is used chronically.

E. Omalizumab

Omalizumab [OH-ma-LIZ-oo-mab] is a recombinant DNA-derived monoclonal antibody that selectively binds to human immunoglobulin E (IgE). This leads to decreased binding of IgE to its receptor on the surface of mast cells and basophils. Reduction in surface-bound IgE limits the release of mediators of the allergic response. *Omalizumab* is indicated for the treatment of moderate to severe persistent asthma in patients who are poorly controlled with conventional therapy. Its use is limited by the high cost, route of administration (subcutaneous), and adverse effect profile. Adverse effects include serious anaphylactic reaction (rare), arthralgias, fever, and rash. Secondary malignancies have been reported.

IV. DRUGS USED TO TREAT CHRONIC OBSTRUCTIVE PULMONARY DISEASE

COPD is a chronic, irreversible obstruction of airflow that is usually progressive. Symptoms include cough, excess mucus production, chest tightness, breathlessness, difficulty sleeping, and fatigue. Although symptoms are similar to asthma, the characteristic **irreversible** airflow obstruction of COPD is one of the most significant differences between the diseases. Smoking is the greatest risk factor for COPD and is directly linked to the progressive decline of lung function as demonstrated by forced expiratory volume in one second (FEV_1). Smoking cessation and/or continued avoidance should be recommended regardless of stage/severity of COPD and age of patient. Drug therapy for COPD is aimed at relief of symptoms and prevention of disease progression. Unfortunately, with currently available care, many patients still experience declining lung function over time.

A. Bronchodilators

Inhaled bronchodilators, including the β_2-adrenergic agonists and anticholinergic agents (*ipratropium* and *tiotropium* [tye-oh-TROE-pee-um]), are the foundation of therapy for COPD (Figure 29.5). These drugs increase airflow, alleviate symptoms, and decrease exacerbation rates. The long-acting agents, LABAs and *tiotropium,* are preferred as first-line treatment of COPD for all patients except those who are at low risk with less symptoms. Combination of both an anticholinergic and a β_2 agonist may be helpful in patients who have inadequate response to a single inhaled bronchodilator.

PATIENT GROUP	RECOMMENDED FIRST CHOICE	ALTERNATIVE CHOICE
A Low risk Less symptoms	Short-acting anticholinergic when necessary or Short-acting β_2 agonist when necessary	Long-acting anticholinergic or Long-acting β_2 agonist or Short-acting β_2 agonist and short-acting anticholinergic
B Low risk More symptoms	Long-acting anticholinergic or Long-acting β_2 agonist	Long-acting anticholinergic and long-acting β_2 agonist
C High risk Less symptoms	Inhaled corticosteroid + long-acting β_2 agonist or Long-acting anticholinergic	Long-acting anticholinergic and long-acting β_2 agonist or Long-acting anticholinergic and PDE-4 inhibitor or Long-acting β_2 agonist and PDE-4 inhibitor
D High risk More symptoms	ICS + long-acting β_2 agonist and/or Long-acting anticholinergic	ICS + long-acting β_2 agonist and long-acting anticholinergic or ICS + long-acting β_2 agonist and PDE-4 inhibitor or Long-acting anticholinergic and long-acting β_2 agonist or Long-acting anticholinergic and PDE-4 inhibitor

COPD = chronic obstructive pulmonary disease, ICS = inhaled corticosteroid, PDE-4 = phosphodiesterase-4
Note: Risk denotes risk of COPD exacerbations.

Figure 29.5
Guidelines for the pharmacologic therapy of stable COPD.

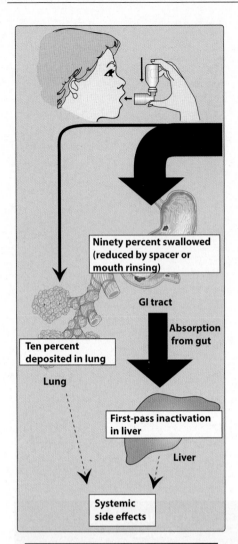

Figure 29.6
Pharmacokinetics of inhaled
glucocorticoids. GI = gastrointestinal.

B. Corticosteroids

The addition of an ICS to a long-acting bronchodilator may improve symptoms, lung function and quality of life in COPD patients with FEV_1 of less than 60% predicted. However, the use of an ICS is associated with an increased risk of pneumonia, and therefore, use should be restricted to these patients. Although often used for acute exacerbations, oral corticosteroids are not recommended for long-term treatment.

C. Other agents

Roflumilast [roe-FLUE-mi-last] is an oral phosphodiesterase-4 inhibitor used to reduce exacerbations in patients with severe chronic bronchitis. Although its activity is not well defined in COPD, it is theorized to reduce inflammation by increasing levels of intracellular cAMP in lung cells. *Roflumilast* is not a bronchodilator and is not indicated for the relief of acute bronchospasm. Its use is limited by common side effects including nausea, vomiting, diarrhea, and headache. As in asthma, the use of *theophylline* has largely been replaced by the more effective and tolerable long-acting bronchodilators.

V. INHALER TECHNIQUE

Appropriate inhaler technique differs between metered-dose inhalers (MDIs) and dry powder inhalers (DPIs), so assessing technique regularly is critical to the success of therapy.

A. Metered-dose inhalers and dry powder inhalers

MDIs have propellants that eject the active medication from the canister. Patients should be instructed to inhale **slowly** and **deeply** just before and throughout actuation of the inhaler to avoid impaction of the medication onto the laryngeal mucosa, rather than the bronchial smooth muscle. A large fraction (typically 80% to 90%) of inhaled glucocorticoids is either deposited in the mouth and pharynx or swallowed (Figure 29.6). The remaining 10% to 20% of a dose of inhaled glucocorticoids that is not swallowed is deposited in the airway. If ICS are inappropriately inhaled, systemic absorption and adverse effects are much more likely. DPIs require a different inhaler technique. Patients should be instructed to inhale **quickly** and **deeply** to optimize drug delivery to the lungs.

B. Spacers

A spacer is a large-volume chamber attached to an MDI. The chamber reduces the velocity of the aerosol before entering the mouth, allowing large drug particles to be deposited in the device. The smaller, higher-velocity drug particles are less likely to be deposited in the mouth and more likely to reach the target airway tissue (Figure 29.7). Spacers improve delivery of inhaled glucocorticoids and are advised for virtually all patients. Patients should be advised to wash and/or rinse spacers to reduce the risk of bacterial or fungal growth that may induce an asthma attack.

VI. DRUGS USED TO TREAT ALLERGIC RHINITIS

Rhinitis is an inflammation of the mucous membranes of the nose and is characterized by sneezing, itchy nose/eyes, watery rhinorrhea, nasal congestion, and sometimes, a nonproductive cough. An attack may be precipitated by inhalation of an allergen (such as dust, pollen, or animal dander). The foreign material interacts with mast cells coated with IgE generated in response to a previous allergen exposure. The mast cells release mediators, such as histamine, leukotrienes, and chemotactic factors that promote bronchiolar spasm and mucosal thickening from edema and cellular infiltration. Antihistamines and/or intranasal corticosteroids are preferred therapies for allergic rhinitis.

A. Antihistamines (H$_1$-receptor blockers)

Antihistamines are useful for the management of symptoms of allergic rhinitis caused by histamine release (sneezing, watery rhinorrhea, itchy eyes/nose). However, they are more effective for prevention of symptoms, rather than treatment once symptoms have begun. Ophthalmic and nasal antihistamine delivery devices are available for more targeted tissue delivery. First-generation antihistamines, such as *diphenhydramine* and *chlorpheniramine*, are usually not preferred due to adverse effects, such as sedation, performance impairment, and other anticholinergic effects (see Chapter 30). The second-generation antihistamines (for example, *fexofenadine*, *loratadine*, *desloratadine*, *cetirizine*, and intranasal *azelastine*) are generally better tolerated. Combinations of antihistamines with decongestants (see below) are effective when congestion is a feature of rhinitis.

B. Corticosteroids

Intranasal corticosteroids, such as *beclomethasone, budesonide, fluticasone, ciclesonide, mometasone,* and *triamcinolone,* are the most effective medications for treatment of allergic rhinitis. They improve sneezing, itching, rhinorrhea, and nasal congestion. Systemic absorption is minimal, and side effects of intranasal corticosteroid treatment are localized. These include nasal irritation, nosebleed, sore throat, and, rarely, candidiasis. To avoid systemic absorption, patients should be instructed **not** to inhale deeply while administering these drugs because the target tissue is the nose, not the lungs or the throat. For patients with chronic rhinitis, improvement may not be seen until 1 to 2 weeks after starting therapy.

C. α-Adrenergic agonists

Short-acting α-adrenergic agonists ("nasal decongestants"), such as *phenylephrine*, constrict dilated arterioles in the nasal mucosa and reduce airway resistance. Longer-acting *oxymetazoline* [OX-i-me-TAZ-oh-leen] is also available. When administered as an aerosol, these drugs have a rapid onset of action and show few systemic effects. Unfortunately, the α-adrenergic agonist intranasal formulations should be used no longer than 3 days due to the risk of rebound nasal congestion (rhinitis medicamentosa). For this reason, the α-adrenergic agents have no place in the long-term treatment of allergic rhinitis. Administration of oral α-adrenergic agonist formulations results in a longer duration of action but also increased systemic effects.

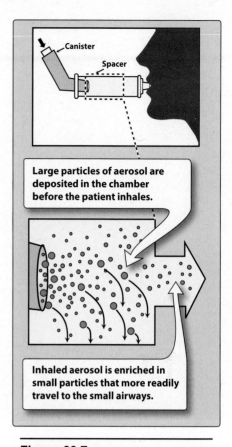

Large particles of aerosol are deposited in the chamber before the patient inhales.

Inhaled aerosol is enriched in small particles that more readily travel to the small airways.

Figure 29.7
Effect of a spacer on the delivery of an inhaled aerosol.

As with intranasal formulations, regular use of oral α-adrenergic agonists (*phenylephrine* and *pseudoephedrine*) alone or in combination with antihistamines is not recommended.

D. Other agents

Intranasal *cromolyn* may be useful in allergic rhinitis, particularly when administered before contact with an allergen. To optimize the therapeutic effect, dosing should begin at least 1 to 2 weeks prior to allergen exposure. A nonprescription (over-the-counter) nasal formulation of *cromolyn* is available. Although potentially inferior to other treatments, some LT antagonists are effective for allergic rhinitis as monotherapy or in combination with other agents. They may be a reasonable option in patients who also have asthma. An intranasal formulation of *ipratropium* is available to treat rhinorrhea associated with allergic rhinitis or the common cold. It does not relieve sneezing or nasal congestion.

VII. DRUGS USED TO TREAT COUGH

Coughing is an important defense mechanism of the respiratory system to irritants and is a common reason for patients to seek medical care. A troublesome cough may represent several etiologies, such as the common cold, sinusitis, and/or an underlying chronic respiratory disease. In some cases, cough may be an effective defense reflex against an underlying bacterial infection and should not be suppressed. Before treating cough, identification of its cause is important to ensure that antitussive treatment is appropriate. The priority should always be to treat the underlying cause of cough when possible.

A. Opioids

Codeine [KOE-deen], an opioid, decreases the sensitivity of cough centers in the central nervous system to peripheral stimuli and decreases mucosal secretion. These therapeutic effects occur at doses lower than those required for analgesia. However, common side effects, such as constipation, dysphoria, and fatigue, still occur. In addition, it has addictive potential (see Chapter 14). *Dextromethorphan* [dextroe-meth-OR-fan] is a synthetic derivative of *morphine* that has no analgesic effects in antitussive doses. In low doses, it has a low addictive profile. However, it is a potential drug of abuse, since it may cause dysphoria at high doses. *Dextromethorphan* has a significantly safer side effect profile than *codeine* and is equally effective for cough suppression. *Guaifenesin* [gwye-FEN-e-sin], an expectorant, is available as a single-ingredient formulation and is also a common ingredient in combination products with *codeine* or *dextromethorphan*.

B. Benzonatate

Unlike the opioids, *benzonatate* [ben-ZOE-na-tate] suppresses the cough reflex through peripheral action. It anesthetizes the stretch receptors located in the respiratory passages, lungs, and pleura. Side effects include dizziness, numbness of the tongue, mouth, and throat. These localized side effects may be particularly problematic if the capsules are broken or chewed and the medication comes in direct contact with the oral mucosa.

Study Questions

Choose the ONE best answer.

29.1 A 12-year-old girl with a childhood history of asthma complained of cough, dyspnea, and wheezing after visiting a riding stable. Her symptoms became so severe that her parents brought her to the emergency room. Which of the following is the most appropriate drug to rapidly reverse her bronchoconstriction?

A. Inhaled fluticasone.

B. Inhaled beclomethasone.

C. Inhaled albuterol.

D. Intravenous propranolol.

E. Oral theophylline.

Correct answer = C. Inhalation of a rapid-acting β_2 agonist, such as albuterol, usually provides immediate bronchodilation. An acute asthmatic crisis often requires intravenous corticosteroids, such as methylprednisolone. Inhaled beclomethasone and fluticasone treat chronic airway inflammation but will not provide any immediate effect. Propranolol is a nonselective β-blocker and would aggravate the patient's bronchoconstriction. Theophylline has been largely replaced with β_2 agonists and is no longer recommended for acute bronchospasm.

29.2 A 9-year-old girl has severe asthma, which required three hospitalizations in the last year. She is now receiving therapy that has greatly reduced the frequency of these severe attacks. Which of the following therapies is most likely responsible for this benefit?

A. Inhaled albuterol.

B. Inhaled ipratropium.

C. Inhaled fluticasone.

D. Oral theophylline.

E. Oral zafirlukast.

Correct answer = C. Administration of a corticosteroid directly to the lung significantly reduces the frequency of severe asthma attacks. This benefit is accomplished with minimal risk of the severe systemic adverse effects of oral corticosteroid therapy. Albuterol is used only to treat acute asthmatic episodes. The other agents may reduce the severity of attacks, but not to the same degree or consistency as fluticasone (or other corticosteroids).

29.3 A 68-year-old male has COPD with moderate airway obstruction. Despite using salmeterol twice daily as prescribed, he reports continued symptoms of shortness of breath with mild exertion. Which one of the following agents would be an appropriate addition to his current therapy?

A. Systemic corticosteroids.

B. Albuterol.

C. Tiotropium.

D. Roflumilast.

E. Theophylline.

Correct answer = C. The addition of an anticholinergic bronchodilator to the LABA salmeterol would be appropriate and provide additional therapeutic benefit. Systemic corticosteroids are used to treat exacerbations in patients with COPD, but not recommended for chronic use. The addition of a SABA (albuterol) is less likely to provide additional benefit since the patient is already using medication with the same mechanism of action. Roflumilast is not indicated as the patient only has moderate airway obstruction. Theophylline is an oral bronchodilator that is beneficial to some patients with stable COPD. However, because of its toxic potential, its use is not routinely recommended.

29.4 A 58-year-old female ceramics worker with a COPD exacerbation has recently been discharged from the hospital. This is the third hospitalization in the past year for this condition, although the patient reports only mild symptoms in between exacerbations. The patient is currently still on the same drug regimen prior to her admission of salmeterol inhalation twice daily and tiotropium inhalation once daily. Her current FEV_1 is below 60%. Which of the following would be an appropriate change in her medication regimen?

A. Chronic systemic corticosteroids.

B. Discontinue the tiotropium.

C. Discontinue the salmeterol.

D. Change the salmeterol to a combination product that includes both a LABA and an inhaled corticosteroid (for example, salmeterol/fluticasone DPI).

E. Theophylline.

Correct answer = D. The addition of an inhaled corticosteroid may provide additional benefit since the patient has significant airway obstruction and frequent exacerbations requiring hospitalization. Systemic corticosteroids are used on a short-term basis to treat exacerbations in patients with COPD but are not recommended for chronic use. It is not routinely recommended to discontinue a long-acting bronchodilator unless the patient experiences an adverse effect or experiences no therapeutic benefit. In this case, the patient reports only mild symptoms in between exacerbations, suggesting she may be benefiting from both bronchodilators. Theophylline is an oral bronchodilator that is beneficial to some patients with stable COPD. However, because of its toxic potential, its use is not routinely recommended.

29.5 A 32-year-old male with a history of opioid addiction presents with symptoms of an upper respiratory system infection for the past 5 days. It is determined to be viral in nature, and no treatment of the underlying infection is appropriate. Which of the following is appropriate symptomatic treatment for this patient's cough?

A. Guaifenesin/dextromethorphan.

B. Guaifenesin/codeine.

C. Cromolyn.

D. Benzonatate.

E. Montelukast.

Correct answer = D. Benzonatate suppresses the cough reflex through peripheral action and has no abuse potential. Dextromethorphan, an opioid derivative, and codeine, an opioid, both have abuse potential. Neither cromolyn nor montelukast is indicated for cough suppression.

29.6 Due to its anti-inflammatory mechanism of action, which of the following medications requires regular administration for the treatment of asthma?

A. Tiotropium MDI.

B. Salmeterol DPI.

C. Mometasone DPI.

D. Albuterol MDI.

Correct answer = C. Inhaled corticosteroids have direct anti-inflammatory properties on the airways and require regular dosing to be effective. Tiotropium is recommended for the treatment of COPD, not asthma. Salmeterol and albuterol are both bronchodilators but do not have anti-inflammatory properties.

29.7 All of the following are preferred antihistamines for the management of allergic rhinitis except:

A. Chlorpheniramine.

B. Fexofenadine.

C. Loratadine.

D. Cetirizine.

E. Intranasal azelastine.

Correct answer = A. Chlorpheniramine is a first-generation antihistamine and is usually not a preferred treatment due to its increased risk of adverse effects of sedation, performance impairment, and other anticholinergic effects. All of the other agents are second-generation antihistamines and are generally better tolerated, making them preferred treatments for allergic rhinitis.

29.8 Which of the following medications inhibits the action of 5-lipoxygenase and consequently the action of leukotriene B_4 and the cysteinyl leukotrienes?

A. Cromolyn.

B. Zafirlukast.

C. Zileuton.

D. Montelukast.

E. Theophylline.

Correct answer = C. Zileuton is the only 5-lipoxygenase inhibitor available. While zafirlukast and montelukast both inhibit the effects of leukotrienes, they do so by blocking the receptor itself. Cromolyn inhibits mast cell degranulation and the release of histamine. Theophylline is a bronchodilator that has no effect on leukotrienes.

29.9 Which of the following describes appropriate inhaler technique for a dry powder inhaler?

A. Inhale slowly and deeply just before and throughout actuation of the inhaler.

B. Use a large-volume chamber (spacer) to decrease deposition of drug in the mouth caused by improper inhaler technique.

C. Inhale quickly and deeply to optimize drug delivery to the lungs.

D. Rinse mouth in a "swish-and-spit" method with water prior to inhaler use to decrease the chance of adverse events.

Correct answer = C. "Quick and deep" inhalation is required for effective use of a DPI. Inhaling "slowly and deeply" and the use of a spacer describe techniques associated with an MDI, not DPI. Mouth rinsing may be appropriate for either type of inhaler if the medication being administered is an inhaled corticosteroid, but this should always be done following inhaler use, not prior to use.

29.10 Which of the following categories of allergic rhinitis medications is most likely to be associated with rhinitis medicamentosa (rebound nasal congestion) with prolonged use?

A. Intranasal corticosteroid.

B. Intranasal decongestant.

C. Leukotriene antagonist.

D. Oral antihistamine.

Correct answer = B. Intranasal decongestants should be used no longer than 3 days due to the risk of rebound nasal congestion (rhinitis medicamentosa). For this reason, the α-adrenergic agents have no place in the long-term treatment of allergic rhinitis.

Antihistamines

30

Thomas A. Panavelil

I. OVERVIEW

Histamine is a chemical messenger mostly generated in mast cells. Histamine, via multiple receptor systems, mediates a wide range of cellular responses, including allergic and inflammatory reactions, gastric acid secretion, and neurotransmission in parts of the brain. Histamine has no clinical applications, but agents that inhibit the action of histamine (antihistamines or histamine receptor blockers) have important therapeutic applications. Figure 30.1 provides a summary of the antihistamines.

A. Location, synthesis, and release of histamine

1. **Location:** Histamine is present in practically all tissues, with significant amounts in the lungs, skin, blood vessels, and GI tract. It is found at high concentration in mast cells and basophils. Histamine functions as a neurotransmitter in the brain. It also occurs as a component of venoms and in secretions from insect stings.

2. **Synthesis:** Histamine is an amine formed by the decarboxylation of the amino acid histidine by the enzyme histidine decarboxylase, which is expressed in cells throughout the body, including neurons, gastric parietal cells, mast cells, and basophils (Figure 30.2). In mast cells, histamine is stored in granules. If histamine is not stored, it is rapidly inactivated by the enzyme amine oxidase.

3. **Release of histamine:** Most often, histamine is just one of several chemical mediators released in response to stimuli. The stimuli for release of histamine from tissues may include destruction of cells as a result of cold, toxins from organisms, venoms from insects and spiders, and trauma. Allergies and anaphylaxis can also trigger significant release of histamine.

B. Mechanism of action

Histamine released in response to certain stimuli exerts its effects by binding to various types of histamine receptors (H_1, H_2, H_3, and H_4). H_1 and H_2 receptors are widely expressed and are the targets of clinically useful drugs. Histamine has a wide range of pharmacologic effects that are mediated by both H_1 and H_2 receptors. For example, the H_1 receptors are important in producing smooth muscle contraction and increasing capillary permeability (Figure 30.3). Histamine promotes vasodilation of small blood vessels by causing the vascular

H₁ ANTIHISTAMINES
Alcaftadine LASTACAFT
Azelastine ASTELIN, OPTIVAR
Bepotastine BEPREVE
Brompheniramine LO-HIST, VAZOL
Cetirizine ZYRTEC
Chlorpheniramine CHLOR-TRIMETON
Clemastine TAVIST ALLERGY
Cyclizine MAREZINE
Cyproheptadine
Desloratadine CLARINEX
Diphenhydramine BENADRYL
Dimenhydrinate DRAMAMINE
Doxylamine UNISOM SLEEPTABS
Emedastine EMADINE
Fexofenadine ALLEGRA
Hydroxyzine VISTARIL, ATARAX
Ketotifen ALAWAY, ZADITOR
Levocetirizine XYZAL
Loratadine CLARITIN
Meclizine BONINE, ANTIVERT
Olopatadine PATANASE, PATANOL
Promethazine PHENERGAN

Figure 30.1
Summary of antihistamines.

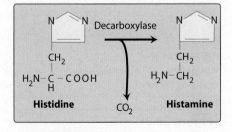

Figure 30.2
Biosynthesis of histamine.

H₁ Receptors

EXOCRINE EXCRETION

Increased production of nasal and bronchial mucus, resulting in respiratory symptoms.

BRONCHIAL SMOOTH MUSCLE

Constriction of bronchioles results in symptoms of asthma and decreased lung capacity.

INTESTINAL SMOOTH MUSCLE

Constriction results in intestinal cramps and diarrhea.

SENSORY NERVE ENDINGS

Causes itching and pain.

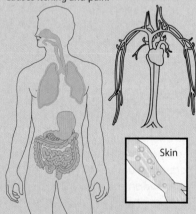

Skin

H₁ and H₂ Receptors

CARDIOVASCULAR SYSTEM

Lowers systemic blood pressure by reducing peripheral resistance. Causes positive chronotropism (mediated by H₂ receptors) and a positive inotropism (mediated by both H₁ and H₂ receptors).

SKIN

Dilation and increased permeability of the capillaries results in leakage of proteins and fluid into the tissues. In the skin, this results in the classic "triple response": wheal formation, reddening due to local vasodilation, and flare ("halo").

H₂ Receptors

STOMACH

Stimulation of gastric hydrochloric acid secretion.

Figure 30.3
Actions of histamine.

endothelium to release nitric oxide. In addition, histamine can enhance the secretion of proinflammatory cytokines in several cell types and in local tissues. Histamine H_1 receptors mediate many pathological processes, including allergic rhinitis, atopic dermatitis, conjunctivitis, urticaria, bronchoconstriction, asthma, and anaphylaxis. Moreover, histamine stimulates the parietal cells in the stomach, causing an increase in acid secretion via the activation of H_2 receptors.

C. Role in allergy and anaphylaxis

The symptoms resulting from intravenous injection of histamine are similar to those associated with anaphylactic shock and allergic reactions. These include contraction of airway smooth muscle, stimulation of secretions, dilation and increased permeability of the capillaries, and stimulation of sensory nerve endings. Symptoms associated with allergy and anaphylactic shock result from the release of certain mediators from their storage sites. Such mediators include histamine, serotonin, leukotrienes, and the eosinophil chemotactic factor of anaphylaxis. In some cases, these mediators cause a localized allergic reaction, producing, for example, actions on the skin or respiratory tract. Under other conditions, these mediators may cause a full-blown anaphylactic response. It is thought that the difference between these two situations results from differences in the sites from which mediators are released and in their rates of release. For example, if the release of histamine is slow enough to permit its inactivation before it enters the bloodstream, a local allergic reaction results. However, if histamine release is too fast for efficient inactivation, a full-blown anaphylactic reaction occurs.

II. H₁ ANTIHISTAMINES

The term antihistamine refers primarily to the classic H_1-receptor blockers. The H_1-receptor blockers can be divided into first- and second-generation drugs (Figure 30.4). The older first-generation drugs are still widely used because they are effective and inexpensive. However, most of these drugs penetrate the CNS and cause sedation. Furthermore, they tend to interact with other receptors, producing a variety of unwanted adverse effects. In contrast, the second-generation agents are specific for peripheral H_1 receptors. Because they are made polar mainly by adding carboxyl groups (for example, *cetirizine* is the carboxylated derivative of *hydroxyzine*), the second-generation agents do not penetrate the blood–brain barrier, causing less CNS depression than the first-generation drugs. Among the second-generation agents, *desloratadine* [des-lor-AH-tah-deen], *fexofenadine* [fex-oh-FEN-a-deen], and *loratadine* [lor-AT-a-deen] show the least sedation (Figure 30.5). *Cetirizine* [seh-TEER-ih-zeen] and *levocetirizine* [lee-voe-seh-TEER-ih-zeen] are partially sedating second-generation agents.

A. Actions

The action of all the H_1-receptor blockers is qualitatively similar. Most of these compounds do not influence the formation or release of histamine. Rather, they block the receptor-mediated response of a target tissue. They are much more effective in preventing symptoms than reversing them once they have occurred. However, most of these agents have additional effects unrelated to their ability to block H₁ receptors. These effects reflect binding of the H₁-receptor antagonists to cholinergic, adrenergic, or serotonin receptors (Figure 30.6). For example, *cyproheptadine* [SYE-proe-HEP-ta-deen] also acts as a serotonin antagonist on the appetite center and is sometimes used off-label as an appetite stimulant and in treating anorgasmy associated with the use of selective serotonin reuptake inhibitors. Antihistamines such as *azelastine* and *ketotifen* also have mast cell–stabilizing effects in addition to their histamine receptor–blocking effects.

B. Therapeutic uses

1. **Allergic and inflammatory conditions:** H₁-receptor blockers are useful in treating and preventing allergic reactions caused by antigens acting on immunoglobulin E antibody. For example, oral antihistamines are the drugs of choice in controlling the symptoms of allergic rhinitis and urticaria because histamine is the principal mediator released by mast cells. Ophthalmic antihistamines, such as *azelastine* [a-ZEL-uh-steen], *olopatadine* [oh-loe-PAT-a-deen], *ketotifen* [kee-toe-TYE-fen], and others (Figure 30.1), are useful for the treatment of allergic conjunctivitis. However, the H₁-receptor blockers are not indicated in treating bronchial asthma, because histamine is only one of several mediators that are responsible for causing bronchial reactions. [Note: *Epinephrine* has actions on smooth muscle that are opposite to those of histamine. It acts via β₂ receptors on smooth muscle, causing cAMP-mediated relaxation. Therefore, *epinephrine* is the drug of choice in treating systemic anaphylaxis and other conditions that involve massive release of histamine.]

2. **Motion sickness and nausea:** Along with the antimuscarinic agent *scopolamine*, certain H₁-receptor blockers, such as *diphenhydramine* [dye-fen-HYE-dra-meen], *dimenhydrinate* [dye-men-HYE-dri-nate] (a chemical combination of *diphenhydramine* and a chlorinated theophylline derivative), *cyclizine* [SYE-kli-zeen], *meclizine* [MEK-li-zeen], and *promethazine* [proe-METH-a-zeen] (Figure 30.4), are the most effective agents for prevention of the symptoms of motion sickness. They are usually not effective if symptoms are already present and, thus, should be taken prior to expected travel. The antihistamines prevent or diminish nausea and vomiting mediated by both the chemoreceptor and vestibular pathways. The antiemetic action of these medications seems to be due to their blockade of central H₁ and M₁ muscarinic receptors. *Meclizine* is also useful for the treatment of vertigo associated with vestibular disorders.

3. **Somnifacients:** Although they are not the medications of choice, many first-generation antihistamines, such as *diphenhydramine* and *doxylamine* [dox-IL-a-meen], have strong sedative properties and are used in the treatment of insomnia (Figure 30.4). These agents are available over-the-counter (OTC), or without a prescription. The use of first-generation H₁ antihistamines is contraindicated in the treatment of individuals working in jobs in which wakefulness is critical. The second-generation antihistamines have no value as somnifacients.

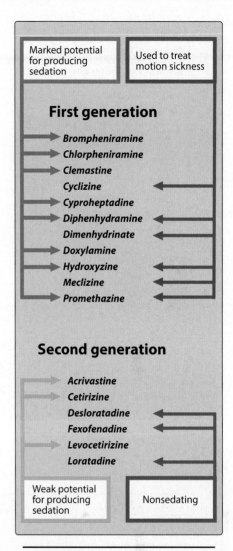

Figure 30.4
Summary of therapeutic advantages and disadvantages of some H₁ histamine receptor–blocking agents.

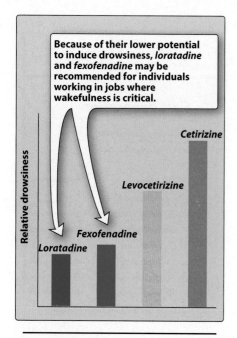

Figure 30.5

Relative potential for causing drowsiness in patients receiving second-generation H₁ antihistamines.

C. Pharmacokinetics

H₁-receptor blockers are well absorbed after oral administration, with maximum serum levels occurring at 1 to 2 hours. The average plasma half-life is 4 to 6 hours, except for that of *meclizine* and the second-generation agents, which is 12 to 24 hours. First-generation H₁-receptor blockers are distributed in all tissues, including the CNS. All first-generation H₁ antihistamines and some second-generation H₁ antihistamines, such as *desloratadine* and *loratadine*, are metabolized by the hepatic cytochrome P450 system. *Levocetirizine* is the active enantiomer of *cetirizine*. *Cetirizine* and *levocetirizine* are excreted largely unchanged in urine, and *fexofenadine* is excreted largely unchanged in feces. After a single oral dose, the onset of action occurs within 1 to 3 hours. The duration of action for many oral antihistamines is 24 hours, allowing once-daily dosing. *Azelastine*, *olopatadine*, *ketotifen*, *alcaftadine* [al-KAF-ta-deen], *bepotastine* [bep-oh-TAS-teen], and *emedastine* [em-e-DAS-teen] are available in ophthalmic formulations that allow for more targeted tissue delivery. *Azelastine* and *olopatadine* have intranasal formulations, as well.

D. Adverse effects

First-generation H₁-receptor blockers have a low specificity, interacting not only with histamine receptors but also with muscarinic cholinergic receptors, α-adrenergic receptors, and serotonin receptors (Figure 30.6). The extent of interaction with these receptors and, as a result, the nature of the side effects varies with the structure of the drug. Some side effects may be undesirable, and others may be of

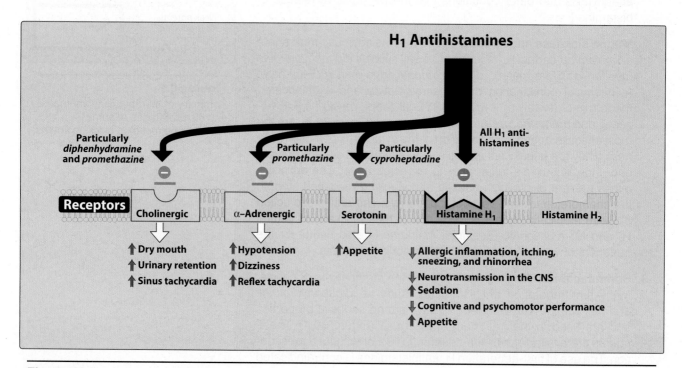

Figure 30.6

Effects of H₁ antihistamines at histamine, adrenergic, cholinergic, and serotonin-binding receptors. Many second-generation antihistamines do not enter the brain and, therefore, show minimal CNS effects.

therapeutic value. Furthermore, the incidence and severity of adverse reactions for a given drug varies between individual subjects.

1. **Sedation:** First-generation H$_1$ antihistamines, such as *chlorpheniramine* [klor-fen-IR-a-meen], *diphenhydramine, hydroxyzine* [hye-DROX-ee-zeen], and *promethazine*, bind to H$_1$ receptors and block the neurotransmitter effect of histamine in the CNS. The most frequently observed adverse reaction is sedation (Figure 30.7). *Diphenhydramine* may cause paradoxical hyperactivity in young children. Other central actions include fatigue, dizziness, lack of coordination, and tremors. Sedation is less common with the second-generation drugs, since they do not readily enter the CNS. Second-generation H$_1$ antihistamines are specific for peripheral H$_1$ receptors.

2. **Other effects:** First-generation antihistamines exert anticholinergic effects, leading not only to dryness in the nasal passage but also to a tendency to dry out the oral cavity. They also may cause blurred vision and retention of urine. The most common adverse reaction associated with second-generation antihistamines is headache. Topical formulations of *diphenhydramine* can cause hypersensitivity reactions such as contact dermatitis when applied to the skin.

3. **Drug interactions:** Interaction of H$_1$-receptor blockers with other drugs can cause serious consequences, such as potentiation of effects of other CNS depressants, including alcohol. Patients taking monoamine oxidase inhibitors (MAOIs) should not take antihistamines because the MAOIs can exacerbate the anticholinergic effects of the antihistamines. In addition, the first-generation antihistamines (*diphenhydramine* and others) with anticholinergic (antimuscarinic) actions may decrease the effectiveness of cholinesterase inhibitors (*donepezil, rivastigmine,* and *galantamine*) in the treatment of Alzheimer's disease.

4. **Overdoses:** Although the margin of safety of H$_1$-receptor blockers is relatively high, and chronic toxicity is rare, acute poisoning is relatively common, especially in young children. The most common and dangerous effects of acute poisoning are those on the CNS, including hallucinations, excitement, ataxia, and convulsions. If untreated, the patient may experience a deepening coma and collapse of the cardiorespiratory system.

III. HISTAMINE H$_2$-RECEPTOR BLOCKERS

Histamine H$_2$-receptor blockers have little, if any, affinity for H$_1$ receptors. Although antagonists of the histamine H$_2$ receptor (H$_2$ antagonists or H$_2$-receptor blockers) block the actions of histamine at all H$_2$ receptors, their chief clinical use is as inhibitors of gastric acid secretion in the treatment of ulcers and heartburn. The four H$_2$-receptor blockers *cimetidine, ranitidine, famotidine,* and *nizatidine* are discussed in Chapter 31.

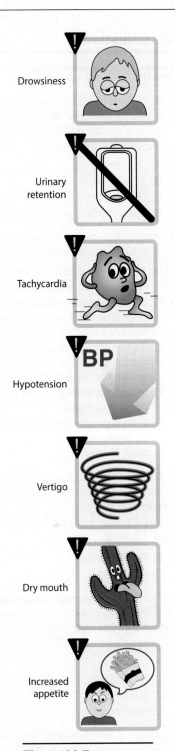

Drowsiness

Urinary retention

Tachycardia

Hypotension

Vertigo

Dry mouth

Increased appetite

Figure 30.7
Some adverse effects observed with antihistamines.
BP = blood pressure.

Study Questions

Choose the ONE best answer.

30.1 A 43-year-old heavy machine operator complains of seasonal allergies. Which one of the following medications would be most appropriate for management of his allergy symptoms?

A. Cyclizine.
B. Doxylamine.
C. Hydroxyzine.
D. Fexofenadine.

Correct answer = D. The use of first-generation H_1 antihistamines is contraindicated in the treatment of pilots and others who must remain alert. Because of its lower potential to induce drowsiness, fexofenadine may be recommended for individuals working in jobs in which wakefulness is critical.

30.2 Which one of the following statements concerning H_1 antihistamines is correct?

A. Second-generation H_1 antihistamines are relatively free of adverse effects.
B. Because of the established long-term safety of first-generation H_1 antihistamines, they are the first choice for allergic rhinitis.
C. The motor coordination involved in driving an automobile is not affected by the use of first-generation H_1 antihistamines.
D. H_1 antihistamines can be used in the treatment of acute anaphylaxis.
E. Both first- and second-generation H_1 antihistamines readily penetrate the blood–brain barrier.

Correct answer = A. Second-generation H_1 antihistamines are preferred over first-generation agents because they are relatively free of adverse effects. Driving performance is adversely affected by first-generation H_1 antihistamines. Epinephrine, not antihistamine, is an acceptable treatment for acute anaphylaxis. Second-generation H_1 antihistamines penetrate the blood–brain barrier to a lesser degree than the first-generation drugs.

30.3 Which of the following medications has the most potential to significantly impair the ability to drive an automobile?

A. Diphenhydramine.
B. Levocetirizine.
C. Fexofenadine.
D. Ranitidine.

Correct answer = A. Diphenhydramine can impair operation of an automobile by causing drowsiness and by impairing accommodation. The other agents do not have this restriction.

30.4 Which of the following histamine receptor antagonists is known to enter the central nervous system readily and is known to be sedative?

A. Hydroxyzine.
B. Cetirizine.
C. Desloratadine.
D. Loratadine.
E. Fexofenadine.

Correct answer = A. Choices B, C, D, and E are all second-generation antihistamines that cross the blood–brain barrier to a much lesser extent than hydroxyzine. Hydroxyzine is the only drug that crosses the blood–brain barrier easily.

30.5 Which of the following statements about histamine receptor antagonists is MOST ACCURATE?

A. Most antihistamines have no antimuscarinic effects.
B. α-Adrenergic effects of antihistamines may cause hypertension.
C. First-generation antihistamines have no sedative side effects.
D. Because of their cholinergic properties, antihistamines may not be effective in the relief of vertigo associated with motion sickness.
E. Headache may be associated with some second-generation antihistamines.

Correct answer = E. Most first-generation antihistamines have α receptor–mediated hypotensive effects, sedative effects, and antimuscarinic (anticholinergic) effects. Second-generation antihistamines have the effects listed in option E.

30.6 A passenger sitting next to you in a plane boasts that he was a famous biochemist. He said he carboxylated a sedating antihistamine, and it is now only partially sedating and is a very well-known drug in the market. Which drug is he talking about?

A. Hydroxyzine.
B. Cetirizine.
C. Diphenhydramine.
D. Doxylamine.
E. Cyproheptadine.

Correct answer = B. Choices A, C, D, and E are first-generation antihistamines and are known to cross the blood–brain barrier. Cetirizine is the carboxylated hydroxyzine.

30.7 Which of the following is an H_1-receptor antagonist that also has serotonin receptor antagonism on the appetite center with the ability to stimulate appetite?

A. Hydroxyzine.
B. Loratadine.
C. Diphenhydramine.
D. Cetirizine.
E. Cyproheptadine.

Correct answer = E. Cyproheptadine has significant serotonin antagonism and is known to increase appetite.

30.8 Your neighbor said she used an H_1 antihistamine that was available over-the-counter (OTC), and it caused her marked drowsiness and dry mouth and she slept quite longer than usual. Which is the most possible drug that she used?

A. Loratadine.
B. Levocetirizine.
C. Diphenhydramine.
D. Fexofenadine.
E. Desloratadine.

Correct answer = C. The only first-generation drug in the list is diphenhydramine. Diphenhydramine and doxylamine, another first-generation antihistamine, are common ingredients in OTC sleep products.

30.9 A patient is going on a deep sea fishing trip and is worried about motion sickness. Which of the following would be the most appropriate?

A. Dimenhydrinate 1 hour prior to departure.
B. Desloratadine 1 hour prior to departure.
C. Doxylamine 1 hour prior to departure.
D. Meclizine at onset of symptoms.

Correct answer = A. Dimenhydrinate and meclizine are both useful for preventing the symptoms of motion sickness. However, they are much more effective in preventing symptoms than treating symptoms once they have started. Therefore, they should be taken prior to expected travel/boating, etc. Desloratadine and doxylamine are not useful for motion sickness.

30.10 A patient has a severe ear infection that is associated with significant vertigo. Which of the following might be helpful?

A. Azelastine.
B. Brompheniramine.
C. Meclizine.
D. Olopatadine.

Correct answer = C. Meclizine is useful for the treatment of vertigo associated with vestibular disorders. Azelastine and olopatadine are ophthalmic or intranasal antihistamines, but they are not useful for symptoms of ear infection. Brompheniramine is a first-generation antihistamine that is mainly used for allergy symptoms.

Gastrointestinal and Antiemetic Drugs

31

Carol Motycka

I. OVERVIEW

This chapter describes drugs used to treat four common medical conditions involving the gastrointestinal (GI) tract: 1) peptic ulcers and gastroesophageal reflux disease (GERD), 2) chemotherapy-induced emesis, 3) diarrhea, and 4) constipation. Many drugs described in other chapters also find application in the treatment of GI disorders. For example, the *meperidine* derivative *diphenoxylate*, which decreases peristaltic activity of the gut, is useful in the treatment of severe diarrhea. Other drugs are used almost exclusively to treat GI tract disorders. For example, H_2-receptor antagonists and proton pump inhibitors (PPIs) are used to heal peptic ulcers.

II. DRUGS USED TO TREAT PEPTIC ULCER DISEASE AND GASTROESOPHAGEAL REFLUX DISEASE

The two main causes of peptic ulcer disease are infection with gram-negative <u>Helicobacter pylori</u> and the use of nonsteroidal anti-inflammatory drugs (NSAIDs). Increased hydrochloric acid (HCl) secretion and inadequate mucosal defense against gastric acid also play a role. Treatment approaches include 1) eradicating the <u>H</u>. <u>pylori</u> infection, 2) reducing secretion of gastric acid with the use of PPIs or H_2-receptor antagonists, and/or 3) providing agents that protect the gastric mucosa from damage, such as *misoprostol* and *sucralfate*. Figure 31.1 summarizes agents that are effective in treating peptic ulcer disease.

A. Antimicrobial agents

Patients with peptic ulcer disease (duodenal or gastric ulcers) who are infected with <u>H</u>. <u>pylori</u> require antimicrobial treatment. Infection with <u>H</u>. <u>pylori</u> is diagnosed via endoscopic biopsy of the gastric mucosa or various noninvasive methods, including serology and urea breath tests (Figure 31.2). Figure 31.3 shows a biopsy sample in which <u>H</u>. <u>pylori</u> is discovered on the gastric mucosa. Eradication of <u>H</u>. <u>pylori</u> results in rapid healing of active ulcers and low recurrence rates (less than 15% compared with 60% to 100% per year for initial ulcers healed with acid-reducing therapy alone). Successful eradication of <u>H</u>. <u>pylori</u> (80% to 90%) is possible with various combinations of antimicrobial drugs. Currently, triple therapy consisting of a PPI combined with

ANTIMICROBIAL AGENTS
Amoxicillin AMOXIL, TRIMOX
Bismuth compounds PEPTO-BISMOL, KAOPECTATE
Clarithromycin BIAXIN
Metronidazole FLAGYL
Tetracycline SUMYCIN

H_2 – HISTAMINE RECEPTOR BLOCKERS
Cimetidine TAGAMET
Famotidine PEPCID
Nizatidine AXID
Ranitidine ZANTAC

PROTON PUMP INHIBITORS (PPIs)
Dexlansoprazole DEXILANT
Esomeprazole NEXIUM
Lansoprazole PREVACID
Omeprazole PRILOSEC
Pantoprazole PROTONIX
Rabeprazole ACIPHEX

PROSTAGLANDINS
Misoprostol CYTOTEC

ANTIMUSCARINIC AGENTS
Dicyclomine BENTYL

ANTACIDS
Aluminum hydroxide ALTERNAGEL
Calcium carbonate TUMS
Magnesium hydroxide MILK OF MAGNESIA
Sodium bicarbonate NUMEROUS

MUCOSAL PROTECTIVE AGENTS
Bismuth subsalicylate PEPTO-BISMOL
Sucralfate CARAFATE

Figure 31.1

Summary of drugs used to treat peptic ulcer disease.

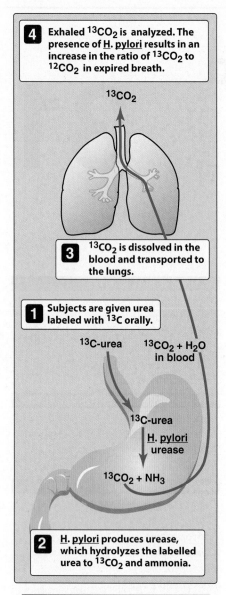

Figure 31.2
Urea breath test, one of several noninvasive methods for detecting presence of <u>Helicobacter</u> <u>pylori</u>.

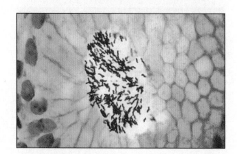

Figure 31.3
<u>Helicobacter</u> <u>pylori</u> in association with gastric mucosa.

amoxicillin (*metronidazole* may be used in *penicillin*-allergic patients) plus *clarithromycin* is the therapy of choice. Quadruple therapy of *bismuth subsalicylate, metronidazole,* and *tetracycline* plus a PPI is another option. Quadruple therapy should be considered in areas with high resistance to *clarithromycin*. This usually results in a 90% or greater eradication rate. Treatment with a single antimicrobial drug is much less effective, results in antimicrobial resistance, and is not recommended. Substitution of antibiotics is also not recommended (that is, do not substitute *ampicillin* for *amoxicillin* or *doxycycline* for *tetracycline*). [Note: GERD (heartburn) is not associated with <u>H</u>. <u>pylori</u> infection and does not respond to antibiotics.]

B. H$_2$-receptor antagonists and regulation of gastric acid secretion

Gastric acid secretion is stimulated by acetylcholine, histamine, and gastrin (Figure 31.4). The receptor-mediated binding of acetylcholine, histamine, or gastrin results in the activation of protein kinases, which in turn stimulates the H$^+$/K$^+$-adenosine triphosphatase (ATPase) proton pump to secrete hydrogen ions in exchange for K$^+$ into the lumen of the stomach. By competitively blocking the binding of histamine to H$_2$ receptors, these agents reduce the secretion of gastric acid. The four drugs used in the United States—*cimetidine* [si-MET-ih-deen], *ranitidine* [ra-NI-ti-deen], *famotidine* [fa-MOE-ti-deen], and *nizatidine* [nye-ZA-ti-deen]—potently inhibit (greater than 90%) basal, food-stimulated, and nocturnal secretion of gastric acid. *Cimetidine* was the first histamine H$_2$-receptor antagonist. However, its utility is limited by its adverse effect profile and drug–drug interactions.

1. **Actions:** The histamine H$_2$-receptor antagonists act selectively on H$_2$ receptors in the stomach, but they have no effect on H$_1$ receptors. They are competitive antagonists of histamine and are fully reversible.

2. **Therapeutic uses:** The use of these agents has decreased with the advent of PPIs.

   a. **Peptic ulcers:** All four agents are equally effective in promoting the healing of duodenal and gastric ulcers. However, recurrence is common if <u>H</u>. <u>pylori</u> is present and the patient is treated with these agents alone. Patients with NSAID-induced ulcers should be treated with PPIs, because these agents heal and prevent future ulcers more effectively than H$_2$ antagonists do.

   b. **Acute stress ulcers:** These drugs are given as an intravenous infusion to prevent and manage acute stress ulcers associated with high-risk patients in intensive care units. However, because tolerance may occur with these agents in this setting, PPIs have gained favor for this indication.

   c. **Gastroesophageal reflux disease (GERD):** Low doses of H$_2$ antagonists, currently available for over-the-counter sale, are effective for the treatment of heartburn (GERD) in only about 50% of patients. H$_2$-receptor antagonists act by stopping acid secretion. Therefore, they may not relieve symptoms for at least

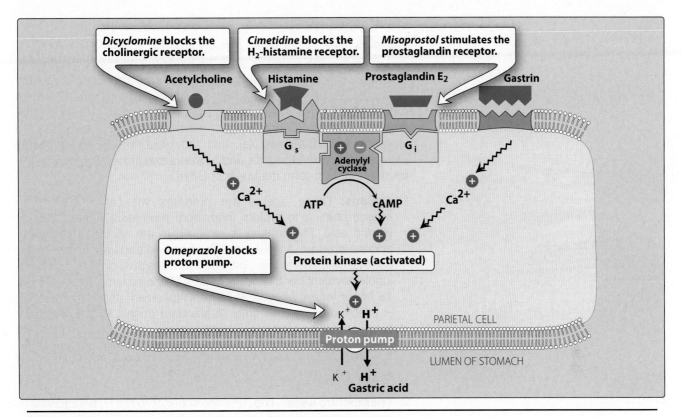

Figure 31.4

Effects of acetylcholine, histamine, prostaglandin E_2, and gastrin on gastric acid secretion by the parietal cells of stomach. G_s and G_i are membrane proteins that mediate the stimulatory or inhibitory effect of receptor coupling to adenylyl cyclase.

45 minutes. Antacids more quickly and efficiently neutralize stomach acid, but their action is only temporary. For these reasons, PPIs are now used preferentially in the treatment of GERD, especially for patients with severe heartburn.

3. **Pharmacokinetics:** After oral administration, the H_2 antagonists distribute widely throughout the body (including into breast milk and across the placenta) and are excreted mainly in urine. *Cimetidine, ranitidine,* and *famotidine* are also available in intravenous formulations. The half-life of all of these agents may be increased in patients with renal dysfunction, and dosage adjustments are needed.

4. **Adverse effects:** In general, the H_2 antagonists are well tolerated. *Cimetidine* can have endocrine effects because it acts as a nonsteroidal antiandrogen. These effects include gynecomastia and galactorrhea (continuous release/discharge of milk). The other agents do not produce the antiandrogenic and prolactin-stimulating effects of *cimetidine*. Other central nervous system effects (such as confusion and altered mentation) occur primarily in elderly patients and after intravenous administration. *Cimetidine* inhibits several cytochrome P450 isoenzymes and can interfere with the metabolism of many other drugs, such as *warfarin, phenytoin,* and *clopidogrel* (Figure 31.5). All H_2 antagonists may reduce the efficacy of drugs that require an acidic environment for absorption, such as *ketoconazole.*

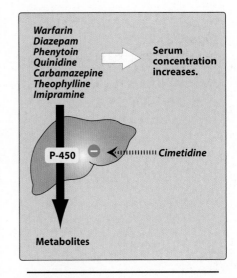

Figure 31.5

Drug interactions with *cimetidine.*

C. PPIs: Inhibitors of the H⁺/K⁺-ATPase proton pump

The PPIs bind to the H^+/K^+-ATPase enzyme system (proton pump) and suppress the secretion of hydrogen ions into the gastric lumen. The membrane-bound proton pump is the final step in the secretion of gastric acid (Figure 31.4). The available PPIs include *dexlansoprazole* [DEX-lan-SO-pra-zole], *esomeprazole* [es-oh-MEH-pra-zole], *lansoprazole* [lan-SO-pra-zole], *omeprazole* [oh-MEH-pra-zole], *pantoprazole* [pan-TOE-pra-zole], and *rabeprazole* [rah-BEH-pra-zole]. *Omeprazole, esomeprazole*, and *lansoprazole* are available over-the-counter for short-term treatment of GERD.

1. **Actions:** These agents are prodrugs with an acid-resistant enteric coating to protect them from premature degradation by gastric acid. The coating is removed in the alkaline duodenum, and the prodrug, a weak base, is absorbed and transported to the parietal cell. There, it is converted to the active drug and forms a stable covalent bond with the H^+/K^+-ATPase enzyme. It takes about 18 hours for the enzyme to be resynthesized, and acid secretion is inhibited during this time. At standard doses, PPIs inhibit both basal and stimulated gastric acid secretion by more than 90%. An oral product containing *omeprazole* combined with *sodium bicarbonate* for faster absorption is also available over the counter and by prescription.

2. **Therapeutic uses:** The PPIs are superior to the H_2 antagonists in suppressing acid production and healing ulcers. Thus, they are the preferred drugs for stress ulcer treatment and prophylaxis and for the treatment of GERD, erosive esophagitis, active duodenal ulcer, and pathologic hypersecretory conditions (for example, Zollinger-Ellison syndrome, in which a gastrin-producing tumor causes hypersecretion of HCl). If a once-daily PPI is only partially effective for GERD symptoms, increasing dosing to twice daily or administering the PPI in the morning and adding an H_2 antagonist in the evening may improve symptom control. If an H_2-receptor antagonist is needed, it should be taken well after the PPI. H_2 antagonists reduce the activity of the proton pump, and PPIs require active pumps to be effective. PPIs also reduce the risk of bleeding from ulcers caused by *aspirin* and other NSAIDs and may be used for prevention or treatment of NSAID-induced ulcers. Finally, they are used with antimicrobial regimens to eradicate H. pylori.

3. **Pharmacokinetics:** All of these agents are effective orally. For maximum effect, PPIs should be taken 30 to 60 minutes before breakfast or the largest meal of the day. [Note: *dexlansoprazole* has a dual delayed release formulation and can be taken without regard to food.] *Esomeprazole, lansoprazole*, and *pantoprazole* are also available in intravenous formulations. Although the plasma half-life of these agents is only a few hours, they have a long duration of action due to covalent bonding with the H^+/K^+-ATPase enzyme. Metabolites of these agents are excreted in urine and feces.

4. **Adverse effects:** The PPIs are generally well tolerated. *Omeprazole* and *esomeprazole* may decrease the effectiveness of *clopidogrel* because they inhibit CYP2C19 and prevent

the conversion of *clopidogrel* to its active metabolite. Although the effect on clinical outcomes is questionable, concomitant use of these PPIs with *clopidogrel* is not recommended because of a possible increased risk of cardiovascular events. PPIs may increase the risk of fractures, particularly if the duration of use is 1 year or greater (Figure 31.6). Prolonged acid suppression with PPIs (and H$_2$ antagonists) may result in low vitamin B$_{12}$ because acid is required for its absorption in a complex with intrinsic factor. Elevated gastric pH may also impair the absorption of *calcium carbonate*. *Calcium citrate* is an effective option for calcium supplementation in patients on acid suppressive therapy, since absorption of the citrate salt is not affected by gastric pH. Diarrhea and <u>Clostridium</u> <u>difficile</u> colitis may occur in community patients receiving PPIs. Patients must be counseled to discontinue PPI therapy and contact their physician if they have diarrhea for several days. Additional adverse effects may include hypomagnesemia and an increased incidence of pneumonia.

D. Prostaglandins

Prostaglandin E, produced by the gastric mucosa, inhibits secretion of acid and stimulates secretion of mucus and bicarbonate (cytoprotective effect). A deficiency of prostaglandins is thought to be involved in the pathogenesis of peptic ulcers. *Misoprostol* [mye-soe-PROST-ole], an analog of prostaglandin E$_1$, is approved for the prevention of NSAID-induced gastric ulcers (Figure 31.7). Prophylactic use of *misoprostol* should be considered in patients who are taking NSAIDs and are at moderate to high risk of NSAID-induced ulcers, such as elderly patients and those with previous ulcers. *Misoprostol* is contraindicated in pregnancy, since it can stimulate uterine contractions and cause miscarriage. Dose-related diarrhea and nausea are the most common adverse effects and limit the use of this agent. Thus, PPIs are preferred agents for the prevention of NSAID-induced ulcers.

E. Antacids

Antacids are weak bases that react with gastric acid to form water and a salt to diminish gastric acidity. Because pepsin (a proteolytic enzyme) is inactive at a pH greater than 4, antacids also reduce pepsin activity.

1. **Chemistry:** Antacid products vary widely in their chemical composition, acid-neutralizing capacity, sodium content, palatability, and price. The efficacy of an antacid depends on its capacity to neutralize gastric HCl and on whether the stomach is full or empty (food delays stomach emptying allowing more time for the antacid to react). Commonly used antacids are combinations of salts of aluminum and magnesium, such as *aluminum hydroxide* and *magnesium hydroxide* [Mg(OH)$_2$]. *Calcium carbonate* [CaCO$_3$] reacts with HCl to form CO$_2$ and CaCl$_2$ and is also a commonly used preparation. Systemic absorption of *sodium bicarbonate* [NaHCO$_3$] can produce transient metabolic alkalosis. Therefore, this antacid is not recommended for long-term use.

2. **Therapeutic uses:** Antacids are used for symptomatic relief of peptic ulcer disease and GERD, and they may also promote

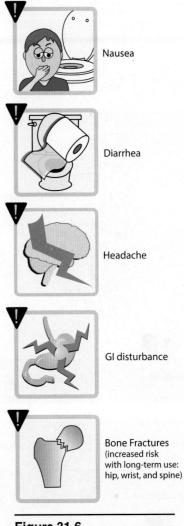

Figure 31.6
Some adverse effects of proton pump therapy.

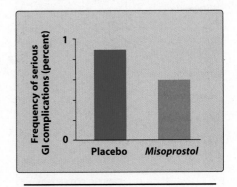

Figure 31.7
Misoprostol reduces serious gastrointestinal (GI) complications in patients with rheumatoid arthritis receiving NSAIDs.

healing of duodenal ulcers. They should be administered after meals for maximum effectiveness. [Note: *Calcium carbonate* preparations are also used as calcium supplements for the treatment of osteoporosis.]

3. **Adverse effects:** *Aluminum hydroxide* tends to cause constipation, whereas *magnesium hydroxide* tends to produce diarrhea. Preparations that combine these agents aid in normalizing bowel function. Absorption of the cations from antacids (Mg^{2+}, Al^{3+}, Ca^{2+}) is usually not a problem in patients with normal renal function; however, accumulation and adverse effects may occur in patients with renal impairment.

F. Mucosal protective agents

Also known as cytoprotective compounds, these agents have several actions that enhance mucosal protection mechanisms, thereby preventing mucosal injury, reducing inflammation, and healing existing ulcers.

1. **Sucralfate:** This complex of *aluminum hydroxide* and sulfated sucrose binds to positively charged groups in proteins of both normal and necrotic mucosa. By forming complex gels with epithelial cells, *sucralfate* [soo-KRAL-fate] creates a physical barrier that protects the ulcer from pepsin and acid, allowing the ulcer to heal. Although *sucralfate* is effective for the treatment of duodenal ulcers and prevention of stress ulcers, its use is limited due to the need for multiple daily dosing and drug–drug interactions. Because it requires an acidic pH for activation, *sucralfate* should not be administered with PPIs, H$_2$ antagonists, or antacids. *Sucralfate* is well tolerated, but it can interfere with the absorption of other drugs by binding to them. This agent does not prevent NSAID-induced ulcers, and it does not heal gastric ulcers.

2. **Bismuth subsalicylate:** This agent is used as a component of quadruple therapy to heal peptic ulcers. In addition to its antimicrobial actions, it inhibits the activity of pepsin, increases secretion of mucus, and interacts with glycoproteins in necrotic mucosal tissue to coat and protect the ulcer.

III. DRUGS USED TO CONTROL CHEMOTHERAPY-INDUCED NAUSEA AND VOMITING

Although nausea and vomiting occur in a variety of conditions (for example, motion sickness, pregnancy, and hepatitis) and are always unpleasant for the patient, the nausea and vomiting produced by chemotherapeutic agents demands especially effective management. Nearly 70% to 80% of patients who undergo chemotherapy experience nausea and/or vomiting. Several factors influence the incidence and severity of chemotherapy-induced nausea and vomiting (CINV), including the specific chemotherapeutic drug (Figure 31.8); the dose, route, and schedule of administration; and patient variables. For example, young patients and women are more susceptible than older patients and men, and 10% to 40% of patients experience nausea and/or vomiting in anticipation of

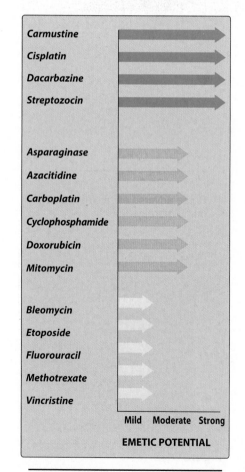

Figure 31.8
Comparison of emetic potential of anticancer drugs.

chemotherapy (anticipatory vomiting). CINV not only affects quality of life but can also lead to rejection of potentially curative chemotherapy. In addition, uncontrolled vomiting can produce dehydration, profound metabolic imbalances, and nutrient depletion.

A. Mechanisms that trigger vomiting

Two brainstem sites have key roles in the vomiting reflex pathway. The chemoreceptor trigger zone (CTZ) is located in the area postrema (a circumventricular structure at the caudal end of the fourth ventricle). It is outside the blood–brain barrier. Thus, it can respond directly to chemical stimuli in the blood or cerebrospinal fluid. The second important site, the vomiting center, which is located in the lateral reticular formation of the medulla, coordinates the motor mechanisms of vomiting. The vomiting center also responds to afferent input from the vestibular system, the periphery (pharynx and GI tract), and higher brainstem and cortical structures. The vestibular system functions mainly in motion sickness.

B. Emetic actions of chemotherapeutic agents

Chemotherapeutic agents can directly activate the medullary CTZ or vomiting center. Several neuroreceptors, including dopamine receptor type 2 and serotonin type 3 (5-HT_3), play critical roles. Often, the color or smell of chemotherapeutic drugs (and even stimuli associated with chemotherapy) can activate higher brain centers and trigger emesis. Chemotherapeutic drugs can also act peripherally by causing cell damage in the GI tract and by releasing serotonin from the enterochromaffin cells of the small intestine. Serotonin activates 5-HT_3 receptors on vagal and splanchnic afferent fibers, which then carry sensory signals to the medulla, leading to the emetic response.

C. Antiemetic drugs

Considering the complexity of the mechanisms involved in emesis, it is not surprising that antiemetics represent a variety of classes (Figure 31.9) and offer a range of efficacies (Figure 31.10). Anticholinergic drugs, especially the muscarinic receptor antagonist *scopolamine* and H_1-receptor antagonists, such as *dimenhydrinate, meclizine,* and *cyclizine,* are very useful in motion sickness but are ineffective against substances that act directly on the CTZ. The major categories of drugs used to control CINV include the following:

1. **Phenothiazines:** The first group of drugs shown to be effective antiemetic agents, phenothiazines, such as *prochlorperazine* [proe-klor-PER-ah-zeen], act by blocking dopamine receptors. *Prochlorperazine* is effective against low or moderately emetogenic chemotherapeutic agents (for example, *fluorouracil* and *doxorubicin*). Although increasing the dose improves antiemetic activity, side effects are dose limiting.

2. **5-HT_3 receptor blockers:** The 5-HT_3 receptor antagonists include *ondansetron* [on-DAN-seh-tron], *granisetron* [gra-NI-seh-tron], *palonosetron* [pa-low-NO-seh-tron], and *dolasetron* [dol-A-seh-tron]. These agents selectively block 5-HT_3 receptors in the periphery (visceral vagal afferent fibers) and in the brain (CTZ).

PHENOTHIAZINES
Prochlorperazine COMPAZINE
5-HT3 SEROTONIN RECEPTOR BLOCKERS
Dolasetron ANZEMET
Granisetron KYTRIL
Ondansetron ZOFRAN
Palonosetron ALOXI
SUBSTITUTED BENZAMIDES
Metoclopramide REGLAN
BUTYROPHENONES
Droperidol
Haloperidol HALDOL
BENZODIAZEPINES
Alprazolam XANAX
Lorazepam ATIVAN
CORTICOSTEROIDS
Dexamethasone DECADRON
Methylprednisolone MEDROL
SUBSTANCE P/NEUROKININ-1 RECEPTOR BLOCKER
Aprepitant EMEND

Figure 31.9
Summary of drugs used to treat CINV.

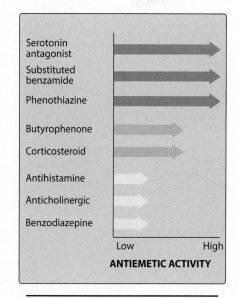

Figure 31.10
Efficacy of antiemetic drugs.

This class of agents is important in treating emesis linked with chemotherapy, largely because of their longer duration of action and superior efficacy. These drugs can be administered as a single dose prior to chemotherapy (intravenously or orally) and are efficacious against all grades of emetogenic therapy. *Ondansetron* and *granisetron* prevent emesis in 50% to 60% of *cisplatin*-treated patients. These agents are also useful in the management of postoperative nausea and vomiting. 5-HT$_3$ antagonists are extensively metabolized by the liver; however, only *ondansetron* requires dosage adjustments in hepatic insufficiency. Elimination is through the urine. Electrocardiographic changes, such as a prolonged QTc interval, can occur with *dolasetron* and high doses of *ondansetron*. For this reason, *dolasetron* is no longer approved for CINV prophylaxis.

3. **Substituted benzamides:** One of several substituted benzamides with antiemetic activity, *metoclopramide* [met-oh-kloe-PRAH-mide] is effective at high doses against the emetogenic *cisplatin,* preventing emesis in 30% to 40% of patients and reducing emesis in the majority of patients. *Metoclopramide* accomplishes this through inhibition of dopamine in the CTZ. Antidopaminergic side effects, including extrapyramidal symptoms, limit long-term high-dose use. *Metoclopramide* was previously used as a prokinetic drug for the treatment of GERD. However, due to the adverse effect profile and the availability of more effective drugs, such as PPIs, it should be reserved for patients with documented gastroparesis.

4. **Butyrophenones:** *Droperidol* [droe-PER-i-doll] and *haloperidol* [hal-oh-PER-i-doll] act by blocking dopamine receptors. The butyrophenones are moderately effective antiemetics. *Droperidol* had been used most often for sedation in endoscopy and surgery, usually in combination with opioids or benzodiazepines. However, it may prolong the QT$_c$ interval and should be reserved for patients with inadequate response to other agents. High-dose *haloperidol* was found to be nearly as effective as high-dose *metoclopramide* in preventing *cisplatin*-induced emesis.

5. **Benzodiazepines:** The antiemetic potency of *lorazepam* [lor-A-ze-pam] and *alprazolam* [al-PRAH-zoe-lam] is low. Their beneficial effects may be due to their sedative, anxiolytic, and amnesic properties. These same properties make benzodiazepines useful in treating anticipatory vomiting. Concomitant use of alcohol should be avoided due to additive CNS depressant effects.

6. **Corticosteroids:** *Dexamethasone* [dex-a-MEH-tha-sone] and *methylprednisolone* [meth-ill-pred-NIH-so-lone], used alone, are effective against mildly to moderately emetogenic chemotherapy. Most frequently, however, they are used in combination with other agents. Their antiemetic mechanism is not known, but it may involve blockade of prostaglandins.

7. **Substance P/neurokinin-1 receptor blocker:** *Aprepitant* [ah-PRE-pih-tant] targets the neurokinin receptor in the brain and blocks the actions of the natural substance. *Aprepitant* is indicated only for highly or moderately emetogenic chemotherapy regimens. It is usually administered orally with *dexamethasone* and

a 5-HT$_3$ antagonist. It undergoes extensive metabolism, primarily by CYP3A4, and it may affect the metabolism of other drugs that are metabolized by this enzyme, such as *warfarin* and oral contraceptives.

8. **Combination regimens:** Antiemetic drugs are often combined to increase antiemetic activity or decrease toxicity (Figure 31.11). Corticosteroids, most commonly *dexamethasone,* increase antiemetic activity when given with high-dose *metoclopramide,* a 5-HT$_3$ antagonist, phenothiazine, butyrophenone, or a benzodiazepine. Antihistamines, such as *diphenhydramine,* are often administered in combination with high-dose *metoclopramide* to reduce extrapyramidal reactions or with corticosteroids to counter *metoclopramide*-induced diarrhea.

IV. ANTIDIARRHEALS

Increased motility of the GI tract and decreased absorption of fluid are major factors in diarrhea. Antidiarrheal drugs include antimotility agents, adsorbents, and drugs that modify fluid and electrolyte transport (Figure 31.12).

A. Antimotility agents

Two drugs that are widely used to control diarrhea are *diphenoxylate* [dye-fen-OX-see-late] and *loperamide* [loe-PER-ah-mide]. Both are analogs of *meperidine* and have opioid-like actions on the gut. They activate presynaptic opioid receptors in the enteric nervous system to inhibit acetylcholine release and decrease peristalsis. At the usual doses, they lack analgesic effects. Because these drugs can contribute to toxic megacolon, they should not be used in young children or in patients with severe colitis.

B. Adsorbents

Adsorbent agents, such as *aluminum hydroxide* and *methylcellulose* [meth-ill-CELL-you-lowse], are used to control diarrhea. Presumably, these agents act by adsorbing intestinal toxins or microorganisms and/or by coating or protecting the intestinal mucosa. They are much less effective than antimotility agents, and they can interfere with the absorption of other drugs.

C. Agents that modify fluid and electrolyte transport

Bismuth subsalicylate, used for traveler's diarrhea, decreases fluid secretion in the bowel. Its action may be due to its salicylate component as well as its coating action. Adverse effects may include black tongue and black stools.

V. LAXATIVES

Laxatives are commonly used for constipation to accelerate the movement of food through the GI tract. These drugs can be classified on the basis of their mechanism of action (Figure 31.13). Laxatives increase the potential for loss of pharmacologic effect of poorly absorbed,

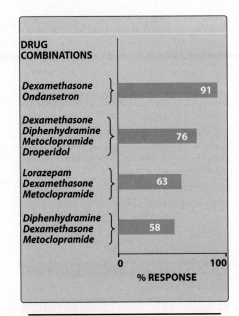

Figure 31.11
Effectiveness of antiemetic activity of some drug combinations against emetic episodes in the first 24 hours after *cisplatin* chemotherapy.

ANTIMOTILITY AGENTS	
Diphenoxylate + atropine LOMOTIL	
Loperamide IMODIUM A-D	
ADSORBENTS	
Aluminum hydroxide ALTERNAGEL	
Methylcellulose CITRUCEL	
AGENTS THAT MODIFY FLUID AND ELECTROLYTE TRANSPORT	
Bismuth subsalicylate PEPTO-BISMOL	

Figure 31.12
Summary of drugs used to treat diarrhea.

IRRITANTS and STIMULANTS

Bisacodyl CORRECTOL, DULCOLAX
Castor oil
Senna EX-LAX, SENOKOT

BULK LAXATIVES

Methylcellulose CITRUCEL
Psyllium METAMUCIL, FIBERALL

SALINE and OSMOTIC LAXATIVES

Magnesium citrate CITROMA
Magnesium hydroxide MILK OF MAGNESIA
Polyethylene glycol MIRALAX, GOLYTELY,
MOVIPREP, NULYTELY, TRILYTE
Lactulose CONSTULOSE, ENULOSE, GENER-
LAC, KRISTALOSE

STOOL SOFTENERS

Docusate COLACE, DOCU-SOFT

LUBRICANT LAXATIVES

Glycerin suppositories
Mineral oil

CHLORIDE CHANNEL ACTIVATORS

Lubiprostone AMITIZA

Figure 31.13
Summary of drugs used to treat
constipation.

delayed-acting, and extended-release oral preparations by accelerating their transit through the intestines. They may also cause electrolyte imbalances when used chronically. Many of these drugs have a risk of dependency for the user.

A. Irritants and stimulants

1. **Senna:** This agent is a widely used stimulant laxative. Its active ingredient is a group of sennosides, a natural complex of anthraquinone glycosides. Taken orally, *senna* causes evacuation of the bowels within 8 to 10 hours. It also causes water and electrolyte secretion into the bowel. In combination products with a *docusate*-containing stool softener, it is useful in treating opioid-induced constipation.

2. **Bisacodyl:** Available as suppositories and enteric-coated tablets, *bisacodyl* is a potent stimulant of the colon. It acts directly on nerve fibers in the mucosa of the colon.

3. **Castor oil:** This agent is broken down in the small intestine to ricinoleic acid, which is very irritating to the stomach and promptly increases peristalsis. Pregnant patients should avoid *castor oil* because it may stimulate uterine contractions.

B. Bulk laxatives

The bulk laxatives include hydrophilic colloids (from indigestible parts of fruits and vegetables). They form gels in the large intestine, causing water retention and intestinal distension, thereby increasing peristaltic activity. Similar actions are produced by *methylcellulose*, psyllium seeds, and bran. They should be used cautiously in patients who are immobile because of their potential for causing intestinal obstruction.

C. Saline and osmotic laxatives

Saline cathartics, such as *magnesium citrate* and *magnesium hydroxide,* are nonabsorbable salts (anions and cations) that hold water in the intestine by osmosis. This distends the bowel, increasing intestinal activity and producing defecation in a few hours. Electrolyte solutions containing *polyethylene glycol* (*PEG*) are used as colonic lavage solutions to prepare the gut for radiologic or endoscopic procedures. *PEG* powder for solution is available as a prescription and also as an over-the-counter laxative and has been shown to cause less cramping and gas than other laxatives. *Lactulose* is a semisynthetic disaccharide sugar that acts as an osmotic laxative. It cannot be hydrolyzed by GI enzymes. Oral doses reach the colon and are degraded by colonic bacteria into lactic, formic, and acetic acids. This increases osmotic pressure, causing fluid accumulation, colon distension, soft stools, and defecation. *Lactulose* is also used for the treatment of hepatic encephalopathy, due to its ability to reduce ammonia levels.

D. Stool softeners (emollient laxatives or surfactants)

Surface-active agents that become emulsified with the stool produce softer feces and ease passage. These include *docusate sodium* and *docusate calcium.* They may take days to become effective and are often used for prophylaxis rather than acute treatment. Stool softeners should not be taken concomitantly with *mineral oil* because of the potential for absorption of the *mineral oil.*

E. Lubricant laxatives

Mineral oil and *glycerin suppositories* are lubricants and act by facilitating the passage of hard stools. *Mineral oil* should be taken orally in an upright position to avoid its aspiration and potential for lipid or lipoid pneumonia.

F. Chloride channel activators

Lubiprostone [loo-bee-PROS-tone], currently the only agent in this class, works by activating chloride channels to increase fluid secretion in the intestinal lumen. This eases the passage of stools and causes little change in electrolyte balance. *Lubiprostone* is used in the treatment of chronic constipation, particularly because tolerance or dependency has not been associated with this drug. Also, drug–drug interactions appear minimal because metabolism occurs quickly in the stomach and jejunum.

Study Questions

Choose the ONE best answer.

31.1 A 68-year-old patient with cardiac failure is diagnosed with ovarian cancer. She begins using cisplatin but becomes nauseous and suffers from severe vomiting. Which of the following medications would be most effective to counteract the emesis in this patient without exacerbating her cardiac problem?

A. Droperidol.

B. Dolasetron.

C. Prochlorperazine.

D. Dronabinol.

E. Palonosetron.

Correct answer = E. Palonosetron is a 5-HT$_3$ antagonist that is effective against drugs with high emetogenic activity, such as cisplatin. Although dolasetron is also in this category, its propensity to affect the heart makes it a poor choice for this patient. Droperidol also affects the heart and now is generally a second-line drug used in combination with opioids or benzodiazepines. The antiemetic effect of prochlorperazine, a phenothiazine, is most beneficial against anticancer drugs with moderate to low emetogenic properties.

31.2 A 45-year-old woman complains of persistent heartburn and an unpleasant, acid-like taste in her mouth. The clinician suspects that she has gastroesophageal reflux disease and advises her to raise the head of her bed 6 to 8 inches, not to eat for several hours before retiring, and to eat smaller meals. Two weeks later, she returns and says the symptoms have subsided slightly but still are a concern. The clinician will likely prescribe which one of the following drugs?

A. An antacid such as aluminum hydroxide.

B. Dicyclomine.

C. An antianxiety agent such as alprazolam.

D. Esomeprazole.

Correct answer = D. It is appropriate to treat this patient with a proton-pump inhibitor (PPI) to reduce acid production and promote healing. An H$_2$-receptor antagonist might also be effective, but the PPIs are preferred. An antacid would decrease gastric acid, but its effects are short lived compared to those of the PPIs and H$_2$-receptor inhibitors. Dicyclomine is an antimuscarinic drug and would decrease acid production, but it is not as effective as the PPIs or the H$_2$-receptor inhibitors. An antianxiety agent might have antiemetic action but would have no effect on the acid production.

31.3 A couple celebrating their 40th wedding anniversary are given a trip to Peru to visit Machu Picchu. Due to past experiences while traveling, they ask their doctor to prescribe an agent for diarrhea. Which of the following would be effective?

A. Omeprazole.
B. Loperamide.
C. Famotidine.
D. Lorazepam.

Correct answer = B. Loperamide is the only drug in this set that has antidiarrheal activity. Omeprazole is a proton-pump inhibitor, famotidine antagonizes the H_2 receptor, and lorazepam is a benzodiazepine that is a sedative and an anxiolytic agent.

31.4 A 27-year-old woman who is 34 weeks pregnant is on bed rest and visits her obstetrician. During the visit, she informs her physician that she has been experiencing mild constipation. Which of the following medications will most likely be recommended to her?

A. Castor oil.
B. Docusate.
C. Mineral oil.
D. Loperamide.

Correct answer = B. Although its effects are not immediate, docusate may be used for mild constipation and is generally considered safe in pregnancy. Castor oil should not be used in pregnancy because of its ability to cause uterine contractions. Mineral oil should not be used in bedridden patients due to the possibility of aspiration. Loperamide is used for diarrhea, not constipation.

31.5 Which of the following drugs has been known to cause discoloration of the tongue?

A. Amoxicillin.
B. Omeprazole.
C. Bismuth compounds.
D. Lubiprostone.

Correct answer = C. Bismuth compounds may cause a black discoloration of the tongue. The other agents have not been associated with this effect.

31.6 A patient is receiving treatment with lorazepam prior to chemotherapy to help reduce her anticipatory nausea and vomiting. Which of the following should generally be avoided in this patient?

A. Docusate.
B. Ondansetron.
C. Polyethylene glycol.
D. Ethanol.

Correct answer = D. Ethanol combined with benzodiazepines, particularly at high doses, may produce unconsciousness, respiratory depression, and even death. The other drugs listed here have not shown a specific drug interaction with benzodiazepines.

31.7 All of the following drugs are generally well tolerated for the treatment of constipation except:

A. Castor oil.
B. Methylcellulose.
C. Polyethylene glycol.
D. Docusate.

Correct answer = A. Castor oil can produce severe cramping, which makes it difficult to tolerate for many, including the elderly. The other three choices are generally well tolerated.

31.8 An elderly woman with a recent history of myocardial infarction is seeking a medication to help treat her occasional heartburn. She is currently taking several medications, including aspirin, clopidogrel, simvastatin, metoprolol, and lisinopril. Which of the following choices should be avoided in this patient?

A. Calcium citrate.
B. Famotidine.
C. Omeprazole.
D. Ranitidine.
E. Calcium carbonate.

Correct answer = C. Omeprazole may possibly decrease the efficacy of clopidogrel because it inhibits the conversion of clopidogrel to its active form.

31.9 Extrapyramidal symptoms (EPS) have been associated with which of the following drugs?

    A. Metoclopramide.

    B. Alprazolam.

    C. Aprepitant.

    D. Loperamide.

Correct answer = A. Only metoclopramide has been associated with EPS. This is due to its ability to inhibit dopamine activity.

31.10 Which of the following medications for gastrointestinal problems is contraindicated in pregnancy?

    A. Calcium carbonate.

    B. Famotidine.

    C. Lansoprazole.

    D. Misoprostol.

Correct answer = D. Misoprostol is contraindicated in pregnancy because it may stimulate uterine contractions. The other medications may be used during pregnancy for the treatment of heartburn (common in pregnancy) or peptic ulcer disease.

Drugs for Urologic Disorders

Katherine Vogel Anderson

32

I. OVERVIEW

Erectile dysfunction (ED) and benign prostatic hyperplasia (BPH) are common urologic disorders in males. ED is the inability to maintain penile erection for the successful performance of sexual activity. ED has many physical and psychological causes, including vascular disease, diabetes, medications, depression, and sequelae to prostatic surgery. It is estimated to affect more than 30 million men in the United States. BPH is nonmalignant enlargement of the prostate, which occurs naturally as men age. As the prostate grows in size, lower urinary tract symptoms develop, which can significantly impact a patient's quality of life. A summary of drugs for ED and BPH is provided in Figure 32.1.

II. DRUGS USED TO TREAT ERECTILE DYSFUNCTION

Therapy for ED includes penile implants, intrapenile injections of *alprostadil*, intraurethral suppositories of *alprostadil*, and oral phosphodiesterase-5 (PDE-5) inhibitors. Because of the efficacy, ease of use, and safety of PDE-5 inhibitors, these drugs are now considered first-line therapy for ED. Four PDE-5 inhibitors (*sildenafil, vardenafil, tadalafil,* and *avanafil*) are approved for the treatment of ED. [Note: *Sildenafil* and *tadalafil* are also indicated to treat pulmonary hypertension, although the dosage regimen differs for this indication.]

A. Phosphodiesterase-5 inhibitors

All four PDE-5 inhibitors, *sildenafil* [sil-DEN-a-fil], *vardenafil* [var-DEN-na-fil], *tadalafil* [ta-DAL-a-fil], and *avanafil* [a-VAN-a-fil], are equally effective in treating ED, and the adverse effect profiles of the drugs are similar. However, these agents differ in the duration of action and the effects of food on drug absorption.

1. **Mechanism of action:** Sexual stimulation results in smooth muscle relaxation of the corpus cavernosum, increasing the inflow of blood (Figure 32.2). The mediator of this response is nitric oxide (NO). NO activates guanylyl cyclase, which forms cyclic guanosine monophosphate (cGMP) from guanosine triphosphate. cGMP produces smooth muscle relaxation through a reduction in the intracellular Ca^{2+} concentration. The duration of action of

DRUGS FOR ERECTILE DYSFUNCTION
Alprostadil MUSE, CAVERJECT, EDEX
Avanafil STENDRA
Sildenafil VIAGRA
Tadalafil CIALIS
Vardenafil LEVITRA, STAXYN

α BLOCKERS
Alfuzosin UROXATRAL
Doxazosin CARDURA
Prazosin MINIPRESS
Silodosin RAPAFLO
Tamsulosin FLOMAX
Terazosin HYTRIN

5 α-REDUCTASE INHIBITORS
Dutasteride AVODART
Finasteride PROPECIA, PROSCAR

Figure 32.1
Summary of drugs used for the treatment of urologic disorders.

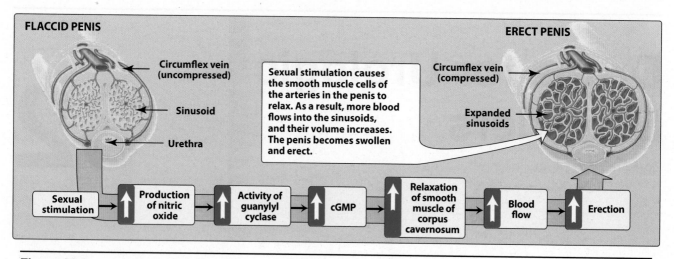

Figure 32.2
Mechanism of penile erection. cGMP = cyclic guanosine monophosphate.

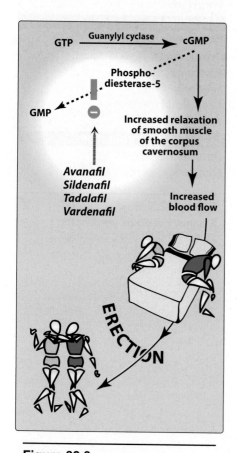

Figure 32.3
Effect of phosphodiesterase inhibitors
on cyclic guanosine monophosphate
(cGMP) levels in the smooth
muscle of the corpus cavernosum.
GTP = guanosine triphosphate.

cyclic nucleotides is controlled by the action of phosphodiester-ase (PDE). At least 11 isozymes of PDE have been characterized. *Sildenafil, vardenafil, tadalafil,* and *avanafil* inhibit PDE-5, the iso-zyme responsible for degradation of cGMP in the corpus caverno-sum. The action of PDE-5 inhibitors is to increase the flow of blood into the corpus cavernosum at any given level of sexual stimulation (Figure 32.3). At recommended doses, PDE-5 inhibitors have no effect in the absence of sexual stimulation.

2. **Pharmacokinetics:** *Sildenafil* and *vardenafil* have similar phar-macokinetic properties. Both drugs should be taken approximately 1 hour prior to anticipated sexual activity, with erectile enhance-ment observed for up to 4 hours after administration. Thus, admin-istration of *sildenafil* and *vardenafil* must be timed appropriately with regard to anticipated sexual activity. The absorption of both drugs is delayed by consumption of a high-fat meal. *Vardenafil* is also available in an orally disintegrating tablet (ODT) formulation, which is not affected by a high-fat meal. However, the bioavail-ability of the ODT formulation may be decreased by water, and therefore the ODT should be placed under the tongue and not administered with liquids. The *vardenafil* ODT provides a higher systemic bioavailability than the *vardenafil* film-coated oral tablet, and these products are not interchangeable. *Tadalafil* has a slower onset of action (Figure 32.4) than *sildenafil* and *vardenafil*, but a significantly longer half-life of approximately 18 hours. As such, it is approved for once-daily dosing (in addition to as-needed dos-ing). This results in enhanced erectile function for up to 36 hours. Furthermore, the absorption of *tadalafil* is not clinically influenced by food. The timing of sexual activity is less critical for *tadalafil* because of its prolonged duration of effect. Of all the PDE-5 inhibi-tors, *avanafil* has the quickest onset of action. It should be taken 30 minutes prior to sexual activity. All PDE-5 inhibitors are metabo-lized by the cytochrome P450 3A4 (CYP3A4) isoenzyme. Dosage adjustments are recommended in patients with hepatic dysfunc-tion. For patients with severe renal dysfunction, the dose of *silde-nafil* and *tadalafil* should be reduced, and daily-dose *tadalafil* and *avanafil* are contraindicated in these patients.

3. **Adverse effects:** The most frequent adverse effects of the PDE-5 inhibitors are headache, flushing, dyspepsia, and nasal congestion. These effects are generally mild, and men with ED rarely discontinue treatment because of side effects. Disturbances in color vision (loss of blue/green discrimination) may occur with PDE-5 inhibitors, probably because of inhibition of PDE-6 (a PDE found in the retina that is important in color vision). *Tadalafil*, however, does not appear to disrupt PDE-6, and reports of changes in color vision have been rare with this medication. The incidence of these reactions appears to be dose dependent. Sudden hearing loss has also been reported with the use of PDE-5 inhibitors, perhaps due to changes in sinus pressure because of vasodilation. *Tadalafil* has been associated with back pain and myalgias, likely because of inhibition of PDE-11, an enzyme found in skeletal muscle. There is an inherent cardiac risk associated with sexual activity. Therefore, PDE-5 inhibitors should be used with caution in patients with a history of cardiovascular disease or those with strong risk factors for cardiovascular disease. PDE-5 inhibitors should not be used more than once per day. All of the PDE-5 inhibitors have the potential to cause priapism (a painful, prolonged erection). Although this is a rare side effect, it is a medical emergency.

4. **Drug interactions:** Because of the ability of PDE-5 inhibitors to potentiate the hypotensive activity of NO, administration of these agents in patients taking any form of organic nitrates (for example, *nitroglycerin* products, *isosorbide dinitrate*, or *isosorbide mononitrate*) is contraindicated. PDE-5 inhibitors may produce additive blood pressure–lowering effects when used in patients taking α-adrenergic antagonists (used to treat hypertension and/or alleviate symptoms associated with BPH). The combination of PDE-5 inhibitors and α-adrenergic antagonists should be used with caution. Patients should be on a stable dose of the α-adrenergic antagonist prior to the initiation of the PDE-5 inhibitor, and the PDE-5 inhibitor should be started at a low dose if this combination is to be used. Doses of PDE-5 inhibitors may need to be reduced in the presence of potent inhibitors of CYP3A4, such as *clarithromycin, ritonavir,* and other protease inhibitors.

B. Alprostadil

Alprostadil [al-PRAHST-uh-dill] is synthetic prostaglandin E1 (PGE1). In the penile tissue, PGE1 allows for relaxation of the smooth muscle in the corpus cavernosum. *Alprostadil* is available as an intraurethral suppository and an injectable formulation. Although PDE-5 inhibitors are considered first-line therapy for the treatment of ED, *alprostadil* may be used for patients who are not candidates for oral therapies. In contrast to oral agents, *alprostadil* acts locally, which may reduce the occurrence of adverse effects.

1. **Mechanism of action:** *Alprostadil* causes smooth muscle relaxation by an unknown mechanism. It is believed that *alprostadil* increases concentrations of cyclic AMP (cAMP) within cavernosal tissue. As a result, protein kinase is activated, allowing trabecular smooth muscle relaxation and dilation of cavernosal arteries. Increased blood flow to the erection chamber compresses venous outflow, so that blood is entrapped and erection may occur.

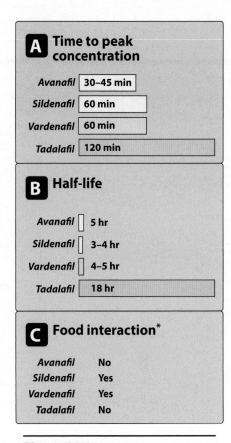

Figure 32.4
Some properties of phosphodiesterase inhibitors.
*Delay in time to reach peak drug concentration when taken with high-fat foods.

2. **Pharmacokinetics:** Systemic absorption of *alprostadil* is minimal. If any *alprostadil* is systemically absorbed, it is quickly metabolized. The onset of action of *alprostadil* is 5 to 10 minutes when given as a urethral suppository and 2 to 25 minutes when administered by injection. The resulting erection may last for 30 to 60 minutes, or longer, depending upon the particular patient.

3. **Adverse effects:** Since *alprostadil* is not systemically absorbed, adverse systemic effects are rare. However, hypotension or headache is a possibility due to PGE1-induced vasodilation. Locally, adverse effects of *alprostadil* include penile pain, urethral pain, and testicular pain. Bleeding from the insertion or injection of *alprostadil* is rare. Hematoma, ecchymosis, and rash are possible from *alprostadil* injection, although these adverse effects are also rare. *Alprostadil* administration may lead to priapism.

III. BENIGN PROSTATIC HYPERPLASIA

Three classes of medications are used to treat BPH: α_1-adrenergic antagonists, 5-α reductase inhibitors, and phosphodiesterase-5 (PDE-5) inhibitors.

A. α1-Adrenergic antagonists

Terazosin [ter-AY-zoe-sin], *doxazosin* [dox-AY-zoe-sin], *tamsulosin* [tam-SUE-loh-sin], *alfuzosin* [al-FUE-zoe-sin], and *silodosin* [sil-oh-DOE-sin] are selective competitive blockers of the α_1 receptor. All five agents are indicated for the treatment of BPH (Figure 32.1). *Prazosin* is an α-blocker that is used off-label in the treatment of BPH. However, current guidelines do not endorse the use of *prazosin* for BPH. Please refer to Chapter 7 for a discussion of α-blockers in the setting of hypertension.

1. **Mechanism of action:** α_{1A} receptors are found in the prostate, α_{1B} receptors are found in the prostate and vasculature, and α_{1D} receptors are found in the vasculature. By blocking the α_{1A} and α_{1B} receptors in the prostate, the α-blockers cause prostatic smooth muscle relaxation, which leads to improved urine flow. *Doxazosin, terazosin,* and *alfuzosin* block α_{1A} and α_{1B} receptors, whereas *tamsulosin* and *silodosin* are more selective for the α_{1A} receptor. Because *doxazosin, terazosin, and alfuzosin* block α_{1B} receptors, these agents decrease peripheral vascular resistance and lower arterial blood pressure by causing relaxation of both arterial and venous smooth muscle. In contrast, *tamsulosin and silodosin* have less of an effect on blood pressure because they are more selective for the prostate-specific α_{1A} receptor. In general, α-blockers cause minimal changes in cardiac output, renal blood flow, and glomerular filtration rate.

2. **Pharmacokinetics:** The α-blockers are well absorbed following oral administration. When taken with food, the absorption of *tamsulosin, alfuzosin*, and *silodosin* is increased. Therefore, for best efficacy, these agents should be taken with meals (typically supper). *Doxazosin, alfuzosin, tamsulosin,* and *silodosin* are metabolized

through the cytochrome P450 (CYP450) system. *Silodosin* is also a substrate for P-glycoprotein (P-gp). *Terazosin* is metabolized in the liver, but not through the CYP system. In general, the α-blockers have a half-life of 8 to 22 hours, with peak effects 1 to 4 hours after administration. *Silodosin* requires dosage adjustment in renal impairment and is contraindicated in patients with severe renal dysfunction.

3. **Adverse effects:** α-Blockers may cause dizziness, a lack of energy, nasal congestion, headache, drowsiness, and orthostatic hypotension (although to a lesser degree than that observed with *phenoxybenzamine* and *phentolamine*). *Tamsulosin* and *silodosin* inhibit the α_{1A} receptors found on the smooth muscle of the prostate. This selectivity accounts for relatively minimal effects on blood pressure, although dizziness and orthostasis may occur. These drugs do not affect male sexual function as severely as *phenoxybenzamine* and *phentolamine*. However, by blocking α receptors in the ejaculatory ducts and impairing smooth muscle contraction, inhibition of ejaculation and retrograde ejaculation have been reported. *Tamsulosin* has a caution about "floppy iris syndrome," a condition in which the iris billows in response to intraoperative eye surgery. Figure 32.5 summarizes some adverse effects observed with α-blockers.

4. **Drug interactions:** Drugs that inhibit CYP3A4 and CYP2D6 (for example, *verapamil, diltiazem*) may increase the plasma concentrations of *doxazosin, alfuzosin, tamsulosin,* and *silodosin,* while drugs that induce the CYP450 system (for example, *carbamazepine, phenytoin,* and *St. John's wort*) may decrease plasma concentrations. *Alfuzosin* may prolong the QT interval, so it should be used with caution with other drugs that cause QT prolongation (for example, class III antiarrhythmics). Since *silodosin* is a substrate for P-gp, drugs that inhibit P-gp, such as *cyclosporine*, may increase *silodosin* concentrations.

B. 5-α reductase inhibitors

Finasteride [fin-AS-ter-ide] and *dutasteride* [doo-TAS-ter-ride] inhibit 5α-reductase. Compared to the α-blockers, which provide patients with relief from BPH symptoms within 7 to 10 days, these agents may take up to 12 months to relieve symptoms.

1. **Mechanism of action:** Both *finasteride* and *dutasteride* inhibit the enzyme 5-α reductase, which is responsible for converting testosterone to the more active dihydrotestosterone (DHT). DHT is an androgen that stimulates prostate growth. By reducing DHT, the prostate shrinks and urine flow improves. Compared to *finasteride,* *dutasteride* is more potent and causes a greater decrease in DHT. In order for the 5-α reductase inhibitors to be effective, the prostate must be enlarged. Thus, it is appropriate to use a 5-α reductase inhibitor in combination with an α-blocker when the prostate is enlarged. Figures 32.6 and 32.7 summarize important differences between these two classes of agents. *Finasteride* and *dutasteride* are also used for alopecia, since a reduction in scalp and serum DHT prevents hair loss.

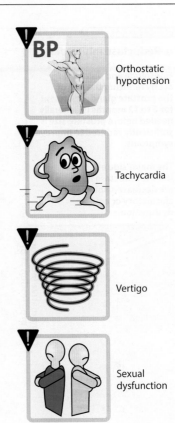

Figure 32.5
Some adverse effects commonly observed with nonselective α-blockers.

Orthostatic hypotension

Tachycardia

Vertigo

Sexual dysfunction

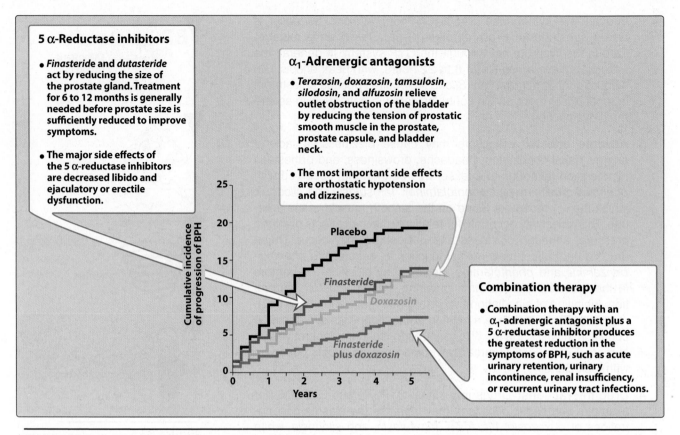

5 α-Reductase inhibitors

- *Finasteride* and *dutasteride* act by reducing the size of the prostate gland. Treatment for 6 to 12 months is generally needed before prostate size is sufficiently reduced to improve symptoms.

- The major side effects of the 5 α-reductase inhibitors are decreased libido and ejaculatory or erectile dysfunction.

α₁-Adrenergic antagonists

- *Terazosin, doxazosin, tamsulosin, silodosin,* and *alfuzosin* relieve outlet obstruction of the bladder by reducing the tension of prostatic smooth muscle in the prostate, prostate capsule, and bladder neck.

- The most important side effects are orthostatic hypotension and dizziness.

Combination therapy

- Combination therapy with an α₁-adrenergic antagonist plus a 5 α-reductase inhibitor produces the greatest reduction in the symptoms of BPH, such as acute urinary retention, urinary incontinence, renal insufficiency, or recurrent urinary tract infections.

Figure 32.6
Therapy for benign prostatic hyperplasia (BPH).

2. **Pharmacokinetics:** Food does not affect the absorption of either agent. Both are highly protein bound. *Finasteride* and *dutasteride* are metabolized by the CYP450 system. The mean plasma elimination half-life of *finasteride* is 6 to 16 hours, while the terminal elimination half-life of *dutasteride* is 5 weeks once steady-state concentrations are achieved, which is typically after 6 months of therapy.

3. **Adverse effects:** The 5-α reductase inhibitors cause sexual side effects, such as decreased ejaculate, decreased libido, ED, gynecomastia, and oligospermia. *Finasteride* and *dutasteride* have

	α₁-ADRENERGIC ANTAGONISTS	5 α-REDUCTASE INHIBITORS
Decrease in prostate size	No	Yes
Peak onset	2–4 weeks	6–12 months
Decrease in PSA	No	Yes
Sexual dysfunction	+	++
Hypotensive effects	++	−
Commonly used drugs	*Tamsulosin* and *alfuzosin*	*Finasteride* and *dutasteride*

Figure 32.7
Comparisons of treatment for BPH. PSA = prostate-specific antigen.

teratogenic potential. Women who are pregnant or of childbearing age should not handle or ingest either agent, as this may lead to serious birth defects involving the genitalia in a male fetus. Although both agents are metabolized by the CYP450 system, drug interactions are rare. It is not ideal to use a 5-α reductase inhibitor with testosterone, since both *finasteride* and *dutasteride* inhibit the conversion of testosterone to its active form, DHT.

C. Phosphodiesterase-5 inhibitor

Tadalafil is the only PDE-5 inhibitor approved for the treatment of BPH. PDE-5 is present in the prostate and bladder. As such, inhibition of PDE-5 by *tadalafil* allows for vasodilation and relaxation of the smooth muscle of the prostate and bladder, which thereby improves symptoms of BPH.

Study Questions

Choose the ONE best answer.

32.1 Which of the following statements is CORRECT regarding the mechanism of action of phosphodiesterase-5 (PDE-5) inhibitors?

A. PDE-5 inhibitors increase prostaglandin production.

B. PDE-5 inhibitors enhance the effect of nitric oxide.

C. PDE-5 inhibitors cause vasoconstriction of the erection chamber.

D. PDE-5 inhibitors antagonize cyclic GMP.

Correct answer = B. PDE-5 inhibitors enhance the effect of nitric oxide by preventing the breakdown of cGMP. PDE-5 inhibitors do not affect prostaglandin production. Although blood is drawn to the erection chamber, PDE-5 inhibitors allow for this via vasodilation, not vasoconstriction. PDE-5 inhibitors prevent the breakdown of cGMP but do not antagonize its action.

32.2 When selecting between the available PDE-5 inhibitors for treatment of ED, which of the following is an important consideration?

A. Tadalafil has the shortest half-life of the PDE-5 inhibitors.

B. Sildenafil should be given with food to increase absorption.

C. Vardenafil ODT doses are not equal to film-coated vardenafil doses.

D. Avanafil should be taken at least 1 hour prior to intercourse.

Correct answer = C. The ODT dosage form of vardenafil provides a high systemic concentration of vardenafil, which is higher than that provided by the film-coated tablets. As such, the doses are not interchangeable. Tadalafil has the longest half-life of all PDE-5 inhibitors. Food may delay sildenafil absorption. Avanafil has the quickest onset of action and may be taken 30 minutes prior to intercourse.

32.3 A patient who is taking a PDE-5 inhibitor for ED is diagnosed with angina. Which of the following antianginal medications would be of particular concern in this patient?

A. Metoprolol.

B. Diltiazem.

C. Amlodipine.

D. Nitroglycerin.

Correct answer = D. Nitrates, when taken with PDE-5 inhibitors, can cause life-threatening hypotension. While metoprolol, diltiazem, and amlodipine may all lower blood pressure, the interaction with PDE-5 inhibitors is not relevant.

32.4 Which of the following BEST describes the mechanism of action of alprostadil?

A. Alprostadil blocks cGMP.

B. Alprostadil blocks nitric oxide.

C. Alprostadil increases PDE-5.

D. Alprostadil increases cAMP.

Correct answer = D. Through an unknown mechanism, alprostadil (a synthetic prostaglandin) increases levels of cAMP, causing smooth muscle relaxation. Alprostadil does not affect cGMP, nitric oxide, or PDE-5.

32.5 Alprostadil is administered locally. Which of the following is CORRECT regarding local administration of alprostadil?

A. Local administration of alprostadil allows for low systemic absorption.
B. Local administration of alprostadil increases the chance of drug interactions.
C. Local administration of alprostadil is accomplished by way of a cream.
D. Local administration of alprostadil causes changes in color vision.

Correct answer = A. Local administration of alprostadil allows for minimal systemic absorption. This makes alprostadil associated with few drug interactions. Alprostadil is administered by injection or urethral suppository, not a cream. Because there is little systemic absorption, and alprostadil does not affect PDE-6, changes in color vision are not likely.

32.6 Which of the following is the BEST description of the mechanism of action of terazosin?

A. Terazosin blocks 5-α reductase.
B. Terazosin blocks α_{1A} receptors.
C. Terazosin blocks PDE-5.
D. Terazosin blocks α_{1A} and α_{1B} receptors.

Correct answer = D. Terazosin blocks both the α_{1A} and α_{1B} receptors. Terazosin does not affect 5-α reductase or PDE-5.

32.7 A patient is worried about starting terazosin because he is very sensitive to side effects of medications. Which of the following adverse effects would be most expected in this patient?

A. Erectile dysfunction.
B. Gynecomastia.
C. Dizziness.
D. Vomiting.

Correct answer = C. Because of the α-blocking properties, terazosin commonly causes dizziness (this may be related to orthostatic hypotension). ED and gynecomastia would be unexpected with α-blockers. While most any drug may cause nausea and vomiting, terazosin is much more likely to cause dizziness.

32.8 Which of the following is an important difference between terazosin and tamsulosin?

A. Terazosin blocks α_{1A} receptors, while tamsulosin blocks α_{1A} and α_{1B} receptors.
B. Terazosin blocks α_{1A} and α_{1B} receptors, while tamsulosin blocks α_{1A} receptors.
C. Terazosin blocks 5-α reductase, while tamsulosin blocks PDE-5.
D. Terazosin must be taken with food, while tamsulosin can be taken on an empty stomach.

Correct answer = B. Tamsulosin is more selective for the α_{1A} receptor, found in the prostate. Terazosin blocks α_{1A}; however, terazosin also blocks α_{1B}. Neither one blocks 5-α reductase nor PDE-5. Tamsulosin should be taken with food, while terazosin does not need to be taken with food.

32.9 Which of the following is CORRECT regarding finasteride?

A. Finasteride is associated with significant hypotension.
B. Finasteride is associated with birth defects.
C. Finasteride is effective within 2 weeks of initiation.
D. Finasteride is renally eliminated.

Correct answer = B. Because finasteride inhibits the conversion of testosterone to its active form, it may cause significant developmental defects in the male genitalia of a developing fetus. As such, it is contraindicated in pregnancy. Unlike the α-blockers, the 5-α reductase inhibitors are not associated with hypotension. Finasteride may take up to 12 months before it is effective. Finally, finasteride is metabolized via CYP450 and is not renally eliminated.

32.10 A 70-year-old male with BPH and an enlarged prostate continues to have urinary symptoms after an adequate trial of tamsulosin. Dutasteride is added to his therapy. In addition to tamsulosin, he is also taking hydrochlorothiazide, testosterone, and vardenafil as needed prior to intercourse. Which of his medications could have an interaction with dutasteride?

A. Hydrochlorothiazide.
B. Tamsulosin.
C. Testosterone.
D. Vardenafil.

Correct answer = C. Because dutasteride prevents the conversion of testosterone to the more active form, DHT, these medications have an interaction. Essentially, dutasteride prevents testosterone from "working." Hydrochlorothiazide does not interfere with the metabolism of dutasteride, and dutasteride does not have any effect on the blood pressure-lowering effects of hydrochlorothiazide. Tamsulosin is appropriate in combination with a 5-α reductase inhibitor when the prostate is enlarged. Vardenafil is only prescribed as needed, and the two drugs do not have a pharmacokinetic interaction.

Drugs for Anemia

33

Katherine Vogel Anderson and Patrick Cogan

I. OVERVIEW

Anemia is defined as a below-normal plasma hemoglobin concentration resulting from a decreased number of circulating red blood cells or an abnormally low total hemoglobin content per unit of blood volume. General signs and symptoms of anemia include fatigue, rapid heartbeat, shortness of breath, pale skin, dizziness, and insomnia. Anemia can be caused by chronic blood loss, bone marrow abnormalities, increased hemolysis, infections, malignancy, endocrine deficiencies, renal failure, and a number of other disease states. A large number of drugs cause toxic effects on blood cells, hemoglobin production, or erythropoietic organs, which, in turn, may cause anemia. Nutritional anemias are caused by dietary deficiencies of substances such as iron, folic acid, and vitamin B_{12} (*cyanocobalamin*) that are necessary for normal erythropoiesis. Individuals with anemia that has a genetic basis, such as sickle cell disease, can benefit from pharmacologic treatment with actions beyond nutritional supplementation, such as *hydroxyurea*. Anemia can be at least temporarily corrected by transfusion of whole blood. A summary of agents used for the treatment of anemias is provided in Figure 33.1.

II. AGENTS USED TO TREAT ANEMIAS

A. Iron

Iron is stored in the intestinal mucosal cells, liver, spleen, and bone marrow as ferritin (an iron–protein complex) until needed by the body. Iron is delivered to the marrow for hemoglobin production by a transport protein, namely transferrin. Iron deficiency results from acute or chronic blood loss, from insufficient intake during periods of accelerated growth in children, and in heavily menstruating or pregnant women. Thus, iron deficiency results from a negative iron balance due to depletion of iron stores and/or inadequate intake, culminating in hypochromic microcytic anemia (due to low iron and small-sized red blood cells). In addition to general signs and symptoms of anemia, iron deficiency anemia may cause pica (hunger for ice, dirt, paper, etc.), koilonychias (upward curvature of the finger and toe nails), and soreness and cracking at the corners of the mouth.

TREATMENT OF ANEMIA
Cyanocobalamin (B₁₂)
Darbepoetin ARANESP
Epoetin alfa EPOGEN, PROCRIT
Folic acid
Iron DEXFERRUM, INFED, OTHERS
TREATMENT OF NEUTROPENIA
Filgrastim NEUPOGEN
Pegfilgrastim NEULASTA
Sargramostim LEUKINE
Tbo-filgrastim GRANIX
TREATMENT OF SICKLE CELL ANEMIA
Hydroxyurea DROXIA, HYDREA
Pentoxifylline TRENTAL

Figure 33.1
Summary of drugs for the treatment of anemia.

1. **Mechanism of action:** Supplementation with elemental iron corrects the iron deficiency. The CDC recommends 150 to 180 mg/day of oral elemental iron administered in divided doses two to three times daily for patients with iron deficiency anemia.

2. **Pharmacokinetics:** Iron is absorbed after oral administration. Acidic conditions in the stomach keep iron in the reduced ferrous form, which is the more soluble form. Iron is then absorbed in the duodenum. [Note: The amount absorbed depends on the current body stores of iron. If iron stores are adequate, less will be absorbed. If stores are low, more iron will be absorbed.] The relative percentage of iron absorbed decreases with increasing doses. For this reason, it is recommended that most people take the prescribed daily iron supplement in two or three divided doses. Some extended-release formulations may be dosed once daily. Oral preparations include *ferrous sulfate*, *ferrous fumarate*, *ferrous gluconate*, *polysaccharide–iron complex*, and *carbonyl iron* formulations. Of these preparations, *ferrous sulfate* is the most commonly used form of iron due to its high content of elemental iron and relatively low cost. The percentage of elemental iron varies in each oral iron preparation (Figure 33.2).

Parenteral formulations of iron, such as *iron dextran*, *sodium ferric gluconate complex*, and *iron sucrose*, are also available. Macrophages phagocytize *iron dextran* and release iron from the dextran molecule. When *iron sucrose* is used, specific exchange mechanisms transfer iron to transferrin. While parenteral administration treats iron deficiency rapidly, oral administration may take several weeks.

IRON FORMULATION	BRAND NAME(S)	ELEMENTAL IRON (%)	NOTES
Ferrous gluconate	Fergon	12	• Less elemental iron, but similar tolerability to *ferrous sulfate*
Ferric ammonium citrate	Iron citrate	18	• Less bioavailable than ferrous salts • Must be reduced to ferrous form in the intestine
Ferrous sulfate	Fer-in-Sol, Feosol	20	• Most common oral iron supplement • Low cost with good effectiveness and tolerability
Ferrous sulfate, anhydrous	Slow-FE	30	• Extended-release formulation of *ferrous sulfate* (once daily dosing) • Higher cost than *ferrous sulfate*
Ferrous fumarate	Ferretts, Ferrimin, Hemocyte	33	• Similar effectiveness and tolerability to *ferrous sulfate* • Almost no taste compared to other iron salts
Carbonyl iron	Icar, Ircon, Renatabs with Iron	100	• Microparticles of purified iron • Dissolves in the stomach to form HCl salt to be absorbed • Less toxic than iron salts due to slower absorption rate (continued iron release for 1 to 2 days)
Polysaccharide-iron complex	Nu-Iron 150, Niferex	100	• Tasteless and odorless • Similar bioavailability to *ferrous sulfate*

Figure 33.2
Characteristics of various iron formulations.

3. Adverse effects: Gastrointestinal (GI) disturbances caused by local irritation (abdominal pain, constipation, diarrhea, etc.) and dark stools are the most common adverse effects of oral iron supplements. Parenteral iron formulations may be used in those who cannot tolerate oral iron. Fatal hypersensitivity and anaphylactoid reactions can occur in patients receiving parenteral iron (mainly *iron dextran* formulations). A test dose should be administered prior to *iron dextran*. Excessive iron can cause toxicities that can be reversed using chelators such as *deferoxamine*.

B. Folic acid (folate)

The primary use of *folic acid* is in treating deficiency states that arise from inadequate levels of the vitamin. *Folate* deficiency may be caused by 1) increased demand (for example, pregnancy and lactation), 2) poor absorption caused by pathology of the small intestine, 3) alcoholism, or 4) treatment with drugs that are dihydrofolate reductase inhibitors (for example, *methotrexate, pyrimethamine,* and *trimethoprim*). In the latter case, the reduced or active form of the vitamin (*folinic acid*—also known as *leucovorin calcium*—available as oral and parenteral formulations) is used for treatment. A primary result of *folic acid* deficiency is megaloblastic anemia (large-sized red blood cells), which is caused by diminished synthesis of purines and pyrimidines. This leads to an inability of erythropoietic tissue to make DNA and, thereby, proliferate (Figure 33.3). [Note: To avoid neurological complications of *vitamin B₁₂* deficiency, it is important to evaluate the basis of the megaloblastic anemia prior to instituting therapy. Both *vitamin B₁₂* and *folate* deficiency can cause similar symptoms.]

Folic acid is well absorbed in the jejunum unless pathology is present. If excessive amounts of the vitamin are ingested, they are excreted in the urine and feces. Oral *folic acid* administration is nontoxic. There have been no substantiated side effects reported. Rare hypersensitivity reactions to parenteral injections have been reported.

C. Cyanocobalamin and hydroxocobalamin (vitamin B₁₂)

Deficiencies of *vitamin B₁₂* can result from either low dietary levels or, more commonly, poor absorption of the vitamin due to the failure of gastric parietal cells to produce intrinsic factor (as in pernicious anemia), or a loss of activity of the receptor needed for intestinal uptake of the vitamin. Intrinsic factor is a glycoprotein produced by the parietal cells of the stomach, and it is required for *vitamin B₁₂* absorption. In patients with bariatric surgery (surgical treatment for obesity), *vitamin B₁₂* supplementation as *cyanocobalamin* [sye-an-oh-koe-BAL-a-min] is required in large oral doses, sublingually or once a month by the parenteral route. Intramuscular *hydroxocobalamin* [hye-drox-oh-koe-BAL-a-min] is now preferred since it has a rapid response, is highly protein bound, and maintains longer plasma levels. Nonspecific malabsorption syndromes or gastric resection can also cause *vitamin B₁₂* deficiency. In addition to general signs and symptoms of anemia, *vitamin B₁₂* deficiency anemia may cause tingling (pins and needles) in the hands and feet, difficulty walking, dementia and, in extreme cases, hallucinations, paranoia, or schizophrenia.

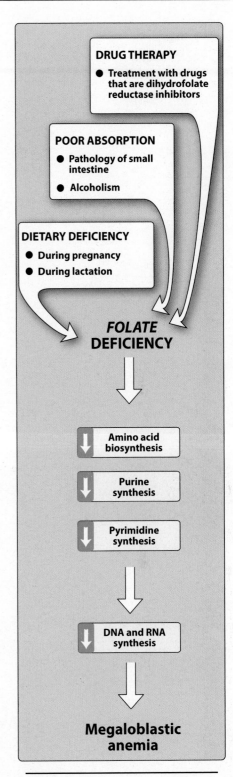

Figure 33.3
Causes and consequences of *folic acid* depletion.

The vitamin may be administered orally (for dietary deficiencies), intramuscularly, or deep subcutaneously (for pernicious anemia). [Note: *Folic acid* administration alone reverses the hematologic abnormality and, thus, masks the *vitamin B$_{12}$* deficiency, which can then proceed to severe neurologic dysfunction and disease. The cause of megaloblastic anemia needs to be determined in order to be specific in terms of treatment. Therefore, megaloblastic anemia should not be treated with *folic acid* alone but, rather, with a combination of *folate* and *vitamin B$_{12}$*.] Therapy must be continued for the remainder of the life of a patient suffering from pernicious anemia. This vitamin is nontoxic even in large doses.

D. Erythropoietin and darbepoetin

Peritubular cells in the kidneys work as sensors that respond to hypoxia and mediate synthesis and release of *erythropoietin* [ee-rith-ro-POI-eh-tin; EPO], a glycoprotein. EPO stimulates stem cells to differentiate into proerythroblasts and promotes the release of reticulocytes from the marrow and initiation of hemoglobin formation. EPO, thus, regulates red blood cell proliferation and differentiation in bone marrow. Human *erythropoietin* (*epoetin alfa*), produced by recombinant DNA technology, is effective in the treatment of anemia caused by end-stage renal disease, anemia associated with human immunodeficiency virus infection, and anemia in bone marrow disorders, anemias of prematurity, and anemias in some cancer patients. *Darbepoetin* [dar-be-POE-e-tin] is a long-acting version of *erythropoietin* that differs from *erythropoietin* by the addition of two carbohydrate chains, which improves its biologic activity. Therefore, *darbepoetin* has decreased clearance and has a half-life about three times that of *epoetin alfa.* Due to their delayed onset of action, these agents have no value in acute treatment of anemia. Supplementation with iron may be required to ensure an adequate response. The protein is usually administered intravenously in renal dialysis patients, but the subcutaneous route is preferred for other indications. These agents are generally well tolerated, but side effects may include elevation in blood pressure and arthralgia in some cases. [Note: The former may be due to increases in peripheral vascular resistance and/or blood viscosity.] When *epoetin alfa* is used to target hemoglobin concentrations more than 11 g/dL, serious cardiovascular events (such as thrombosis and severe hypertension), increased risk of death, shortened time to tumor progression, and decreased survival have been observed. The recommendations for all patients receiving *epoetin alfa* or *darbepoetin* include a minimum effective dose that does not exceed a hemoglobin level of 12 g/dL, and the hemoglobin should not rise by more than 1 g/dL over a 2-week period. Additionally, if the hemoglobin level exceeds 10 g/dL, doses of *epoetin alfa* or *darbepoetin* should be reduced or treatment should be discontinued.

III. AGENTS USED TO TREAT NEUTROPENIA

Myeloid growth factors or granulocyte colony–stimulating factors (G-CSF), such as *filgrastim* [fil-GRAS-tim], *tbo-filgrastim*, and *pegfilgrastim* [peg-fil-GRAS-tim], and granulocyte–macrophage colony–stimulating factors

(GM-CSF), such as *sargramostim* [sar-GRA-moe-stim], stimulate granulocyte production in the marrow to increase the neutrophil counts and reduce the duration of severe neutropenia. These agents are typically used prophylactically to reduce risk of neutropenia following chemotherapy and bone marrow transplantation. *Filgrastim* and *sargramostim* can be dosed either subcutaneously or intravenously, whereas *tbo-filgrastim* and *pegfilgrastim* are dosed subcutaneously only. The main difference between the available agents lies in the frequency of dosing. *Filgrastim, tbo-filgrastim*, and *sargramostim* are dosed once a day beginning 24 to 72 hours after chemotherapy, until the absolute neutrophil count (ANC) reaches 5000 to 10,000/µL. *Pegfilgrastim* is a pegylated form of G-CSF, resulting in a much longer half-life when compared to the other agents. As such, it is given as a single dose 24 hours after chemotherapy, rather than once daily. Monitoring of ANC is typically not necessary with *pegfilgrastim*. There is no evidence to show superiority of one agent over another in terms of efficacy, safety, or tolerability. Bone pain is a common adverse effect with these agents.

IV. AGENTS USED TO TREAT SICKLE CELL DISEASE

A. Hydroxyurea

Clinical trials have shown that *hydroxyurea* [high-DROX-ee-YOUR-ee-ah] can reduce the frequency of painful sickle cell crises (Figure 33.4). *Hydroxyurea* is also used off-label to treat chronic myelogenous leukemia and polycythemia vera. In sickle cell disease, the drug apparently increases fetal hemoglobin levels, thus diluting the abnormal hemoglobin S (HbS). This process takes several months. Polymerization of HbS is delayed in treated patients, so that painful crises are not caused by sickled cells blocking capillaries and causing tissue anoxia. Important side effects of *hydroxyurea* include bone marrow suppression and cutaneous vasculitis. It is important that *hydroxyurea* is administered under the supervision of a physician experienced in the treatment of sickle cell disease.

B. Pentoxifylline

Pentoxifylline [pen-tox-IH-fi-leen] is a methylxanthine derivative that has been called a "rheologic modifier." It increases the deformability of red blood cells (improves erythrocyte flexibility) and reduces the viscosity of blood. This decreases total systemic vascular resistance, improves blood flow, and enhances tissue oxygenation in patients with peripheral vascular disease. It is indicated to treat intermittent claudication, where it can modestly control function and symptoms. Unlabeled uses include improving psychopathological symptoms in patients with cerebrovascular insufficiency. It has been studied in diabetic angiopathies, transient ischemic attacks, leg ulcers, sickle cell anemias, strokes, and Raynaud's phenomenon. It is available in extended-release tablets and is taken three times a day with food. Adverse reactions are mainly GI in nature and are lessened by administration with food.

Figure 33.5 provides a summary of medications used in the management of anemia.

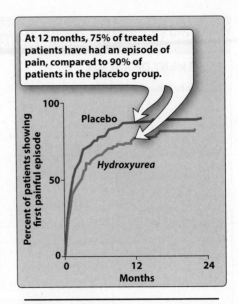

At 12 months, 75% of treated patients have had an episode of pain, compared to 90% of patients in the placebo group.

Figure 33.4
Effect of treatment with *hydroxyurea* on the percentage of sickle cell patients experiencing first painful episode.

MEDICATION	ADVERSE EFFECTS	DRUG INTERACTIONS	MONITORING PARAMETERS
TREATMENT OF ANEMIA			
Cyanocobalamin/B₁₂	Injection site pain Arthralgia Dizziness Headache Nasopharyngitis Anaphylaxis	Proton pump inhibitors—may decrease oral absorption of vitamin B₁₂	Vitamin B₁₂ Folate Iron
Erythropoietin/epoetin alfa	Edema Pruritus Nausea/Vomiting Hypertension CVA Thrombosis	*Darbepoietin alfa*—duplication of therapy can lead to increase adverse events	H/H Serum ferritin Blood pressure
Darbepoetin alfa	Edema Dyspnea Hypertension CVA Thrombosis	*Epoetin alfa*—duplication of therapy can lead to increase adverse events	H/H Serum ferritin Blood pressure
Folic acid	Bad taste in mouth Nausea Confusion Irritability	*Cholestyramine*—may interfere with absorption	CBC Serum folate
Iron	Pruritus N/V/D Headache Anaphylaxis	*Deferoxamine*—chelates iron *Dimercaprol*—chelates iron	H/H Serum iron TIBC Transferrin Reticulocyte count
TREATMENT OF SICKLE CELL ANEMIA			
Hydroxyurea	Myelosuppression Skin ulcer Secondary leukemia	HIV medications—*hydroxyurea* can decrease CD4 counts Salicylates—increase bleeding risk *Probenecid*—↑ uric acid	CBC
Pentoxifylline	Nausea/Vomiting Thrombocytopenia Jaundice Anaphylaxis	*Ketorolac* (contraindicated)—increased bleeding risk *Ginkgo biloba*—increased antiplatelet effect	CBC

CVA=cerebrovascular accident, H/H=hemoglobin and hematocrit, CBC=complete blood count, N/V/D=nausea/vomiting/diarrhea, TIBC=total iron binding capacity

Figure 33.5
Medications for the management of anemia.

Study Questions

Choose the ONE best answer.

33.1 All of the following are classifications of dietary deficiencies causing nutritional anemia except:

A. Vitamin B₁₂ (cyanocobalamin).
B. Folic acid.
C. Vitamin D.
D. Iron.

Correct answer = C. Vitamin D deficiency does exist, but this does not cause anemia in patients. Vitamin B₁₂, folic acid, and iron deficiencies all contribute to anemia.

33.2 Which of the following iron supplements contains the highest percentage of elemental iron?

A. Ferrous sulfate.
B. Carbonyl iron.
C. Ferrous gluconate.
D. Ferric ammonium citrate.

Correct answer = B. Ferrous sulfate contains 20% (or 30% in the anhydrous formulation), ferrous gluconate contains 12% elemental iron, and ferric ammonium citrate contains 18% elemental iron. These are all well below the percent of elemental iron in carbonyl iron, which contains 100% elemental iron.

33.3 A 56-year-old female is discovered to have megaloblastic anemia. Her past medical history is significant for alcoholism. Which of the following would be the best treatment option for this patient?

A. Oral vitamin B_{12}.
B. Parenteral vitamin B_{12}.
C. Oral folate.
D. Oral vitamin B_{12} with oral folate.

Correct answer = D. The patient has a history of alcoholism, which would suggest folic acid deficiency anemia. However, folic acid administration alone reverses the hematologic abnormality and masks possible vitamin B_{12} deficiency, which can then proceed to severe neurologic dysfunction and disease. The cause of megaloblastic anemia needs to be determined in order to be specific in terms of treatment. Therefore, megaloblastic anemia should not be treated with folic acid alone but, rather, with a combination of folate and vitamin B_{12}.

33.4 A 60-year-old female presents to her primary care physician complaining of dizziness and fatigue. Following laboratory testing, the patient is diagnosed with iron deficiency anemia, and oral iron supplementation is needed. Which of the following would be the most appropriate dosing regimen for the patient?

A. Ferrous fumarate 325 mg once daily.
B. Ferrous gluconate 256 mg once daily.
C. Polysaccharide–iron complex 150 mg two to three times daily.
D. Ferrous sulfate 325 mg two to three times daily.

Correct answer = D. The recommended dose of iron supplementation in iron deficiency anemia is typically about 150 mg of elemental iron in two to three divided doses. Extended-release formulations (such as polysaccharide–iron complex) may be dosed once daily. Ferrous sulfate 325 mg contains approximately 65 mg of elemental iron, ferrous fumarate 325 mg contains about 107 mg elemental iron, ferrous gluconate 256 mg contains approximately 30 mg elemental iron, and polysaccharide–iron complex 150 mg contains 150 mg elemental iron.

33.5 A 63-year-old female patient with anemia secondary to chronic kidney disease and a hemoglobin level of 8.6 g/dL is treated with epoetin alfa. Eight days after the initial dose of epoetin alfa, the patient's hemoglobin is 11.3 mg/dL. Why is it appropriate to discontinue treatment with epoetin alfa?

A. Treatment goals of hemoglobin greater than 12 g/dL and a rise in hemoglobin of greater than 1 g/dL in a 2-week period are associated with cardiovascular events and decreased survival.
B. The patient has not responded to the epoetin alfa and therefore requires treatment with a different agent for her anemia.
C. Epoetin alfa is less effective than darbepoetin alfa, and treatment with epoetin alfa should be transitioned to darbepoetin to receive maximum benefit.
D. Epoetin alfa is not indicated for treatment of anemia secondary to chronic kidney disease.

Correct answer = A. Answer B is incorrect because the patient has responded to the epoetin alfa, as the patient's hemoglobin has increased following its administration. Answer C is incorrect because there is no clear evidence to claim that either agent is more effective than the other in treatment of anemia. Answer D is incorrect because epoetin alfa is indicated for the treatment of anemia secondary to chronic kidney disease.

33.6 Which of the following might be beneficial to reduce the frequency of painful crises in a patient with sickle cell disease?

A. Epoetin alfa.
B. Filgrastim.
C. Hydroxyurea.
D. Sargramostim.

Correct answer = C. Clinical evidence supports the use of hydroxyurea for reducing the frequency and severity of painful sickle cell crises during the course of sickle cell disease. Epoetin alfa helps increase hemoglobin and red blood cell production in anemias secondary to chronic kidney disease, HIV, bone marrow disorders, and other disorders. Filgrastim and sargramostim stimulate granulocyte production in the marrow to increase the neutrophil counts and reduce the duration of severe neutropenia.

Drugs for Dermatologic Disorders

Thomas A. Panavelil

34

I. OVERVIEW

The skin is the largest organ system of the body. It has many essential functions including serving as a protective barrier, helping to regulate temperature, offering defense against infections and toxic chemicals, serving as a source of vitamin D, and providing sensation to touch, temperature, sexual pleasure, and pain. Skin disorders, such as acne and dermatitis, are among the top reasons that patients seek medical attention. Pharmacological approaches to correct skin abnormalities, including infections, can be administered topically or systemically, depending on the nature and extent of the disorder. This chapter discusses drugs that are used for the treatment of common skin disorders including acne, bacterial infections, ectoparasitic infections, psoriasis, and others. Drugs for acne vulgaris and topical antibacterials are summarized in Figure 34.1. [Note: Agents for fungal infections of the skin are covered in the chapter on antifungals (see Chapter 42).]

II. TOPICAL PREPARATIONS

The skin is composed of two main layers, the epidermis and the dermis (Figure 34.2). The epidermis itself is composed of many layers and serves as a defense against pathogens. The outermost layer of the epidermis, the stratum corneum, consists of a lipophilic keratinous layer of skin. The dermis is located between the epidermis and the subcutaneous tissue, and it is composed of connective tissue. It also contains specialized structures such as sweat glands, sebaceous glands, hair follicles, and blood vessels.

Use of topical agents for treatment of dermatologic disorders is not only convenient but also minimizes systemic adverse effects. Topical agents may be formulated as sprays, powders, lotions, creams, pastes, packed dressings, ointments, and aerated foams. The bioavailability of these agents and the ability to retain therapeutic effect on the skin involve factors such as the vehicle (water or oil based) and the physical methods used to localize them, such as the use of a patch formulation. The therapeutic efficacy of topical agents is dependent on the thickness of the stratum corneum, the drug concentration and permeability, frequency of

ACNE VULGARIS AGENTS
Adapalene DIFFERIN
Azelaic acid AZELEX
Benzoyl peroxide VARIOUS
Isotretinoin VARIOUS
Tazarotene TAZORAC
Tretinoin RETIN-A

TOPICAL ANTIBACTERIAL AGENTS
Bacitracin
Clindamycin CLEOCIN T
Dapsone ACZONE
Erythromycin BENZAMYCIN
Gentamicin
Mupirocin BACTROBAN
Neomycin (with *bacitracin* and *polymyxin B*) TRIPLE ANTIBIOTIC
Retapamulin ALTABAX

Figure 34.1
Summary of drugs for acne and topical antibacterials.

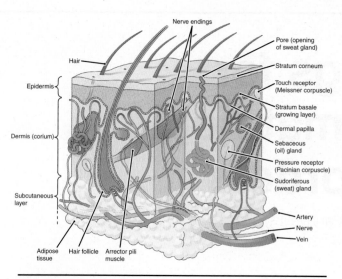

Figure 34.2
Cross section of the skin.

dosing, and other factors such as age and health of the skin. Lipophilic agents are more readily absorbed than those that are hydrophilic.

III. AGENTS FOR ACNE

Acne vulgaris (common acne) is a common skin disorder that is characterized by pimples, comedones, pustules, and sometimes nodules and scarring (Figure 34.3). Comedones are clogged hair follicles (pores) in the skin, which can be open (blackhead) or closed (whitehead). Acne occurs due to alterations in pilosebaceous units—skin structures that contain a hair follicle and a sebaceous (oil) gland. Androgens stimulate sebaceous glands, thereby producing sebum that leads to follicular keratinization and obstruction. Propionibacterium acnes, part of the normal skin flora, can enter the clogged pore and multiply, causing redness and inflammation and leading to papillary, pustulary, and cystic acne. Treatments for acne help to reduce sebum production or control P. acnes. [Note: Use of oral contraceptives may help decrease circulating levels of free androgen and reduce symptoms of acne (see Chapter 26).]

A. Retinoids

Retinoids are derivatives of vitamin A that are highly effective in the treatment of acne, as well as other skin conditions such as psoriasis and photoaging. *Tretinoin* [TRET-in-oin] and *isotretinoin* [eye-so-TRET-i-noyn] are first-generation retinoids that are used for the management of acne. Third-generation retinoids include *adapalene* [a-DAP-a-leen] and *tazarotene* [ta-ZAR-oh-teen]. Third-generation agents are less irritating and more effective than first-generation retinoids and are considered first-line therapy for comedonal and inflammatory acne. These agents are applied topically, with the exception of *isotretinoin*, which is an oral drug. Due to the adverse effect profile, use of *isotretinoin* should be reserved for severe cystic acne.

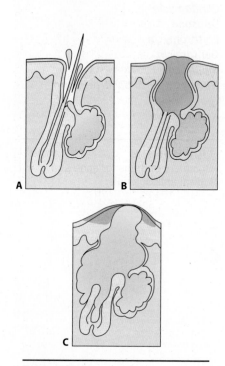

Figure 34.3
Acne vulgaris. **A.** Normal sebaceous gland and hair follicle. **B.** Comedone formation. **C.** Pustule formation.

1. **Mechanism of action:** Retinoids influence a wide variety of biological activities, including cellular proliferation and differentiation, immune function, inflammation, and sebum production. Unlike the first-generation agents, the third-generation agents do not influence sebum production. They are comedolytic and anti-inflammatory. The molecular actions of retinoids are mediated through nucleic retinoic acid receptors. Once bound to the receptors, retinoids function as transcription factors that enhance initiation of transcription (Figure 34.4).

2. **Adverse effects:** Irritation, dryness, and skin peeling are all complications with the use of retinoids. Photosensitivity is also an adverse effect, and patients should be cautioned to wear sunscreen. Other adverse effects include dry mucous membranes and dry eyes. Suicide or suicide attempts have been associated with the use of oral *isotretinoin*. There is a very high risk of birth defects if pregnancy occurs while taking *isotretinoin*, and this drug as well as other retinoids are contraindicated in pregnancy.

B. Benzoyl peroxide

Benzoyl peroxide [BEN-zoyl per-OX-ide] is considered the first-line agent for mild to moderate acne with no inflammation. The mechanism of action includes antiseptic effects against P. acnes as well as opening of the pores. *Benzoyl peroxide* is a topical agent that is available in many over-the-counter acne treatment products, as well as some prescription products. Dry skin, peeling, and irritation are local adverse effects.

C. Salicylic acid

Topical *salicylic* [sal-i-SIL-ik] *acid*, a β-hydroxy acid, penetrates the pilosebaceous unit and works as an exfoliant to clear comedones. Its comedolytic effects are not as pronounced as those of the retinoids. The drug has mild anti-inflammatory activity and is keratolytic at higher concentrations. *Salicylic acid* is used as a treatment for mild acne and is available in many over-the-counter facial washes and medicated treatment pads. Mild skin peeling, dryness, and local irritation are adverse effects.

D. Azelaic acid

Azelaic [aze-eh-LAY-ik] *acid*, a dicarboxylic acid, has antibacterial activity against P. acnes as well as anti-inflammatory actions. *Azelaic acid* normalizes keratinization and is anticomedogenic. It is available as a topical preparation for the treatment of mild to moderate inflammatory acne. It is generally well tolerated, with mild skin irritation as the most common adverse effect.

E. Antibiotics

As noted above, P. acnes is a gram-positive rod that is associated with inflammatory lesions in acne. For moderate to severe acne with inflammatory lesions, use of topical or oral antibiotics is useful for inhibition of P. acnes. Topical formulations of *erythromycin* and *clindamycin* (preferred) are available. These agents may be combined with

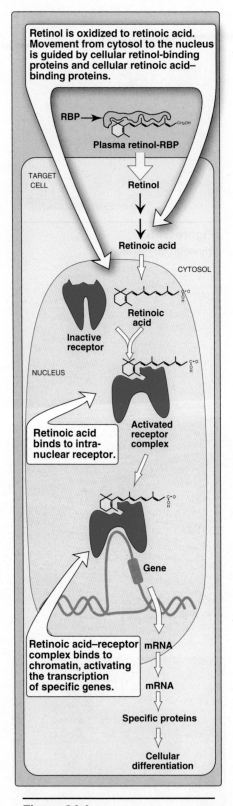

Figure 34.4
Action of retinoids. Note: Retinoic acid complex is a dimer but is shown as a monomer for simplicity. RBP = retinol-binding protein.

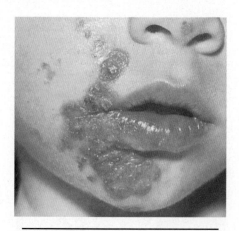

Figure 34.5
Impetigo on the face.

benzoyl peroxide or the retinoids for better effectiveness. *Dapsone*, a synthetic sulfone (see Chapter 41), is available as a topical gel that treats acne. Its mechanism of action in the treatment of acne is unknown. [Note: *Metronidazole* as a topical agent is useful in adult acne, also known as rosacea.] Oral antibiotics commonly used for the management of moderate to severe acne include *minocycline*, *doxycycline*, and *erythromycin*. *Erythromycin* is used infrequently due to gastrointestinal adverse effects. Each of these agents is covered in more detail in the chapters on anti-infective therapy.

IV. TOPICAL ANTIBACTERIAL AGENTS

Organisms such as staphylococci and streptococci can cause folliculitis, abscesses, fasciitis, cellulitis, impetigo, and many pus-forming infections. Several gram-positive and gram-negative bacteria cause infections that are not limited to the skin and may cause serious diseases, since they can spread and become systemic infections.

A. Gram-positive infections

Bacitracin [bas-i-TRAY-sin] is a peptide antibiotic active against many gram-positive organisms. It is used mainly in topical formulations; if used systemically, it is toxic. *Bacitracin* is mostly used for the prevention of skin infections after burns or minor scrapes. It is frequently found in combination products with *neomycin* and/or *polymyxin* (see below). *Mupirocin* [mue-PIR-oh-sin] is a protein synthesis inhibitor that is useful in treating impetigo (a contagious skin infection caused by streptococci or staphylococci; Figure 34.5) and other serious gram-positive skin infections, including infections caused by *methicillin*-resistant Staphylococcus aureus. *Retapamulin* [RE-te-PAM-ue-lin] is a newer protein synthesis inhibitor that treats impetigo. Adverse effects are minimal with these agents and usually consist of mild local skin reactions.

B. Gram-negative infections

Polymyxin [paw-lee-MIX-in] *B* is a cyclic hydrophobic peptide that disrupts the bacterial cell membrane of gram-negative organisms. As noted above, it is commonly combined with *neomycin* and *bacitracin* ("triple antibiotic") in topical products used for the prevention of skin infections after minor skin trauma. *Neomycin* [nee-oh-MY-sin] in combination with other agents and also *gentamicin* can be used to treat skin infections caused by gram-negative organisms such as Pseudomonas, E. coli, and Klebsiella sp. Topical use of these agents rarely causes systemic side effects. Rare adverse reactions such as allergic dermatitis and other sensitivities occur with *neomycin*.

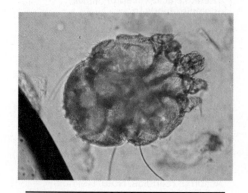

Figure 34.6
Scabies mite.

V. AGENTS USED IN ECTOPARASITIC INFECTIONS

Ectoparasites are parasites that live on the skin of animals from which they derive nutrition. Pediculosis (infestation with lice) and scabies (caused by Sarcoptes scabiei, human mite; Figure 34.6) are common ectoparasitic infections. Lice infestations may be caused by Pediculus capitis (head louse),

Pediculus corporis (body louse), or Pthirus pubis (pubic or crab louse). Treatments for ectoparasitic infections are outlined in Figure 34.7. Lindane [LIN-dane] is a cyclohexane derivative that is available as a cream or shampoo. Lindane is toxic when absorbed by the parasite and is an effective pediculicide (kills lice) and scabicide. Permethrin [per-METH-rin] is a synthetic pyrethroid that is neurotoxic to lice (1% non-prescription) and is effective in 5% concentration by prescription to treat scabies. Permethrin is preferred over lindane for the treatment of lice and scabies, since lindane can cause neurotoxicity. [Note: Oral iver-mectin (see Chapter 44) is an alternative treatment for lice and sca-bies]. Synergized pyrethrins (pyrethrins [pye-REE-thrins] with piperonyl butoxide [pye-PER-oh-nil bue-TOX-ide]) is a nonprescription product approved to treat head and pubic lice. Pyrethrins are pesticides and piperonyl butoxide prevents the lice from metabolizing the pyrethrins, thereby enhancing their effect. Due to a low risk of toxicity, this agent is considered a first-line treatment for pediculosis. Crotamiton [crow-TA-mi-ton] is a scabicide and has antipruritic functions. Its mechanism of action is unknown.

VI. AGENTS FOR PIGMENTATION DISORDERS

Agents for pigmentation disorders include hydroquinone and methox-salen, which are used for the treatment of hyperpigmented skin conditions and vitiligo, respectively (Figure 34.7).

A. Hydroquinone

Hydroquinone [HYE-droe-KWIN-one] is a topical skin whitening agent that reduces hyperpigmentation associated with freckles and melasma. It is often used in combination with topical retinoids to treat the signs of photoaging. The mechanism of action of hydroquinone is inhibition of the tyrosinase enzyme required for melanin synthesis. Hydroquinone lightens the skin temporarily and is commonly used as a 4% prepara-tion. It should not be used in higher concentrations, or in excessive quantities for an extended duration, as it is associated with possible carcinogenicity. Local skin irritation is the most common adverse effect. Monobenzone [mon-oh-BEN-zone], the benzyl ether of hydroquinone, is sometimes used to even out the skin discoloration associated with vitiligo (depigmentation disorder of the skin; Figure 34.8). The drug may cause permanent depigmentation and is no longer available in many markets.

B. Methoxsalen

Methoxsalen [meth-OX-ah-len] is a photoactive substance (psoralen) that stimulates melanocytes and is used as a repigmentation agent for patients with vitiligo. It must be photoactivated by UV radiation to form a DNA adduct inhibiting DNA replication by a method called PUVA (psoralen plus UVA radiation). Methoxsalen inhibits cell pro-liferation and promotes cell differentiation of epithelial cells. Topical methoxsalen may be used for small patches of vitiligo, and oral ther-apy is used for more widespread disease. Because of the possibili-ties for aging of the skin and possible carcinogenicity, it is used with caution.

ECTOPARASITICIDES
Crotamiton EURAX
Lindane
Permethrin ELIMITE, NIX
Pyrethrins RID

AGENTS FOR PIGMENTATION DISORDERS
Hydroquinone VARIOUS
Methoxsalen OXSORALEN

AGENTS FOR PSORIASIS
Acitretin SORIATANE
Calcipotriene DOVONEX, SORILUX
Calcitriol VECTICAL
Tazarotene TAZORAC

KERATOLYTIC AGENTS
Coal tar OXIPOR, SCYTERA
Salicylic acid SALEX

TRICHOGENIC AGENTS
Finasteride PROPECIA
Minoxidil ROGAINE

Figure 34.7
Summary of agents for selected dermatologic disorders.

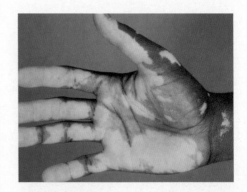

Figure 34.8
The palm is frequently affected by vitiligo.

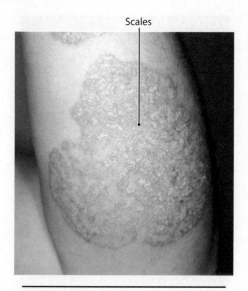
Scales

Figure 34.9
Psoriasis. A large, scaly, erythematous plaque.

VII. DRUGS FOR PSORIASIS

Psoriasis is a skin disease that presents with erythematous scaling plaques (Figure 34.9). It manifests with increased epidermal cell proliferation. Psoriasis appears to have both genetic factors and T-cell–mediated immune components. The majority of patients have mild to moderate psoriasis, and this can be managed with topical treatments including retinoids, vitamin D analogues, keratolytic agents (Figure 34.7), and corticosteroids. More severe cases require systemic therapy with phototherapy (*methoxsalen* followed by UVA or UVB alone), *methotrexate*, *cyclosporine*, or biologic response modifiers (for example, *etanercept*, *adalimumab*; see Chapters 36, 46, and 47).

A. Retinoids

Tazarotene is a topical retinoid used for the treatment of plaque psoriasis. Adverse effects are similar to other retinoids. *Acitretin* [a-si-TRE-tin] is a second-generation retinoid used orally in the treatment of pustular forms of psoriasis. It is a metabolite of *etretinate* (no longer available), which has a half-life of 120 days. Since ingestion of ethanol can increase transesterification of *acitretin* to *etretinate*, ethanol is contraindicated with this agent. Like other retinoids, *acitretin* is teratogenic and women must avoid pregnancy for at least 3 years after the use of this drug (due to the long duration of teratogenic potential). Cheilitis, pruritus, peeling skin, and hyperlipidemia are common adverse effects.

B. Vitamin D analogues

Calcipotriene [cal-sih-poh-TRY-een] and *calcitriol* [kal-si-TRYE-ol] are synthetic vitamin D_3 derivatives used topically to treat plaque psoriasis. They inhibit keratinocyte proliferation and increase keratinocyte differentiation. Their therapeutic effectiveness does not appear to decrease upon continued use. Transient elevations in calcium levels have been reported in some patients. Adverse effects include itching, dryness, burning irritation, and erythema.

C. Keratolytic agents

Keratolytic agents such as *coal tar* and *salicylic acid* are effective in localized psoriasis, especially on the scalp. They improve corticosteroid penetration. *Coal tar* inhibits excessive skin cell proliferation and may also have anti-inflammatory effects. Because it is cosmetically unappealing, *coal tar* may have a low acceptance rate among patients and, consequently, its use has been largely supplanted by the newer topical agents.

VIII. TOPICAL CORTICOSTEROIDS

Corticosteroids (glucocorticoids) have immunosuppressive and anti-inflammatory properties. Topical corticosteroids are used for the treatment of psoriasis, eczema, contact dermatitis, and other skin conditions manifested by itching and inflammation. They are administered locally and via topical and intralesional routes. Corticosteroids work via intracellular

LOW STRENGTH	INTERMEDIATE STRENGTH	HIGH STRENGTH	VERY HIGH STRENGTH
Alclometasone dipropionate 0.05% (c, o)	Betamethasone dipropionate 0.05% (c)	Amcinonide 0.1% (c, l, o)	Betamethasone dipropionate 0.05% (o, g)
Clocortolone pivalate 0.1% (c) Fluocinolone acetonide 0.01% solution (s)	Desonide 0.05% (c, l, o)	Betamethasone dipropionate, augmented 0.05% (c, l)	Clobetasol propionate 0.05% (c, g, o)
Hydrocortisone base or acetate 0.25% to 2.5% (o, c)	Desoximetasone 0.05% (c)	Desoximetasone 0.05% (o)	Diflorasone diacetate 0.05% (o)
Triamcinolone acetonide 0.025% (c, l, o)	Fluocinolone acetonide 0.025% (c, o)	Diflorasone diacetate 0.05% (o, c)	Fluocinonide 0.1% (c)
	Flurandrenolide 0.025 to 0.5% (c, o)	Fluocinonide 0.05% (c, g, o, s)	Flurandrenolide 0.05% (l)
	Fluticasone propionate 0.005% to 0.05% (o, c)	Halcinonide 0.1% (c, o)	Halobetasol 0.05% (c, o)
	Hydrocortisone butyrate 0.1% (c, o, s)	Triamcinolone acetonide 0.5% (c, o)	
	Hydrocortisone valerate 0.2% (c, o)		
	Mometasone furoate 0.1% (c, o, l)		
	Triamcinolone acetonide 0.1% to 0.2% (c, o)		

c = cream, g = gel, l= lotion, o= ointment, s=solution

Figure 34.10
Potency of various topical corticosteroids.

receptors and initiate several transcriptions and translations leading to their multiple effects. The actions include inhibitory effects on the arachidonic acid cascade, depression of production of many cytokines, and effects on inflammatory cells (see Chapter 27). In psoriasis, they inhibit epidermal cell mitosis. Numerous topical corticosteroids are available, with varying potencies and multiple vehicles of delivery (Figure 34.10). Tachyphylaxis (decrease in response after repetitive use, tolerance) can occur with continuous use. Substitution of a different corticosteroid or less frequent use can minimize tolerance. Adverse effects include skin atrophy (thinning of the skin), striae, purpura, acneiform eruptions, dermatitis, local infections, and hypopigmentation. In children, potent agents applied to a large surface area can cause systemic toxicity, including depression of the hypothalamic–pituitary–adrenal axis and growth retardation.

IX. TRICHOGENIC AGENTS

Minoxidil [min-OX-i-dil] and *finasteride* [fih-NAH-steh-ride] are trichogenic agents that are indicated for the treatment of androgenic alopecia ("male pattern baldness"). *Minoxidil*, originally used as a systemic antihypertensive, was noted to have the adverse effect of increased hair growth. This adverse effect was turned into a therapeutic application in the treatment of alopecia. For hair loss, the drug is available as a nonprescription topical foam or solution. As a topical therapy, it does not cause systemic hypotension. *Minoxidil* is effective at halting hair loss in both men and women and may produce hair growth in some patients. Although the mechanism of action is not fully known, it is believed to act, at least in part, by shortening the rest phase of the hair cycle. The drug must be used continuously to maintain effects on hair growth.

Finasteride is an oral 5-α reductase inhibitor that blocks conversion of testosterone to the potent androgen 5-α dihydrotestosterone (DHT). High levels of DHT can cause the hair follicle to miniaturize and atrophy. *Finasteride* decreases scalp and serum DHT concentrations, thus inhibiting a key factor in the etiology of androgenic alopecia. [Note: *Finasteride* is used in higher doses for the treatment of benign prostatic hyperplasia (see Chapter 32).] Adverse effects include decreased libido, decreased ejaculation, and erectile dysfunction. The drug should not be used or handled in pregnancy, as it can cause hypospadias in a male fetus. Like *minoxidil*, use must be continued to maintain therapeutic benefits.

Study Questions

Choose the ONE best answer.

34.1 Which of the following is correct regarding the use of isotretinoin in the treatment of acne?

   A. Isotretinoin is given intravenously in the treatment of acne.
   B. Isotretinoin acts primarily on the membrane receptors.
   C. If given in high dosages, isotretinoin can indirectly increase the concentration of <u>Propionibacterium acnes</u> bacteria.
   D. Isotretinoin activates prostaglandin E_2 and collagenase, which causes the adverse effect of inflammation.
   E. Isotretinoin is contraindicated in pregnancy due to its high risk of birth defects.

Correct answer = E. Retinoic acids play an important role in mammalian embryogenesis. Excessive amounts of retinoid have been shown to cause teratogenicity, and the exact molecular mechanism is not known.

34.2 A 3-year-old boy has contracted scabies from his playmate at the daycare center. Which of the following would be the most appropriate treatment?

   A. Azelaic acid.
   B. Mupirocin.
   C. Permethrin.
   D. Triple antibiotic ointment.

Correct answer = C. Permethrin is a topical scabicide that is preferred due to its lower risk of neurotoxicity. Azelaic acid is a topical treatment for acne. Mupirocin and triple antibiotic ointment are used for the treatment of bacterial infections and would not be appropriate for scabies.

34.3 Which of the following drugs is taken orally before using UVA radiation in the treatment of severe cases of psoriasis?

   A. Methoxsalen.
   B. Hydroquinone.
   C. Finasteride.
   D. Minoxidil.
   E. Tazarotene.

Correct answer = A. In severe cases of psoriasis, methoxsalen is taken orally followed by UVA phototherapy. Other drugs are not options for treating severe cases of psoriasis. Hydroquinone is a topical depigmenting agent used for the treatment of photoaging. Finasteride is an oral drug for the treatment of alopecia, and minoxidil is a topical drug for alopecia. Tazarotene is a topical agent indicated for the treatment of acne or psoriasis.

34.4 Which of the following is correct regarding trichogenic agents?

    A. Minoxidil is known to decrease the microcirculation surrounding the follicle, thus decreasing cutaneous blood flow.

    B. A frequent adverse effect of topical minoxidil is orthostatic hypotension.

    C. Finasteride inhibits the 5-α reductase enzyme that controls the production of DHT from testosterone.

    D. An adverse effect associated with finasteride is increased libido.

    E. Only 6 months of finasteride is necessary for a lifelong benefit.

Correct answer = C. Androgenic alopecia is associated with DHT concentrations, and finasteride is known to inhibit the 5-α reductase enzyme required for the formation of DHT from testosterone. Continuous use of finasteride is needed to maintain therapeutic benefit for alopecia. Finasteride can decrease libido.

Drugs for Bone Disorders

Karen Whalen

35

I. OVERVIEW

Osteoporosis, Paget disease, and osteomalacia are disorders of the bone. Osteoporosis is characterized by progressive loss of bone mass and skeletal fragility. Patients with osteoporosis have an increased risk of fractures, which can cause significant morbidity. Osteoporosis occurs in older men and women but is most pronounced in postmenopausal women. Paget disease is a disorder of bone remodeling that results in disorganized bone formation and enlarged or misshapen bones. Unlike osteoporosis, Paget disease is usually limited to one or a few bones. Patients may experience bone pain, bone deformities, or fractures. Osteomalacia is softening of the bones that is most often attributed to vitamin D deficiency. [Note: Osteomalacia in children is referred to as rickets]. As osteoporosis is more common, drug therapy for osteoporosis is the focus of this chapter (Figure 35.1).

II. BONE REMODELING

Throughout life, bone is continuously remodeled, with about 10% of the adult skeleton replaced each year. The purpose of bone remodeling is to remove and replace damaged bone and to maintain calcium homeostasis. Osteoclasts are cells that break down bone, a process known as bone resorption. Following bone resorption, osteoblasts or bone-building cells synthesize new bone. Crystals of calcium phosphate known as hydroxyapatite are deposited in the new bone matrix during the process of bone mineralization. Bone mineralization is essential for bone strength. Lastly, bone enters a resting phase until the cycle of remodeling begins again. Bone loss occurs when bone resorption exceeds bone formation during the remodeling process. Figure 35.2 shows changes in bone morphology seen in osteoporosis.

III. TREATMENT OF OSTEOPOROSIS

Nondrug strategies to reduce bone loss in postmenopausal women include adequate dietary intake of calcium and vitamin D, weight-bearing exercise, and smoking cessation. In addition, patients at risk for osteoporosis should avoid drugs that increase bone loss such as glucocorticoids. [Note: Use of glucocorticoids (for example, prednisone 5 mg/day

DRUGS FOR OSTEOPOROSIS
Alendronate FOSAMAX, BINOSTO
Calcitonin FORTICAL, MIACALCIN
Denosumab PROLIA
Ibandronate BONIVA
Risedronate ACTONEL, ATELVIA
Raloxifene EVISTA
Teriparatide FORTEO
Zoledronic acid RECLAST, ZOMETA
DRUGS FOR DISORDERS OF BONE REMODELING
Etidronate
Pamidronate
Tiludronate SKELID

Figure 35.1
Summary of drugs used in the treatment of osteoporosis and other bone disorders.

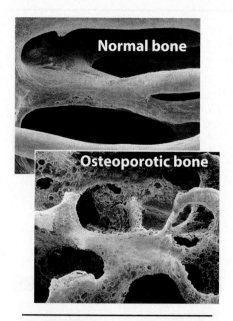

Figure 35.2
Changes in bone morphology seen
in osteoporosis.

| Aluminum antacids |
| Anticonvulsants (e.g., *phenytoin*) |
| Aromatase inhibitors |
| *Furosemide* |
| Glucocorticoids |
| *Heparin* |
| *Medroxyprogesterone acetate* |
| Proton pump inhibitors |
| Selective serotonin reuptake inhibitors |
| Thiazolidinediones |
| Thyroid (excessive replacement) |

Figure 35.3
Drugs that can contribute to bone
loss or increased fracture risk.

or equivalent) for 3 months or more is a significant risk factor for
osteoporosis.] Figure 35.3 outlines drugs that are associated with bone
loss or increased fracture risk. Pharmacologic therapy for osteoporosis
is warranted in postmenopausal women and men aged 50 years or over
who have a previous osteoporotic fracture, a bone mineral density that
is 2.5 standard deviations or more below that of a young adult, or a low
bone mass with a high probability of future fractures.

A. Bisphosphonates

Bisphosphonates including *alendronate* [a-LEND-row-nate], *ibandronate* [eye-BAN-dro-nate], *risedronate* [rih-SED-row-nate], and *zoledronic*
[zole-DROE-nick] *acid* are preferred agents for prevention and treatment of postmenopausal osteoporosis. These bisphosphonates, along
with *etidronate* [e-TID-row-nate], *pamidronate* [pah-MID-row-nate], and
tiludronate [till-UH-droe-nate], comprise an important drug group used
for the treatment of bone disorders such as osteoporosis and Paget
disease, as well as for treatment of bone metastases and hypercalcemia
of malignancy.

1. **Mechanism of action:** Bisphosphonates decrease osteoclastic
   bone resorption mainly through an increase in osteoclastic apoptosis (programmed cell death) and inhibition of the cholesterol bio-
   synthetic pathway important for osteoclast function. The decrease
   in osteoclastic bone resorption results in a small increase in bone
   mass and a decreased risk of fractures in patients with osteoporosis. The beneficial effects of *alendronate* persist over several years
   of therapy (Figure 35.4), but discontinuation results in a gradual
   loss of effects.

2. **Pharmacokinetics:** The oral bisphosphonates *alendronate*, *risedronate*, and *ibandronate* are dosed on a daily, weekly, or monthly
   basis depending on the drug (Figure 35.5). Absorption after oral
   administration is poor, with less than 1% of the dose absorbed. Food
   and other medications significantly interfere with absorption of oral
   bisphosphonates, and specific guidelines for administration should
   be followed to maximize absorption (Figure 35.5). Bisphosphonates
   are rapidly cleared from the plasma, primarily because they avidly
   bind to hydroxyapatite in the bone. Once bound to bone, they are
   cleared over a period of hours to years. Elimination is primarily via
   the kidney, and bisphosphonates should be avoided in severe renal
   impairment. For patients unable to tolerate oral bisphosphonates,
   intravenous *ibandronate* and *zoledronic acid* are alternatives.

3. **Adverse effects:** These include diarrhea, abdominal pain, and
   musculoskeletal pain. *Alendronate*, *risedronate*, and *ibandronate*
   are associated with esophagitis and esophageal ulcers. To minimize esophageal irritation, patients should remain upright after
   taking oral bisphosphonates. Osteonecrosis of the jaw has been
   reported with bisphosphonates but is usually associated with
   higher intravenous doses used for hypercalcemia of malignancy.
   Although uncommon, use of bisphosphonates may be associated with atypical fractures. The risk of atypical fractures may
   increase with long-term use of bisphosphonate therapy. *Etidronate*
   is the only bisphosphonate that causes osteomalacia following

long-term, continuous administration. Figure 35.6 shows relative potencies of the bisphosphonates.

B. Selective estrogen receptor modulators

Lower estrogen levels after menopause promote proliferation and activation of osteoclasts, and bone mass can decline rapidly. Estrogen replacement is effective for the prevention of postmenopausal bone loss. However, since estrogen may increase the risk of endometrial cancer (when used without a progestin in women with an intact uterus), breast cancer, stroke, venous thromboembolism, and coronary events, it is no longer recommended as a primary preventive therapy for osteoporosis. *Raloxifene* [rah-LOX-ih-feen] is a selective estrogen receptor modulator approved for the prevention and treatment of osteoporosis. It has estrogen-like effects on bone and estrogen antagonist effects on breast and endometrial tissue. It is an alternative for postmenopausal osteoporosis in women who are intolerant to bisphosphonates. *Raloxifene* increases bone density without increasing the risk of endometrial cancer. In addition, it decreases the risk of invasive breast cancer and also reduces levels of total and low-density lipoprotein cholesterol. Adverse effects include hot flashes, leg cramps, and a risk of venous thromboembolism similar to estrogen.

C. Calcitonin

Salmon *calcitonin* [cal-SIH-toe-nin] is indicated for the treatment of osteoporosis in women who are at least 5 years postmenopausal. The drug reduces bone resorption, but it is less effective than bisphosphonates. A unique property of *calcitonin* is the relief of pain associated with osteoporotic fracture. Therefore, *calcitonin* may be beneficial in patients with a recent vertebral fracture. It is available in intranasal and parenteral formulations, but the parenteral formulation is rarely used for the treatment of osteoporosis. Common adverse effects of intranasal administration include rhinitis and other nasal symptoms. Resistance to *calcitonin*

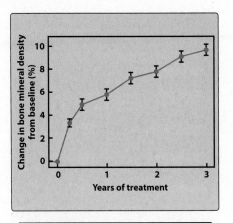

Figure 35.4
Effect of *alendronate* therapy on the bone mineral density of the lumbar spine.

BISPHOSPHONATE	FORMULATION	DOSING FREQUENCY
Alendronate	Oral tablet	Daily or weekly
Ibandronate	Oral tablet Intravenous	Daily or monthly Every 3 months
Risedronate	Oral tablet Oral delayed-release tablet	Daily or weekly Twice monthly or monthly
Zoledronic acid	Intravenous	Yearly

DOSING INSTRUCTIONS FOR ORAL BISPHOSPHONATES

- Take with 6 to 8 ounces of plain water only
  [Note: Take *risedronate* delayed-release tablet with at least 4 ounces of plain water]

- Take at least 30 minutes (60 minutes for *ibandronate*) BEFORE other food, drink, or medications
  [Note: Take *risedronate* delayed-release tablet immediately AFTER breakfast]

- Remain upright and do not lie down or recline for at least 30 minutes (60 minutes for *ibandronate*) after taking

Figure 35.5
Dosage formulations and instructions for administration of bisphosphonates for the treatment of osteoporosis.

Bisphosphonate	Antiresorptive activity
Etidronate	1
Tiludronate	10
Pamidronate	100
Alendronate	1000
Risedronate	5000
Ibandronate	10,000
Zoledronic acid	10,000

Figure 35.6
Antiresorptive activity of some bisphosphonates.

has been observed with long-term use in Paget disease. Because of a potential increased risk of malignancy with *calcitonin*, this agent should be reserved for patients intolerant of other drugs for osteoporosis.

D. Denosumab

Denosumab [den-OH-sue-mab] is a monoclonal antibody that targets receptor activator of nuclear factor kappa-B ligand and inhibits osteoclast formation and function. *Denosumab* is approved for the treatment of postmenopausal osteoporosis in women at high risk of fracture. It is administered via subcutaneous injection every 6 months. *Denosumab* has been associated with an increased risk of infections, dermatological reactions, hypocalcemia, osteonecrosis of the jaw, and atypical fractures. It should be reserved for women at high risk of fracture and those who are intolerant of or unresponsive to other osteoporosis therapies.

E. Teriparatide

Teriparatide [ter-ih-PAR-a-tide] is a recombinant form of human parathyroid hormone that is administered subcutaneously daily for the treatment of osteoporosis. *Teriparatide* is the first approved treatment for osteoporosis that stimulates bone formation. Other drugs for osteoporosis inhibit bone resorption. *Teriparatide* promotes bone formation by stimulating osteoblastic activity. *Teriparatide* has been associated with an increased risk of osteosarcoma in rats. The safety and efficacy of this agent have not been evaluated beyond 2 years. *Teriparatide* should be reserved for patients at high risk of fractures and those who have failed or cannot tolerate other osteoporosis therapies.

Study Questions

Choose the ONE best answer.

35.1 Which of the following is correct regarding the pharmacokinetics of the bisphosphonates?

    A. Bisphosphonates are well absorbed after oral administration.

    B. Food or other medications greatly impair absorption of bisphosphonates.

    C. Bisphosphonates are mainly metabolized via the cytochrome P450 system.

    D. Elimination half-life of bisphosphonates ranges from 4 to 6 hours.

> Correct answer = B. Food and other medications do decrease absorption of bisphosphonates, which are already poorly absorbed (less than 1%) after oral administration. Bisphosphonates are cleared from the plasma by binding to bone and being cleared by the kidney (not metabolized by the CYP450 system). The elimination half-life may be years.

35.2 OP is a 65-year-old female who has been diagnosed with postmenopausal osteoporosis. She has no history of fractures and no other pertinent medical conditions. Which of the following would be most appropriate for management of her osteoporosis?

    A. Alendronate.

    B. Calcitonin.

    C. Denosumab.

    D. Raloxifene.

    E. Teriparatide.

> Correct answer = A. Bisphosphonates are first-line therapy for osteoporosis in postmenopausal women without contraindications. Calcitonin and raloxifene are alternatives but may be less efficacious (especially for nonvertebral fractures). Teriparatide and denosumab should be reserved for patients at high risk or those who fail other therapies.

35.3 TT is a 55-year-old female who has been diagnosed with postmenopausal osteoporosis. She has a past medical history of ethanol abuse, alcoholic liver disease, erosive esophagitis, and hypothyroidism. Which of the following would be the primary reason oral bisphosphonates should be used with caution in this patient?

A. Age.
B. Erosive esophagitis.
C. Liver disease.
D. Thyroid disease.

Correct answer = B. Bisphosphonates are known to cause esophageal irritation and should be used with caution in a patient with a history of erosive esophagitis. Age is not a factor for consideration in bisphosphonate use. Liver disease is not a contraindication to bisphosphonate use, since bisphosphonates are mainly cleared via the kidney. Thyroid disease is not a contraindication to bisphosphonate use, although overaggressive replacement of thyroid may contribute to osteoporosis.

35.4 VS is a 70-year-old female who is being started on ibandronate once monthly for the treatment of osteoporosis. Which of the following is important to communicate to this patient?

A. Take this medication with orange juice to increase absorption.
B. Take this medication after meals to minimize stomach upset.
C. Remain upright for at least 60 minutes after taking this medication.
D. Adverse effects may include blood clots and leg cramps.

Correct answer = C. Patients need to remain upright for 60 minutes after ibandronate (30 minutes for other bisphosphonates). Ibandronate should be given on an empty stomach with plain water only. Bisphosphonates, unlike raloxifene, are not associated with blood clots and leg cramps.

Anti-inflammatory, Antipyretic, and Analgesic Agents

36

Eric Dietrich, Nicholas Carris, and Thomas A. Panavelil

I. OVERVIEW

Inflammation is a normal, protective response to tissue injury caused by physical trauma, noxious chemicals, or microbiologic agents. Inflammation is the body's effort to inactivate or destroy invading organisms, remove irritants, and set the stage for tissue repair. When healing is complete, the inflammatory process usually subsides. However, inappropriate activation of the immune system can result in inflammation, leading to immune-mediated diseases such as rheumatoid arthritis (RA). Normally, the immune system can differentiate between self and nonself. In RA, white blood cells (WBCs) view the synovium (tissue that nourishes cartilage and bone) as nonself and initiate an inflammatory attack. WBC activation leads to stimulation of T lymphocytes (the cell-mediated part of the immune system), which recruit and activate monocytes and macrophages. These cells secrete proinflammatory cytokines, including tumor necrosis factor (TNF)-α and interleukin (IL)-1, into the synovial cavity. The release of cytokines then causes 1) increased cellular infiltration into the endothelium due to release of histamines, kinins, and vasodilatory prostaglandins; 2) increased production of C-reactive protein by hepatocytes (a marker for inflammation); 3) increased production and release of proteolytic enzymes by chondrocytes (cells that maintain cartilage), leading to degradation of cartilage and joint space narrowing; 4) increased osteoclast activity (osteoclasts regulate bone breakdown), resulting in focal bone erosions and bone demineralization around joints; and 5) systemic manifestations in certain organs such as the heart. In addition to T-lymphocyte activation, B lymphocytes are also involved and produce rheumatoid factor (inflammatory marker) and other autoantibodies with the purpose of maintaining inflammation. These defensive reactions cause progressive tissue injury, resulting in joint damage and erosions, functional disability, significant pain, and reduction in quality of life. Pharmacotherapy in the management of RA includes anti-inflammatory and/or immunosuppressive agents that modulate/reduce the inflammatory process, with the goals of reducing inflammation and pain, and halting or slowing disease progression. The agents to be discussed (Figure 36.1) include nonsteroidal

NSAIDs
Aspirin BAYER, BUFFERIN, ECOTRIN
Celecoxib CELEBREX
Diclofenac CATAFLAM, FLECTOR, PENNSAID, VOLTAREN
Diflunisal DOLOBID
Etodolac
Fenoprofen NALFON
Flurbiprofen ANSAID
Ibuprofen ADVIL, MOTRIN
Indomethacin INDOCIN
Ketorolac ACULAR, ACUVAIL, TORADOL
Ketoprofen
Meclofenamate
Mefenamic acid PONSTEL
Meloxicam MOBIC
Methyl salicylate WINTERGREEN OIL
Nabumetone
Naproxen ALEVE, ANAPROX, NAPROSYN
Oxaprozin DAYPRO
Piroxicam FELDENE
Salsalate
Sulindac CLINORIL
Tolmetin TOLMETIN SODIUM

OTHER ANALGESICS
Acetaminophen (Paracetamol) OFIRMEV, TYLENOL

Figure 36.1
Summary of anti-inflammatory drugs. NSAIDs = nonsteroidal anti-inflammatory drugs; COX = cyclooxygenase. (Figure continues on next page.)

447

Figure 36.1 (Continued)
Summary of anti-inflammatory drugs.

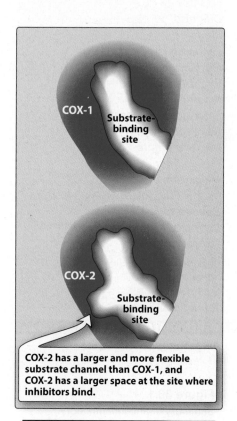

COX-2 has a larger and more flexible substrate channel than COX-1, and COX-2 has a larger space at the site where inhibitors bind.

Figure 36.2
Structural differences in active sites of cyclooxygenase (COX)-1 and COX-2.

anti-inflammatory drugs (NSAIDs) and *celecoxib* (cyclooxygenase-2 inhibitor), *acetaminophen*, and disease-modifying antirheumatic drugs (DMARDs). Additionally, agents used for the treatment of gout and migraine headache are reviewed.

II. PROSTAGLANDINS

The NSAIDs act by inhibiting the synthesis of prostaglandins. Thus, an understanding of NSAIDs requires comprehension of the actions and biosynthesis of prostaglandins—unsaturated fatty acid derivatives containing 20 carbons that include a cyclic ring structure. [Note: These compounds are sometimes referred to as eicosanoids; "eicosa" refers to the 20 carbon atoms.]

A. Role of prostaglandins as local mediators

Prostaglandins and related compounds are produced in minute quantities by virtually all tissues. They generally act locally on the tissues in which they are synthesized, and they are rapidly metabolized to inactive products at their sites of action. Therefore, the prostaglandins do not circulate in the blood in significant concentrations. Thromboxanes and leukotrienes are related lipids that are synthesized from the same precursors as the prostaglandins.

B. Synthesis of prostaglandins

Arachidonic acid is the primary precursor of the prostaglandins and related compounds. Arachidonic acid is present as a component of the phospholipids of cell membranes. Free arachidonic acid is released from tissue phospholipids by the action of phospholipase A_2 via a process controlled by hormones and other stimuli. There are two major pathways in the synthesis of the eicosanoids from arachidonic acid, the cyclooxygenase and the lipoxygenase pathways.

1. **Cyclooxygenase pathway:** All eicosanoids with ring structures (that is, the prostaglandins, thromboxanes, and prostacyclins) are synthesized via the cyclooxygenase pathway. Two related isoforms of the cyclooxygenase enzymes have been described. Cyclooxygenase-1 (COX-1) is responsible for the physiologic production of prostanoids, whereas cyclooxygenase-2 (COX-2) causes the elevated production of prostanoids that occurs in sites of chronic disease and inflammation. COX-1 is a constitutive enzyme that regulates normal cellular processes, such as gastric cytoprotection, vascular homeostasis, platelet aggregation, and reproductive and kidney functions. COX-2 is constitutively expressed in tissues such as the brain, kidney, and bone. Its expression at other sites is increased during states of chronic inflammation. Differences in binding site shape have permitted the development of selective COX-2 inhibitors (Figure 36.2). Another distinguishing characteristic of COX-2 is that its expression is induced by inflammatory mediators like TNF-α and IL-1 but can also be pharmacologically inhibited by glucocorticoids (Figure 36.3), which may contribute to the significant anti-inflammatory effects of these drugs.

2. **Lipoxygenase pathway:** Alternatively, several lipoxygenases can act on arachidonic acid to form leukotrienes (Figure 36.3).

Antileukotriene drugs, such as *zileuton*, *zafirlukast*, and *montelukast*, are treatment options for asthma (see Chapter 29).

C. Actions of prostaglandins

Many of the actions of prostaglandins are mediated by their binding to a wide variety of distinct cell membrane receptors that operate via G-coupled proteins. Prostaglandins and their metabolites, produced endogenously in tissues, act as local signals that fine-tune the response of a specific cell type. Their functions vary widely, depending on the tissue and the specific enzymes within the pathway that are available at that particular site. For example, the release of thromboxane A$_2$ (TXA$_2$) from platelets during tissue injury triggers the recruitment of new platelets for aggregation, as well as local vasoconstriction. However, prostacyclin (PGI$_2$), produced by endothelial cells, has opposite effects, inhibiting platelet aggregation and producing vasodilation. The net effect on platelets and blood vessels depends on the balance of these two prostanoids.

D. Therapeutic uses of prostaglandins

Prostaglandins have a major role in modulating pain, inflammation, and fever. They also control many physiological functions, such as acid secretion and mucus production in the gastrointestinal (GI) tract, uterine contractions, and renal blood flow. Prostaglandins are also among the chemical mediators that are released in allergic and inflammatory processes. Therefore, they find use for a number of disorders discussed below.

E. Alprostadil

Alprostadil [al-PROS-ta-dil] is a PGE$_1$ that is naturally produced in tissues such as seminal vesicles and cavernous tissues, in the placenta, and in the ductus arteriosus of the fetus. Therapeutically, *alprostadil* can be used to treat erectile dysfunction or to keep the ductus arteriosus open in neonates with congenital heart conditions until surgery is possible. PGE$_1$ maintains the patency of the ductus arteriosus during pregnancy. The ductus closes soon after delivery to allow normal blood circulation between the lungs and the heart. Infusion of the drug maintains the ductus open as it naturally occurs during pregnancy, allowing time until surgical correction is possible. The use of *alprostadil* for erectile dysfunction is discussed in Chapter 32.

F. Lubiprostone

Lubiprostone [loo-bee-PROS-tone] is a PGE$_1$ derivative indicated for the treatment of chronic idiopathic constipation, opioid-induced constipation, and irritable bowel syndrome with constipation. It stimulates chloride channels in the luminal cells of the intestinal epithelium, thereby increasing intestinal fluid secretion (see Chapter 31). Nausea and diarrhea are the most common side effects of *lubiprostone* (Figure 36.4). Nausea can be decreased if taken with food.

G. Misoprostol

Misoprostol [mye-soe-PROST-ole], a PGE$_1$ analog, is used to protect the mucosal lining of the stomach during chronic NSAID treatment. *Misoprostol* interacts with prostaglandin receptors on parietal cells within

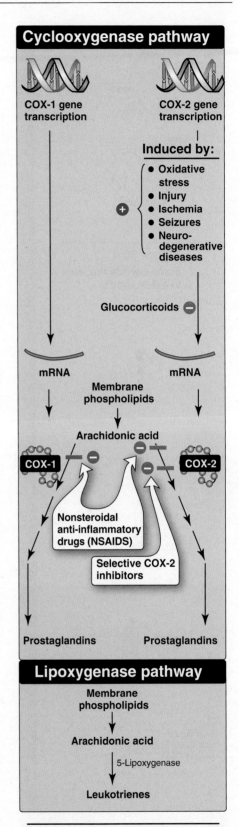

Figure 36.3
Synthesis of prostaglandins and leukotrienes. COX = cyclooxygenase.

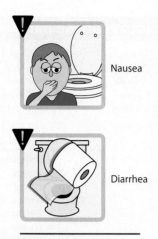

Figure 36.4
Some adverse reactions
to *lubiprostone*.

the stomach, reducing gastric acid secretion. Furthermore, *misoprostol* has a GI cytoprotective effect by stimulating mucus and bicarbonate production. This combination of effects decreases the incidence of gastric ulcers caused by NSAIDs. [Note: There is a combination product containing *diclofenac* and *misoprostol*.] *Misoprostol* is also used off-label in obstetric settings for labor induction, since it increases uterine contractions by interacting with prostaglandin receptors in the uterus. *Misoprostol* has the potential risk to induce abortion in pregnant women. Therefore, the drug is contraindicated during pregnancy. Its use is limited by common side effects including diarrhea and abdominal pain.

H. Prostaglandin $F_{2\alpha}$ analogs

Bimatoprost [bih-MAT-o-prost], *latanoprost* [la-TAN-oh-prost], *tafluprost* [TAF-loo-prost], and *travoprost* [TRA-voe-prost] are $PGF_{2\alpha}$ analogs that are indicated for the treatment of open-angle glaucoma. By binding to prostaglandin receptors, they increase uveoscleral outflow, reducing intraocular pressure. They are administered as ophthalmic solutions once a day and are as effective as *timolol* or better in reducing intraocular pressure. *Bimatoprost* increases eyelash prominence, length, and darkness and is approved for the treatment of eyelash hypotrichosis. Ocular reactions include blurred vision, iris color change (increased brown pigmentation), increased number and pigment of eyelashes, ocular irritation, and foreign body sensation.

I. Prostacyclin (PGI_2) analogs

Epoprostenol [ee-poe-PROST-en-ol], the pharmaceutical form of naturally occurring prostacyclin, and the synthetic analogs of prostacyclin (*iloprost* [EYE-loe-prost] and *treprostinil* [tre-PROS-ti-nil]) are potent pulmonary vasodilators that are used for the treatment of pulmonary arterial hypertension. These drugs mimic the effects of prostacyclin in endothelial cells, producing a significant reduction in pulmonary arterial resistance with a subsequent increase in cardiac index and oxygen delivery. These agents all have a short half-life. *Epoprostenol* and *treprostinil* are administered as a continuous intravenous infusion, and *treprostinil* may also be administered orally or via inhalation or subcutaneous infusion. Inhaled *iloprost* requires frequent dosing due to the short half-life (Figure 36.5). Dizziness, headache, flushing, and fainting are the most common adverse effects (Figure 36.6). Bronchospasm and cough can also occur after inhalation of *iloprost*.

III. NONSTEROIDAL ANTI-INFLAMMATORY DRUGS

The NSAIDs are a group of chemically dissimilar agents that differ in their antipyretic, analgesic, and anti-inflammatory activities. The class includes derivatives of salicylic acid (*aspirin* [AS-pir-in], *diflunisal* [dye-FLOO-ni-sal], *salsalate* [SAL-sa-late]), propionic acid (*ibuprofen* [eye-bue-PROE-fen], *fenoprofen* [fen-oh-PROE-fen], *flurbiprofen* [flure-BI-proe-fen], *ketoprofen* [kee-toe-PROE-fen], *naproxen* [na-PROX-en], *oxaprozin* [ox-a-PROE-zin]), acetic acid (*diclofenac* [dye-KLOE-fen-ak], *etodolac* [ee-toe-DOE-lak], *indomethacin* [in-doe-METH-a-sin], *ketorolac* [kee-toe-ROLE-ak], *nabumetone* [na-BUE-me-tone], *sulindac* [sul-IN-dak], *tolmetin* [TOLE-met-in]), enolic acid (*meloxicam* [mel-OKS-i-kam], *piroxicam* [peer-OX-i-kam]), fenamates (*mefenamic* [me-fe-NAM-ik]

Iloprost
nebulizer
7–9 times
per day

Metabolites of
***iloprost* are**
excreted in
urine (68%) and
feces (12%)

Iloprost

Figure 36.5
Administration and fate of *iloprost*.

acid, meclofenamate [me-kloe-fen-AM-ate]), and the selective COX-2 inhibitor (*celecoxib* [sel-e-KOX-ib]). They act primarily by inhibiting the cyclooxygenase enzymes that catalyze the first step in prostanoid biosynthesis. This leads to decreased prostaglandin synthesis with both beneficial and unwanted effects. [Note: Differences in safety and efficacy of the NSAIDs may be explained by relative selectivity for the COX-1 or COX-2 enzyme. Inhibition of COX-2 is thought to lead to the anti-inflammatory and analgesic actions of NSAIDs, while inhibition of COX-1 is responsible for prevention of cardiovascular events and most adverse events.]

A. Aspirin and other NSAIDs

Aspirin can be thought of as a traditional NSAID, but it exhibits anti-inflammatory activity only at relatively high doses that are rarely used. It has gained much more usage at lower doses for the prevention of cardiovascular events such as stroke and myocardial infarction (MI). *Aspirin* is often differentiated from other NSAIDs, since it is an irreversible inhibitor of cyclooxygenase activity.

1. **Mechanism of action:** *Aspirin* is a weak organic acid that irreversibly acetylates (and, thus, inactivates) cyclooxygenase (Figure 36.7). The other NSAIDs are all reversible inhibitors of cyclooxygenase. The NSAIDs, including *aspirin*, have three major therapeutic actions: they reduce inflammation (anti-inflammatory), pain (analgesic effect), and fever (antipyretic effect; Figure 36.8). However, as outlined below, not all NSAIDs are equally effective in each of these actions.

   a. **Anti-inflammatory actions:** Cyclooxygenase inhibition diminishes the formation of prostaglandins and, thus, modulates aspects of inflammation in which prostaglandins act as mediators. NSAIDs inhibit inflammation in arthritis, but they neither arrest the progression of the disease nor induce remission.

   b. **Analgesic action:** PGE_2 is thought to sensitize nerve endings to the action of bradykinin, histamine, and other chemical mediators released locally by the inflammatory process. Thus, by decreasing PGE_2 synthesis, the sensation of pain can be decreased. As COX-2 is expressed during times of inflammation and injury, it is thought that inhibition of this enzyme is responsible for the analgesic activity of NSAIDs. No single NSAID has demonstrated superior efficacy over another, and all agents are generally considered to have equivalent efficacy. The NSAIDs are used mainly for the management of mild to moderate pain arising from musculoskeletal disorders. One exception is *ketorolac*, which can be used for more severe pain but for only a short duration.

   c. **Antipyretic action:** Fever occurs when the set-point of the anterior hypothalamic thermoregulatory center is elevated. This can be caused by PGE_2 synthesis, which is stimulated when endogenous fever-producing agents (pyrogens), such as cytokines, are released from WBCs that are activated by infection, hypersensitivity, malignancy, or inflammation. The NSAIDs lower body temperature in patients with fever by impeding PGE_2 synthesis and release. These agents essentially reset the "thermostat"

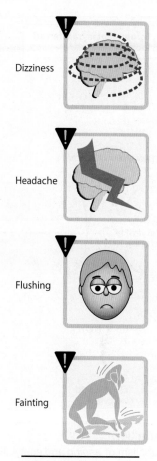

Dizziness

Headache

Flushing

Fainting

Figure 36.6
Some adverse reactions to *iloprost*.

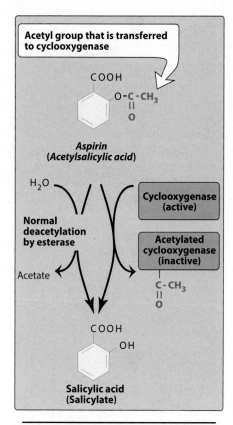

Figure 36.7
Metabolism of *aspirin* and acetylation of cyclooxygenase by *aspirin*.

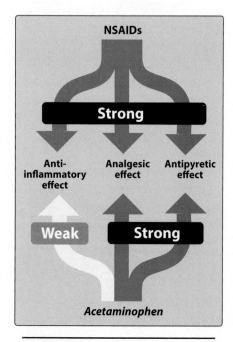

Figure 36.8
Actions of nonsteroidal anti-inflammatory drugs (NSAIDs) and *acetaminophen*.

toward normal. This rapidly lowers the body temperature of febrile patients by increasing heat dissipation as a result of peripheral vasodilation and sweating. NSAIDs have no effect on normal body temperature.

2. Therapeutic uses:

a. Anti-inflammatory and analgesic uses: NSAIDs are used in the treatment of osteoarthritis, gout, and RA. These agents are also used to treat common conditions (for example, headache, arthralgia, myalgia, and dysmenorrhea) requiring analgesia. Combinations of opioids and NSAIDs may be effective in treating pain caused by malignancy. Furthermore, the addition of NSAIDs may lead to an opioid-sparing effect, allowing for lower doses of opioids to be utilized. The salicylates exhibit analgesic activity at lower doses. Only at higher doses do these drugs show anti-inflammatory activity (Figure 36.9). For example, two 325-mg *aspirin* tablets administered four times daily produce analgesia, whereas 12 to 20 tablets per day produce both analgesic and anti-inflammatory activity.

b. Antipyretic uses: *Aspirin*, *ibuprofen*, and *naproxen* may be used to treat fever. [Note: *Aspirin* should be avoided in patients less than 20 years old with viral infections, such as varicella (chickenpox) or influenza, to prevent Reye syndrome (a syndrome that can cause fulminating hepatitis with cerebral edema, often leading to death).]

c. Cardiovascular applications: *Aspirin* is used to inhibit platelet aggregation. Low-dose *aspirin* inhibits COX-1–mediated production of TXA_2, thereby reducing TXA_2-mediated vasoconstriction and platelet aggregation and the subsequent risk of cardiovascular events. Low doses (doses less than 325 mg; many classify it as doses of 75 to 162 mg—commonly 81 mg) of *aspirin* are used prophylactically to 1) reduce the risk of recurrent cardiovascular events and/or death in patients with previous MI or unstable angina pectoris, 2) reduce the risk of recurring transient ischemic attacks (TIAs) and stroke or death in those who have had a prior TIA or stroke, and 3) reduce the risk of cardiovascular events or death in high-risk patients such as those with chronic stable angina or diabetes. As *aspirin* irreversibly inhibits COX-1 (Figure 36.10) the antiplatelet effects persist for the life of the platelet. Chronic use of low doses allows for continued inhibition as new platelets are generated. *Aspirin* is also used acutely to reduce the risk of death in acute MI and in patients undergoing certain revascularization procedures.

d. External applications: *Salicylic acid* is used topically to treat acne, corns, calluses, and warts. *Methyl salicylate* ("oil of wintergreen") is used externally as a cutaneous counterirritant in liniments, such as arthritis creams and sports rubs.

3. Pharmacokinetics:

a. Aspirin: After oral administration, *aspirin* is rapidly deacetylated by esterases in the body, thereby producing salicylate. Unionized salicylates are passively absorbed mostly from the upper small intestine (dissolution of the tablets is favored at the higher pH of the gut). Salicylates (except for *diflunisal*) cross both the blood–brain barrier and the placenta and are absorbed through intact skin (especially *methyl salicylate*). Salicylate is converted by the liver to water-soluble conjugates that are rapidly cleared by the kidney, resulting in first-order elimination and a serum half-life of 3.5 hours. At anti-inflammatory dosages (more than 4 g/day), the hepatic metabolic pathway becomes saturated, and zero-order kinetics are observed, leading to a half-life of 15 hours or more (Figure 36.11). Being an organic acid, salicylate is secreted into the urine and can affect uric acid excretion. At low doses of *aspirin* (less than 2 g/day), uric acid secretion is decreased, whereas at high doses, uric acid secretion may be unchanged or increased. Therefore, *aspirin* is avoided in gout or in patients taking *probenecid*.

b. **Other NSAIDs:** Most NSAIDs are well absorbed after oral administration and circulate highly bound to plasma proteins. The majority are metabolized by the liver, mostly to inactivate metabolites. Few (for example, *nabumetone* and *sulindac*) have active metabolites. Elimination of active drug and metabolites is primarily via the urine.

4. **Adverse events:** Because of the associated adverse events below, it is preferable to use NSAIDs at the lowest effective dose for the shortest duration possible.

a. **Gastrointestinal:** The most common adverse effects of NSAIDs are GI related, ranging from dyspepsia to bleeding. Normally, production of prostacyclin (PGI_2) inhibits gastric acid secretion, and PGE_2 and $PGF_{2\alpha}$ stimulate synthesis of protective mucus in both the stomach and small intestine. Agents that inhibit COX-1 reduce beneficial levels of these prostaglandins, resulting in increased gastric acid secretion, diminished mucus protection, and increased risk for GI bleeding and ulceration. Agents with a higher relative selectivity for COX-1 may have a higher risk for GI events compared to those with a lower relative selectivity for COX-1 (that is, higher COX-2 selectivity). NSAIDs should be taken with food or fluids to diminish GI upset. If NSAIDs are used in patients with a high risk for GI events, proton pump inhibitors or *misoprostol* should be used concomitantly to prevent NSAID-induced ulcers (see Chapter 31).

b. **Increased risk of bleeding (antiplatelet effect):** TXA_2 enhances platelet aggregation, whereas PGI_2 decreases it. *Aspirin* irreversibly inhibits COX-1–mediated TXA_2 formation, while other NSAIDs reversibly inhibit the production of TXA_2. Because platelets lack nuclei, they cannot synthesize new enzyme when inhibited by *aspirin*, and the lack of thromboxane persists for the lifetime of the platelet (3 to 7 days). Because of the decrease in TXA_2 production, platelet aggregation (the first step in thrombus formation) is reduced, producing an antiplatelet effect with a prolonged bleeding time. For this reason, *aspirin* is often held, or not given, at least 1 week prior to surgery. NSAIDs other than *aspirin* are not utilized for their antiplatelet effect but can still prolong bleeding time. [Note: As agents become more COX-2 selective, they are

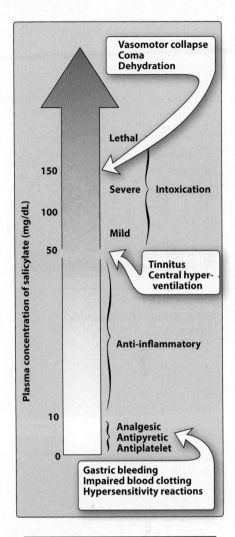

Figure 36.9
Dose-dependent effects of salicylate.

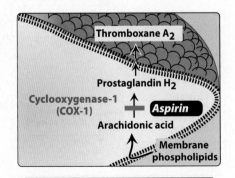

Figure 36.10
Aspirin irreversibly inhibits platelet cyclooxygenase-1.

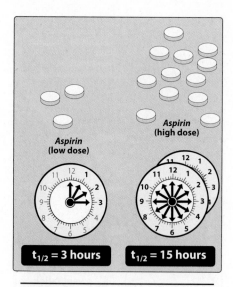

Figure 36.11
Effect of dose on the half-life of *aspirin*.

expected to have less effect on platelet inhibition and bleeding time.] NSAIDs can also block *aspirin* binding to cyclooxygenase when used concomitantly. Patients who take *aspirin* for cardioprotection should avoid concomitant NSAID use if possible.

c. **Actions on the kidney:** NSAIDs prevent the synthesis of PGE_2 and PGI_2, prostaglandins that are responsible for maintaining renal blood flow (Figure 36.12). Decreased synthesis of prostaglandins can result in retention of sodium and water and may cause edema in some patients. Patients with a history of heart failure or kidney disease are at particularly high risk. These effects can also mitigate the beneficial effects of antihypertensive medications.

d. **Cardiac effects:** Agents such as *aspirin*, with a very high degree of COX-1 selectivity, have shown a cardiovascular protective effect thought to be due to a reduction in the production of TXA_2. Agents with higher relative COX-2 selectivity have been associated with an increased risk for cardiovascular events, possibly by decreasing PGI_2 production mediated by COX-2. An increased risk for cardiovascular events, including MI and stroke, has been associated with all NSAIDs except *aspirin*. Use of NSAIDs, other than *aspirin*, is discouraged in patients with established cardiovascular disease. For patients with cardiovascular disease in whom NSAID treatment cannot be avoided, *naproxen* appears to be the least likely to be harmful. NSAID use should be limited to the lowest dose possible for the shortest duration.

e. **Other side effects:** NSAIDs are inhibitors of cyclooxygenases and, therefore, inhibit the synthesis of prostaglandins but not of leukotrienes. For this reason, NSAIDs should be used with caution in patients with asthma, as inhibition of prostaglandin synthesis can cause a shift toward leukotriene production and, therefore, increase the risk of exacerbations of asthma. Central nervous system (CNS) adverse events, such as headache,

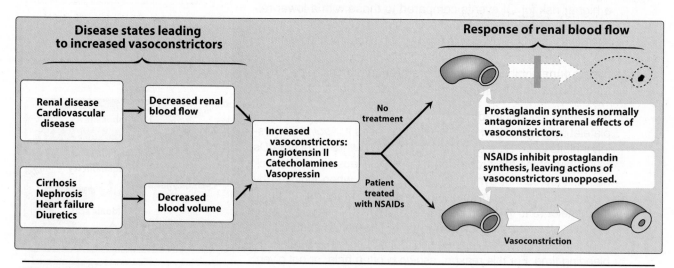

Figure 36.12
Renal effect of NSAIDs inhibition of prostaglandin synthesis. NSAIDs = nonsteroidal anti-inflammatory drugs.

tinnitus, and dizziness, may occur. Approximately 15% of patients taking *aspirin* experience hypersensitivity reactions. Symptoms of true allergy include urticaria, bronchoconstriction, and angioedema. Fatal anaphylactic shock is rare. Patients with severe hypersensitivity to *aspirin* should avoid using NSAIDs.

f. **Drug interactions:** Salicylate is roughly 80% to 90% plasma protein bound (albumin) and can be displaced from protein-binding sites, resulting in increased concentration of free salicylate. Alternatively, *aspirin* can displace other highly protein-bound drugs, such as *warfarin, phenytoin,* or *valproic acid,* resulting in higher free concentrations of these agents (Figure 36.13).

g. **Toxicity:** Salicylate intoxication may be mild or severe. The mild form is called salicylism and is characterized by nausea, vomiting, marked hyperventilation, headache, mental confusion, dizziness, and tinnitus (ringing or roaring in the ears). When large doses of salicylate are administered, severe salicylate intoxication may result (Figure 36.9). Restlessness, delirium, hallucinations, convulsions, coma, respiratory and metabolic acidosis, and death from respiratory failure may occur. Children are particularly prone to salicylate intoxication. Ingestion of as little as 10 g of *aspirin* can cause death in children.

h. **Pregnancy:** Most NSAIDs are pregnancy risk category C in the first two trimesters. [Note: *Acetaminophen* is preferred if analgesic or antipyretic effects are needed during pregnancy.] In the third trimester, NSAIDs should generally be avoided due to the risk of premature closure of the ductus arteriosus.

B. Celecoxib

Celecoxib [SEL-e-KOX-ib], a selective COX-2 inhibitor, is significantly more selective for inhibition of COX-2 than COX-1 (Figure 36.14). Unlike the inhibition of COX-1 by *aspirin* (which is rapid and irreversible), the inhibition of COX-2 is reversible.

1. **Therapeutic uses:** *Celecoxib* is approved for the treatment of RA, osteoarthritis, and acute mild to moderate pain. *Celecoxib* has similar efficacy to NSAIDs in the treatment of pain.

2. **Pharmacokinetics:** *Celecoxib* is readily absorbed after oral administration. It is extensively metabolized in the liver by cytochrome P450 (CYP2C9) and is excreted in feces and urine. The half-life is about 11 hours, and the drug may be dosed once or twice daily. The dosage should be reduced in those with moderate hepatic impairment, and *celecoxib* should be avoided in patients with severe hepatic or renal disease.

3. **Adverse effects:** Headache, dyspepsia, diarrhea, and abdominal pain are the most common adverse effects. *Celecoxib*, when used without concomitant *aspirin* therapy, is associated with less GI bleeding and dyspepsia than other NSAIDs. However, this benefit is lost when *aspirin* is added to *celecoxib* therapy. Patients who are at high risk of ulcers and require *aspirin* for cardiovascular prevention should avoid the use of *celecoxib*. Like other NSAIDs, the

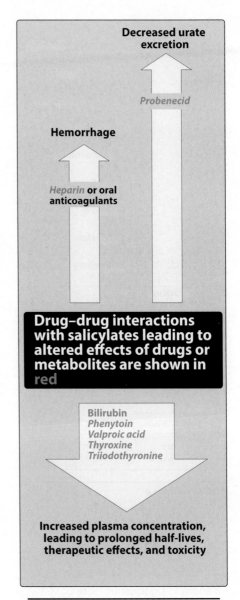

Figure 36.13
Drugs interacting with salicylates.

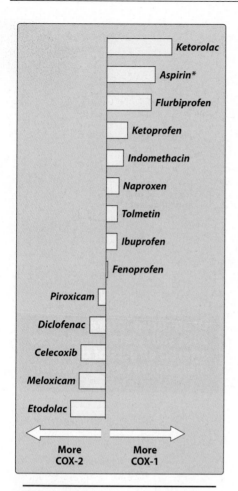

Figure 36.14
Relative selectivity of some commonly used NSAIDs. Data shown as the logarithm of their ratio of IC_{80} (drug concentration to achieve 80% inhibition of cyclooxygenase). *Aspirin* graphed for IC_{50} value due to it showing significantly more COX-1 selectivity at lower doses and graph using higher concentrations does not accurately reflect the usage or selectivity of *aspirin*.

drug has a similar risk for cardiovascular events. *Celecoxib* should be used with caution in patients who are allergic to sulfonamides. Patients who have had anaphylactoid reactions to *aspirin* or nonselective NSAIDs may be at risk for similar effects with *celecoxib*. Inhibitors of CYP2C9, such as *fluconazole* and *fluvastatin*, may increase serum levels of *celecoxib*.

Figure 36.15 summarizes some of the therapeutic advantages and disadvantages of members of the NSAID family.

IV. ACETAMINOPHEN

Acetaminophen [a-SEET-a-MIN-oh-fen] (*N*-acetyl-*p*-aminophenol or APAP) inhibits prostaglandin synthesis in the CNS. This explains its antipyretic and analgesic properties. *Acetaminophen* has less effect on cyclo-oxygenase in peripheral tissues (due to peripheral inactivation), which accounts for its weak anti-inflammatory activity. *Acetaminophen* does not affect platelet function or increase bleeding time. It is not considered to be an NSAID.

A. Therapeutic uses

Acetaminophen is a suitable substitute for the analgesic and antipyretic effects of NSAIDs for those patients with gastric complaints/ risks, in those whom a prolongation of bleeding time is not desirable, as well as those who do not require the anti-inflammatory action of NSAIDs. *Acetaminophen* is the analgesic/antipyretic of choice for children with viral infections or chickenpox (due to the risk of Reye syndrome with *aspirin*).

B. Pharmacokinetics

Acetaminophen is rapidly absorbed from the GI tract. A significant first-pass metabolism occurs in the luminal cells of the intestine and in the hepatocytes. Under normal circumstances, *acetaminophen* is conjugated in the liver to form inactive glucuronidated or sulfated metabolites. A portion of *acetaminophen* is hydroxylated to form *N*-acetyl-*p*-benzoquinoneimine, or NAPQI, a highly reactive metabolite that can react with sulfhydryl groups and cause liver damage. At normal doses of *acetaminophen*, NAPQI reacts with the sulfhydryl group of glutathione, which is produced by the liver, forming a nontoxic substance (Figure 36.16). *Acetaminophen* and its metabolites are excreted in urine. The drug is also available in intravenous and rectal formulations.

C. Adverse effects

At normal therapeutic doses, *acetaminophen* is virtually free of significant adverse effects. With large doses of *acetaminophen*, the available glutathione in the liver becomes depleted, and NAPQI reacts with the sulfhydryl groups of hepatic proteins, forming covalent bonds (Figure 36.16). Hepatic necrosis, a very serious and potentially life-threatening condition, can result. Patients with hepatic disease, viral hepatitis, or a history of alcoholism are at higher risk of *acetaminophen*-induced hepatotoxicity. [Note: *N-acetylcysteine*, which contains sulfhydryl groups to which the toxic metabolite can bind, is an antidote

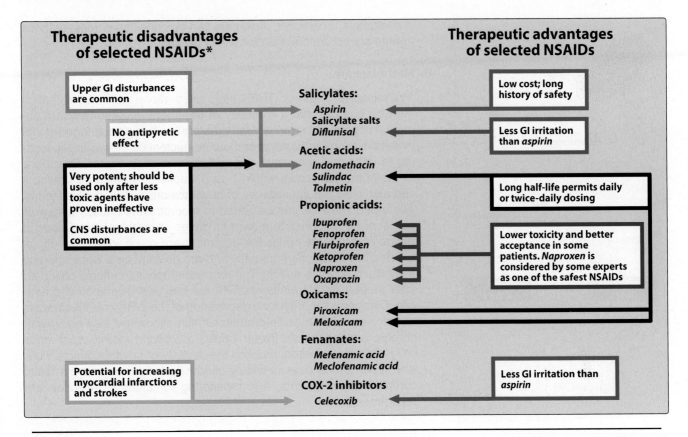

Figure 36.15
Summary of nonsteroidal anti-inflammatory agents (NSAIDs). GI = gastrointestinal; CNS = central nervous system; COX-2 = cyclooxygenase-2. *As a group, with the exception of *aspirin*, these drugs may have the potential to increase risk of myocardial infarction and stroke.

in cases of overdose (see Chapter 48).] *Acetaminophen* should be avoided in patients with severe hepatic impairment.

V. DISEASE-MODIFYING ANTIRHEUMATIC DRUGS

DMARDs are used in the treatment of RA and have been shown to slow the course of the disease, induce remission, and prevent further destruction of the joints and involved tissues. When a patient is diagnosed with RA, DMARDs should be started within 3 months to help stop the progression of the disease at the earlier stages. NSAIDs or corticosteroids may also be used for relief of symptoms if needed.

A. Choice of drug

No one DMARD is efficacious and safe in every patient, and trials of several different drugs may be necessary. Monotherapy may be initiated with any of the DMARDs (*methotrexate, leflunomide, hydroxychloroquine,* or *sulfasalazine*) for patients with low disease activity. For patients with moderate to high disease activity or inadequate response to monotherapy, combination DMARD therapy (usually *methotrexate* based) or use of anti-TNF drugs (*adalimumab, certolizumab, etanercept, golimumab,* and *infliximab*) may be needed. For patients with more established disease, use of other biologic therapies

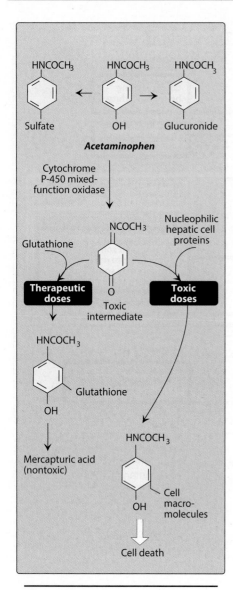

Figure 36.16
Metabolism of *acetaminophen*.

(for example, *abatacept, rituximab*) can be considered. Most of these agents are contraindicated for use in pregnant women.

B. Methotrexate

Methotrexate [meth-oh-TREX-ate], used alone or in combination therapy, has become a mainstay of treatment in patients with rheumatoid or psoriatic arthritis. *Methotrexate* is a folic acid antagonist that inhibits cytokine production and purine nucleotide biosynthesis, leading to immunosuppressive and anti-inflammatory effects. Response to *methotrexate* occurs within 3 to 6 weeks of starting treatment; it can also slow the appearance of new erosions within involved joints. The other DMARDs can be added to *methotrexate* therapy if there is partial or no response to maximum doses of *methotrexate*. Doses of *methotrexate* required for RA treatment are much lower than those needed in cancer chemotherapy and are given once a week, thereby minimizing adverse effects. The most common side effects observed after *methotrexate* treatment of RA are mucosal ulceration and nausea. Cytopenias (particularly depression of the WBC count), cirrhosis of the liver, and an acute pneumonia-like syndrome may occur with chronic administration. [Note: Taking *leucovorin* (*folinic acid*) once daily after *methotrexate* reduces the severity of adverse effects. *Folic acid* taken on off-days is widely used.] Periodic liver enzyme tests, complete blood counts, and monitoring for signs of infection are recommended.

C. Hydroxychloroquine

Hydroxychloroquine [hye-drox-ee-KLOR-oh-kwin] is used for early, mild RA, often combined with *methotrexate*. This agent is also used in the treatment of lupus and malaria. Its mechanism of action in autoimmune disorders is unknown, and onset of effects takes 6 weeks to 6 months. *Hydroxychloroquine* has less effects on the liver and immune system than other DMARDs; however, it may cause ocular toxicity, including irreversible retinal damage and corneal deposits. It may also cause CNS disturbances, GI upset, and skin discoloration and eruptions.

D. Leflunomide

Leflunomide [le-FLOO-no-mide] is an immunomodulatory agent that preferentially causes cell arrest of the autoimmune lymphocytes through its action on dihydroorotate dehydrogenase (DHODH). Activated proliferating lymphocytes require constant DNA synthesis to proliferate. Pyrimidines and purines are the building blocks of DNA, and DHODH is necessary for pyrimidine synthesis. After biotransformation, *leflunomide* becomes a reversible inhibitor of DHODH (Figure 36.17). *Leflunomide* is approved for the treatment of RA. It can be used as monotherapy or in combination with *methotrexate*. The most common adverse effects are headache, diarrhea, and nausea. Other untoward effects are weight loss, allergic reactions, including a flu-like syndrome, skin rash, alopecia, and hypokalemia. It is not recommended in patients with liver disease, because of a risk of hepatotoxicity. Monitoring parameters include signs of infection, complete blood counts, and liver enzymes.

E. Minocycline

Minocycline [mi-noe-SYE-kleen], a tetracycline antibiotic, is considered to be a DMARD. Although *minocycline* has been shown to be effective in the treatment of early RA, it is generally not utilized as first-line therapy. *Minocycline* can be used as monotherapy or in combination with other DMARDs.

F. Sulfasalazine

Sulfasalazine [sul-fa-SAH-la-zeen] is also used for early, mild RA in combination with *methotrexate* and/or *hydroxychloroquine*. Onset of activity is 1 to 3 months, and it is associated with leukopenia. Its mechanism of action in treating RA is unclear.

G. Glucocorticoids

Glucocorticoids (see Chapter 27) are potent anti-inflammatory drugs that are commonly used in patients with RA to provide symptomatic relief and bridge the time until DMARDs are effective. Timely dose reductions and cessation are necessary to avoid adverse effects associated with long-term use.

VI. BIOLOGIC THERAPIES IN RHEUMATOID ARTHRITIS

IL-1 and TNF-α are proinflammatory cytokines involved in the pathogenesis of RA. When secreted by synovial macrophages, IL-1 and TNF-α stimulate synovial cells to proliferate and synthesize collagenase, thereby degrading cartilage, stimulating bone resorption, and inhibiting proteoglycan synthesis. The TNF-α inhibitors (*adalimumab, certolizumab, etanercept, golimumab*, and *infliximab*) have been shown to decrease signs and symptoms of RA, reduce progression of structural damage, and improve physical function. Clinical response can be seen within 2 weeks of therapy. As with DMARDs, the decision to continue or stop a biological agent can often be made within 3 months after initiation of therapy. If a patient has failed therapy with one TNF-α inhibitor, a trial with a different TNF-α inhibitor or a non-TNF biologic therapy (*abatacept, rituximab, tocilizumab, tofacitinib*) is appropriate. TNF-α inhibitors can be administered with any of the other drugs for RA, except for the non-TNF biologic therapies (due to increased risk of infection).

Patients receiving TNF-α inhibitors are at increased risk for infections (tuberculosis and sepsis), fungal opportunistic infections, and pancytopenia. Live vaccinations should not be administered while on TNF-α inhibitor therapy. These agents should be used very cautiously in those with heart failure, as they can cause and/or worsen preexisting heart failure. An increased risk of lymphoma and other cancers has been observed with the use of TNF-α inhibitors. Characteristics of the TNF-α inhibitors and other biologic therapies are outlined below.

A. Adalimumab

Adalimumab [a-dal-AYE-mu-mab] is a recombinant monoclonal antibody that binds to TNF-α, thereby interfering with endogenous TNF-α

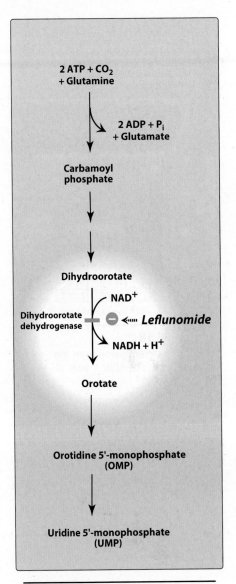

Figure 36.17
Site of action of *leflunomide*.

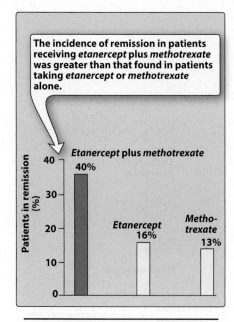

Figure 36.18
Incidence of remission from the symptoms of RA after 1 year of therapy.

activity by blocking its interaction with cell surface receptors. This agent is indicated for treatment of moderate to severe RA, either as monotherapy or in combination with *methotrexate*. It is also indicated for psoriatic arthritis, ankylosing spondylitis, and Crohn disease. *Adalimumab* is administered subcutaneously weekly or every other week. It may cause headache, nausea, agranulocytosis, rash, reaction at the injection site, or increased risk of infections, such as urinary tract infections, upper respiratory tract infections, and sinusitis.

B. Certolizumab pegol

Certolizumab [ser-toe-LIZ-oo-mab] is a unique TNF-α blocker that contains a Fab fragment of a humanized antibody and is a potent neutralizer of TNF-α biological actions. It is combined with polyethylene glycol (pegylated) and is administered every 2 weeks via subcutaneous injection. It has similar indications to *adalimumab*. Adverse effects are similar to other TNF-α inhibitors.

C. Etanercept

Etanercept [ee-TAN-er-cept] is a genetically engineered, soluble, recombinant, fully human receptor fusion protein that binds to TNF-α, thereby blocking its interaction with cell surface TNF-α receptors. This agent is approved for use in patients with moderate to severe RA, either alone or in combination with *methotrexate*. It is also approved for use in ankylosing spondylitis and psoriasis. The combination of *etanercept* and *methotrexate* is more effective than *methotrexate* or *etanercept* alone in retarding the RA disease process, improving function, and achieving remission (Figure 36.18). *Etanercept* is given subcutaneously twice a week. The drug is generally well tolerated. As with all TNF-α inhibitors, it can increase the risk for infections, malignancy, and new or worsening heart failure.

D. Golimumab

Golimumab [goe-LIM-ue-mab] neutralizes the biological activity of TNF-α by binding to it and blocking its interaction with cell surface receptors. This compound is administered subcutaneously once a month in combination with *methotrexate* or other nonbiologic DMARDs. *Golimumab* may increase hepatic enzymes. Reactivation of hepatitis B may occur in chronic carriers. As with other TNF-α inhibitors, this drug may increase the risk of malignancies and serious infections.

E. Infliximab

Infliximab [in-FLIX-i-mab] is a chimeric monoclonal antibody composed of human and murine regions. The antibody binds specifically to human TNF-α and inhibits binding with its receptors. *Infliximab* is approved for use in combination with *methotrexate* in patients with RA who have had inadequate response to *methotrexate* monotherapy. This agent is not indicated for monotherapy, as this leads to the development of anti-*infliximab* antibodies, resulting in reduced efficacy. Additional indications include plaque psoriasis, psoriatic arthritis, ulcerative colitis, ankylosing spondylitis, and Crohn disease. *Infliximab* is administered as an IV infusion every 8 weeks. Infusion site reactions, such as fever, chills, pruritus, and urticaria, may occur. Infections (for example, pneumonia, cellulitis, and activation of latent tuberculosis), leukopenia, and neutropenia have also been reported.

F. Abatacept

T lymphocytes need two interactions to become activated: 1) the antigen-presenting cell (that is, macrophages or B cells) must interact with the receptor on the T cell and 2) the CD80/CD86 protein on the antigen-presenting cell must interact with the CD28 protein on the T cell. *Abatacept* [a-BAT-ah-cept] is a soluble recombinant fusion protein that competes with CD28 for binding on CD80/CD86 protein, thereby preventing full T-cell activation. This agent is indicated for patients with moderate to severe RA who have had an inadequate response to DMARDs or TNF-α inhibitors. *Abatacept* is administered as an IV infusion every 4 weeks. Common adverse effects include headache, upper respiratory infections, nasopharyngitis, and nausea. Concurrent use with TNF-α inhibitors is not recommended due to increased risk of serious infections.

G. Rituximab

B lymphocytes are derived from the bone marrow and are necessary for efficient immune response. In RA, however, B cells can perpetuate the inflammatory process in the synovium by 1) activating T lymphocytes, 2) producing autoantibodies and rheumatoid factor, and 3) producing proinflammatory cytokines, such as TNF-α and IL-1. *Rituximab* [ri-TUK-si-mab] is a genetically engineered chimeric murine/human monoclonal antibody directed against the CD20 antigen found on the surface of normal and malignant B lymphocytes, resulting in B-cell depletion. This agent is indicated for use in combination with *methotrexate* for patients with moderate to severe RA who have had an inadequate response to TNF-α inhibitors. *Rituximab* is administered as an intravenous infusion every 16 to 24 weeks. To reduce the severity of infusion reactions, *methylprednisolone* is administered 30 minutes prior to each infusion. Infusion reactions (urticaria, hypotension, and angioedema) are the most common complaints with this agent and typically occur during the first infusion.

H. Tocilizumab

Tocilizumab [toe-si-LIZ-ue-mab] is a monoclonal antibody that inhibits the actions of IL-6 by blocking the IL-6 receptor. *Tocilizumab* is administered as an intravenous infusion every 4 weeks. The drug can be used as monotherapy or in combination with *methotrexate* or other nonbiologic DMARDs for patients with moderate to severe RA.

I. Tofacitinib

Janus kinases are intracellular enzymes that modulate immune cell activity in response to the binding of inflammatory mediators to the cellular membrane. Cytokines, growth factors, interferons, ILs, and erythropoietin can lead to an increase in Janus kinase activity and activation of the immune system. *Tofacitinib* [toe-fa-SYE-ti-nib] is an oral inhibitor of Janus kinases indicated for the treatment of moderate to severe RA in patients who have had an inadequate response

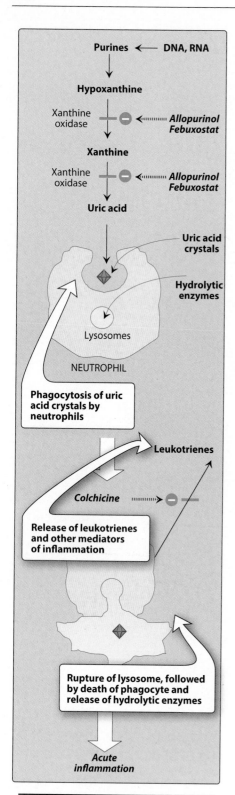

Figure 36.19
Role of uric acid in the inflammation of gout.

or intolerance to *methotrexate*. Metabolism of *tofacitinib* is mediated primarily by CYP3A4, and dosage adjustments may be required if the drug is taken with potent inhibitors or inducers of this isoenzyme. Hemoglobin concentrations must be greater than 9 g/dL to start *tofacitinib* and must be monitored during therapy due to the risk for anemia. Likewise, lymphocyte and neutrophil counts should be checked prior to initiation of therapy and monitored during treatment. *Tofacitinib* treatment may also increase the risk for secondary malignancy, opportunistic infections, renal, or hepatic dysfunction.

J. Anakinra

IL-1 is induced by inflammatory stimuli and mediates a variety of immunologic responses, including degradation of cartilage and stimulation of bone resorption. *Anakinra* [an-a-KIN-ra] is an IL-1 receptor antagonist. *Anakinra* treatment leads to a modest reduction in the signs and symptoms of moderate to severe RA in patients who have failed one or more DMARDs. This agent is associated with neutropenia and is infrequently used in the treatment of RA.

VII. DRUGS USED FOR THE TREATMENT OF GOUT

Gout is a metabolic disorder characterized by high levels of uric acid in the blood (hyperuricemia). Hyperuricemia can lead to deposition of sodium urate crystals in tissues, especially the joints and kidney. Hyperuricemia does not always lead to gout, but gout is always preceded by hyperuricemia. The deposition of urate crystals initiates an inflammatory process involving the infiltration of granulocytes that phagocytize the urate crystals (Figure 36.19). The cause of hyperuricemia is an imbalance between overproduction of uric acid and/or the inability of the patient to excrete it via renal elimination. Most therapeutic strategies for gout involve lowering the uric acid level below the saturation point (6 mg/dL), thus preventing the deposition of urate crystals. This can be accomplished by interfering with uric acid synthesis or increasing uric acid excretion.

A. Treatment of acute gout

Acute gout attacks can result from a number of conditions, including excessive alcohol consumption, a diet rich in purines, and kidney disease. NSAIDs, corticosteroids, or *colchicine* are effective alternatives for the management of acute gouty arthritis. *Indomethacin* is considered the classic NSAID of choice, although all NSAIDs are likely to be effective in decreasing pain and inflammation. Intra-articular administration of corticosteroids (when only one or two joints are affected) is also appropriate in the acute setting, with systemic corticosteroid therapy for more widespread joint involvement. Patients are candidates for prophylactic urate-lowering therapy if they have more than two attacks per year or they have chronic kidney disease, kidney stones, or tophi (deposit of urate crystals in the joints, bones, cartilage, or other body structures).

B. Treatment of chronic gout

Urate-lowering therapy for chronic gout aims to reduce the frequency of attacks and complications of gout. Treatment strategies include the use of xanthine oxidase inhibitors to reduce the synthesis of uric acid or use of uricosuric drugs to increase its excretion. Xanthine oxidase inhibitors (*allopurinol, febuxostat*) are first-line urate-lowering agents. Uricosuric agents (*probenecid*) may be used in patients who are intolerant to xanthine oxidase inhibitors or fail to achieve adequate response with those agents. [Note: Initiation of urate-lowering therapy can precipitate an acute gout attack due to rapid changes in serum urate concentrations. Medications for the prevention of an acute gout attack (low-dose *colchicine*, NSAIDs, or corticosteroids) should be initiated with urate-lowering therapy and continued for at least 6 months.]

C. Colchicine

Colchicine [KOL-chi-seen], a plant alkaloid, is used for the treatment of acute gouty attacks. It is neither a uricosuric nor an analgesic agent, although it relieves pain in acute attacks of gout.

1. **Mechanism of action:** *Colchicine* binds to tubulin, a microtubular protein, causing its depolymerization. This disrupts cellular functions, such as the mobility of granulocytes, thus decreasing their migration into the affected area. Furthermore, *colchicine* blocks cell division by binding to mitotic spindles.

2. **Therapeutic uses:** The anti-inflammatory activity of *colchicine* is specific for gout, usually alleviating the pain of acute gout within 12 hours. [Note: *Colchicine* must be administered within 36 hours of onset of attack to be effective.] NSAIDs have largely replaced *colchicine* in the treatment of acute gouty attacks for safety reasons. *Colchicine* is also used as a prophylactic agent to prevent acute attacks of gout in patients initiating urate-lowering therapy.

3. **Pharmacokinetics:** *Colchicine* is administered orally and is rapidly absorbed from the GI tract. *Colchicine* is recycled in the bile and is excreted unchanged in feces or urine.

4. **Adverse effects:** *Colchicine* may cause nausea, vomiting, abdominal pain, and diarrhea (Figure 36.20). Chronic administration may lead to myopathy, neutropenia, aplastic anemia, and alopecia. The drug should not be used in pregnancy, and it should be used with caution in patients with hepatic, renal, or cardiovascular disease. Dosage adjustments are required in patients taking CYP3A4 inhibitors, like *clarithromycin*, *itraconazole*, and protease inhibitors. For patients with severe renal impairment, the dose should be reduced.

D. Allopurinol

Allopurinol [al-oh-PURE-i-nole], a xanthine oxidase inhibitor, is a purine analog. It reduces the production of uric acid by competitively inhibiting the last two steps in uric acid biosynthesis that are catalyzed by xanthine oxidase (Figure 36.19).

1. **Therapeutic uses:** *Allopurinol* is an effective urate-lowering therapy in the treatment of gout and hyperuricemia secondary to other conditions, such as that associated with certain malignancies (those in which large amounts of purines are produced, particularly after chemotherapy) or in renal disease.

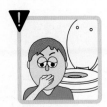
Nausea

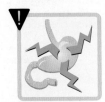
GI disturbance

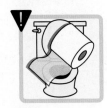
Diarrhea

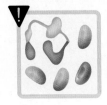
Agranulocytosis
Aplastic anemia

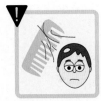
Alopecia

Figure 36.20
Some adverse effects of *colchicine*. GI = gastrointestinal.

2. **Pharmacokinetics:** *Allopurinol* is completely absorbed after oral administration. The primary metabolite is alloxanthine (oxypurinol), which is also a xanthine oxidase inhibitor with a half-life of 15 to 18 hours. Thus, effective inhibition of xanthine oxidase can be maintained with once-daily dosage. The drug and its active metabolite are excreted in the feces and urine. The dosage should be reduced if the creatinine clearance is less than 50 mL/min.

3. **Adverse effects:** *Allopurinol* is well tolerated by most patients. Hypersensitivity reactions, especially skin rashes, are the most common adverse reactions. The risk is increased in those with reduced renal function. Because acute attacks of gout may occur more frequently during the first several months of therapy, *colchicine*, NSAIDs, or corticosteroids can be administered concurrently. *Allopurinol* interferes with the metabolism of *6-mercaptopurine*, the immunosuppressant *azathioprine*, and *theophylline*, requiring a reduction in dosage of these drugs.

E. Febuxostat

Febuxostat [feb-UX-oh-stat], a xanthine oxidase inhibitor, is structurally unrelated to *allopurinol*; however, it has the same indications. In addition, the same drug interactions with *6-mercaptopurine*, *azathioprine*, and *theophylline* apply. Its adverse effect profile is similar to that of *allopurinol*, although the risk for rash and hypersensitivity reactions may be reduced. *Febuxostat* does not have the same degree of renal elimination as *allopurinol* and thus requires less adjustment in those with reduced renal function.

F. Probenecid

Probenecid [proe-BEN-a-sid] is a uricosuric drug. It is a weak organic acid that promotes renal clearance of uric acid by inhibiting the urate-anion exchanger in the proximal tubule that mediates urate reabsorption. At therapeutic doses, it blocks proximal tubular reabsorption of uric acid. *Probenecid* blocks the tubular secretion of *penicillin* and is sometimes used to increase levels of β-lactam antibiotics. It also inhibits the excretion of *methotrexate*, *naproxen*, *ketoprofen*, and *indomethacin*. *Probenecid* should be avoided if the creatinine clearance is less than 50 mL/min.

G. Pegloticase

Pegloticase [peg-LOE-ti-kase] is a recombinant form of the enzyme urate oxidase or uricase. It acts by converting uric acid to allantoin, a water-soluble nontoxic metabolite that is excreted primarily by the kidneys. *Pegloticase* is indicated for patients with gout who fail treatment with standard therapies such as xanthine oxidase inhibitors. It is administered as an IV infusion every 2 weeks.

VIII. DRUGS USED TO TREAT HEADACHE

The most common types of headaches are migraine, tension-type, and cluster headaches. Migraine can usually be distinguished from cluster headaches and tension-type headaches by its characteristics as shown

	MIGRAINE	CLUSTER	TENSION TYPE
Family history	Yes	No	Yes
Sex	Females more often than males	Males more often than females	Females more often than males
Onset	Variable	During sleep	Under stress
Location	Usually unilateral	Behind or around one eye	Bilateral in band around head
Character and severity	Pulsating, throbbing	Excruciating, sharp, steady	Dull, persistent, tightening
Duration	2–72 hours per episode	15–90 minutes per episode	30 minutes to 7 days per episode
Associated symptoms	Visual auras, sensitivity to light and sound, pale facial appearance, nausea and vomiting	Unilateral or bilateral sweating, facial flushing, nasal congestion, lacrimation, pupillary changes	Mild intolerance to light and noise, anorexia

Figure 36.21
Characteristics of migraine, cluster, and tension-type headaches.

in Figure 36.21. Migraines, for example, present as a pulsatile, throbbing pain, whereas cluster headaches present as excruciating, sharp, steady pain. This is in contrast to tension-type headaches, which present as dull pain, with a persistent, tightening feeling in the head. Patients with severe migraine headaches report one to five attacks per month of moderate to severe pain, usually unilateral. The headaches significantly affect quality of life and result in considerable health care costs. Management of headaches involves avoidance of headache triggers (for example, alcohol, chocolate, and stress) and use of abortive treatments for acute headaches, as well as prophylactic therapy in patients with frequent or severe migraines (Figure 36.22).

A. Types of migraine

There are two main types of migraine headaches. The first, migraine without aura, is a severe, unilateral, pulsating headache that typically lasts from 2 to 72 hours. These headaches are often aggravated by physical activity and are accompanied by nausea, vomiting, photophobia (hypersensitivity to light), and phonophobia (hypersensitivity to sound). The majority of patients with migraine do not have aura. In the second type, migraine with aura, the headache is preceded by neurologic symptoms called auras, which can be visual, sensory, and/or cause speech or motor disturbances. Most commonly, these prodromal symptoms are visual (flashes, zigzag lines, and glare), occurring approximately 20 to 40 minutes before headache pain begins. In the 15% of migraine patients whose headache is preceded by an aura, the aura itself allows diagnosis. The headache in migraines with or without auras is similar. Women are threefold more likely than men to experience either type of migraine.

TRIPTANS
Almotriptan AXERT
Eletriptan RELPAX
Frovatriptan FROVA
Naratriptan AMERGE
Rizatriptan MAXALT
Sumatriptan IMITREX, ALSUMA
Zolmitriptan ZOMIG

ERGOTS
Dihydroergotamine MIGRANAL, VARIOUS

NSAIDs
Aspirin BAYER, BUFFERIN, ECOTRIN
Ibuprofen ADVIL, MOTRIN
Indomethacin INDOCIN
Ketorolac TORADOL
Naproxen ALEVE, ANAPROX, NAPROSYN

PROPHYLACTIC AGENTS
Anticonvulsants
Beta-blockers
Calcium channel blockers
Tricyclic antidepressants

Figure 36.22
Summary of drugs used to treat migraine headache.

B. Biologic basis of migraine headaches

The first manifestation of migraine with aura is a spreading depression of neuronal activity accompanied by reduced blood flow in the most posterior part of the cerebral hemisphere. This hypoperfusion gradually spreads forward over the surface of the cortex to other contiguous areas of the brain. The vascular alteration is accompanied by functional changes. The hypoperfusion persists throughout the aura and well into the headache phase. Patients who have migraine without aura do not show hypoperfusion. However, the pain of both types of migraine may be due to extracranial and intracranial arterial vasodilation, which leads to release of neuroactive molecules, such as substance P, neurokinin A, and calcitonin gene–related peptide.

C. Symptomatic treatment of acute migraine

Acute treatments can be classified as nonspecific (symptomatic) or migraine specific. Nonspecific treatment includes analgesics such as NSAIDs and antiemetics (for example, *prochlorperazine*) to control vomiting. Opioids are reserved as rescue medication when other treatments of a severe migraine attack are not successful. Specific migraine therapy includes triptans and ergot alkaloids, which are 5-HT$_{1B/1D}$ receptor and 5-HT$_{1D}$ receptor agonists, respectively. It has been proposed that activation of 5-HT$_1$ receptors by these agents leads either to vasoconstriction or to inhibition of the release of proinflammatory neuropeptides on the trigeminal nerve innervating cranial blood vessels.

1. **Triptans:** This class of drugs includes *almotriptan* [al-moe-TRIP-tan], *eletriptan* [el-e-TRIP-tan], *frovatriptan* [froe-va-TRIP-tan], *naratriptan* [nar-a-TRIP-tan], *rizatriptan* [rye-za-TRIP-tan], *sumatriptan* [soo-ma-TRIP-tan], and *zolmitriptan* [zole-ma-TRIP-tan]. *Sumatriptan* was the first available triptan, and is the prototype of this class. These agents rapidly and effectively abort or markedly reduce the severity of migraine headaches in about 70% of patients. The triptans are serotonin agonists, acting at a subgroup of serotonin receptors found on small peripheral nerves that innervate the intracranial vasculature. The nausea that occurs with *dihydroergotamine* and the vasoconstriction caused by *ergotamine* (see below) are much less pronounced with the triptans. *Sumatriptan* is given subcutaneously, intranasally, or orally (*sumatriptan* is also available in a combination product with *naproxen*). *Zolmitriptan* is available orally and by nasal spray. [Note: All other agents are taken orally.] The onset of the parenteral drug *sumatriptan* is about 20 minutes, compared with 1 to 2 hours when the drug is administered orally. The drug has a short duration of action, with an elimination half-life of 2 hours. Headache commonly recurs within 24 to 48 hours after a single dose of drug, but in most patients, a second dose is effective in aborting the headache. *Frovatriptan* is the longest-acting triptan, with a half-life of more than 24 hours. Individual responses to triptans vary, and a trial of more than one triptan may be necessary

before treatment is successful. Elevation of blood pressure and other cardiac events have been reported with triptan use. Therefore, triptans should not be administered to patients with risk factors for coronary artery disease without performing a cardiac evaluation prior to administration. Other adverse events with the use of triptans include pain and pressure sensations in the chest, neck, throat, and jaw. Dizziness and malaise have also been seen with the use of triptans.

2. **Ergot alkaloids:** *Ergotamine* [er-GOT-a-meen] and *dihydroergotamine* [dye-hye-droe-er-GOT-a-meen], a semisynthetic derivative of *ergotamine*, are ergot alkaloids approved for the treatment of migraine headaches. The action of the ergot alkaloids is complex, with ability to bind to 5-HT$_1$ receptors, α receptors, and dopamine receptors. 5-HT$_1$ receptors located on intracranial blood vessels are targets that cause vasoconstriction with the use of these agents. *Ergotamine* is currently available sublingually and is mostly effective when used in the early stages of the migraine. It is also available as an oral tablet or suppository containing both *ergotamine* and caffeine. *Ergotamine* is used with strict daily and weekly dosage limits due to its ability to cause dependence and rebound headaches. *Dihydroergotamine* is administered intravenously or intranasally and has an efficacy similar to that of *sumatriptan*. The use of *dihydroergotamine* is limited to severe cases of migraines. Nausea is a common adverse effect. *Ergotamine* and *dihydroergotamine* are contraindicated in patients with angina and peripheral vascular disease because they are significant vasoconstrictors.

D. Prophylaxis for migraine headache

Therapy to prevent migraine is indicated if the attacks occur two or more times a month and if the headaches are severe or complicated by serious neurologic signs. β-Blockers are the drugs of choice for migraine prophylaxis (Figure 36.23). *Propranolol* and other β-blockers, such as *metoprolol, atenolol, and nadolol*, have been shown to be effective. The calcium channel blocker *verapamil* is an alternative. Anticonvulsants (*divalproex*) and antidepressants (tricyclics) have also shown effectiveness in preventing migraine. Antidepressants are especially useful for migraine prophylaxis in patients with comorbid depression.

E. Drugs for tension and cluster headache

Analgesics such as NSAIDs (for example, *naproxen* and *ibuprofen*), *acetaminophen*, and *aspirin* are used for symptomatic relief of tension headaches. *Acetaminophen* and/or *aspirin* may also be combined with caffeine. [Note: Caffeine is believed to increase the central effectiveness of *acetaminophen* and *aspirin*.] *Butalbital*, a barbiturate, in combination with *acetaminophen* or *aspirin* with or without caffeine is also used in tension headaches. Inhalation of 100% oxygen and triptans (especially *sumatriptan*) are used as first-line abortive strategies for cluster headache.

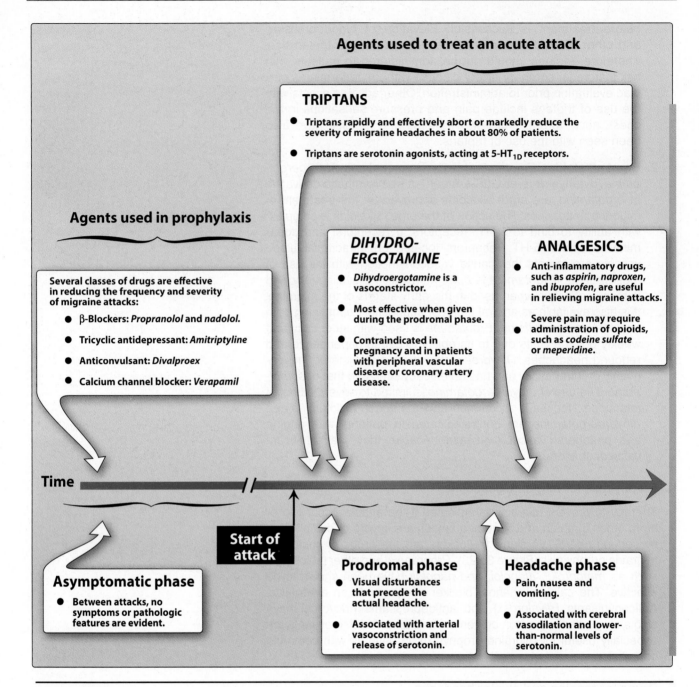

Figure 36.23
Drugs useful in the treatment and prophylaxis of migraine headaches.

Study Questions

Choose the ONE best answer.

36.1 A 64-year-old male presents with mild to moderate musculoskeletal back pain after playing golf. He states he has tried acetaminophen and that it did not help. His past medical history includes diabetes, hypertension, hyperlipidemia, gastric ulcer (resolved), and coronary artery disease. Which of the following is the most appropriate NSAID regimen to treat this patient's pain?

A. Celecoxib.

B. Indomethacin and omeprazole.

C. Naproxen and omeprazole.

D. Naproxen.

Correct answer = C. This patient is at high risk of future ulcers, due to the history of gastric ulcer. Therefore, using a regimen that includes an agent that is more COX-2 selective or a proton pump inhibitor is warranted. Therefore, D is incorrect. Choices A and B are incorrect because this patient has significant cardiovascular risk and a history of coronary artery disease. Naproxen is thought of as the safest NSAID regarding cardiovascular disease, though it still can present risks. Therefore, C is correct as it uses the first-choice NSAID with the GI protection of a proton pump inhibitor.

36.2 Which of the following correctly represents the mechanism of action of tofacitinib in the treatment of RA?

A. TNF-α inhibitor.

B. Inhibitor of Janus kinases.

C. IL-6 receptor blocker.

D. Dihydrofolate reductase inhibitor.

Correct answer = B. Methotrexate inhibits dihydrofolate reductase. Etanercept is a TNF-α inhibitor. An IL-6 inhibitor is tocilizumab. Tofacitinib is an inhibitor of Janus kinase 1, 3, and, to a lesser extent, 2.

36.3 A 64-year-old male presents with signs and symptoms of an acute gouty flare. His doctor wishes to treat him accordingly to improve his symptoms. Which of the following strategies would be the LEAST likely to acutely improve his gout symptoms and pain?

A. Naproxen.

B. Colchicine.

C. Probenecid.

D. Prednisone.

Correct answer = C. Probenecid is a uricosuric agent indicated to lower serum urate levels to prevent gout attacks. It is not indicated during acute gout flares and should not be started until after the resolution of an acute attack. Naproxen, colchicine, and prednisone all represent viable treatment options that acutely reduce pain and inflammation associated with acute gout attacks.

36.4 Which of the following drugs for headache is contraindicated in patients with peripheral vascular disease?

A. Ergotamine.

B. Aspirin.

C. Acetaminophen.

D. Naproxen

E. Ibuprofen.

Correct answer = A. Ergotamine is contraindicated in peripheral vascular disease since it is a significant vasoconstrictor.

Principles of Antimicrobial Therapy

Jamie Kisgen

37

I. OVERVIEW

Antimicrobial therapy takes advantage of the biochemical differences that exist between microorganisms and human beings. Antimicrobial drugs are effective in the treatment of infections because of their selective toxicity; that is, they have the ability to injure or kill an invading microorganism without harming the cells of the host. In most instances, the selective toxicity is relative rather than absolute, requiring that the concentration of the drug be carefully controlled to attack the microorganism, while still being tolerated by the host.

II. SELECTION OF ANTIMICROBIAL AGENTS

Selection of the most appropriate antimicrobial agent requires knowing 1) the organism's identity, 2) the organism's susceptibility to a particular agent, 3) the site of the infection, 4) patient factors, 5) the safety of the agent, and 6) the cost of therapy. However, some patients require empiric therapy (immediate administration of drug(s) prior to bacterial identification and susceptibility testing).

A. Identification of the infecting organism

Characterizing the organism is central to selection of the proper drug. A rapid assessment of the nature of the pathogen can sometimes be made on the basis of the Gram stain, which is particularly useful in identifying the presence and morphologic features of microorganisms in body fluids that are normally sterile (blood, serum, cerebrospinal fluid [CSF], pleural fluid, synovial fluid, peritoneal fluid, and urine). However, it is generally necessary to culture the infective organism to arrive at a conclusive diagnosis and determine the susceptibility to

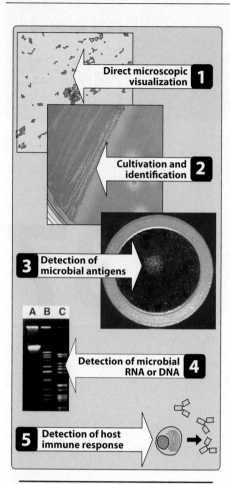

Figure 37.1
Some laboratory techniques that are useful in the diagnosis of microbial diseases.

antimicrobial agents. Thus, it is essential to obtain a sample culture of the organism prior to initiating treatment. Otherwise, it is impossible to differentiate whether a negative culture is due to the absence of organisms or is a result of antimicrobial effects of administered antibiotic. Definitive identification of the infecting organism may require other laboratory techniques, such as detection of microbial antigens, DNA, or RNA, or an inflammatory or host immune response to the microorganism (Figure 37.1).

B. Empiric therapy prior to identification of the organism

Ideally, the antimicrobial agent used to treat an infection is selected after the organism has been identified and its drug susceptibility established. However, in the critically ill patient, such a delay could prove fatal, and immediate empiric therapy is indicated.

1. **Timing:** Acutely ill patients with infections of unknown origin—for example, a neutropenic patient (one who is predisposed to infections due to a reduction in neutrophils) or a patient with meningitis (acute inflammation of the membranes covering the brain and spinal cord)—require immediate treatment. If possible, therapy should be initiated after specimens for laboratory analysis have been obtained but before the results of the culture and sensitivity are available.

2. **Selecting a drug:** Drug choice in the absence of susceptibility data is influenced by the site of infection and the patient's history (for example, previous infections, age, recent travel history, recent antimicrobial therapy, immune status, and whether the infection was hospital- or community-acquired). Broad-spectrum therapy may be indicated initially when the organism is unknown or polymicrobial infections are likely. The choice of agent(s) may also be guided by known association of particular organisms in a given clinical setting. For example, gram-positive cocci in the spinal fluid of a newborn infant is unlikely to be Streptococcus pneumoniae and most likely to be Streptococcus agalactiae (a group B streptococci), which is sensitive to *penicillin G*. By contrast, gram-positive cocci in the spinal fluid of a 40-year-old patient are most likely to be S. pneumoniae. This organism is frequently resistant to *penicillin G* and often requires treatment with a high-dose third-generation cephalosporin (such as *ceftriaxone*) or *vancomycin*.

C. Determining antimicrobial susceptibility of infective organisms

After a pathogen is cultured, its susceptibility to specific antibiotics serves as a guide in choosing antimicrobial therapy. Some pathogens, such as Streptococcus pyogenes and Neisseria meningitidis, usually have predictable susceptibility patterns to certain antibiotics. In contrast, most gram-negative bacilli, enterococci, and staphylococcal species often show unpredictable susceptibility patterns and require susceptibility testing to determine appropriate antimicrobial therapy. The minimum inhibitory and bactericidal concentrations of a drug can be experimentally determined (Figure 37.2).

1. **Bacteriostatic versus bactericidal drugs:** Antimicrobial drugs are classified as either bacteriostatic or bactericidal. Bacteriostatic drugs arrest the growth and replication of bacteria at serum

(or urine) levels achievable in the patient, thus limiting the spread of infection until the immune system attacks, immobilizes, and eliminates the pathogen. If the drug is removed before the immune system has scavenged the organisms, enough viable organisms may remain to begin a second cycle of infection. Bactericidal drugs kill bacteria at drug serum levels achievable in the patient. Because of their more aggressive antimicrobial action, bactericidal agents are often the drugs of choice in seriously ill and immunocompromised patients. Figure 37.3 shows a laboratory experiment in which the growth of bacteria is arrested by the addition of a bacteriostatic agent. Note that viable organisms remain even in the presence of the bacteriostatic drug. In contrast, addition of a bactericidal agent kills bacteria, and the total number of viable organisms decreases. Although practical, this classification may be too simplistic because it is possible for an antibiotic to be bacteriostatic for one organism and bactericidal for another. For example, *linezolid* is bacteriostatic against <u>Staphylococcus</u> <u>aureus</u> and enterococci but is bactericidal against most strains of <u>S. pneumoniae</u>.

2. **Minimum inhibitory concentration:** The minimum inhibitory concentration (MIC) is the lowest antimicrobial concentration that prevents visible growth of an organism after 24 hours of incubation. This serves as a quantitative measure of in vitro susceptibility and is commonly used in practice to streamline therapy. Computer automation has improved the accuracy and decreased the turnaround time for determining MIC results and is the most common approach used by clinical laboratories.

3. **Minimum bactericidal concentration:** The minimum bactericidal concentration (MBC) is the lowest concentration of antimicrobial agent that results in a 99.9% decline in colony count after overnight broth dilution incubations (Figure 37.2). [Note: The MBC is rarely determined in clinical practice due to the time and labor requirements.]

D. Effect of the site of infection on therapy: the blood–brain barrier

Adequate levels of an antibiotic must reach the site of infection for the invading microorganisms to be effectively eradicated. Capillaries with varying degrees of permeability carry drugs to the body tissues. Natural barriers to drug delivery are created by the structures of the capillaries of some tissues, such as the prostate, testes, placenta, the vitreous body of the eye, and the central nervous system (CNS). Of particular significance are the capillaries in the brain, which help to create and maintain the blood–brain barrier. This barrier is formed by the single layer of endothelial cells fused by tight junctions that impede entry from the blood to the brain of virtually all molecules, except those that are small and lipophilic. The penetration and concentration of an antibacterial agent in the CSF are particularly influenced by the following:

1. **Lipid solubility of the drug:** The lipid solubility of a drug is a major determinant of its ability to penetrate into the brain. Lipid-soluble drugs, such as *chloramphenicol* and *metronidazole*, have significant penetration into the CNS, whereas β-lactam

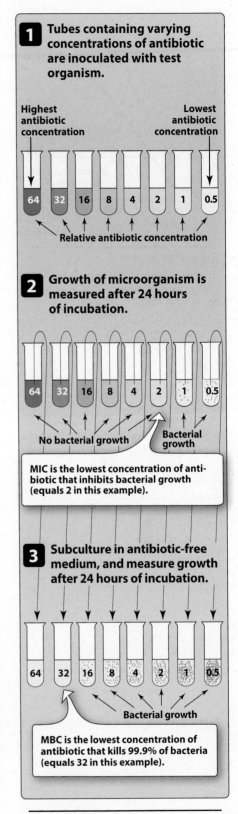

Figure 37.2

Determination of minimum inhibitory concentration (MIC) and minimum bactericidal concentration (MBC) of an antibiotic.

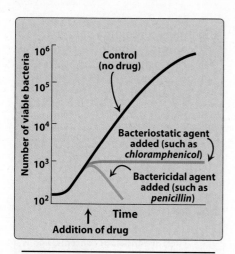

Figure 37.3
Effects of bactericidal and bacteriostatic drugs on the growth of bacteria in vitro.

antibiotics, such as *penicillin*, are ionized at physiologic pH and have low solubility in lipids. They therefore have limited penetration through the intact blood–brain barrier under normal circumstances. In infections such as meningitis in which the brain becomes inflamed, the barrier does not function as effectively, and local permeability is increased. Some β-lactam antibiotics can enter the CSF in therapeutic amounts when the meninges are inflamed.

2. **Molecular weight of the drug:** A compound with a low molecular weight has an enhanced ability to cross the blood–brain barrier, whereas compounds with a high molecular weight (for example, *vancomycin*) penetrate poorly, even in the presence of meningeal inflammation.

3. **Protein binding of the drug:** A high degree of protein binding of a drug restricts its entry into the CSF. Therefore, the amount of free (unbound) drug in serum, rather than the total amount of drug present, is important for CSF penetration.

E. Patient factors

In selecting an antibiotic, attention must be paid to the condition of the patient. For example, the status of the patient's immune system, kidneys, liver, circulation, and age must be considered. In women, pregnancy or breast-feeding also affects selection of the antimicrobial agent.

1. **Immune system:** Elimination of infecting organisms from the body depends on an intact immune system, and the host defense system must ultimately eliminate the invading organisms. Alcoholism, diabetes, HIV infection, malnutrition, autoimmune diseases, pregnancy, or advanced age can affect a patient's immunocompetence, as can immunosuppressive drugs. High doses of bactericidal agents or longer courses of treatment may be required to eliminate infective organisms in these individuals.

2. **Renal dysfunction:** Poor kidney function may cause accumulation of certain antibiotics. Dosage adjustment prevents drug accumulation and therefore adverse effects. Serum creatinine levels are frequently used as an index of renal function for adjustment of drug regimens. However, direct monitoring of serum levels of some antibiotics (for example, *vancomycin*, aminoglycosides) is preferred to identify maximum and/or minimum values to prevent potential toxicities. [Note: The number of functional nephrons decreases with age. Thus, elderly patients are particularly vulnerable to accumulation of drugs eliminated by the kidneys.]

3. **Hepatic dysfunction:** Antibiotics that are concentrated or eliminated by the liver (for example, *erythromycin* and *doxycycline*) must be used with caution when treating patients with liver dysfunction.

4. **Poor perfusion:** Decreased circulation to an anatomic area, such as the lower limbs of a diabetic patient, reduces the amount of antibiotic that reaches that area, making these infections difficult to treat.

5. **Age:** Renal or hepatic elimination processes are often poorly developed in newborns, making neonates particularly vulnerable to the toxic effects of *chloramphenicol* and sulfonamides. Young children should not be treated with tetracyclines or quinolones, which affect bone growth and joints, respectively. Elderly patients may have decreased renal or liver function, which may alter the pharmacokinetics of certain antibiotics.

6. **Pregnancy and lactation:** Many antibiotics cross the placental barrier or enter the nursing infant via the breast milk. Figure 37.4 summarizes the U.S. Food and Drug Administration (FDA) risk categories of antibiotic use during pregnancy. The drug examples listed in Figure 37.4 are not all inclusive but merely represent an example from each category. Although the concentration of an antibiotic in breast milk is usually low, the total dose to the infant may be sufficient to produce detrimental effects.

7. **Risk factors for multidrug-resistant organisms:** Infections with multidrug-resistant pathogens need broader antibiotic coverage when initiating empiric therapy. Common risk factors for infection with these pathogens include prior antimicrobial therapy in the preceding 90 days, hospitalization for greater than 2 days within the preceding 90 days, current hospitalization exceeding 5 days, high frequency of resistance in the community or local hospital unit (assessed using hospital antibiograms), and immunosuppressive diseases and/or therapies.

F. Safety of the agent

Antibiotics such as the penicillins are among the least toxic of all drugs because they interfere with a site or function unique to the growth of microorganisms. Other antimicrobial agents (for example, *chloramphenicol*) have less specificity and are reserved for life-threatening infections because of the potential for serious toxicity to the patient. [Note: Safety is related not only to the inherent nature of the drug but also to patient factors that can predispose to toxicity.]

G. Cost of therapy

Often several drugs may show similar efficacy in treating an infection but vary widely in cost. For example, treatment of *methicillin*-resistant <u>Staphylococcus</u> <u>aureus</u> (MRSA) generally includes one of the following: *vancomycin, clindamycin, daptomycin,* or *linezolid.* Although choice of therapy usually centers on the site of infection, severity of the illness, and ability to take oral medications, it is also important to consider the cost of the medication. Figure 37.5 illustrates the relative cost of commonly used drugs for staphylococcal infections.

III. ROUTE OF ADMINISTRATION

The oral route of administration is appropriate for mild infections that can be treated on an outpatient basis. In addition, economic pressures have prompted the use of oral antibiotic therapy in all but the most serious

CATE-GORY	DESCRIPTION	DRUG
A	No human fetal risk or remote possibility of fetal harm	
B	No controlled studies show human risk; animal studies suggest potential toxicity	β-Lactams β-Lactams with inhibitors Cephalosporins *Aztreonam* *Clindamycin* *Erythromycin* *Azithromycin* *Metronidazole* *Nitrofurantoin* *Sulfonamides*
C	Animal fetal toxicity demonstrated; human risk undefined	*Chloramphenicol* *Fluoroquinolones* *Clarithromycin* *Trimethoprim* *Vancomycin* *Gentamicin* *Trimethoprim-sulfa-methoxazole*
D	Human fetal risk present, but benefits may outweigh risks	Tetracyclines Aminoglycosides (except *genta-micin*)
X	Human fetal risk clearly outweighs benefits; contraindicated in pregnancy	

Figure 37.4
FDA categories of antimicrobials and fetal risk.

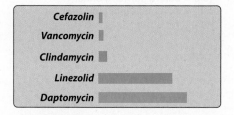

Figure 37.5
Relative cost of some drugs used for the treatment of <u>Staphylococcus aureus</u>.

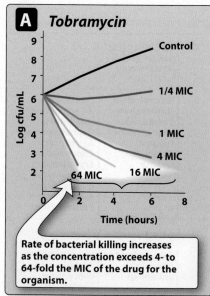

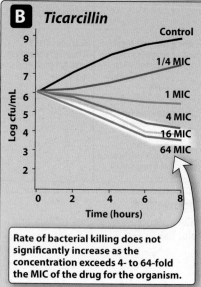

Figure 37.6
A. Significant dose-dependent killing effect shown by *tobramycin*. **B.** Nonsignificant dose-dependent killing effect shown by *ticarcillin*. (cfu = colony-forming units; MIC = minimum inhibitory concentration.)

infectious diseases. In hospitalized patients requiring intravenous therapy initially, the switch to oral agents should occur as soon as possible. However, some antibiotics, such as *vancomycin*, the aminoglycosides, and *amphotericin B* are so poorly absorbed from the gastrointestinal (GI) tract that adequate serum levels cannot be obtained by oral administration. Parenteral administration is used for drugs that are poorly absorbed from the GI tract and for treatment of patients with serious infections, for whom it is necessary to maintain higher serum concentrations of antimicrobial agents.

IV. DETERMINANTS OF RATIONAL DOSING

Rational dosing of antimicrobial agents is based on their pharmacodynamics (the relationship of drug concentrations to antimicrobial effects) and pharmacokinetic properties (the absorption, distribution, metabolism, and elimination of the drug). Three important properties that have a significant influence on the frequency of dosing are concentration-dependent killing, time-dependent killing, and postantibiotic effect (PAE). Utilizing these properties to optimize antibiotic dosing regimens can improve clinical outcomes and possibly decrease the development of resistance.

A. Concentration-dependent killing

Certain antimicrobial agents, including aminoglycosides and *daptomycin*, show a significant increase in the rate of bacterial killing as the concentration of antibiotic increases from 4- to 64-fold the MIC of the drug for the infecting organism (Figure 37.6A). Giving drugs that exhibit this concentration-dependent killing by a once-a-day bolus infusion achieves high peak levels, favoring rapid killing of the infecting pathogen.

B. Time-dependent (concentration-independent) killing

In contrast, β-lactams, glycopeptides, macrolides, *clindamycin*, and *linezolid* do not exhibit concentration-dependent killing (Figure 37.6B). The clinical efficacy of these antimicrobials is best predicted by the percentage of time that blood concentrations of a drug remain above the MIC. This effect is sometimes called concentration-independent or time-dependent killing. For example, dosing schedules for the penicillins and cephalosporins that ensure blood levels greater than the MIC for 50% and 60% of the time, respectively, provide the most clinical efficacy. Therefore, extended (generally 3 to 4 hours) or continuous (24 hours) infusions can be utilized instead of intermittent dosing (generally 30 minutes) to achieve prolonged time above the MIC and kill more bacteria.

C. Postantibiotic effect

The PAE is a persistent suppression of microbial growth that occurs after levels of antibiotic have fallen below the MIC. Antimicrobial drugs exhibiting a long PAE (for example, aminoglycosides and fluoroquinolones) often require only one dose per day, particularly against gram-negative bacteria.

V. CHEMOTHERAPEUTIC SPECTRA

In this book, the clinically important bacteria have been organized into eight groups based on Gram stain, morphology, and biochemical or other characteristics. They are represented as a color-coded list (Figure 37.7A). The ninth section of the list is labeled "Other," and it is used to represent any organism not included in one of the other eight categories. In this chapter, the list is used to illustrate the spectra of bacteria for which a particular class of antibiotics is therapeutically effective.

A. Narrow-spectrum antibiotics

Chemotherapeutic agents acting only on a single or a limited group of microorganisms are said to have a narrow spectrum. For example, *isoniazid* is active only against <u>Mycobacterium</u> <u>tuberculosis</u> (Figure 37.7B).

B. Extended-spectrum antibiotics

Extended spectrum is the term applied to antibiotics that are modified to be effective against gram-positive organisms and also against a significant number of gram-negative bacteria. For example, *ampicillin* is considered to have an extended spectrum because it acts against gram-positive and some gram-negative bacteria (Figure 37.7C).

C. Broad-spectrum antibiotics

Drugs such as *tetracycline*, fluoroquinolones and carbapenems affect a wide variety of microbial species and are referred to as broad-spectrum antibiotics (Figure 37.7D). Administration of broad-spectrum antibiotics can drastically alter the nature of the normal bacterial flora and precipitate a superinfection due to organisms such as <u>Clostridium</u> <u>difficile</u>, the growth of which is normally kept in check by the presence of other colonizing microorganisms.

VI. COMBINATIONS OF ANTIMICROBIAL DRUGS

It is therapeutically advisable to treat patients with a single agent that is most specific to the infecting organism. This strategy reduces the possibility of superinfections, decreases the emergence of resistant organisms, and minimizes toxicity. However, some situations require combinations of antimicrobial drugs. For example, the treatment of tuberculosis benefits from drug combinations.

A. Advantages of drug combinations

Certain combinations of antibiotics, such as β-lactams and aminoglycosides, show synergism; that is, the combination is more effective than either of the drugs used separately. Because such synergism among antimicrobial agents is rare, multiple drugs used in combination are only indicated in special situations (for example, when an infection is of unknown origin or in the treatment of enterococcal endocarditis).

B. Disadvantages of drug combinations

A number of antibiotics act only when organisms are multiplying. Thus, coadministration of an agent that causes bacteriostasis plus a second

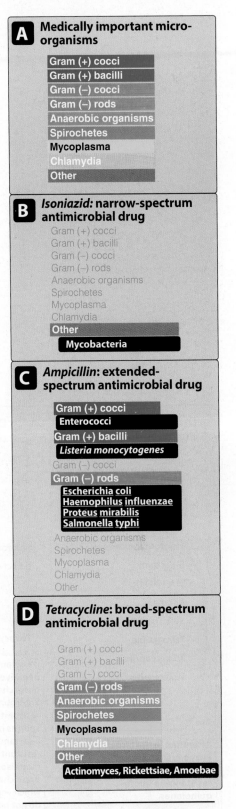

Figure 37.7
A. Color-coded representation of medically important microorganisms. **B.** *Isoniazid*, a narrow-spectrum antimicrobial agent. **C.** *Ampicillin*, an extended-spectrum antimicrobial agent. **D.** *Tetracycline*, a broad-spectrum antimicrobial agent.

agent that is bactericidal may result in the first drug interfering with the action of the second. For example, bacteriostatic tetracycline drugs may interfere with the bactericidal effects of penicillins and cephalosporins. Another concern is the risk of selection pressure and the development of antibiotic resistance by giving unnecessary combination therapy.

VII. DRUG RESISTANCE

Bacteria are considered resistant to an antibiotic if the maximal level of that antibiotic that can be tolerated by the host does not halt their growth. Some organisms are inherently resistant to an antibiotic. For example, most gram-negative organisms are inherently resistant to *vancomycin*. However, microbial species that are normally responsive to a particular drug may develop more virulent or resistant strains through spontaneous mutation or acquired resistance and selection. Some of these strains may even become resistant to more than one antibiotic.

A. Genetic alterations leading to drug resistance

Acquired antibiotic resistance requires the temporary or permanent gain or alteration of bacterial genetic information. Resistance develops due to the ability of DNA to undergo spontaneous mutation or to move from one organism to another (Figure 37.8).

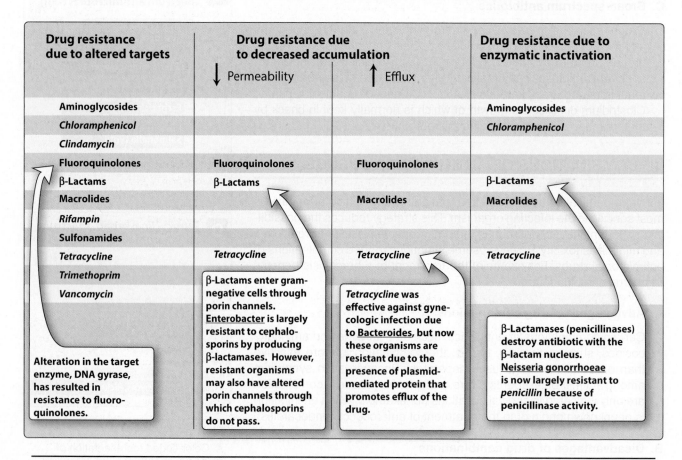

Figure 37.8
Some mechanisms of resistance to antibiotics.

B. Altered expression of proteins in drug-resistant organisms

Drug resistance is mediated by a variety of mechanisms, such as an alteration in an antibiotic target site, lowered penetrability of the drug due to decreased permeability, increased efflux of the drug, or presence of antibiotic-inactivating enzymes (Figure 37.8).

1. **Modification of target sites:** Alteration of an antibiotic's target site through mutation can confer resistance to one or more related antibiotics. For example, <u>S. pneumoniae</u> resistance to β-lactam antibiotics involves alterations in one or more of the major bacterial penicillin-binding proteins, resulting in decreased binding of the antibiotic to its target.

2. **Decreased accumulation:** Decreased uptake or increased efflux of an antibiotic can confer resistance because the drug is unable to attain access to the site of its action in sufficient concentrations to injure or kill the organism. For example, gram-negative organisms can limit the penetration of certain agents, including β-lactam antibiotics, as a result of an alteration in the number and structure of porins (channels) in the outer membrane. Also, the presence of an efflux pump can limit levels of a drug in an organism, as seen with tetracyclines.

3. **Enzymatic inactivation:** The ability to destroy or inactivate the antimicrobial agent can also confer resistance on microorganisms. Examples of antibiotic-inactivating enzymes include 1) β-lactamases ("penicillinases") that hydrolytically inactivate the β-lactam ring of penicillins, cephalosporins, and related drugs; 2) acetyltransferases that transfer an acetyl group to the antibiotic, inactivating *chloramphenicol* or aminoglycosides; and 3) esterases that hydrolyze the lactone ring of macrolides.

VIII. PROPHYLACTIC USE OF ANTIBIOTICS

Certain clinical situations, such as dental procedures and surgeries, require the use of antibiotics for the prevention rather than for the treatment of infections (Figure 37.9). Because the indiscriminate use of antimicrobial agents can result in bacterial resistance and superinfection, prophylactic use is restricted to clinical situations in which the benefits outweigh the potential risks. The duration of prophylaxis should be closely observed to prevent the unnecessary development of antibiotic resistance.

IX. COMPLICATIONS OF ANTIBIOTIC THERAPY

Even though antibiotics are selectively toxic to an invading organism, it does not protect the host against adverse effects. For example, the drug may produce an allergic response or may be toxic in ways unrelated to the antimicrobial activity.

A. Hypersensitivity

Hypersensitivity or immune reactions to antimicrobial drugs or their metabolic products frequently occur. For example, the penicillins, despite their almost absolute selective microbial toxicity, can cause serious hypersensitivity problems, ranging from urticaria (hives) to anaphylactic

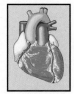

1 Pretreatment may prevent streptococcal infections in patients with a history of rheumatic heart disease. Patients may require years of treatment.

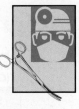

2 Pretreating of patients undergoing dental extractions who have implanted prosthetic devices, such as artificial heart valves, prevents seeding of the prosthesis.

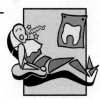

3 Pretreatment may prevent tuberculosis or meningitis among individuals who are in close contact with infected patients.

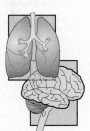

4 Treatment prior to most surgical procedures can decrease the incidence of infection afterwards. Effective prophylaxis is directed against the most likely organism, not eradication of every potential pathogen.

Figure 37.9
Some clinical situations in which prophylactic antibiotics are indicated.

shock. Patients with a documented history of Stevens-Johnson syndrome (SJS) or toxic epidermal necrolysis reaction to an antibiotic should *never* be rechallenged, not even for antibiotic desensitization.

B. Direct toxicity

High serum levels of certain antibiotics may cause toxicity by directly affecting cellular processes in the host. For example, aminoglycosides can cause ototoxicity by interfering with membrane function in the auditory hair cells.

C. Superinfections

Drug therapy, particularly with broad-spectrum antimicrobials or combinations of agents, can lead to alterations of the normal microbial flora of the upper respiratory, oral, intestinal, and genitourinary tracts, permitting the overgrowth of opportunistic organisms, especially fungi or resistant bacteria. These infections usually require secondary treatments using specific anti-infective agents.

X. SITES OF ANTIMICROBIAL ACTIONS

Antimicrobial drugs can be classified in a number of ways: 1) by their chemical structure (for example, β-lactams or aminoglycosides), 2) by their mechanism of action (for example, cell wall synthesis inhibitors), or 3) by their activity against particular types of organisms (for example, bacteria, fungi, or viruses). Chapters 37 through 40 are organized by the mechanisms of action of the drug (Figure 37.10), and Chapters 41 through 45 are organized according to the type of organisms affected by the drug.

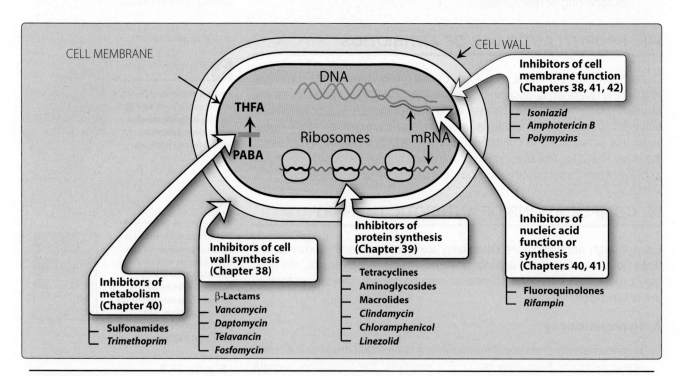

Figure 37.10
Classification of some antimicrobial agents by their sites of action. (THFA = tetrahydrofolic acid; PABA = *p*-aminobenzoic acid.)

Study Questions

Choose the ONE best answer.

37.1 A 24-year-old pregnant female presents to the urgent care clinic with fever, frequency, and urgency. She is diagnosed with a urinary tract infection (UTI). Based on potential harm to the fetus, which of the following medications should be avoided in treating her UTI?

A. Nitrofurantoin.
B. Amoxicillin.
C. Cephalexin.
D. Tobramycin.

> Correct answer = D. Tobramycin (an aminoglycoside) is considered a pregnancy risk category D drug which means there is chance for potential harm to the fetus. Nitrofurantoin, amoxicillin (a penicillin), and cephalexin (a cephalosporin) are considered category B.

37.2 Which of the following is the primary method of β-lactam resistance with <u>Streptococcus</u> <u>pneumoniae</u>?

A. Modification of target site.
B. Decreased drug levels due to changes in permeability.
C. Decreased drug levels due to an efflux pump.
D. Enzymatic inactivation.

> Correct answer = A. <u>S.</u> <u>pneumoniae</u> resistance to β-lactam antibiotics involves alteration in one or more of the major penicillin-binding proteins.

37.3 Which of the following agents is considered a narrow-spectrum antibiotic?

A. Ceftriaxone.
B. Ciprofloxacin.
C. Isoniazid.
D. Imipenem.

> Correct answer = C. Isoniazid is only active against <u>Mycobacterium</u> <u>tuberculosis</u>, while ceftriaxone, ciprofloxacin, and imipenem are considered broad spectrum due to their activity against multiple types of bacteria and risk for developing a superinfection.

37.4 Which of the following antibiotics exhibits concentration-dependent killing?

A. Clindamycin.
B. Linezolid.
C. Vancomycin.
D. Daptomycin.

> Correct answer = D. Clindamycin, linezolid, and vancomycin exhibit time-dependent killing, while daptomycin works best in a concentration-dependent fashion.

37.5 Which of the following antibiotics exhibits a long post-antibiotic effect that permits once-daily dosing?

A. Gentamicin.
B. Penicillin G.
C. Vancomycin.
D. Aztreonam.

> Correct answer = A. Aminoglycosides, including gentamicin, possess a long post-antibiotic effect, especially when given as a high dose every 24 hours. Penicillin G, clindamycin, and vancomycin have a relatively short postantibiotic effect and require frequent dosing to maintain activity.

37.6 A 58-year-old male with a history of hepatitis C, cirrhosis, and ascites presents with spontaneous bacterial peritonitis. Which of the following antibiotics requires close monitoring and dosing adjustment in this patient given his liver disease?

A. Penicillin G.
B. Tobramycin.
C. Erythromycin.
D. Vancomycin.

> Correct answer = C. Erythromycin is metabolized by the liver and should be used with caution in patients with hepatic impairment. Penicillin G, tobramycin, and vancomycin are primarily eliminated by the kidneys.

37.7 Which of the following antibiotics is considered safe to use in neonates?

    A. Chloramphenicol.

    B. Sulfamethoxazole/trimethoprim.

    C. Tetracycline.

    D. Penicillin G.

> Correct answer = D. Chloramphenicol and sulfonamides (sulfamethoxazole) can cause toxic effects in newborns due to poorly developed renal and hepatic elimination processes. Tetracycline can have effects on bone growth and development and should be avoided in newborns and young children. Penicillin G is safe and effective in this population.

37.8 All of the following factors influence the penetration and concentration of an antibacterial agent in the cerebrospinal fluid except:

    A. Lipid solubility of the drug.

    B. Minimum inhibitory concentration of the drug.

    C. Protein binding of the drug.

    D. Molecular weight of the drug.

> Correct answer = B. Although the minimum inhibitory concentration will impact the effectiveness of the drug against a given bacteria, it does not affect the ability of a drug to penetrate into the brain. The lipid solubility, protein binding, and molecular weight all determine the likelihood of a drug to penetrate the blood–brain barrier and concentrate in the brain.

37.9 A 72-year-old male presents with fever, cough, malaise, and shortness of breath. His chest x-ray shows bilateral infiltrates consistent with pneumonia. Bronchial wash cultures reveal Pseudomonas aeruginosa sensitive to cefepime. Which of the following is the best dosing scheme for cefepime based on the drug's time-dependent bactericidal activity?

    A. 1 g every 6 hours given over 30 minutes.

    B. 2 g every 12 hours given over 3 hours.

    C. 4 g every 24 hours given over 30 minutes.

    D. 4 g given as continuous infusion over 24 hours.

> Correct answer = D. The clinical efficacy of cefepime is based on the percentage of time that the drug concentration remains above the MIC. A continuous infusion would allow for the greatest amount of time above the MIC compared to intermittent (30 minutes) and prolonged infusions (3 to 4 hours).

37.10 Which of the following adverse drug reactions precludes a patient from being rechallenged with that drug in the future?

    A. Itching/rash from penicillin.

    B. Stevens-Johnson syndrome from sulfamethoxazole–trimethoprim.

    C. Gastrointestinal (GI) upset from clarithromycin.

    D. Clostridium difficile superinfection from moxifloxacin.

> Correct answer = B. Stevens-Johnson syndrome is a severe idiosyncratic reaction that can be life threatening, and these patients should never be rechallenged with the offending agent. Itching/rash is a commonly reported reaction in patients receiving penicillins but is not life threatening. A patient may be rechallenged if the benefits outweigh the risk (for example, pregnant patient with syphilis) or the patient could be exposed through a desensitization procedure. GI upset is a common side effect of clarithromycin but is not due to an allergic reaction. Moxifloxacin is a broad-spectrum antibiotic that can inhibit the normal flora of the GI tract, increasing the risk for the development of superinfections like C. difficile. This is not an allergic reaction, and the patient can be rechallenged; however, the patient might be at risk for developing C. difficile infection again.

Cell Wall Inhibitors

38

Jamie Kisgen

I. OVERVIEW

Some antimicrobial drugs selectively interfere with synthesis of the bacterial cell wall—a structure that mammalian cells do not possess. The cell wall is composed of a polymer called peptidoglycan that consists of glycan units joined to each other by peptide cross-links. To be maximally effective, inhibitors of cell wall synthesis require actively proliferating microorganisms. They have little or no effect on bacteria that are not growing and dividing. The most important members of this group of drugs are the β-lactam antibiotics (named after the β-lactam ring that is essential to their activity), *vancomycin*, and *daptomycin*. Figure 38.1 shows the classification of agents affecting cell wall synthesis.

II. PENICILLINS

The penicillins are among the most widely effective and the least toxic drugs known, but increased resistance has limited their use. Members of this family differ from one another in the R substituent attached to the 6-aminopenicillanic acid residue (Figure 38.2). The nature of this side chain affects the antimicrobial spectrum, stability to stomach acid, cross-hypersensitivity, and susceptibility to bacterial degradative enzymes (β-lactamases).

A. Mechanism of action

The penicillins interfere with the last step of bacterial cell wall synthesis (transpeptidation or cross-linkage), resulting in exposure of the osmotically less stable membrane. Cell lysis can then occur, either through osmotic pressure or through the activation of autolysins. These drugs are bactericidal and work in a time-dependent fashion. Penicillins are only effective against rapidly growing organisms that synthesize a peptidoglycan cell wall. Consequently, they are inactive against organisms devoid of this structure, such as mycobacteria, protozoa, fungi, and viruses.

1. **Penicillin-binding proteins:** Penicillins also inactivate numerous proteins on the bacterial cell membrane. These penicillin-binding proteins (PBPs) are bacterial enzymes involved in the synthesis of the cell wall and in the maintenance of the morphologic features of the bacterium. Exposure to these antibiotics can therefore not only

PENICILLINS
Amoxicillin AMOXIL
Ampicillin PRINCIPEN
Dicloxacillin DYNAPEN
Nafcillin
Oxacillin
Penicillin G PFIZERPEN
Penicillin V
Piperacillin
Ticarcillin

CEPHALOSPORINS
Cefaclor CECLOR
Cefadroxil DURACEF
Cefazolin KEFZOL
Cefdinir OMNICEF
Cefepime MAXIPIME
Cefixime SUPRAX
Cefotaxime CLAFORAN
Cefotetan CEFOTAN
Cefoxitin MEFOXIN
Cefprozil CEFZIL
Ceftaroline TEFLARO
Ceftazidime FORTAZ
Ceftibuten CEDAX
Ceftizoxime CEFIZOX
Ceftriaxone ROCEPHIN
Cefuroxime CEFTIN
Cephalexin KEFLEX

CARBAPENEMS
Doripenem DORIBAX
Ertapenem INVANZ
Imipenem/cilastatin PRIMAXIN
Meropenem MERREM

MONOBACTAMS
Aztreonam AZACTAM

Figure 38.1
Summary of antimicrobial agents affecting cell wall synthesis. (Figure continues on next page.)

β-LACTAMASE INHIBITOR + ANTIBIOTIC COMBINATIONS

Clavulanic acid + amoxicillin
AUGMENTIN

Clavulanic acid + ticarcillin TIMENTIN

Sulbactam + ampicillin UNASYN

Tazobactam + piperacillin ZOSYN

OTHER ANTIBIOTICS

Colistin COLOMYCIN, COLY-MYCIN M

Daptomycin CUBICIN

Fosfomycin MONUROL

Polymyxin B AEROSPORIN

Telavancin VIBATIV

Vancomycin VANCOCIN

Figure 38.1 (Continued)
Summary of antimicrobial agents affecting cell wall synthesis.

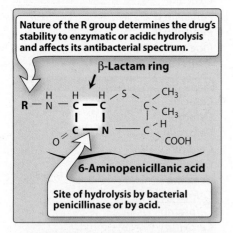

Figure 38.2
Structure of β-lactam antibiotics.

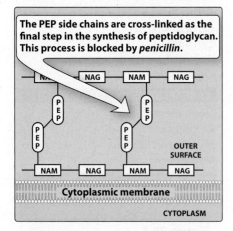

Figure 38.3
Bacterial cell wall of gram-positive bacteria. (NAM = *N*-acetylmuramic acid; NAG = *N*-acetylglucosamine; PEP = cross-linking peptide.)

prevent cell wall synthesis but also lead to morphologic changes or lysis of susceptible bacteria. The number of PBPs varies with the type of organism. Alterations in some of these PBPs provide the organism with resistance to the penicillins. [Note: *Methicillin*-resistant <u>Staphylococcus</u> <u>aureus</u> (MRSA) arose because of such an alteration.]

2. **Inhibition of transpeptidase:** Some PBPs catalyze formation of the cross-linkages between peptidoglycan chains (Figure 38.3). Penicillins inhibit this transpeptidase-catalyzed reaction, thus hindering the formation of cross-links essential for cell wall integrity.

3. **Production of autolysins:** Many bacteria, particularly the gram-positive cocci, produce degradative enzymes (autolysins) that participate in the normal remodeling of the bacterial cell wall. In the presence of a penicillin, the degradative action of the autolysins proceeds in the absence of cell wall synthesis. Thus, the antibacterial effect of a penicillin is the result of both inhibition of cell wall synthesis and destruction of the existing cell wall by autolysins.

B. Antibacterial spectrum

The antibacterial spectrum of the various penicillins is determined, in part, by their ability to cross the bacterial peptidoglycan cell wall to reach the PBPs in the periplasmic space. Factors that determine the susceptibility of PBPs to these antibiotics include the size, charge, and hydrophobicity of the particular β-lactam antibiotic. In general, gram-positive microorganisms have cell walls that are easily traversed by penicillins, and, therefore, in the absence of resistance, they are susceptible to these drugs. Gram-negative microorganisms have an outer lipopolysaccharide membrane surrounding the cell wall that presents a barrier to the water-soluble penicillins. However, gram-negative bacteria have proteins inserted in the lipopolysaccharide layer that act as water-filled channels (called porins) to permit transmembrane entry.

1. **Natural penicillins:** Natural penicillins (*penicillin G* and *penicillin V*) are obtained from fermentations of the fungus <u>Penicillium</u> <u>chrysogenum</u>. Semisynthetic penicillins, such as *amoxicillin* and *ampicillin* (also known as aminopenicillins), are created by chemically attaching different R groups to the 6-aminopenicillanic acid nucleus. *Penicillin* [pen-i-SILL-in] *G* (*benzyl-penicillin*) is the cornerstone of therapy for infections caused by a number of gram-positive and gram-negative cocci, gram-positive bacilli, and spirochetes (Figure 38.4). Penicillins are susceptible to inactivation by β-lactamases (penicillinases) that are produced by the resistant bacteria. Despite widespread use and increase in resistance to many types of bacteria, *penicillin* remains the drug of choice for the treatment of gas gangrene (<u>Clostridium</u> <u>perfringens</u>) and syphilis (<u>Treponema</u> <u>pallidum</u>). *Penicillin V* has a similar spectrum to that of *penicillin G*, but it is not used for treatment of bacteremia because of its poor oral absorption. *Penicillin V* is more acid stable than *penicillin G* and is often employed orally in the treatment of infections.

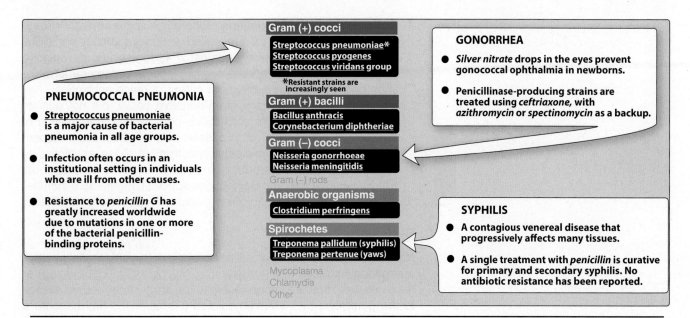

Figure 38.4
Typical therapeutic applications of *penicillin G.*

2. **Antistaphylococcal penicillins:** *Methicillin* [meth-i-SILL-in], *nafcillin* [naf-SILL-in], *oxacillin* [ox-a-SILL-in], and *dicloxacillin* [dye-klox-a-SILL-in] are β-lactamase (penicillinase)-resistant penicillins. Their use is restricted to the treatment of infections caused by penicillinase-producing staphylococci, including *methicillin*-sensitive Staphylococcus aureus (MSSA). [Note: Because of its toxicity (interstitial nephritis), *methicillin* is not used clinically in the United States except in laboratory tests to identify resistant strains of S. aureus. MRSA is currently a source of serious community and nosocomial (hospital-acquired) infections and is resistant to most commercially available β-lactam antibiotics.] The penicillinase-resistant penicillins have minimal to no activity against gram-negative infections.

3. **Extended-spectrum penicillins:** *Ampicillin* [am-pi-SILL-in] and *amoxicillin* [a-mox-i-SILL-in] have an antibacterial spectrum similar to that of *penicillin G* but are more effective against gram-negative bacilli (Figure 38.5A). *Ampicillin* (with or without the addition of *gentamicin*) is the drug of choice for the gram-positive bacillus Listeria monocytogenes and susceptible enterococcal species. These extended-spectrum agents are also widely used in the treatment of respiratory infections, and *amoxicillin* is employed prophylactically by dentists in high-risk patients for the prevention of bacterial endocarditis. Resistance to these antibiotics is now a major clinical problem because of inactivation by plasmid-mediated penicillinases. [Note: Escherichia coli and Haemophilus influenzae are frequently resistant.] Formulation with a β-lactamase inhibitor, such as *clavulanic acid* or *sulbactam*, protects *amoxicillin* or *ampicillin,* respectively, from enzymatic hydrolysis and extends their antimicrobial spectra. For example, without the β-lactamase inhibitor, MSSA is resistant to *ampicillin* and *amoxicillin.*

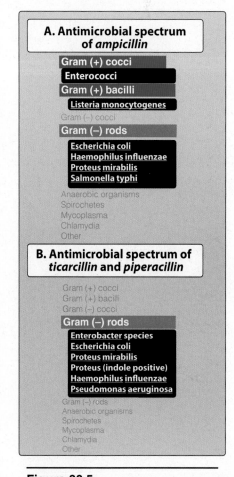

Figure 38.5
Antimicrobial activity of *ampicillin* **(A)** and the antipseudomonal penicillins **(B)**.

4. Antipseudomonal penicillins: *Piperacillin* [pip-er-a-SILL-in] and *ticarcillin* [tye-kar-SILL-in] are called antipseudomonal penicillins because of their activity against <u>Pseudomonas</u> <u>aeruginosa</u> (Figure 38.5B). These agents are available in parenteral formulations only. *Piperacillin* is the most potent of these antibiotics. They are effective against many gram-negative bacilli, but not against <u>Klebsiella</u> because of its constitutive penicillinase. Formulation of *ticarcillin* or *piperacillin* with *clavulanic acid* or *tazobactam*, respectively, extends the antimicrobial spectrum of these antibiotics to include penicillinase-producing organisms (for example, most Enterobacteriaceae and <u>Bacteroides</u> species). Figure 38.6 summarizes the stability of the penicillins to acid or the action of penicillinase.

C. Resistance

Natural resistance to the penicillins occurs in organisms that either lack a peptidoglycan cell wall (for example, <u>Mycoplasma</u> <u>pneumoniae</u>) or have cell walls that are impermeable to the drugs. Acquired resistance to the penicillins by plasmid-mediated β-lactamases has become a significant clinical problem. Multiplication of resistant strains leads to increased dissemination of the resistance genes. By obtaining resistance plasmids, bacteria may acquire one or more of the following properties, thus allowing survival in the presence of β-lactam antibiotics.

1. β-Lactamase activity: This family of enzymes hydrolyzes the cyclic amide bond of the β-lactam ring, which results in loss of bactericidal activity (Figure 38.2). They are the major cause of resistance to the penicillins and are an increasing problem. β-Lactamases either are constitutive, mostly produced by the bacterial chromosome or, more commonly, are acquired by the transfer of plasmids. Some of the β-lactam antibiotics are poor substrates for β-lactamases and resist hydrolysis, thus retaining their activity against β-lactamase–producing organisms. [Note: Certain organisms may have chromosome-associated β-lactamases that are inducible by β-lactam antibiotics (for example, second and third generation cephalosporins).] Gram-positive organisms secrete β-lactamases extracellularly, whereas gram-negative bacteria inactivate β-lactam drugs in the periplasmic space.

2. Decreased permeability to the drug: Decreased penetration of the antibiotic through the outer cell membrane of the bacteria prevents the drug from reaching the target PBPs. The presence of an efflux pump can also reduce the amount of intracellular drug (for example, <u>Klebsiella</u> <u>pneumoniae</u>).

3. Altered PBPs: Modified PBPs have a lower affinity for β-lactam antibiotics, requiring clinically unattainable concentrations of the drug to effect inhibition of bacterial growth. This explains MRSA resistance to most commercially available β-lactams.

D. Pharmacokinetics

1. Administration: The route of administration of a β-lactam antibiotic is determined by the stability of the drug to gastric acid and by the severity of the infection.

a. **Routes of administration:** The combination of *ampicillin* with *sulbactam, ticarcillin* with *clavulanic acid,* and *piperacillin* with *tazobactam*, and the antistaphylococcal penicillins *nafcillin* and *oxacillin* must be administered intravenously (IV) or intramuscularly (IM). *Penicillin V, amoxicillin*, and *dicloxacillin* are available only as oral preparations. Others are effective by the oral, IV, or IM routes (Figure 38.6). [Note: The combination of *amoxicillin* with *clavulanic acid* is only available in an oral formulation in the United States].

b. **Depot forms:** *Procaine penicillin G* and *benzathine penicillin G* are administered IM and serve as depot forms. They are slowly absorbed into the circulation and persist at low levels over a long time period.

2. **Absorption:** Most of the penicillins are incompletely absorbed after oral administration, and they reach the intestine in sufficient amounts to affect the composition of the intestinal flora. Food decreases the absorption of all the penicillinase-resistant penicillins because as gastric emptying time increases, the drugs are destroyed by stomach acid. Therefore, they should be taken on an empty stomach.

3. **Distribution:** The β-lactam antibiotics distribute well throughout the body. All the penicillins cross the placental barrier, but none have been shown to have teratogenic effects. However, penetration into bone or cerebrospinal fluid (CSF) is insufficient for therapy unless these sites are inflamed (Figures 38.7 and 38.8). [Note: Inflamed meninges are more permeable to the penicillins, resulting in an increased ratio of the drug in the CSF compared to the serum.] Penicillin levels in the prostate are insufficient to be effective against infections.

4. **Metabolism:** Host metabolism of the β-lactam antibiotics is usually insignificant, but some metabolism of *penicillin G* may occur in patients with impaired renal function.

5. **Excretion:** The primary route of excretion is through the organic acid (tubular) secretory system of the kidney as well as by glomerular filtration. Patients with impaired renal function must have dosage regimens adjusted. *Nafcillin* and *oxacillin* are exceptions to the rule. They are primarily metabolized in the liver and do not require dose adjustment for renal insufficiency. *Probenecid* inhibits the secretion of penicillins by competing for active tubular secretion via the organic acid transporter and, thus, can increase blood levels. The penicillins are also excreted in breast milk.

E. Adverse reactions

Penicillins are among the safest drugs, and blood levels are not monitored. However, adverse reactions may occur (Figure 38.9).

1. **Hypersensitivity:** Approximately 5% percent of patients have some kind of reaction, ranging from rashes to angioedema (marked swelling of the lips, tongue, and periorbital area) and anaphylaxis. Cross-allergic reactions occur among the β-lactam antibiotics.

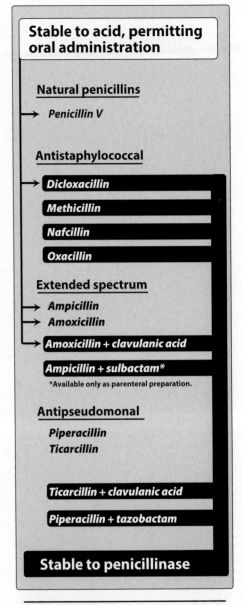

Stable to acid, permitting oral administration

Natural penicillins
→ Penicillin V

Antistaphylococcal
→ Dicloxacillin
Methicillin
Nafcillin
Oxacillin

Extended spectrum
→ Ampicillin
→ Amoxicillin
Amoxicillin + clavulanic acid
Ampicillin + sulbactam*
*Available only as parenteral preparation.

Antipseudomonal
Piperacillin
Ticarcillin

Ticarcillin + clavulanic acid
Piperacillin + tazobactam

Stable to penicillinase

Figure 38.6
Stability of the penicillins to acid or the action of penicillinase.

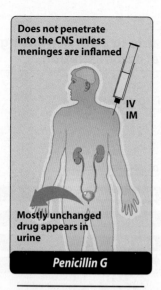

Figure 38.7
Administration and fate of *penicillin*. (CNS = central nervous system.)

To determine whether treatment with a β-lactam is safe when an allergy is noted, patient history regarding severity of previous reaction is essential.

2. **Diarrhea:** Diarrhea is a common problem that is caused by a disruption of the normal balance of intestinal microorganisms. It occurs to a greater extent with those agents that are incompletely absorbed and have an extended antibacterial spectrum. Pseudomembranous colitis from Clostridium difficile and other organisms may occur with penicillin use.

3. **Nephritis:** Penicillins, particularly *methicillin*, have the potential to cause acute interstitial nephritis. [Note: *Methicillin* is therefore no longer used clinically.]

4. **Neurotoxicity:** The penicillins are irritating to neuronal tissue, and they can provoke seizures if injected intrathecally or if very high blood levels are reached. Epileptic patients are particularly at risk due to the ability of penicillins to cause GABAergic inhibition.

5. **Hematologic toxicities:** Decreased coagulation may be observed with high doses of *piperacillin*, *ticarcillin*, and *nafcillin* (and, to some extent, with *penicillin G*). Cytopenias have been associated with therapy of greater than 2 weeks, and therefore, blood counts should be monitored weekly for such patients.

III. CEPHALOSPORINS

The cephalosporins are β-lactam antibiotics that are closely related both structurally and functionally to the penicillins. Most cephalosporins are produced semisynthetically by the chemical attachment of side chains to 7-aminocephalosporanic acid. Cephalosporins have the same mode of action as penicillins, and they are affected by the same resistance mechanisms. However, they tend to be more resistant than the penicillins to certain β-lactamases.

A. Antibacterial spectrum

Cephalosporins have been classified as first, second, third, fourth, and advanced generation, based largely on their bacterial susceptibility patterns and resistance to β-lactamases (Figure 38.10). [Note: Commercially available cephalosporins are ineffective against MRSA, L. monocytogenes, C. difficile, and the enterococci.]

1. **First generation:** The first-generation cephalosporins act as *penicillin G* substitutes. They are resistant to the staphylococcal penicillinase (that is, they cover MSSA) and also have activity against Proteus mirabilis, E. coli, and K. pneumoniae.

2. **Second generation:** The second-generation cephalosporins display greater activity against three additional gram-negative organisms: H. influenzae, Enterobacter aerogenes, and some Neisseria species, whereas activity against gram-positive organisms is weaker. Antimicrobial coverage of the cephamycins (*cefotetan*

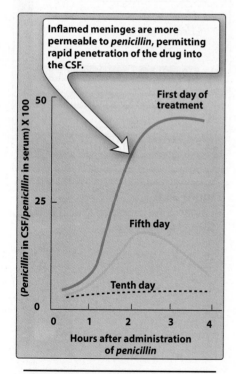

Figure 38.8
Enhanced penetration of *penicillin* into the cerebral spinal fluid (CSF) during inflammation.

[sef-oh-TEE-tan] and *cefoxitin* [sef-OX-i-tin]) also includes anaerobes (for example, <u>Bacteroides fragilis</u>). They are the only cephalosporins commercially available with appreciable activity against gram-negative anaerobic bacteria. However, neither drug is first line because of the increasing prevalence of resistance among <u>B</u>. <u>fragilis</u> to both agents.

3. **Third generation:** These cephalosporins have assumed an important role in the treatment of infectious diseases. Although they are less potent than first-generation cephalosporins against MSSA, the third-generation cephalosporins have enhanced activity against gram-negative bacilli, including those mentioned above, as well as most other enteric organisms plus <u>Serratia</u> <u>marcescens</u>. *Ceftriaxone* [sef-trye-AKS-own] and *cefotaxime* [sef-oh-TAKS-eem] have become agents of choice in the treatment of meningitis. *Ceftazidime* [sef-TA-zi-deem] has activity against <u>P</u>. <u>aeruginosa</u>; however, resistance is increasing and use should be evaluated on a case-by-case basis. Third-generation cephalosporins must be used with caution, as they are associated with significant "collateral damage," essentially meaning the induction and spread of antimicrobial resistance. [Note: Fluoroquinolone use is also associated with collateral damage.]

4. **Fourth generation:** *Cefepime* [SEF-eh-peem] is classified as a fourth-generation cephalosporin and must be administered parenterally. *Cefepime* has a wide antibacterial spectrum, with activity against streptococci and staphylococci (but only those that are *methicillin* susceptible). *Cefepime* is also effective against aerobic gram-negative organisms, such as <u>Enterobacter</u> species, <u>E</u>. <u>coli</u>, <u>K</u>. <u>pneumoniae</u>, <u>P</u>. <u>mirabilis</u>, and <u>P</u>. <u>aeruginosa</u>. When selecting an antibiotic that is active against <u>P</u>. <u>aeruginosa</u>, clinicians should refer to their local antibiograms (laboratory testing for the sensitivity of an isolated bacterial strain to different antibiotics) for direction.

5. **Advanced generation:** *Ceftaroline* [sef-TAR-oh-leen] is a broad-spectrum, advanced-generation cephalosporin that is administered IV as a prodrug, *ceftaroline fosamil*. It is the only commercially available β-lactam in the United States with activity against MRSA and is indicated for the treatment of complicated skin and skin structure infections and community-acquired pneumonia. The unique structure allows *ceftaroline* to bind to PBP2a found with MRSA and PBP2x found with <u>Streptococcus</u> <u>pneumoniae</u>. In addition to its broad gram-positive activity, it also has similar gram-negative activity to the third-generation cephalosporin *ceftriaxone*. Important gaps in coverage include <u>P</u>. <u>aeruginosa</u>, extended-spectrum β-lactamase (ESBL)-producing Enterobacteriaceae, and <u>Acinetobacter</u> <u>baumannii</u>. The twice-daily dosing regimen also limits its use outside of an institutional setting.

B. Resistance

Mechanisms of bacterial resistance to the cephalosporins are essentially the same as those described for the penicillins. [Note: Although they are not susceptible to hydrolysis by the staphylococcal

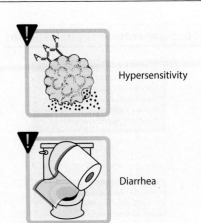

Hypersensitivity

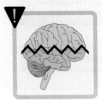

Diarrhea

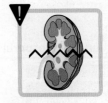

Nephritis

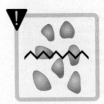

Neurotoxicity

Hematologic toxicities

Figure 38.9
Summary of the adverse effects of *penicillin*.

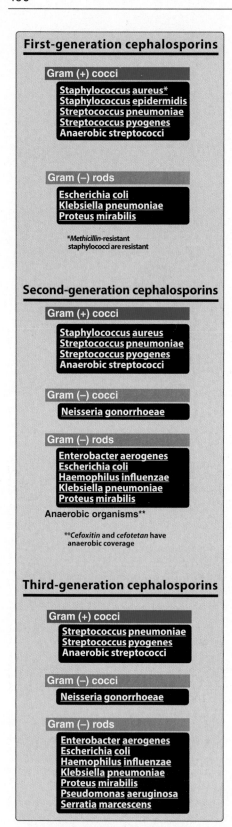

Figure 38.10
Summary of therapeutic applications of cephalosporins.

penicillinase, cephalosporins may be susceptible to ESBLs. Organisms such as E. coli and K. pneumoniae are particularly associated with ESBLs.]

C. Pharmacokinetics

1. **Administration:** Many of the cephalosporins must be administered IV or IM (Figure 38.11) because of their poor oral absorption. Exceptions are noted in Figure 38.12.

2. **Distribution:** All cephalosporins distribute very well into body fluids. However, adequate therapeutic levels in the CSF, regardless of inflammation, are achieved with only a few cephalosporins. For example, *ceftriaxone* and *cefotaxime* are effective in the treatment of neonatal and childhood meningitis caused by H. influenzae. *Cefazolin* [se-FA-zo-lin] is commonly used as a single prophylaxis dose prior to surgery because of its 1.8-hour half-life and its activity against penicillinase-producing S. aureus. *Cefazolin* is effective for most surgical procedures, including orthopedic surgery because of its ability to penetrate bone. All cephalosporins cross the placenta.

3. **Elimination:** Cephalosporins are eliminated through tubular secretion and/or glomerular filtration (Figure 38.11). Therefore, doses must be adjusted in cases of renal dysfunction to guard against accumulation and toxicity. One exception is *ceftriaxone*, which is excreted through the bile into the feces and, therefore, is frequently employed in patients with renal insufficiency.

D. Adverse effects

Like the penicillins, the cephalosporins are generally well tolerated. However, allergic reactions are a concern. Patients who have had an anaphylactic response, Stevens-Johnson syndrome, or toxic epidermal necrolysis to penicillins should not receive cephalosporins. Cephalosporins should be avoided or used with caution in individuals with penicillin allergy. Current data suggest that the cross-reactivity between penicillin and cephalosporins is around 3% to 5% and is determined by the similarity in the side chain, not the β-lactam structure. The highest rate of allergic cross-sensitivity is between penicillin and first-generation cephalosporins.

IV. OTHER β-LACTAM ANTIBIOTICS

A. Carbapenems

Carbapenems are synthetic β-lactam antibiotics that differ in structure from the penicillins in that the sulfur atom of the thiazolidine ring (Figure 38.2) has been externalized and replaced by a carbon atom (Figure 38.13). *Imipenem* [i-mi-PEN-em], *meropenem* [mer-oh-PEN-em], *doripenem* [dore-i-PEN-em], and *ertapenem* [er-ta-PEN-em] are the drugs of this group currently available. *Imipenem* is compounded with *cilastatin* to protect it from metabolism by renal dehydropeptidase.

1. **Antibacterial spectrum:** *Imipenem* resists hydrolysis by most β-lactamases, but not the metallo-β-lactamases. This drug plays a role in empiric therapy because it is active against β-lactamase–producing gram-positive and gram-negative organisms, anaerobes, and P. aeruginosa (although other pseudomonal strains are resistant and resistant strains of P. aeruginosa have been reported to arise during therapy). *Meropenem* and *doripenem* have antibacterial activity similar to that of *imipenem* (Figure 38.14). Unlike other carbapenems, *ertapenem* lacks coverage against P. aeruginosa, Enterococcus species, and Acinetobacter species.

2. **Pharmacokinetics:** *Imipenem/cilastatin* and *meropenem* are administered IV and penetrate well into body tissues and fluids, including the CSF when the meninges are inflamed. *Meropenem* is known to reach therapeutic levels in bacterial meningitis even without inflammation. They are excreted by glomerular filtration. *Imipenem* undergoes cleavage by a dehydropeptidase found in the brush border of the proximal renal tubule. This enzyme forms an inactive metabolite that is potentially nephrotoxic. Compounding the *imipenem* with *cilastatin* protects the parent drug and, thus, prevents the formation of the toxic metabolite. The other carbapenems do not require coadministration of *cilastatin*. *Ertapenem* can be administered via IV or IM injection once

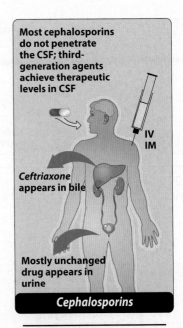

Figure 38.11
Administration and fate of the cephalosporins.
(CSF = cerebrospinal fluid.)

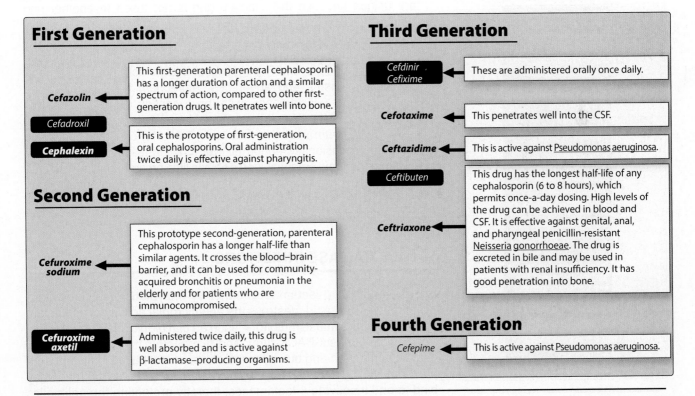

First Generation

Cefazolin ← This first-generation parenteral cephalosporin has a longer duration of action and a similar spectrum of action, compared to other first-generation drugs. It penetrates well into bone.

Cefadroxil

Cephalexin ← This is the prototype of first-generation, oral cephalosporins. Oral administration twice daily is effective against pharyngitis.

Second Generation

Cefuroxime sodium ← This prototype second-generation, parenteral cephalosporin has a longer half-life than similar agents. It crosses the blood–brain barrier, and it can be used for community-acquired bronchitis or pneumonia in the elderly and for patients who are immunocompromised.

Cefuroxime axetil ← Administered twice daily, this drug is well absorbed and is active against β-lactamase–producing organisms.

Third Generation

Cefdinir Cefixime ← These are administered orally once daily.

Cefotaxime ← This penetrates well into the CSF.

Ceftazidime ← This is active against Pseudomonas aeruginosa.

Ceftibuten

Ceftriaxone ← This drug has the longest half-life of any cephalosporin (6 to 8 hours), which permits once-a-day dosing. High levels of the drug can be achieved in blood and CSF. It is effective against genital, anal, and pharyngeal penicillin-resistant Neisseria gonorrhoeae. The drug is excreted in bile and may be used in patients with renal insufficiency. It has good penetration into bone.

Fourth Generation

Cefepime ← This is active against Pseudomonas aeruginosa.

Figure 38.12
Therapeutic advantages of some clinically useful cephalosporins. [Note: Drugs that can be administered orally are shown in reverse type. More useful drugs shown in **bold**.]. **(CSF = cerebrospinal fluid.)**

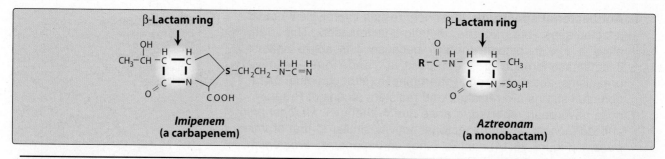

Figure 38.13
Structural features of *imipenem* and *aztreonam*.

daily. [Note: Doses of these agents must be adjusted in patients with renal insufficiency.]

3. **Adverse effects:** *Imipenem/cilastatin* can cause nausea, vomiting, and diarrhea. Eosinophilia and neutropenia are less common than with other β-lactams. High levels of *imipenem* may provoke seizures; however, the other carbapenems are less likely to do so.

B. Monobactams

The monobactams, which also disrupt bacterial cell wall synthesis, are unique because the β-lactam ring is not fused to another ring (Figure 38.13). *Aztreonam* [az-TREE-oh-nam], which is the only commercially available monobactam, has antimicrobial activity directed primarily against gram-negative pathogens, including the Enterobacteriaceae and P. aeruginosa. It lacks activity against gram-positive organisms and anaerobes. *Aztreonam* is resistant to the action of most β-lactamases, with the exception of the ESBLs. It is administered either IV or IM and can accumulate in patients with renal failure. *Aztreonam* is relatively nontoxic, but it may cause phlebitis, skin rash and, occasionally, abnormal liver function tests. This drug has a low immunogenic potential, and it shows little cross-reactivity with antibodies induced by other β-lactams. Thus, this drug may offer a safe alternative for treating patients who are allergic to other penicillins, cephalosporins, or carbapenems.

V. β-LACTAMASE INHIBITORS

Hydrolysis of the β-lactam ring, either by enzymatic cleavage with a β-lactamase or by acid, destroys the antimicrobial activity of a β-lactam antibiotic. β-Lactamase inhibitors, such as *clavulanic* [cla-vue-LAN-ick] *acid, sulbactam* [sul-BACK-tam], and *tazobactam* [ta-zoh-BACK-tam], contain a β-lactam ring but, by themselves, do not have significant antibacterial activity or cause any significant adverse effects. Instead, they bind to and inactivate β-lactamases, thereby protecting the antibiotics that are normally substrates for these enzymes. The β-lactamase inhibitors are therefore formulated in combination with β-lactamase–sensitive

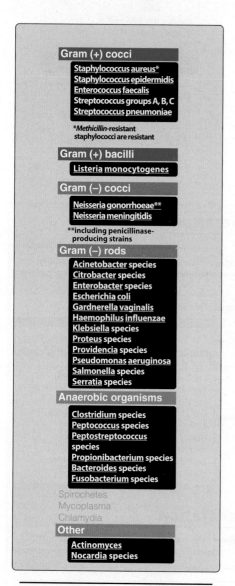

Figure 38.14
Antimicrobial spectrum of *imipenem*.

antibiotics. For example, Figure 38.15 shows the effect of *clavulanic acid* and *amoxicillin* on the growth of β-lactamase–producing E. coli. [Note: *Clavulanic acid* alone is nearly devoid of any antibacterial activity.]

VI. VANCOMYCIN

Vancomycin [van-koe-MYE-sin] is a tricyclic glycopeptide that has become increasingly important in the treatment of life-threatening MRSA and *methicillin*-resistant Staphylococcus epidermidis (MRSE) infections, as well as enterococcal infections (Figure 38.16). With the emergence of resistant strains, it is important to curtail the increase in *vancomycin*-resistant bacteria (for example, Enterococcus faecium and Enterococcus faecalis) by restricting the use of *vancomycin* to the treatment of serious infections caused by β-lactam resistant, gram-positive microorganisms or gram-positive infections in patients who have a serious allergy to the β-lactams. Intravenous *vancomycin* is used in individuals with prosthetic heart valves and in patients undergoing implantation with prosthetic devices, especially in those hospitals where there are high rates of MRSA or MRSE. Serum drug concentrations (troughs) are commonly measured to monitor and adjust dosages for safety and efficacy. *Vancomycin* is not absorbed after oral administration, so the use of the oral formulation is limited to the treatment of severe antibiotic-associated C. difficile colitis.

VII. DAPTOMYCIN

Daptomycin [DAP-toe-mye-sin] is a bactericidal concentration-dependent cyclic lipopeptide antibiotic that is an alternative to other agents, such as *linezolid* and *quinupristin/dalfopristin,* for treating infections caused by resistant gram-positive organisms, including MRSA and *vancomycin*-resistant enterococci (VRE) (Figure 38.17). *Daptomycin* is indicated for the treatment of complicated skin and skin structure infections and bacteremia caused by S. aureus, including those with right-sided infective endocarditis. Efficacy of treatment with *daptomycin* in left-sided endocarditis has not been demonstrated. Additionally, *daptomycin* is inactivated by pulmonary surfactants; thus, it should *never* be used in the treatment of pneumonia.

VIII. TELAVANCIN

Telavancin [tel-a-VAN-sin] is a bactericidal concentration-dependent semisynthetic lipoglycopeptide antibiotic that is a synthetic derivative of *vancomycin.* Like *vancomycin, telavancin* inhibits bacterial cell wall synthesis. Moreover, *telavancin* exhibits an additional mechanism of action similar to that of *daptomycin,* which involves disruption of the bacterial cell membrane due to the presence of a lipophilic side chain moiety. It is an alternative to *vancomycin, daptomycin,* and *linezolid,* in treating complicated skin and skin structure infections by

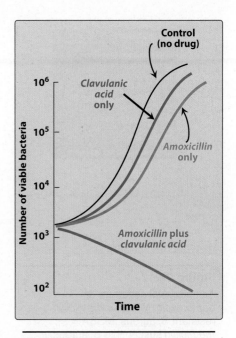

Figure 38.15
The in vitro growth of Escherichia coli in the presence of *amoxicillin,* with and without *clavulanic acid.*

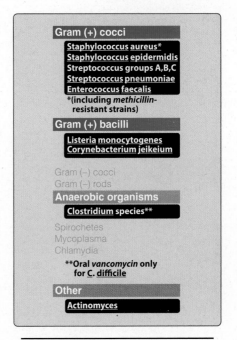

Figure 38.16
Antimicrobial spectrum of *vancomycin.*

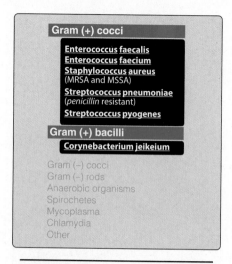

Figure 38.17
Antimicrobial spectrum of *daptomycin*. MRSA = *methicillin* resistant S. aureus; MSSA = *methicillin* susceptible S. aureus.

resistant gram-positive organisms (including MRSA). It is also an agent of last choice for hospital-acquired and ventilator-associated bacterial pneumonia when alternative treatments are not suitable. The use of *telavancin* in clinical practice is limited by significant adverse effects (for example, renal impairment), interaction with anticoagulation laboratory assays, risk of fetal harm in pregnant women, and interaction with medications that can prolong the QT_c interval (for example, fluoroquinolones, azole antifungals, macrolides). Figure 38.18 provides a comparison of important characteristics of *vancomycin*, *daptomycin*, and *telavancin*.

IX. FOSFOMYCIN

Fosfomycin [fos-foe-MYE-sin] is a bactericidal synthetic derivative of phosphonic acid. It blocks cell wall synthesis by inhibiting the enzyme UDP-*N*-acetylglucosamine enolpyruvyl transferase, which catalyzes the first step in peptidoglycan synthesis. It is indicated for urinary tract infections caused by E. coli or E. faecalis. Due to its unique structure and mechanism of action, cross resistance with other antimicrobial agents is unlikely. *Fosfomycin* is rapidly absorbed after oral administration and distributes well to the kidneys, bladder, and prostate. The drug is excreted in its active form in the urine and feces. It maintains high concentrations in the urine over several days, allowing for a one-time dose for the treatment of urinary tract infections. [Note: A parenteral formulation is available in select countries and has been used for the treatment of systemic infections.] The most commonly reported adverse effects include diarrhea, vaginitis, nausea, and headache.

X. POLYMYXINS

The polymyxins are cation polypeptides that bind to phospholipids on the bacterial cell membrane of gram-negative bacteria. They have a detergent-like effect that disrupts cell membrane integrity, leading to leakage of cellular components and ultimately cell death. Polymyxins are concentration-dependent bactericidal agents with activity against most clinically important gram-negative bacteria, including P. aeruginosa, E. coli, K. pneumoniae, Acinetobacter species, and Enterobacter species. However, alterations in the cell membrane lipid polysaccharides allow many species of Proteus and Serratia to be intrinsically resistant. Only two forms of polymyxin are in clinical use today, *polymyxin B* and *colistin (polymyxin E)*. *Polymyxin B* is available in parenteral, ophthalmic, otic, and topical preparations. *Colistin* is only available as a prodrug, *colistimethate sodium*, which is administered IV or inhaled via a nebulizer. The use of these drugs has been limited for a long time, due to the increased risk of nephrotoxicity and neurotoxicity (for example, slurred speech, muscle weakness) when used systemically. However, with the increase in gram-negative resistance, they have seen a resurgence in use and are now commonly used as salvage therapy for patients with multidrug-resistant infections. Careful dosing and monitoring of adverse effects are important to maximize the safety and efficacy of these agents.

	VANCOMYCIN	*DAPTOMYCIN*	*TELAVANCIN*
Mechanism of Action	Inhibits synthesis of bacterial cell wall phospholipids as well as peptidoglycan polymerization	Causes rapid depolarization of the cell membrane, inhibits intracellular synthesis of DNA, RNA, and protein	Inhibits bacterial cell wall synthesis; disrupts cell membrane
Pharmacodynamics	Time dependent Bactericidal	Concentration dependent Bactericidal	Concentration dependent Bactericidal
Common Antibacterial Spectrum	Activity limited to gram-positive organisms: <u>Staphylococcus aureus</u> (including MRSA), <u>Streptococcus pyogenes</u>, <u>S. agalactiae</u>, penicillin-resistant <u>S. pneumoniae</u>, <u>Corynebacterium jeikeium</u>, *vancomycin*-susceptible <u>Enterococcus faecalis</u>, and <u>E. faecium</u>		
Unique Antibacterial Spectrum	<u>Clostridium difficile</u> (oral only)	*Vancomycin*-resistant <u>E. faecalis</u> and <u>E. faecium</u> (VRE)	Some isolates of *vancomycin*-resistant enterococci (VRE)
Route	IV/PO	IV	IV
Typical Administration Time	60- to 90-minute IV infusion	2-minute IV push 30-minute IV infusion	60-minute IV infusion
Pharmacokinetics	Renal elimination Normal half-life: 6–10 hours Dose is adjusted based on renal function and serum trough levels	Renal elimination Normal half-life: 7–8 hours Dose is adjusted based on renal function	Renal elimination Normal half-life: 7–9 hours Dose is adjusted based on renal function
Unique Adverse Effects	Infusion related reactions due to histamine release: Fever, chills, phlebitis, flushing (red man syndrome); dose-related ototoxicity and nephrotoxicity	Myalgias, elevated hepatic transaminases and creatine phosphokinases (check weekly), and rhabdomyolysis (consider holding HMG-CoA reductase inhibitors [statins] while on therapy)	Taste disturbances, foamy urine, QTc prolongation, interferes with coagulation labs (PT/INR, aPTT, ACT), not recommended in pregnancy (box warning recommends pregnancy test prior to initiation)
Key Learning Points	Drug of choice for severe MRSA infections; oral form only used for <u>C. difficile</u> infection; resistance can be caused by plasmid-mediated changes in permeability to the drug or by decreased binding of *vancomycin* to receptor molecules; monitor serum trough concentrations for safety and efficacy	*Daptomycin* is inactivated by pulmonary surfactants and should never be used in the treatment of pneumonia	Use with caution in patients with baseline renal dysfunction (CrCl < 50 mL/min) due to higher rates of treatment failure and mortality in clinical studies; any necessary coagulation labs should be drawn just prior to the *telavancin* dose to avoid interaction

Figure 38.18
Side-by-side comparison of *vancomycin*, *daptomycin*, and *telavancin*.

Study Questions

Choose the ONE best answer.

38.1 A 45-year-old male presented to the hospital 3 days ago with severe cellulitis and a large abscess on his left leg. Incision and drainage were performed on the abscess, and cultures revealed methicillin-resistant <u>Staphylococcus aureus</u>. Which of the following would be the most appropriate treatment option for once-daily outpatient intravenous therapy?

A. Ertapenem.

B. Ceftaroline.

C. Daptomycin.

D. Piperacillin/tazobactam.

Correct answer = C. Daptomycin is approved for skin and skin structure infections caused by MRSA and is given once daily. A and D are incorrect because they do not cover MRSA. Ceftaroline covers MRSA, but it must be given twice daily.

38.2 Which of the following adverse effects is associated with daptomycin?

A. Ototoxicity.

B. Red man syndrome.

C. QT$_c$ prolongation.

D. Rhabdomyolysis.

> Correct answer = D. Ototoxicity and red man syndrome are associated with vancomycin. QTc prolongation is associated with telavancin. Myalgias and rhabdomyolysis have been reported with daptomycin therapy and require patient education and monitoring.

38.3 A 72-year-old male is admitted to the hospital from a nursing home with severe pneumonia. He was recently discharged from the hospital 1 week ago after open heart surgery. The patient has no known allergies. Which of the following regimens is most appropriate for empiric coverage of methicillin-resistant Staphylococcus aureus and Pseudomonas aeruginosa in this patient?

A. Vancomycin + cefepime + ciprofloxacin.

B. Vancomycin + cefazolin + ciprofloxacin.

C. Telavancin + cefepime + ciprofloxacin.

D. Daptomycin + cefepime + ciprofloxacin.

> Correct answer = A. Vancomycin provides adequate coverage against MRSA, and cefepime and ciprofloxacin provide adequate empiric coverage of Pseudomonas. B is incorrect because cefazolin does not have activity against Pseudomonas. C is incorrect because telavancin should be avoided if possible with drugs that prolong the QTc interval, in this case ciprofloxacin. Daptomycin is inactivated by pulmonary surfactant and should not be used for pneumonia.

38.4 A 23-year-old male presents with acute appendicitis that ruptures shortly after admission. He is taken to the operating room for surgery, and postsurgical cultures reveal Escherichia coli and Bacteroides fragilis, susceptibilities pending. Which of the following provides adequate empiric coverage of these two pathogens?

A. Cefepime.

B. Piperacillin/tazobactam.

C. Aztreonam.

D. Ceftaroline.

> Correct answer = B. While all of these agents cover most strains of E. coli, piperacillin/tazobactam is the only drug on this list that provides coverage against Bacteroides species.

38.5 A 68-year-old male presents from a nursing home with fever, increased urinary frequency and urgency, and mental status changes. He has a penicillin allergy of anaphylaxis. Which of the following β-lactams is the most appropriate choice for gram-negative coverage of this patient's urinary tract infection?

A. Cefepime.

B. Ertapenem.

C. Aztreonam.

D. Ceftaroline.

> Correct answer = C. Based on the severity of the allergic reaction, aztreonam is the choice of all the β-lactams. Although cross-reactivity with cephalosporins and carbapenems is low, the risk rarely outweighs the benefit in these cases.

38.6 A 25-year-old male presents to the urgent care center with a painless sore on his genitals that started 1 to 2 weeks ago. He reports unprotected sex with a new partner about a month ago. A blood test confirms the patient has Treponema pallidum. Which of the following is the drug of choice for the treatment of this patient's infection as a single dose?

A. Benzathine penicillin G.

B. Ceftriaxone.

C. Aztreonam.

D. Vancomycin.

> Correct answer = A. A single treatment with penicillin is curative for primary and secondary syphilis. No antibiotic resistance has been reported, and it remains the drug of choice unless the patient has a severe allergic reaction.

38.7 A 20-year-old female presents to the emergency room with headache, stiff neck, and fever for 2 days and is diagnosed with meningitis. Which of the following agents is the best choice for the treatment of meningitis in this patient?

A. Cefazolin.
B. Cefdinir.
C. Cefotaxime.
D. Cefuroxime axetil.

Correct answer = C. Cefotaxime is the only drug on this list with adequate CSF penetration to treat meningitis. Cefdinir and cefuroxime axetil are only available orally, and cefazolin CSF penetration and spectrum of coverage against S. pneumoniae are not likely adequate to treat meningitis.

38.8 Which of the following cephalosporins has activity against gram-negative anaerobic pathogens like Bacteroides fragilis?

A. Cefoxitin.
B. Cefepime.
C. Ceftriaxone.
D. Cefazolin.

Correct answer = A. The cephamycins (cefoxitin and cefotetan) are the only cephalosporins with in vitro activity against anaerobic gram-negative pathogens. Cefepime, ceftriaxone, and cefazolin have no appreciable activity against Bacteroides fragilis.

38.9 In which of the following cases would it be appropriate to use telavancin?

A. A 29-year-old pregnant female with ventilator-associated pneumonia.
B. A 76-year-old male with hospital-acquired pneumonia also receiving amiodarone for atrial fibrillation.
C. A 36-year-old male with cellulitis and abscess growing MRSA.
D. A 72-year-old female with a diabetic foot infection growing MRSA who has moderate renal dysfunction.

Correct answer = C. A is not a good option due to the potential of telavancin harming the fetus. Option B is not a good choice because the patient is on amiodarone, and telavancin can cause QT_c prolongation. Option D is not an appropriate choice because the patient has baseline renal dysfunction and telavancin should be avoided unless benefit outweighs the risk. Option C is the best choice in this case since it is approved for skin and skin structure infections, and the patient has no apparent contraindication.

38.10 An 18-year-old female presents to the urgent care clinic with urinary frequency, urgency, and fever for the past 3 days. Based on symptoms and a urinalysis, she is diagnosed with a urinary tract infection. Cultures reveal Enterococcus faecalis that is pan sensitive. Which of the following is an appropriate oral option to treat the urinary tract infection in this patient?

A. Cephalexin.
B. Vancomycin.
C. Cefdinir.
D. Amoxicillin.

Correct answer = D. Option A and C are incorrect because enterococci are inherently resistant to all cephalosporins. Option B is incorrect because oral vancomycin is not absorbed and would not reach the urinary tract in sufficient quantities to treat a urinary tract infection. Option D is the best choice, as amoxicillin is well absorbed orally and concentrates in the urine.

Protein Synthesis Inhibitors

39

Nathan R. Unger and Timothy P. Gauthier

I. OVERVIEW

A number of antibiotics exert their antimicrobial effects by targeting bacterial ribosomes and inhibiting bacterial protein synthesis. Bacterial ribosomes differ structurally from mammalian cytoplasmic ribosomes and are composed of 30S and 50S subunits (mammalian ribosomes have 40S and 60S subunits). In general, selectivity for bacterial ribosomes minimizes potential adverse consequences encountered with the disruption of protein synthesis in mammalian host cells. However, high concentrations of drugs such as *chloramphenicol* or the tetracyclines may cause toxic effects as a result of interaction with mitochondrial mammalian ribosomes, since the structure of mitochondrial ribosomes more closely resembles bacterial ribosomes. Figure 39.1 summarizes the protein synthesis inhibitors discussed in this chapter.

II. TETRACYCLINES

Tetracyclines consist of four fused rings with a system of conjugated double bonds. Substitutions on these rings alter the individual pharmacokinetics and spectrum of antimicrobial activity.

A. Mechanism of action

Tetracyclines enter susceptible organisms via passive diffusion and also by an energy-dependent transport protein mechanism unique to the bacterial inner cytoplasmic membrane. Tetracyclines concentrate intracellularly in susceptible organisms. The drugs bind reversibly to the 30S subunit of the bacterial ribosome. This action prevents binding of tRNA to the mRNA–ribosome complex, thereby inhibiting bacterial protein synthesis (Figure 39.2).

B. Antibacterial spectrum

The tetracyclines are bacteriostatic antibiotics effective against a wide variety of organisms, including gram-positive and gram-negative bacteria, protozoa, spirochetes, mycobacteria, and atypical species (Figure 39.3). They are commonly used in the treatment of acne and Chlamydia infections (*doxycycline*).

TETRACYCLINES
Demeclocycline DECLOMYCIN
Doxycycline VIBRAMYCIN
Minocycline MINOCIN
Tetracycline

GLYCYLCYCLINES
Tigecycline TYGACIL

AMINOGLYCOSIDES
Amikacin
Gentamicin GARAMYCIN
Neomycin NEO-FRADIN
Streptomycin
Tobramycin TOBREX

MACROLIDES/KETOLIDES
Azithromycin ZITHROMAX
Clarithromycin BIAXIN
Erythromycin VARIOUS
Telithromycin KETEK

MACROCYCLIC
Fidaxomicin DIFICID

LINCOSAMIDES
Clindamycin CLEOCIN

OXAZOLIDINONES
Linezolid ZYVOX

OTHERS
Chloramphenicol CHLOROMYCETIN
Quinupristin/Dalfopristin SYNERCID

Figure 39.1
Summary of protein synthesis inhibitors.

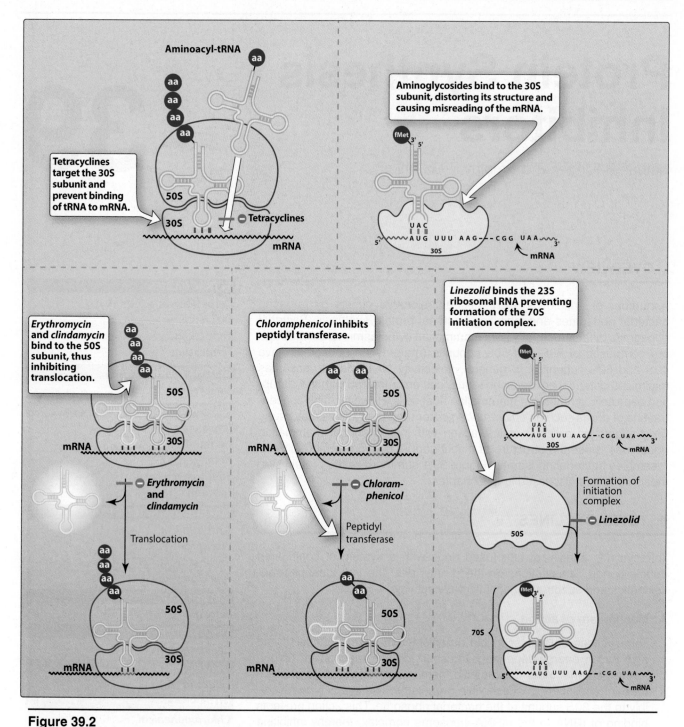

Figure 39.2
Mechanisms of action of the various protein synthesis inhibitors. aa = amino acid.

C. Resistance

The most commonly encountered naturally occurring resistance to tetracyclines is an efflux pump that expels drug out of the cell, thus preventing intracellular accumulation. Other mechanisms of bacterial resistance to tetracyclines include enzymatic inactivation of the drug and production of bacterial proteins that prevent tetracyclines from

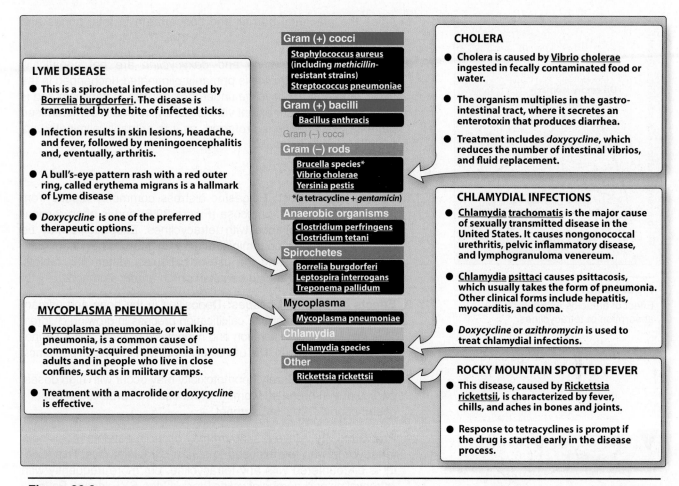

LYME DISEASE

- This is a spirochetal infection caused by <u>Borrelia burgdorferi</u>. The disease is transmitted by the bite of infected ticks.

- Infection results in skin lesions, headache, and fever, followed by meningoencephalitis and, eventually, arthritis.

- A bull's-eye pattern rash with a red outer ring, called erythema migrans is a hallmark of Lyme disease

- *Doxycycline* is one of the preferred therapeutic options.

MYCOPLASMA PNEUMONIAE

- <u>Mycoplasma pneumoniae</u>, or walking pneumonia, is a common cause of community-acquired pneumonia in young adults and in people who live in close confines, such as in military camps.

- Treatment with a macrolide or *doxycycline* is effective.

Gram (+) cocci
<u>Staphylococcus aureus</u> (including *methicillin-resistant strains*)
<u>Streptococcus pneumoniae</u>

Gram (+) bacilli
<u>Bacillus anthracis</u>

Gram (–) cocci

Gram (–) rods
<u>Brucella species</u>*
<u>Vibrio cholerae</u>
<u>Yersinia pestis</u>
*(a tetracycline + *gentamicin*)

Anaerobic organisms
<u>Clostridium perfringens</u>
<u>Clostridium tetani</u>

Spirochetes
<u>Borrelia burgdorferi</u>
<u>Leptospira interrogans</u>
<u>Treponema pallidum</u>

Mycoplasma
<u>Mycoplasma pneumoniae</u>

Chlamydia
<u>Chlamydia species</u>

Other
<u>Rickettsia rickettsii</u>

CHOLERA

- Cholera is caused by <u>Vibrio cholerae</u> ingested in fecally contaminated food or water.

- The organism multiplies in the gastrointestinal tract, where it secretes an enterotoxin that produces diarrhea.

- Treatment includes *doxycycline*, which reduces the number of intestinal vibrios, and fluid replacement.

CHLAMYDIAL INFECTIONS

- <u>Chlamydia trachomatis</u> is the major cause of sexually transmitted disease in the United States. It causes nongonococcal urethritis, pelvic inflammatory disease, and lymphogranuloma venereum.

- <u>Chlamydia psittaci</u> causes psittacosis, which usually takes the form of pneumonia. Other clinical forms include hepatitis, myocarditis, and coma.

- *Doxycycline* or *azithromycin* is used to treat chlamydial infections.

ROCKY MOUNTAIN SPOTTED FEVER

- This disease, caused by <u>Rickettsia rickettsii</u>, is characterized by fever, chills, and aches in bones and joints.

- Response to tetracyclines is prompt if the drug is started early in the disease process.

Figure 39.3
Typical therapeutic applications of tetracyclines.

binding to the ribosome. Resistance to one tetracycline does not confer universal resistance to all tetracyclines.

D. Pharmacokinetics

1. **Absorption:** Tetracyclines are adequately absorbed after oral ingestion (Figure 39.4). Administration with dairy products or other substances that contain divalent and trivalent cations (for example, magnesium and aluminum antacids or iron supplements) decreases absorption, particularly for *tetracycline* [tet-rah-SYE-kleen], due to the formation of nonabsorbable chelates (Figure 39.5). Both *doxycycline* [dox-i-SYE-kleen] and *minocycline* [min-oh-SYE-kleen] are available as oral and intravenous (IV) preparations.

2. **Distribution:** The tetracyclines concentrate well in the bile, liver, kidney, gingival fluid, and skin. Moreover, they bind to tissues undergoing calcification (for example, teeth and bones) or to tumors that have a high calcium content. Penetration into most body fluids is adequate. Only *minocycline* and *doxycycline* achieve therapeutic levels in the cerebrospinal fluid (CSF). *Minocycline* also achieves high levels in saliva and tears, rendering it useful in eradicating the meningococcal carrier state. All tetracyclines

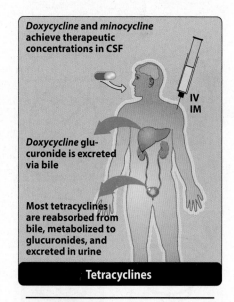

Doxycycline and *minocycline* achieve therapeutic concentrations in CSF

IV
IM

Doxycycline glucuronide is excreted via bile

Most tetracyclines are reabsorbed from bile, metabolized to glucuronides, and excreted in urine

Tetracyclines

Figure 39.4
Administration and fate of tetracyclines. CSF = cerebrospinal fluid.

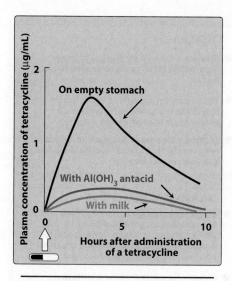

Figure 39.5
Effect of antacids and milk on the absorption of tetracyclines.

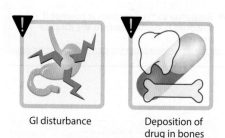

GI disturbance   Deposition of
                        drug in bones
                        and teeth

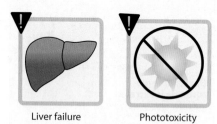

Liver failure   Phototoxicity

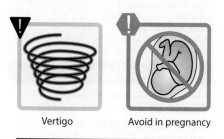

Vertigo   Avoid in pregnancy

Figure 39.6
Some adverse effects of tetracyclines.

cross the placental barrier and concentrate in fetal bones and dentition.

3. **Elimination:** *Tetracycline* and *doxycycline* are not hepatically metabolized. *Tetracycline* is primarily eliminated unchanged in the urine, whereas *minocycline* undergoes hepatic metabolism and is eliminated to a lesser extent via the kidney. In renally compromised patients, *doxycycline* is preferred, as it is primarily eliminated via the bile into the feces.

E. Adverse effects

1. **Gastric discomfort:** Epigastric distress commonly results from irritation of the gastric mucosa (Figure 39.6) and is often responsible for noncompliance with tetracyclines. Esophagitis may be minimized through coadministration with food (other than dairy products) or fluids and the use of capsules rather than tablets. [Note: *Tetracycline* should be taken on an empty stomach.]

2. **Effects on calcified tissues:** Deposition in the bone and primary dentition occurs during the calcification process in growing children. This may cause discoloration and hypoplasia of teeth and a temporary stunting of growth. The use of tetracyclines is limited in pediatrics.

3. **Hepatotoxicity:** Rarely hepatotoxicity may occur with high doses, particularly in pregnant women and those with preexisting hepatic dysfunction or renal impairment.

4. **Phototoxicity:** Severe sunburn may occur in patients receiving a tetracycline who are exposed to sun or ultraviolet rays. This toxicity is encountered with any tetracycline, but more frequently with *tetracycline* and *demeclocycline* [dem-e-kloe-SYE-kleen]. Patients should be advised to wear adequate sun protection.

5. **Vestibular dysfunction:** Dizziness, vertigo, and tinnitus may occur particularly with *minocycline,* which concentrates in the endolymph of the ear and affects function. *Doxycycline* may also cause vestibular dysfunction.

6. **Pseudotumor cerebri:** Benign, intracranial hypertension characterized by headache and blurred vision may occur rarely in adults. Although discontinuation of the drug reverses this condition, it is not clear whether permanent sequelae may occur.

7. **Contraindications:** The tetracyclines should not be used in pregnant or breast-feeding women or in children less than 8 years of age.

III. GLYCYLCYCLINES

Tigecycline [tye-ge-SYE-kleen], a derivative of *minocycline*, is the first available member of the glycylcycline antimicrobial class. It is indicated for the treatment of complicated skin and soft tissue infections, as well as complicated intra-abdominal infections.

A. Mechanism of action

Tigecycline exhibits bacteriostatic action by reversibly binding to the 30S ribosomal subunit and inhibiting protein synthesis.

B. Antibacterial spectrum

Tigecycline exhibits broad-spectrum activity that includes *methicillin*-resistant staphylococci (MRSA), multidrug-resistant streptococci, vancomycin-resistant enterococci (VRE), extended-spectrum β-lactamase–producing gram-negative bacteria, Acinetobacter baumannii, and many anaerobic organisms. However, *tigecycline* is not active against Morganella, Proteus, Providencia, or Pseudomonas species.

C. Resistance

Tigecycline was developed to overcome the recent emergence of tetracycline class–resistant organisms that utilize efflux pumps and ribosomal protection to confer resistance. However, resistance is seen and is primarily attributed to overexpression of efflux pumps.

D. Pharmacokinetics

Following IV infusion, *tigecycline* exhibits a large volume of distribution. It penetrates tissues well but has low plasma concentrations. Consequently, *tigecycline* is a poor option for bloodstream infections. The primary route of elimination is biliary/fecal. No dosage adjustments are necessary for patients with renal impairment. However, a dose reduction is recommended in severe hepatic dysfunction.

E. Adverse effects

Tigecycline is associated with significant nausea and vomiting. Acute pancreatitis, including fatality, has been reported with therapy. Elevations in liver enzymes and serum creatinine may also occur. Other adverse effects are similar to those of the tetracyclines and include photosensitivity, pseudotumor cerebri, discoloration of permanent teeth when used during tooth development, and fetal harm when administered in pregnancy. *Tigecycline* may decrease the clearance of *warfarin* and increase prothrombin time. Therefore, the international normalized ratio should be monitored closely when *tigecycline* is coadministered with *warfarin*.

IV. AMINOGLYCOSIDES

Aminoglycosides are used for the treatment of serious infections due to aerobic gram-negative bacilli. However, their clinical utility is limited by serious toxicities. The term "aminoglycoside" stems from their structure—two amino sugars joined by a glycosidic linkage to a central hexose nucleus. Aminoglycosides are derived from either Streptomyces sp. (have -*mycin* suffixes) or Micromonospora sp. (end in -*micin*).

A. Mechanism of action

Aminoglycosides diffuse through porin channels in the outer membrane of susceptible organisms. These organisms also have an oxygen-dependent system that transports the drug across the cytoplasmic membrane. Inside the cell, they bind the 30S ribosomal subunit, where they interfere with assembly of the functional ribosomal

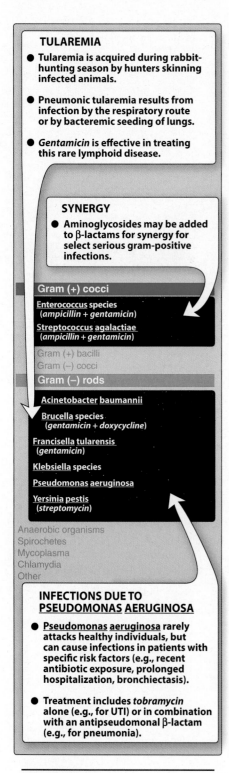

Figure 39.7
Typical therapeutic applications of aminoglycosides.

apparatus and/or cause the 30S subunit of the completed ribosome to misread the genetic code (Figure 39.2). Antibiotics that disrupt protein synthesis are generally bacteriostatic; however, aminoglycosides are unique in that they are bactericidal. The bactericidal effect of aminoglycosides is concentration dependent; that is, efficacy is dependent on the maximum concentration (C_{max}) of drug above the minimum inhibitory concentration (MIC) of the organism. For aminoglycosides, the target C_{max} is eight to ten times the MIC. They also exhibit a postantibiotic effect (PAE), which is continued bacterial suppression after drug levels fall below the MIC. The larger the dose, the longer the PAE. Because of these properties, extended interval dosing (a single large dose given once daily) is now more commonly utilized than divided daily doses. This reduces the risk of nephrotoxicity and increases convenience.

B. Antibacterial spectrum

The aminoglycosides are effective for the majority of aerobic gram-negative bacilli, including those that may be multidrug resistant, such as Pseudomonas aeruginosa, Klebsiella pneumoniae, and Enterobacter sp. Additionally, aminoglycosides are often combined with a β-lactam antibiotic to employ a synergistic effect, particularly in the treatment of Enterococcus faecalis and Enterococcus faecium infective endocarditis. Some therapeutic applications of four commonly used aminoglycosides—amikacin [am-i-KAY-sin], gentamicin [jen-ta-MYE-sin], tobramycin [toe-bra-MYE-sin], and streptomycin [strep-toe-MYE-sin]—are shown in Figure 39.7.

C. Resistance

Resistance to aminoglycosides occurs via: 1) efflux pumps, 2) decreased uptake, and/or 3) modification and inactivation by plasmid-associated synthesis of enzymes. Each of these enzymes has its own aminoglycoside specificity; therefore, cross-resistance cannot be presumed. [Note: Amikacin is less vulnerable to these enzymes than other antibiotics in this group.]

D. Pharmacokinetics

1. **Absorption:** The highly polar, polycationic structure of the aminoglycosides prevents adequate absorption after oral administration. Therefore, all aminoglycosides (except neomycin [nee-oh-MYE-sin]) must be given parenterally to achieve adequate serum levels (Figure 39.8). [Note: Neomycin is not given parenterally due to severe nephrotoxicity. It is administered topically for skin infections or orally for bowel preparation prior to colorectal surgery.]

2. **Distribution:** All the aminoglycosides have similar pharmacokinetic properties. Due to their hydrophilicity, tissue concentrations may be subtherapeutic, and penetration into most body fluids is variable. [Note: Due to low distribution into fatty tissue, the aminoglycosides are dosed based on lean body mass, not actual body weight.] Concentrations in CSF are inadequate, even in the presence of inflamed meninges. For central nervous system infections, the intrathecal (IT) route may be utilized. All aminoglycosides cross the placental barrier and may accumulate in fetal plasma and amniotic fluid.

3. **Elimination:** More than 90% of the parenteral aminoglycosides are excreted unchanged in the urine (Figure 39.8). Accumulation occurs in patients with renal dysfunction, and dose adjustments are required.

E. Adverse effects

Therapeutic drug monitoring of *gentamicin*, *tobramycin*, and *amikacin* plasma levels is imperative to ensure adequacy of dosing and to minimize dose-related toxicities (Figure 39.9). The elderly are particularly susceptible to nephrotoxicity and ototoxicity.

1. **Ototoxicity:** Ototoxicity (vestibular and auditory) is directly related to high peak plasma levels and the duration of treatment. The antibiotic accumulates in the endolymph and perilymph of the inner ear. Deafness may be irreversible and has been known to affect developing fetuses. Patients simultaneously receiving concomitant ototoxic drugs, such as *cisplatin* or loop diuretics, are particularly at risk. Vertigo (especially in patients receiving *streptomycin*) may also occur.

2. **Nephrotoxicity:** Retention of the aminoglycosides by the proximal tubular cells disrupts calcium-mediated transport processes. This results in kidney damage ranging from mild, reversible renal impairment to severe, potentially irreversible, acute tubular necrosis.

3. **Neuromuscular paralysis:** This adverse effect is associated with a rapid increase in concentrations (for example, high doses infused over a short period.) or concurrent administration with neuromuscular blockers. Patients with myasthenia gravis are particularly at risk. Prompt administration of *calcium gluconate* or *neostigmine* can reverse the block that causes neuromuscular paralysis.

4. **Allergic reactions:** Contact dermatitis is a common reaction to topically applied *neomycin*.

V. MACROLIDES AND KETOLIDES

The macrolides are a group of antibiotics with a macrocyclic lactone structure to which one or more deoxy sugars are attached. *Erythromycin* [er-ith-roe-MYE-sin] was the first of these drugs to find clinical application, both as a drug of first choice and as an alternative to *penicillin* in individuals with an allergy to β-lactam antibiotics. *Clarithromycin* [kla-rith-roe-MYE-sin] (a methylated form of *erythromycin*) and *azithromycin* [a-zith-roe-MYE-sin] (having a larger lactone ring) have some features in common with, and others that improve upon, *erythromycin*. *Telithromycin* [tel-ith-roe-MYE-sin], a semisynthetic derivative of *erythromycin*, is the first "ketolide" antimicrobial agent. Ketolides and macrolides have similar antimicrobial coverage. However, the ketolides are active against many macrolide-resistant gram-positive strains.

A. Mechanism of action

The macrolides bind irreversibly to a site on the 50S subunit of the bacterial ribosome, thus inhibiting translocation steps of protein

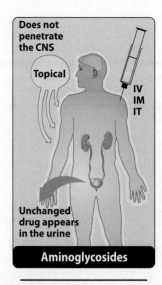

Figure 39.8
Administration and fate of aminoglycosides. CNS = central nervous system.

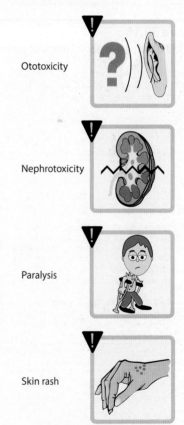

Ototoxicity

Nephrotoxicity

Paralysis

Skin rash

Figure 39.9
Some adverse effects of aminoglycosides.

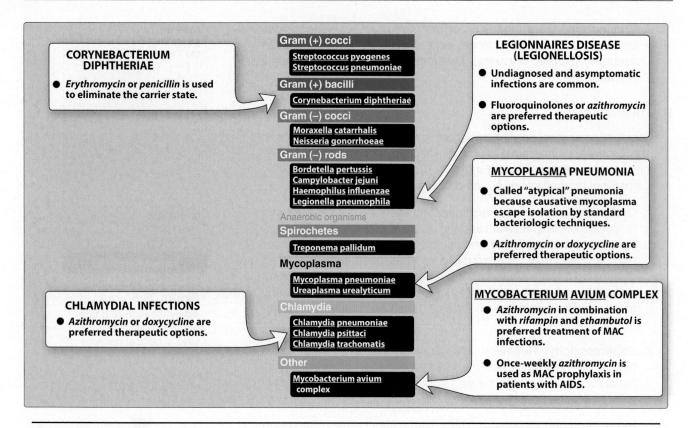

Figure 39.10
Typical therapeutic applications of macrolides.

synthesis (Figure 39.2). They may also interfere with other steps, such as transpeptidation. Generally considered to be bacteriostatic, they may be bactericidal at higher doses. Their binding site is either identical to or in close proximity to that for *clindamycin* and *chloramphenicol*.

B. Antibacterial spectrum

1. **Erythromycin:** This drug is effective against many of the same organisms as *penicillin G* (Figure 39.10). Therefore, it may be used in patients with *penicillin* allergy.

2. **Clarithromycin:** *Clarithromycin* has activity similar to *erythromycin,* but it is also effective against Haemophilus influenzae. Its activity against intracellular pathogens, such as Chlamydia, Legionella, Moraxella, Ureaplasma species and Helicobacter pylori, is higher than that of *erythromycin*.

3. **Azithromycin:** Although less active against streptococci and staphylococci than *erythromycin, azithromycin* is far more active against respiratory infections due to H. influenzae and Moraxella catarrhalis. Extensive use of *azithromycin* has resulted in growing Streptococcus pneumoniae resistance. *Azithromycin* is the preferred therapy for urethritis caused by Chlamydia trachomatis. Mycobacterium avium is preferentially treated with a macrolide-containing regimen, including *clarithromycin* or *azithromycin*.

4. Telithromycin: This drug has an antimicrobial spectrum similar to that of *azithromycin*. Moreover, the structural modification within ketolides neutralizes the most common resistance mechanisms (methylase-mediated and efflux-mediated) that make macrolides ineffective.

C. Resistance

Resistance to macrolides is associated with: 1) the inability of the organism to take up the antibiotic, 2) the presence of efflux pumps, 3) a decreased affinity of the 50S ribosomal subunit for the antibiotic, resulting from the methylation of an adenine in the 23S bacterial ribosomal RNA in gram-positive organisms, and 4) the presence of plasmid-associated *erythromycin* esterases in gram-negative organisms such as Enterobacteriaceae. Resistance to *erythromycin* has been increasing, thereby limiting its clinical use (particularly for <u>S</u>. <u>pneumoniae</u>). Both *clarithromycin* and *azithromycin* share some cross-resistance with *erythromycin,* but *telithromycin* may be effective against macrolide-resistant organisms.

D. Pharmacokinetics

1. **Administration:** The *erythromycin* base is destroyed by gastric acid. Thus, either enteric-coated tablets or esterified forms of the antibiotic are administered. All are adequately absorbed upon oral administration (Figure 39.11). *Clarithromycin, azithromycin,* and *telithromycin* are stable in stomach acid and are readily absorbed. Food interferes with the absorption of *erythromycin* and *azithromycin* but can increase that of *clarithromycin. Erythromycin* and *azithromycin* are available in IV formulations.

2. **Distribution:** *Erythromycin* distributes well to all body fluids except the CSF. It is one of the few antibiotics that diffuses into prostatic fluid, and it also accumulates in macrophages. All four drugs concentrate in the liver. *Clarithromycin, azithromycin,* and *telithromycin* are widely distributed in the tissues. *Azithromycin* concentrates in neutrophils, macrophages, and fibroblasts, and serum levels are low. It has the longest half-life and the largest volume of distribution of the four drugs (Figure 39.12).

3. **Elimination:** *Erythromycin* and *telithromycin* are extensively metabolized hepatically. They inhibit the oxidation of a number of drugs through their interaction with the cytochrome P450 system. Interference with the metabolism of drugs, such as *theophylline*, statins, and numerous antiepileptics, has been reported for *clarithromycin*.

4. **Excretion:** *Erythromycin* and *azithromycin* are primarily concentrated and excreted in the bile as active drugs (Figure 39.11). Partial reabsorption occurs through the enterohepatic circulation. In contrast, *clarithromycin* and its metabolites are eliminated by the kidney as well as the liver. The dosage of this drug should be adjusted in patients with renal impairment.

E. Adverse effects

1. **Gastric distress and motility:** Gastric upset is the most common adverse effect of the macrolides and may lead to poor patient

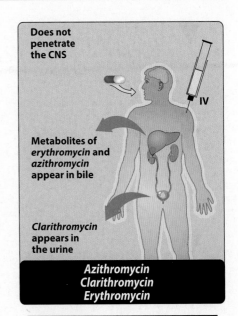

Does not penetrate the CNS

IV

Metabolites of *erythromycin* and *azithromycin* appear in bile

***Clarithromycin* appears in the urine**

Azithromycin
Clarithromycin
Erythromycin

Figure 39.11
Administration and fate of the macrolide antibiotics. CNS = central nervous system.

	Erythro-mycin	Clarithro-mycin	Azithro-mycin	Telithro-mycin
Oral absorption	Yes	Yes	Yes	Yes
Half-life (hours)	2	3.5	>40	10
Conversion to an active metabolite	No	Yes	Yes	Yes
Percent excretion in urine	15	50	12	13

Figure 39.12
Some properties of the macrolide antibiotics.

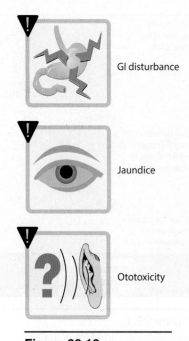

Figure 39.13
Some adverse effects of
macrolide antibiotics.

compliance (especially with *erythromycin*). *Clarithromycin* and *azithromycin* seem to be better tolerated (Figure 39.13). Higher doses of *erythromycin* lead to smooth muscle contractions that result in the movement of gastric contents to the duodenum, an adverse effect sometimes used therapeutically for the treatment of gastroparesis or postoperative ileus.

2. **Cholestatic jaundice:** This side effect occurs especially with the estolate form (not used in the United States) of *erythromycin*; however, it has been reported with other formulations.

3. **Ototoxicity:** Transient deafness has been associated with *erythromycin,* especially at high dosages. *Azithromycin* has also been associated with irreversible sensorineural hearing loss.

4. **Contraindications:** Patients with hepatic dysfunction should be treated cautiously with *erythromycin, telithromycin,* or *azithromycin,* because these drugs accumulate in the liver. Severe hepatotoxicity with *telithromycin* has limited its use, given the availability of alternative therapies. Additionally, macrolides and ketolides may prolong the QT_c interval and should be used with caution in those patients with proarrhythmic conditions or concomitant use of proarrhythmic agents.

5. **Drug interactions:** *Erythromycin, telithromycin,* and *clarithromycin* inhibit the hepatic metabolism of a number of drugs, which can lead to toxic accumulation of these compounds (Figure 39.14). An interaction with *digoxin* may occur. In this case, the antibiotic eliminates a species of intestinal flora that ordinarily inactivates *digoxin,* thus leading to greater reabsorption of the drug from the enterohepatic circulation.

VI. FIDAXOMICIN

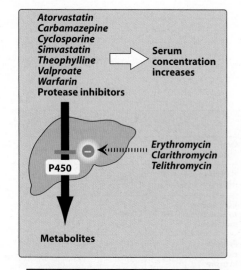

Figure 39.14
Inhibition of the cytochrome
P450 system by *erythromycin,*
clarithromycin, and *telithromycin.*

Fidaxomicin [fye-DAX-oh-MYE-sin] is a macrocyclic antibiotic with a structure similar to the macrolides; however, it has a unique mechanism of action. *Fidaxomicin* acts on the sigma subunit of RNA polymerase, thereby disrupting bacterial transcription, terminating protein synthesis, and resulting in cell death in susceptible organisms. *Fidaxomicin* has a very narrow spectrum of activity limited to gram-positive aerobes and anaerobes. While it possesses activity against staphylococci and enterococci, it is used primarily for its bactericidal activity against <u>Clostridium difficile</u>. Due to the unique target site, cross-resistance with other antibiotic classes has not been documented. Following oral administration, *fidaxomicin* has minimal systemic absorption and primarily remains within the gastrointestinal tract. This is ideal for the treatment of <u>C. difficile</u> infection, which occurs in the gut. This characteristic also likely contributes to the low rate of adverse effects. The most common adverse effects include nausea, vomiting, and abdominal pain. Hypersensitivity reactions including angioedema, dyspnea, and pruritus have occurred. *Fidaxomicin* should be used with caution in patients with a macrolide allergy, as they may be at increased risk for hypersensitivity. Anemia and neutropenia have been observed infrequently.

VII. CHLORAMPHENICOL

The use of *chloramphenicol* [klor-am-FEN-i-kole], a broad-spectrum antibiotic, is restricted to life-threatening infections for which no alternatives exist.

A. Mechanism of action

Chloramphenicol binds reversibly to the bacterial 50S ribosomal subunit and inhibits protein synthesis at the peptidyl transferase reaction (Figure 39.2). Due to some similarity of mammalian mitochondrial ribosomes to those of bacteria, protein and ATP synthesis in these organelles may be inhibited at high circulating *chloramphenicol* levels, producing bone marrow toxicity. [Note: The oral formulation of *chloramphenicol* was removed from the US market due to this toxicity.]

B. Antibacterial spectrum

Chloramphenicol is active against many types of microorganisms including chlamydiae, rickettsiae, spirochetes, and anaerobes. The drug is primarily bacteriostatic, but depending on the dose and organism, it may be bactericidal.

C. Resistance

Resistance is conferred by the presence of enzymes that inactivate *chloramphenicol*. Other mechanisms include decreased ability to penetrate the organism and ribosomal binding site alterations.

D. Pharmacokinetics

Chloramphenicol is administered intravenously and is widely distributed throughout the body. It reaches therapeutic concentrations in the CSF. *Chloramphenicol* primarily undergoes hepatic metabolism to an inactive glucuronide, which is secreted by the renal tubule and eliminated in the urine. Dose reductions are necessary in patients with liver dysfunction or cirrhosis. It is also secreted into breast milk and should be avoided in breastfeeding mothers.

E. Adverse effects

1. **Anemias:** Patients may experience dose-related anemia, hemolytic anemia (seen in patients with glucose-6-phosphate dehydrogenase deficiency), and aplastic anemia. [Note: Aplastic anemia is independent of dose and may occur after therapy has ceased.]

2. **Gray baby syndrome:** Neonates have a low capacity to glucuronidate the antibiotic, and they have underdeveloped renal function. Therefore, neonates have a decreased ability to excrete the drug, which accumulates to levels that interfere with the function of mitochondrial ribosomes. This leads to poor feeding, depressed breathing, cardiovascular collapse, cyanosis (hence the term "gray baby"), and death. Adults who have received very high doses of the drug can also exhibit this toxicity.

3. **Drug interactions:** *Chloramphenicol* inhibits some of the hepatic mixed-function oxidases and, thus, blocks the metabolism of drugs such as *warfarin* and *phenytoin,* thereby elevating their concentrations and potentiating their effects.

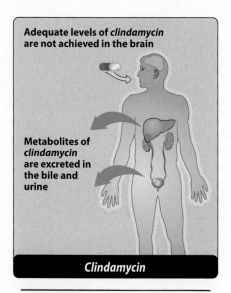

Adequate levels of *clindamycin* are not achieved in the brain

Metabolites of *clindamycin* are excreted in the bile and urine

Clindamycin

Figure 39.15
Administration and fate of *clindamycin*.

VIII. CLINDAMYCIN

Clindamycin [klin-da-MYE-sin] has a mechanism of action that is the same as that of *erythromycin*. *Clindamycin* is used primarily in the treatment of infections caused by gram-positive organisms, including MRSA and streptococcus, and anaerobic bacteria. Resistance mechanisms are the same as those for *erythromycin*, and cross-resistance has been described. C. difficile is always resistant to *clindamycin*, and the utility of *clindamycin* for gram-negative anaerobes (for example, Bacteroides *sp.*) is decreasing due to increasing resistance. *Clindamycin* is available in both IV and oral formulations, but use of the oral form is limited by gastrointestinal intolerance. It distributes well into all body fluids including bone, but exhibits poor entry into the CSF. *Clindamycin* undergoes extensive oxidative metabolism to inactive products and is primarily excreted into the bile. Low urinary elimination limits its clinical utility for urinary tract infections (Figure 39.15). Accumulation has been reported in patients with either severe renal impairment or hepatic failure. In addition to skin rashes, the most common adverse effect is diarrhea, which may represent a serious pseudomembranous colitis caused by overgrowth of C. difficile. Oral administration of either *metronidazole* or *vancomycin* is usually effective in the treatment of C. difficile.

IX. QUINUPRISTIN/DALFOPRISTIN

Quinupristin/dalfopristin [KWIN-yoo-pris-tin/DAL-foh-pris-tin] is a mixture of two streptogramins in a ratio of 30 to 70, respectively. Due to significant adverse effects, the drug is normally reserved for the treatment of severe *vancomycin*-resistant Enterococcus faecium (VRE) in the absence of other therapeutic options.

A. Mechanism of action

Each component of this combination drug binds to a separate site on the 50S bacterial ribosome. *Dalfopristin* disrupts elongation by interfering with the addition of new amino acids to the peptide chain. *Quinupristin* prevents elongation similar to the macrolides and causes release of incomplete peptide chains. Thus, they synergistically interrupt protein synthesis. The combination drug is bactericidal and has a long PAE.

B. Antibacterial spectrum

The combination drug is active primarily against gram-positive cocci, including those resistant to other antibiotics. Its primary use is in the treatment of E. faecium infections, including VRE strains, for which it is bacteriostatic. The drug is not effective against E. faecalis.

C. Resistance

Enzymatic processes commonly account for resistance to these agents. For example, the presence of a ribosomal enzyme that methylates the target bacterial 23S ribosomal RNA site can interfere in *quinupristin* binding. In some cases, the enzymatic modification can change the action from bactericidal to bacteriostatic. Plasmid-associated acetyltransferase inactivates *dalfopristin*. An active efflux pump can also decrease levels of the antibiotics in bacteria.

D. Pharmacokinetics

Quinupristin/dalfopristin is injected intravenously (the drug is incompatible with a saline medium). The combination drug is particularly useful for intracellular organisms (for example, VRE) due to its excellent penetration of macrophages and neutrophils. Levels in the CSF are low. Both compounds undergo hepatic metabolism, with excretion mainly in the feces.

E. Adverse effects

Venous irritation commonly occurs when *quinupristin/dalfopristin* is administered through a peripheral rather than a central line. Hyperbilirubinemia occurs in about 25% of patients, resulting from a competition with the antibiotic for excretion. Arthralgia and myalgia have been reported when higher doses are used. *Quinupristin/dalfopristin* inhibits the cytochrome P450 (CYP3A4) isoenzyme, and concomitant administration with drugs that are metabolized by this pathway may lead to toxicities.

X. LINEZOLID

Linezolid [lih-NEH-zo-lid] is a synthetic oxazolidinone developed to combat resistant gram-positive organisms, such as *methicillin*-resistant Staphylococcus aureus, VRE, and *penicillin*-resistant streptococci.

A. Mechanism of action

Linezolid binds to the bacterial 23S ribosomal RNA of the 50S subunit, thereby inhibiting the formation of the 70S initiation complex (Figure 39.2).

B. Antibacterial spectrum

The antibacterial action of *linezolid* is directed primarily against gram-positive organisms, such as staphylococci, streptococci, and enterococci, as well as *Corynebacterium* species and Listeria monocytogenes (Figure 39.16). It is also moderately active against Mycobacterium tuberculosis and may be used against drug-resistant strains. However, its main clinical use is against drug-resistant gram-positive organisms. Like other agents that interfere with bacterial protein synthesis, *linezolid* is bacteriostatic. However, it is bactericidal against streptococci. *Linezolid* is an alternative to *daptomycin* for infections caused by VRE. Use of *linezolid* for the treatment of MRSA bacteremia is not recommended.

C. Resistance

Resistance primarily occurs via reduced binding at the target site. Reduced susceptibility and resistance have been reported in S. aureus and Enterococcus sp. Cross-resistance with other protein synthesis inhibitors does not occur.

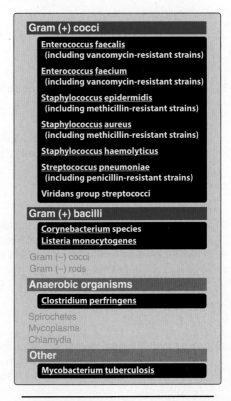

Figure 39.16
Antimicrobial spectrum of *linezolid*.

D. Pharmacokinetics

Linezolid is completely absorbed after oral administration. An IV preparation is also available. The drug is widely distributed throughout the body. Although the metabolic pathway of linezolid has not been fully determined, it is known that it is metabolized via oxidation to two inactive metabolites. The drug is excreted both by renal and nonrenal routes. No dose adjustments are required for renal or hepatic dysfunction.

E. Adverse effects

The most common adverse effects are gastrointestinal upset, nausea, diarrhea, headache, and rash. Thrombocytopenia has been reported, mainly in patients taking the drug for longer than 10 days. *Linezolid* possesses nonselective monoamine oxidase activity and may lead to serotonin syndrome if given concomitantly with large quantities of tyramine-containing foods, selective serotonin reuptake inhibitors, or monoamine oxidase inhibitors. The condition is reversible when the drug is discontinued. Irreversible peripheral neuropathies and optic neuritis (causing blindness) have been associated with greater than 28 days of use, limiting utility for extended-duration treatments.

Study Questions

Choose the ONE best answer.

39.1 Which of the following antibiotic combinations is inappropriate based on antagonism at the same site of action?

   A. Clindamycin and erythromycin.
   B. Doxycycline and amoxicillin.
   C. Tigecycline and azithromycin.
   D. Ciprofloxacin and amoxicillin.

> Correct answer = A. Clindamycin and erythromycin share the same site of action on the 50S ribosomal subunit and may result in antagonism, rendering both drugs ineffective. They also share cross-resistance.

39.2 Children younger than 8 years of age should not receive tetracyclines because these agents:

   A. Cause rupture of tendons.
   B. Deposit in tissues undergoing calcification.
   C. Do not cross into the cerebrospinal fluid.
   D. Can cause aplastic anemia.

> Correct answer = B. Tetracyclines are contraindicated in this age group because they are deposited in tissues undergoing calcification, such as teeth and bone, and can stunt growth. Ciprofloxacin can interfere in cartilage formation and cause rupture of tendons and is also contraindicated in children, but it is a fluoroquinolone. Tetracyclines can cross into the cerebrospinal fluid. They do not cause aplastic anemia, a property usually associated with chloramphenicol.

39.3 A 30-year-old pregnant female has cellulitis caused by MRSA. Which of the following antibiotics would be the most appropriate option for outpatient therapy?

   A. Doxycycline.
   B. Clindamycin.
   C. Quinupristin/dalfopristin.
   D. Tigecycline.

> Correct answer = B. Clindamycin is the safest option for the treatment of MRSA in a pregnant patient. Doxycycline and tigecycline can cross the placenta and can cause harm to the fetus. Moreover, quinupristin/dalfopristin and tigecycline are only available intravenously and would not be appropriate for home antibiotic therapy for the given indication.

39.4 A patient is being discharged from the hospital on a 3-week course of clindamycin. Which of the following potential adverse effects should be discussed with her?

   A. Hyperbilirubinemia.
   B. Nephrotoxicity.
   C. Clostridium difficile diarrhea.
   D. Pseudotumor cerebri.

> Correct answer = C. Clindamycin, among other antibiotics, is associated with the development of C. difficile and pseudomembranous colitis due to disruption of normal gut flora, particularly with prolonged therapy. Hyperbilirubinemia is associated with quinupristin/dalfopristin, nephrotoxicity is associated with aminoglycosides, and pseudotumor cerebri can occur with tetracyclines.

Quinolones, Folic Acid Antagonists, and Urinary Tract Antiseptics

40

Timothy P. Gauthier and Nathan R. Unger

I. FLUOROQUINOLONES

Nalidixic acid is the predecessor to all fluoroquinolones, a class of man-made antibiotics. Over 10,000 fluoroquinolone analogs have been synthesized, including several with wide clinical applications. Fluoroquinolones in use today typically offer greater efficacy, a broader spectrum of antimicrobial activity, and a better safety profile than their predecessors. Unfortunately, fluoroquinolone use has been closely tied to Clostridium difficile infection and the spread of antimicrobial resistance in many organisms (for example, *methicillin* resistance in staphylococci). The unfavorable effects of fluoroquinolones on the induction and spread of antimicrobial resistance are sometimes referred to as "collateral damage," a term which is also associated with third-generation cephalosporins (for example, *ceftazidime*). The fluoroquinolones and other antibiotics discussed in this chapter are listed in Figure 40.1.

A. Mechanism of action

Fluoroquinolones enter bacteria through porin channels and exhibit antimicrobial effects on DNA gyrase (bacterial topoisomerase II) and bacterial topoisomerase IV. Inhibition of DNA gyrase results in relaxation of supercoiled DNA, promoting DNA strand breakage. Inhibition of topoisomerase IV impacts chromosomal stabilization during cell division, thus interfering with the separation of newly replicated DNA. In gram-negative organisms (for example, Pseudomonas aeruginosa), the inhibition of DNA gyrase is more significant than that of topoisomerase IV, whereas in gram-positive organisms (for example, Streptococcus pneumoniae), the opposite is true. Agents with higher affinity for topoisomerase IV (for example, *ciprofloxacin*) should not be used for S. pneumoniae infections, while those with more topoisomerase II activity (for example, *moxifloxacin*) should not be used for P. aeruginosa infections.

FLUOROQUINOLONES
Ciprofloxacin CIPRO
Levofloxacin LEVAQUIN
Moxifloxacin AVELOX
Nalidixic acid
Norfloxacin NOROXIN
Ofloxacin
INHIBITORS OF FOLATE SYNTHESIS
Mafenide SULFAMYLON
Silver sulfadiazine SILVADENE
Sulfasalazine AZULFIDINE
INHIBITORS OF FOLATE REDUCTION
Pyrimethamine DARAPRIM
Trimethoprim
COMBINATION OF INHIBITORS OF FOLATE SYNTHESIS AND REDUCTION
Cotrimoxazole (trimethoprim + sulfamethoxazole) BACTRIM
URINARY TRACT ANTISEPTICS
Methenamine MANDELAMINE, HIPREX
Nitrofurantoin MACROBID

Figure 40.1
Summary of drugs described in this chapter.

B. Antimicrobial spectrum

Fluoroquinolones are bactericidal and exhibit area under the curve/minimum inhibitory concentration (AUC/MIC)–dependent killing. Bactericidal activity is more pronounced as serum drug concentrations increase to approximately 30-fold the MIC of the bacteria. In general, fluoroquinolones are effective against gram-negative organisms (Escherichia coli, P. aeruginosa, Haemophilus influenzae), atypical organisms (Legionellaceae, Chlamydiaceae), gram-positive organisms (streptococci), and some mycobacteria (Mycobacterium tuberculosis). Fluoroquinolones are typically not used for the treatment of Staphylococcus aureus or enterococcal infections. They are not effective against syphilis and have limited utility against Neisseria gonorrhoeae due to disseminated resistance worldwide. Levofloxacin and moxifloxacin are sometimes referred to as "respiratory fluoroquinolones," because they have excellent activity against S. pneumoniae, which is a common cause of community-acquired pneumonia (CAP). Moxifloxacin also has activity against many anaerobes. Fluoroquinolones are commonly considered alternatives for patients with a documented severe β-lactam allergy.

Fluoroquinolones may be classified into "generations" based on their antimicrobial targets. The nonfluorinated quinolone nalidixic acid is considered to be first generation, with a narrow spectrum of susceptible organisms. Ciprofloxacin and norfloxacin are second generation because of their activity against aerobic gram-negative and atypical bacteria. In addition, these fluoroquinolones exhibit significant intracellular penetration, allowing therapy for infections in which a bacterium spends part or all of its life cycle inside a host cell (for example, chlamydia, mycoplasma, and mycobacteria). Levofloxacin is classified as third generation because of its increased activity against gram-positive bacteria. Lastly, the fourth generation includes only moxifloxacin because of its activity against anaerobic and gram-positive organisms.

C. Examples of clinically useful fluoroquinolones

1. **Norfloxacin:** Norfloxacin [nor-FLOX-a-sin] is infrequently prescribed due to poor oral bioavailability and a short half-life. It is effective in treating nonsystemic infections, such as urinary tract infections (UTIs), prostatitis, and infectious diarrhea (unlabeled use).

2. **Ciprofloxacin:** Ciprofloxacin [sip-row-FLOX-a-sin] is effective in the treatment of many systemic infections caused by gram-negative bacilli (Figure 40.2). Of the fluoroquinolones, it has the best activity against P. aeruginosa and is commonly used in cystic fibrosis patients for this indication. With 80% bioavailability, the intravenous and oral formulations are frequently interchanged. Traveler's diarrhea caused by E. coli as well as typhoid fever caused by Salmonella typhi can be effectively treated with ciprofloxacin. Ciprofloxacin is also used as a second-line agent in the treatment of tuberculosis. Although typically dosed twice daily, an extended-release formulation is available for once-daily dosing, which may improve patient adherence to treatment.

3. **Levofloxacin:** Levofloxacin [leave-oh-FLOX-a-sin] is the L-isomer of ofloxacin [oh-FLOX-a-sin] and has largely replaced it clinically.

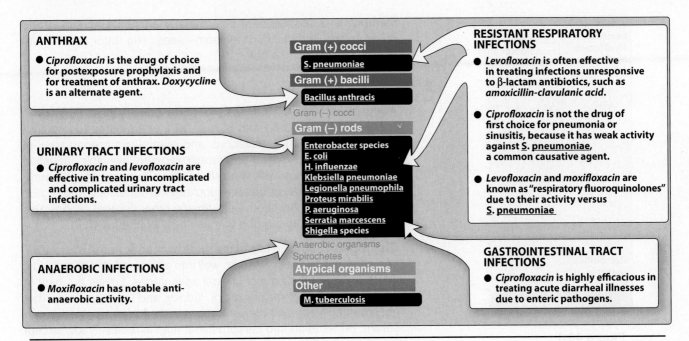

Figure 40.2
Typical therapeutic applications of fluoroquinolones.

Due to its broad spectrum of activity, *levofloxacin* is utilized in a wide range of infections, including prostatitis, skin infections, CAP, and nosocomial pneumonia. Unlike *ciprofloxacin*, *levofloxacin* has excellent activity against S. pneumoniae respiratory infections. *Levofloxacin* has 100% bioavailability and is dosed once daily.

4. **Moxifloxacin:** *Moxifloxacin* [mox-ee-FLOX-a-sin] not only has enhanced activity against gram-positive organisms (for example, S. pneumoniae) but also has excellent activity against many anaerobes, although resistance to Bacteroides fragilis has been reported. It has poor activity against P. aeruginosa. *Moxifloxacin* does not concentrate in urine and is not indicated for the treatment of UTIs.

D. Resistance

Although plasmid-mediated resistance or resistance via enzymatic degradation is not of great concern, high levels of fluoroquinolone resistance have emerged in gram-positive and gram-negative bacteria, primarily due to chromosomal mutations. Cross-resistance exists among the quinolones. The mechanisms responsible for this resistance include the following:

1. **Altered target:** Chromosomal mutations in bacterial genes (for example, gyrA or parC) have been associated with a decreased affinity for fluoroquinolones at their site of action. Both topoisomerase IV and DNA gyrase may undergo mutations.

2. **Decreased accumulation:** Reduced intracellular concentration is linked to 1) porin channels and 2) efflux pumps. The former involves a decreased number of porin proteins in the outer

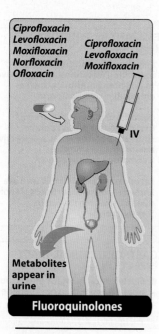

Figure 40.3
Administration and fate
of the fluoroquinolones.

membrane of the resistant cell, thereby impairing access of the drugs to the intracellular topoisomerases. The latter mechanism pumps drug out of the cell.

E. Pharmacokinetics

1. **Absorption:** Only 35% to 70% of orally administered *norfloxacin* is absorbed, compared with 80% to 99% of the other fluoroquinolones (Figure 40.3). Intravenous and ophthalmic preparations of *ciprofloxacin*, *levofloxacin*, and *moxifloxacin* are available. Ingestion of fluoroquinolones with *sucralfate*, aluminum- or magnesium-containing antacids, or dietary supplements containing iron or zinc can reduce the absorption. Calcium and other divalent cations also interfere with the absorption of these agents (Figure 40.4).

2. **Distribution:** Binding to plasma proteins ranges from 10% to 40%. The fluoroquinolones distribute well into all tissues and body fluids, which is one of their major clinical advantages. Levels are high in bone, urine (except *moxifloxacin*), kidney, and prostatic tissue (but not prostatic fluid), and concentrations in the lungs exceed those in serum. Penetration into cerebrospinal fluid is relatively low except for *ofloxacin*. Fluoroquinolones also accumulate in macrophages and polymorphonuclear leukocytes, thus having activity against intracellular organisms.

3. **Elimination:** Most fluoroquinolones are excreted renally. Therefore, dosage adjustments are needed in renal dysfunction. *Moxifloxacin* is excreted primarily by the liver, and no dose adjustment is required for renal impairment.

F. Adverse reactions

In general, these agents are well tolerated (Figure 40.5). Like most antibiotics, the most common adverse effects of fluoroquinolones are nausea, vomiting, and diarrhea. Headache and dizziness or light-headedness may occur. Thus, patients with central nervous system (CNS) disorders, such as epilepsy, should be treated cautiously with these drugs. Peripheral neuropathy and glucose dysregulation (hypoglycemia and hypoglycemia) have also been noted. Fluoroquinolones can cause phototoxicity, and patients taking these agents should be advised to use sunscreen and avoid excess exposure to sunlight. If phototoxicity occurs, discontinuation of the drug is advisable. Articular cartilage erosion (arthropathy) has been observed in immature animals exposed to fluoroquinolones. Therefore, these agents should be avoided in pregnancy and lactation and in children under 18 years of age. [Note: Careful monitoring is indicated in children with cystic fibrosis who receive fluoroquinolones for acute pulmonary exacerbations.] An increased risk of tendinitis or tendon rupture may also occur with systemic fluoroquinolone use. *Moxifloxacin* and other fluoroquinolones may prolong the QT_c interval and, thus, should not be used in patients who are predisposed to arrhythmias or those who are taking other medications that cause QT prolongation. *Ciprofloxacin* can increase serum levels of *theophylline* by inhibiting its metabolism (Figure 40.6). Quinolones may also raise the serum levels of *warfarin*, *caffeine*, and *cyclosporine*.

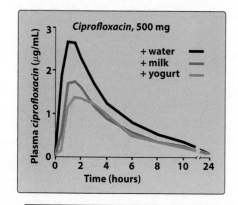

Figure 40.4
Effect of dietary calcium on the absorption of *ciprofloxacin*.

II. OVERVIEW OF THE FOLATE ANTAGONISTS

Enzymes requiring folate-derived cofactors are essential for the synthesis of purines and pyrimidines (precursors of RNA and DNA) and other compounds necessary for cellular growth and replication. Therefore, in the absence of folate, cells cannot grow or divide. To synthesize the critical folate derivative, tetrahydrofolic acid, humans must first obtain preformed folate in the form of folic acid from the diet. In contrast, many bacteria are impermeable to folic acid and other folates and, therefore, must rely on their ability to synthesize folate de novo. The sulfonamides (sulfa drugs) are a family of antibiotics that inhibit de novo synthesis of folate. A second type of folate antagonist—*trimethoprim*—prevents microorganisms from converting dihydrofolic acid to tetrahydrofolic acid, with minimal effect on the ability of human cells to make this conversion. Thus, both sulfonamides and *trimethoprim* interfere with the ability of an infecting bacterium to perform DNA synthesis. Combining the sulfonamide *sulfamethoxazole* with *trimethoprim* (the generic name for the combination is *cotrimoxazole*) provides a synergistic combination.

III. SULFONAMIDES

The sulfa drugs are seldom prescribed alone except in developing countries, where they are still employed because of their low cost and efficacy.

A. Mechanism of action

In many microorganisms, dihydrofolic acid is synthesized from *p*-aminobenzoic acid (PABA), pteridine, and glutamate (Figure 40.7). All the sulfonamides currently in clinical use are synthetic analogs of PABA. Because of their structural similarity to PABA, the sulfonamides compete with this substrate for the bacterial enzyme, dihydropteroate synthetase. They thus inhibit the synthesis of bacterial dihydrofolic acid and, thereby, the formation of its essential cofactor forms. The sulfa drugs, including *cotrimoxazole*, are bacteriostatic.

B. Antibacterial spectrum

Sulfa drugs are active against select Enterobacteriaceae in the urinary tract and Nocardia infections. In addition, *sulfadiazine* [sul-fa-DYE-a-zeen] in combination with the dihydrofolate reductase inhibitor *pyrimethamine* [py-ri-METH-a-meen] is the preferred treatment for toxoplasmosis. *Sulfadoxine* in combination with *pyrimethamine* is used as an antimalarial drug (see Chapter 43).

C. Resistance

Bacteria that can obtain folate from their environment are naturally resistant to these drugs. Acquired bacterial resistance to the sulfa drugs can arise from plasmid transfers or random mutations. [Note: Organisms resistant to one member of this drug family are resistant to all.] Resistance is generally irreversible and may be due to 1) an altered dihydropteroate synthetase, 2) decreased cellular permeability to sulfa drugs, or 3) enhanced production of the natural substrate, PABA.

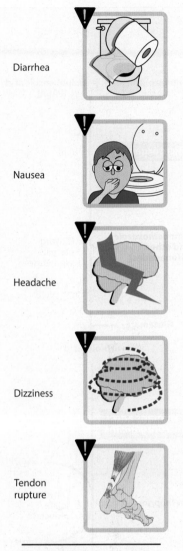

Diarrhea

Nausea

Headache

Dizziness

Tendon rupture

Figure 40.5
Some adverse reactions to fluoroquinolones.

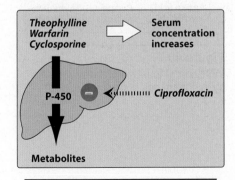

Figure 40.6
Drug interactions with fluoroquinolones.

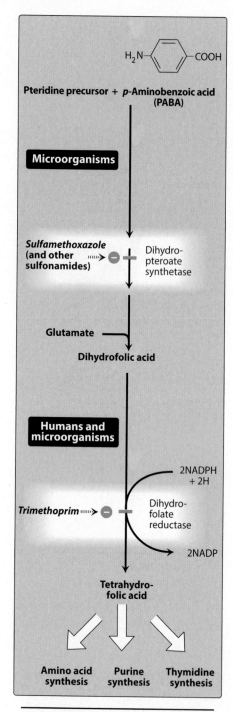

Figure 40.7
Inhibition of tetrahydrofolate synthesis by sulfonamides and *trimethoprim*.

D. Pharmacokinetics

1. **Absorption:** After oral administration, most sulfa drugs are well absorbed (Figure 40.8). An exception is *sulfasalazine* [sul-fa-SAL-a-zeen]. It is not absorbed when administered orally or as a suppository and, therefore, is reserved for treatment of chronic inflammatory bowel disease (for example, ulcerative colitis). [Note: Local intestinal flora split *sulfasalazine* into sulfapyridine and 5-aminosalicylate, with the latter exerting the anti-inflammatory effect. Absorption of sulfapyridine can lead to toxicity in patients who are slow acetylators.] Intravenous sulfonamides are generally reserved for patients who are unable to take oral preparations. Because of the risk of sensitization, sulfa drugs are not usually applied topically. However, in burn units, creams of *silver sulfadiazine* [sul-fa-DYE-ah-zeen] or *mafenide* [mah-FEN-ide] *acetate* (α-amino-p-toluenesulfonamide) have been effective in reducing burn-associated sepsis because they prevent colonization of bacteria. [Note: *Silver sulfadiazine* is preferred because *mafenide* produces pain on application and its absorption may contribute to acid–base disturbances.]

2. **Distribution:** Sulfa drugs are bound to serum albumin in the circulation, where the extent of binding depends on the ionization constant (pK_a) of the drug. In general, the smaller the pK_a value, the greater the binding. Sulfa drugs distribute throughout the bodily fluids and penetrate well into cerebrospinal fluid—even in the absence of inflammation. They can also pass the placental barrier and enter fetal tissues.

3. **Metabolism:** The sulfa drugs are acetylated and conjugated primarily in the liver. The acetylated product is devoid of antimicrobial activity but retains the toxic potential to precipitate at neutral or acidic pH. This causes crystalluria ("stone formation"; see below) and, therefore, potential damage to the kidney.

4. **Excretion:** Sulfa drugs are eliminated by glomerular filtration and secretion and require dose adjustments for renal dysfunction. Sulfonamides may be eliminated in breast milk.

E. Adverse effects

1. **Crystalluria:** Nephrotoxicity may develop as a result of crystalluria (Figure 40.9). Adequate hydration and alkalinization of urine can prevent the problem by reducing the concentration of drug and promoting its ionization.

2. **Hypersensitivity:** Hypersensitivity reactions, such as rashes, angioedema or Stevens-Johnson syndrome, may occur. When patients report previous sulfa allergies, it is paramount to acquire a description of the reaction to direct appropriate therapy.

3. **Hematopoietic disturbances:** Hemolytic anemia is encountered in patients with glucose-6-phosphate dehydrogenase (G6PD) deficiency. Granulocytopenia and thrombocytopenia can also occur. Fatal reactions have been reported from associated agranulocytosis, aplastic anemia, and other blood dyscrasias.

4. **Kernicterus:** This disorder may occur in newborns, because sulfa drugs displace bilirubin from binding sites on serum albumin. The bilirubin is then free to pass into the CNS, because the blood–brain barrier is not fully developed.

5. **Drug potentiation:** Transient potentiation of the anticoagulant effect of *warfarin* results from the displacement from binding sites on serum albumin. Serum *methotrexate* levels may also rise through its displacement.

6. **Contraindications:** Due to the danger of kernicterus, sulfa drugs should be avoided in newborns and infants less than 2 months of age, as well as in pregnant women at term. Sulfonamides should not be given to patients receiving *methenamine*, since they can crystallize in the presence of formaldehyde produced by this agent (Figure 40.10).

IV. TRIMETHOPRIM

Trimethoprim [try-METH-oh-prim], a potent inhibitor of bacterial dihydrofolate reductase, exhibits an antibacterial spectrum similar to that of the sulfonamides. *Trimethoprim* is most often compounded with *sulfamethoxazole* [sul-fa-meth-OX-a-zole], producing the combination called *cotrimoxazole*.

A. Mechanism of action

The active form of folate is the tetrahydro derivative that is formed through reduction of dihydrofolic acid by dihydrofolate reductase. This enzymatic reaction (Figure 40.7) is inhibited by *trimethoprim*, leading to a decreased availability of the tetrahydrofolate cofactors required for purine, pyrimidine, and amino acid synthesis. The bacterial reductase has a much stronger affinity for *trimethoprim* than does the mammalian enzyme, which accounts for the selective toxicity of the drug.

B. Antibacterial spectrum

The antibacterial spectrum of *trimethoprim* is similar to that of *sulfamethoxazole*. However, *trimethoprim* is 20- to 50-fold more potent than the sulfonamides. *Trimethoprim* may be used alone in the treatment of UTIs and in the treatment of bacterial prostatitis (although fluoroquinolones are preferred).

C. Resistance

Resistance in gram-negative bacteria is due to the presence of an altered dihydrofolate reductase that has a lower affinity for *trimethoprim*. Efflux pumps and decreased permeability to the drug may play a role.

D. Pharmacokinetics

Trimethoprim is rapidly absorbed following oral administration. Because the drug is a weak base, higher concentrations of *trimethoprim* are achieved in the relatively acidic prostatic and vaginal fluids. The drug is widely distributed into body tissues and fluids, including

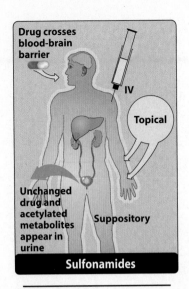

Figure 40.8
Administration and fate of the sulfonamides.

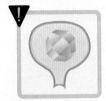
Crystalluria

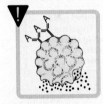
Hypersensitivity

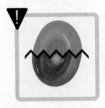
Hemolytic anemia

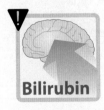
Kernicterus

Figure 40.9
Some adverse reactions to sulfonamides.

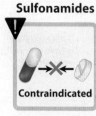

Sulfonamides

Contraindicated

Methenamine

Figure 40.10
Contraindication for sulfonamide treatment.

penetration into the cerebrospinal fluid. *Trimethoprim* undergoes some *O*-demethylation, but 60% to 80% is renally excreted unchanged.

E. Adverse effects

Trimethoprim can produce the effects of folic acid deficiency. These effects include megaloblastic anemia, leukopenia, and granulocytopenia, especially in pregnant patients and those having very poor diets. These blood disorders may be reversed by the simultaneous administration of *folinic acid*, which does not enter bacteria.

V. COTRIMOXAZOLE

The combination of *trimethoprim* with *sulfamethoxazole*, called *cotrimoxazole* [co-try-MOX-a-zole], shows greater antimicrobial activity than equivalent quantities of either drug used alone (Figure 40.11). The combination was selected because of the synergistic activity and the similarity in the half-lives of the two drugs.

A. Mechanism of action

The synergistic antimicrobial activity of *cotrimoxazole* results from its inhibition of two sequential steps in the synthesis of tetrahydrofolic acid. *Sulfamethoxazole* inhibits the incorporation of PABA into dihydrofolic acid precursors, and *trimethoprim* prevents reduction of dihydrofolate to tetrahydrofolate (Figure 40.7).

B. Antibacterial spectrum

Cotrimoxazole has a broader spectrum of antibacterial action than the sulfa drugs alone (Figure 40.12). It is effective in treating UTIs and respiratory tract infections, as well as Pneumocystis jirovecii pneumonia (PCP), toxoplasmosis, and *ampicillin-* or *chloramphenicol*-resistant salmonella infections. It has activity against MRSA and can be particularly useful for community-acquired skin and soft tissue infections caused by this organism. It is the drug of choice for infections caused by susceptible Nocardia species and Stenotrophomonas maltophilia.

C. Resistance

Resistance to the *trimethoprim–sulfamethoxazole* combination is less frequently encountered than resistance to either of the drugs alone, because it requires that the bacterium have simultaneous resistance to both drugs. Significant resistance has been documented in a number of clinically relevant organisms, including E. coli and MRSA.

D. Pharmacokinetics

Cotrimoxazole is generally administered orally (Figure 40.13). Intravenous administration may be utilized in patients with severe pneumonia caused by PCP. Both agents distribute throughout the body. *Trimethoprim* concentrates in the relatively acidic milieu of prostatic fluids, and this accounts for the use of *trimethoprim–sulfamethoxazole* in the treatment of prostatitis. *Cotrimoxazole* readily crosses the blood–brain barrier. Both parent drugs and their metabolites are excreted in the urine.

Trimethoprim and sulfamethoxazole together (*cotrimoxazole*) show greater inhibition of bacterial growth.

Number of bacteria (arbitrary units)

100

50

0

0   5   10

Hours

No drug

Trimethoprim alone

Sulfamethoxazole alone

Both drugs

Figure 40.11
Synergism between *trimethoprim* and *sulfamethoxazole* inhibits growth of E. coli.

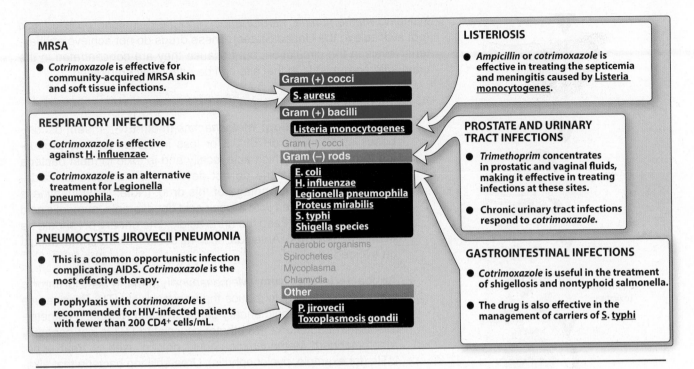

MRSA

● *Cotrimoxazole* is effective for community-acquired MRSA skin and soft tissue infections.

RESPIRATORY INFECTIONS

● *Cotrimoxazole* is effective against <u>H. influenzae</u>.

● *Cotrimoxazole* is an alternative treatment for <u>Legionella pneumophila</u>.

<u>PNEUMOCYSTIS JIROVECII</u> PNEUMONIA

● This is a common opportunistic infection complicating AIDS. *Cotrimoxazole* is the most effective therapy.

● Prophylaxis with *cotrimoxazole* is recommended for HIV-infected patients with fewer than 200 CD4+ cells/mL.

Gram (+) cocci
<u>S. aureus</u>
Gram (+) bacilli
<u>Listeria</u> <u>monocytogenes</u>
Gram (−) cocci
Gram (−) rods
<u>E. coli</u>
<u>H. influenzae</u>
<u>Legionella pneumophila</u>
<u>Proteus</u> <u>mirabilis</u>
<u>S. typhi</u>
<u>Shigella</u> species
Anaerobic organisms
Spirochetes
Mycoplasma
Chlamydia
Other
<u>P. jirovecii</u>
<u>Toxoplasmosis gondii</u>

LISTERIOSIS

● *Ampicillin* or *cotrimoxazole* is effective in treating the septicemia and meningitis caused by <u>Listeria monocytogenes</u>.

PROSTATE AND URINARY TRACT INFECTIONS

● *Trimethoprim* concentrates in prostatic and vaginal fluids, making it effective in treating infections at these sites.

● Chronic urinary tract infections respond to *cotrimoxazole*.

GASTROINTESTINAL INFECTIONS

● *Cotrimoxazole* is useful in the treatment of shigellosis and nontyphoid salmonella.

● The drug is also effective in the management of carriers of <u>S. typhi</u>

Figure 40.12
Typical therapeutic applications of *cotrimoxazole* (*sulfamethoxazole* plus *trimethoprim*).

E. Adverse effects

Reactions involving the skin are very common and may be severe in the elderly (Figure 40.14). Nausea and vomiting are the most common gastrointestinal adverse effects. Glossitis and stomatitis have been observed. Hyperkalemia may occur, especially with higher doses. Megaloblastic anemia, leukopenia, and thrombocytopenia may occur and have been fatal. The hematologic effects may be reversed by the concurrent administration of *folinic acid*, which protects the patient and does not enter the microorganism. Hemolytic anemia may occur in patients with G6PD deficiency due to the *sulfamethoxazole* component. Immunocompromised patients with PCP frequently show drug-induced fever, rashes, diarrhea, and/or pancytopenia. Prolonged prothrombin times (increased INR) in patients receiving both *sulfamethoxazole* and *warfarin* have been reported, and increased monitoring is recommended when the drugs are used concurrently. The plasma half-life of *phenytoin* may be increased due to inhibition of its metabolism. *Methotrexate* levels may rise due to displacement from albumin-binding sites by *sulfamethoxazole*.

VI. URINARY TRACT ANTISEPTICS/ANTIMICROBIALS

UTIs are prevalent in women of child-bearing age and in the elderly population. <u>E. coli</u> is the most common pathogen, causing about 80% of uncomplicated upper and lower UTIs. <u>Staphylococcus</u> <u>saprophyticus</u> is the second most common bacterial pathogen causing UTIs. In addition to *cotrimoxazole* and the quinolones previously mentioned, UTIs may be treated with any one of a group of agents called urinary tract antiseptics,

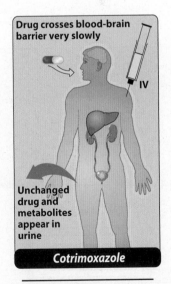

Drug crosses blood-brain barrier very slowly

IV

Unchanged drug and metabolites appear in urine

Cotrimoxazole

Figure 40.13
Administration and fate of *cotrimoxazole*.

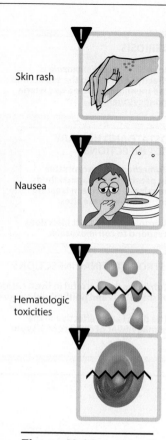

Skin rash

Nausea

Hematologic
toxicities

Figure 40.14
Some adverse reactions
to *cotrimoxazole*.

including *methenamine*, *nitrofurantoin*, and the quinolone *nalidixic acid* (not available in the United States). These drugs do not achieve antibacterial levels in the circulation, but because they are concentrated in the urine, microorganisms at that site can be effectively eradicated.

A. Methenamine

1. **Mechanism of action:** *Methenamine* [meth-EN-a-meen] decomposes at an acidic pH of 5.5 or less in the urine, thus producing formaldehyde, which acts locally and is toxic to most bacteria (Figure 40.15). Bacteria do not develop resistance to formaldehyde, which is an advantage of this drug. [Note: *Methenamine* is frequently formulated with a weak acid (for example, mandelic acid or hippuric acid) to keep the urine acidic. The urinary pH should be maintained below 6. Antacids, such as *sodium bicarbonate*, should be avoided.]

2. **Antibacterial spectrum:** *Methenamine* is primarily used for chronic suppressive therapy to reduce the frequency of UTIs. Routine use in patients with chronic urinary catheterization to reduce catheter-associated bacteriuria or catheter-associated UTI is not generally recommended. *Methenamine* should not be used to treat upper UTIs (for example, pyelonephritis). Urea-splitting bacteria that alkalinize the urine, such as <u>Proteus</u> species, are usually resistant to the action of *methenamine*.

3. **Pharmacokinetics:** *Methenamine* is administered orally. In addition to formaldehyde, ammonium ions are produced in the bladder. Because the liver rapidly metabolizes ammonia to form urea, *methenamine* is contraindicated in patients with hepatic insufficiency, as ammonia can accumulate. *Methenamine* is distributed throughout the body fluids, but no decomposition of the drug occurs at pH 7.4. Thus, systemic toxicity does not occur, and the drug is eliminated in the urine.

4. **Adverse effects:** The major side effect of *methenamine* is gastrointestinal distress, although at higher doses, albuminuria, hematuria, and rashes may develop. *Methenamine mandelate* is contraindicated in patients with renal insufficiency, because mandelic acid may precipitate. [Note: Sulfonamides, such as *cotrimoxazole*, react with formaldehyde and must not be used concomitantly with *methenamine*. The combination increases the risk of crystalluria and mutual antagonism.]

B. Nitrofurantoin

Nitrofurantoin [nye-troe-FYOOR-an-toyn] sensitive bacteria reduce the drug to a highly active intermediate that inhibits various enzymes and damages bacterial DNA. It is useful against <u>E. coli</u>, but other common urinary tract gram-negative bacteria may be resistant. Gram-positive cocci (for example, <u>S. saprophyticus</u>) are typically susceptible. Hemolytic anemia may occur with *nitrofurantoin* use in patients with G6PD deficiency. Other adverse effects include gastrointestinal disturbances, acute pneumonitis, and neurologic problems. Interstitial pulmonary fibrosis has occurred in patients who take *nitrofurantoin* chronically. The drug should not be used in patients with significant renal impairment or women who are 38 weeks or more pregnant.

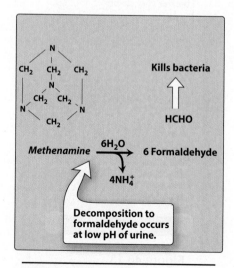

Figure 40.15
Formation of formaldehyde from
methenamine at acid pH.

Study Questions

Choose the ONE best answer.

40.1 A 32-year-old male presents to an outpatient clinic with a 5-day history of productive cough, purulent sputum, and shortness of breath. He is diagnosed with community-acquired pneumonia (CAP). It is noted that this patient has a severe ampicillin allergy (anaphylaxis). Which of the following would be an acceptable treatment for this patient?

    A. Levofloxacin.
    B. Ciprofloxacin.
    C. Penicillin VK.
    D. Nitrofurantoin.

> Correct answer = A. Streptococcus pneumoniae is a common cause of CAP, and the respiratory fluoroquinolones levofloxacin and moxifloxacin provide good coverage. Ciprofloxacin does not cover S. pneumoniae well and is a poor choice for treatment of CAP. Penicillin would be a poor choice due to allergy. Nitrofurantoin has no clinical utility for respiratory tract infections.

40.2 A 22-year-old female presents with a 2-day history of dysuria with increased urinary frequency and urgency. A urine culture and urinalysis are done. She is diagnosed with a urinary tract infection (UTI) caused by E. coli. All of the following would be considered appropriate therapy for this patient except:

    A. Levofloxacin.
    B. Cotrimoxazole.
    C. Moxifloxacin.
    D. Nitrofurantoin.

> Correct answer = C. Moxifloxacin does not concentrate in the urine and would be ineffective for treatment of a UTI. All other answers are viable alternatives, and the resistance profile for the E. coli can be utilized to direct therapy.

40.3 Which of the following drugs is correctly matched with the appropriate adverse effect?

    A. Levofloxacin—hyperkalemia.
    B. Nitrofurantoin—pulmonary fibrosis.
    C. Cotrimoxazole—hepatic encephalopathy.
    D. Methenamine—nystagmus.

> Correct answer = B. Hyperkalemia may be caused by cotrimoxazole, not fluoroquinolones. Hepatic encephalopathy may be related to therapy with methenamine in patients with hepatic insufficiency. Nystagmus is not associated with methenamine therapy.

40.4 Cotrimoxazole would be expected to provide coverage for all of the following organisms except:

    A. Pseudomonas aeruginosa.
    B. Community-acquired MRSA.
    C. Nocardia asteroides.
    D. Stenotrophomonas maltophilia.

> Correct answer = A. Cotrimoxazole is generally the drug of choice for answers C and D. It is also an excellent option for treatment of community-acquired MRSA skin and soft tissue infections.

Antimycobacterial Drugs

41

Charles A. Peloquin and Eric Egelund

I. OVERVIEW

Mycobacteria are rod-shaped aerobic bacilli that multiple slowly, every 18 to 24 hours in vitro. Their cell walls contain mycolic acids, which give the genus its name. Mycolic acids are very long-chain, β-hydroxylated fatty acids. Mycobacteria produce highly lipophilic cell walls that stain poorly with Gram stain. Once stained, the bacilli are not decolorized easily by acidified organic solvents. Hence, the organisms are called "acid-fast bacilli." Mycobacterial infections classically result in the formation of slow-growing, granulomatous lesions that cause tissue destruction anywhere in the body.

Mycobacterium tuberculosis can cause latent tuberculosis infection (LTBI) and the disease known as tuberculosis (TB). [Note: In LTBI, the patient is infected with M. tuberculosis but does not have any signs or symptoms of active TB disease.] TB is the leading infectious cause of death worldwide, and over 2 billion people already have been infected (roughly 10 million are in the United States). Increasing in frequency are diseases caused by nontuberculosis mycobacteria (NTM). These species include M. avium-intracellulare, M. chelonae, M. abscessus, M. kansasii, and M. fortuitum. Finally, M. leprae causes leprosy.

TB treatment generally includes four first-line drugs (Figure 41.1). Second-line drugs are typically less effective, more toxic, and less extensively studied. They are used for patients who cannot tolerate the first-line drugs or who are infected with resistant TB. No drugs are specifically developed for NTM infections. Macrolides, rifamycins, and aminoglycosides are frequently included, but NTM regimens vary widely by organism.

II. CHEMOTHERAPY FOR TUBERCULOSIS

M. tuberculosis is slow growing and requires treatment for months to years. LTBI can be treated for 9 months with isoniazid (INH) monotherapy or with 12 once-weekly doses of INH (900 mg) and rifapentine (900 mg). In contrast, active TB disease must be treated with several drugs. Treatment for drug-susceptible TB lasts for at least 6 months, while treatment of multidrug-resistant TB (MDR-TB) typically lasts for about 2 years.

DRUGS USED TO TREAT TUBERCULOSIS
Ethambutol MYAMBUTOL
Isoniazid
Pyrazinamide
Rifabutin MYCOBUTIN
Rifampin RIFADIN
Rifapentine PRIFTIN

DRUGS USED TO TREAT TUBERCULOSIS (2nd line)
Aminoglycosides
Aminosalicylic acid PASER
Bedaquiline SIRTURO
Capreomycin CAPASTAT
Cycloserine SEROMYCIN
Ethionamide TRECATOR
Fluoroquinolones
Macrolides

DRUGS USED TO TREAT LEPROSY
Clofazimine LAMPRENE
Dapsone
Rifampin (Rifampicin) RIFADIN

Figure 41.1
Summary of drugs used to treat mycobacterial infections.

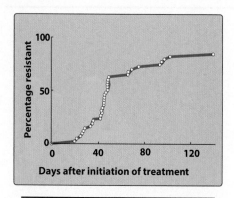

Figure 41.2
Cumulative percentage of strains of
<u>Mycobacterium</u> <u>tuberculosis</u> showing
resistance to *streptomycin*.

A. Strategies for addressing drug resistance

Populations of <u>M</u>. <u>tuberculosis</u> contain small numbers of organisms
that are naturally resistant to a particular drug. Under selective pressure from inadequate treatment, especially from monotherapy, these
resistant TB can emerge as the dominant population. Figure 41.2
shows that resistance develops rapidly in patients given only *streptomycin*. Multidrug therapy is employed to suppress these resistant
organisms. The first-line drugs *isoniazid*, *rifampin*, *ethambutol*, and
pyrazinamide are preferred because of their high efficacy and acceptable incidence of toxicity. *Rifabutin* or *rifapentine* may replace *rifampin*
under certain circumstances. Active disease always requires treatment with multidrug regimens, and preferably three or more drugs
with proven in vitro activity against the isolate. Although clinical
improvement can occur in the first several weeks of treatment, therapy is continued much longer to eradicate persistent organisms and
to prevent relapse.

Standard short-course chemotherapy for tuberculosis includes
isoniazid, *rifampin*, *ethambutol*, and *pyrazinamide* for 2 months (the
intensive phase), followed by *isoniazid* and *rifampin* for 4 months
(the continuation phase; Figure 41.3). Once susceptibility data are
available, the drug regimen can be individually tailored. Second-
line regimens for MDR-TB (TB resistant to at least *isoniazid* and
rifampin) normally include an aminoglycoside (*streptomycin*, *kanamycin*, or *amikacin*) or *capreomycin* (all injectable agents), a fluoroquinolone (typically *levofloxacin* or *moxifloxacin*), any first-line
drugs that remain active, and one or more of the following: *cycloserine*, *ethionamide*, or *p-aminosalicylic acid*. For extensively drug-
resistant TB (XDR-TB), *clofazimine*, *linezolid*, and other drugs may
be employed empirically.

Patient adherence can be low when multidrug regimens last for 6
months or longer. One successful strategy for achieving better treatment completion rates is directly observed therapy, also known as
DOT. Patients take their medications while being watched by a member of the health care team. DOT has been shown to decrease drug
resistance and to improve cure rates. Most public health departments
offer DOT services.

B. Isoniazid

Isoniazid [eye-so-NYE-a-zid], along with *rifampin*, is one of the two
most important TB drugs.

1. **Mechanism of action:** *Isoniazid* is a prodrug activated by a
   mycobacterial catalase–peroxidase (KatG). *Isoniazid* targets the
   enzymes acyl carrier protein reductase (InhA) and β-ketoacyl-ACP
   synthase (KasA), which are essential for the synthesis of mycolic
   acid. Inhibiting mycolic acid leads to a disruption in the bacterial
   cell wall.

2. **Antibacterial spectrum:** *Isoniazid* is specific for treatment of
   <u>M</u>. <u>tuberculosis</u>, although <u>M</u>. <u>kansasii</u> may be susceptible at higher
   drug concentrations. Most NTM are resistant to *INH*. The drug
   is particularly effective against rapidly growing bacilli and is also
   active against intracellular organisms.

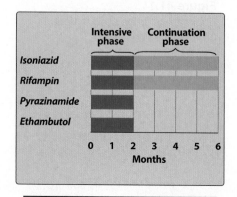

Figure 41.3
One of several recommended
multidrug schedules for the treatment
of tuberculosis.

3. **Resistance:** Resistance follows chromosomal mutations, including 1) mutation or deletion of KatG (producing mutants incapable of prodrug activation), 2) varying mutations of the acyl carrier proteins, or 3) overexpression of the target enzyme InhA. Cross-resistance may occur between *isoniazid* and *ethionamide*.

4. **Pharmacokinetics:** *Isoniazid* is readily absorbed after oral administration. Absorption is impaired if *isoniazid* is taken with food, particularly high-fat meals. The drug diffuses into all body fluids, cells, and caseous material (necrotic tissue resembling cheese that is produced in tuberculous lesions). Drug concentrations in the cerebrospinal fluid (CSF) are similar to those in the serum. *Isoniazid* undergoes *N*-acetylation and hydrolysis, resulting in inactive products. [Note: *Isoniazid* acetylation is genetically regulated, with the fast acetylators exhibiting a 90-minute serum half-life, as compared to 3 to 4 hours for slow acetylators (Figure 41.4).] Excretion is through glomerular filtration and secretion, predominantly as metabolites (Figure 41.5). Slow acetylators excrete more of the parent compound.

5. **Adverse effects:** Hepatitis is the most serious adverse effect associated with *isoniazid*. If hepatitis goes unrecognized, and if *isoniazid* is continued, it can be fatal. The incidence increases with age (greater than 35 years old), among patients who also take *rifampin*, or among those who drink alcohol daily. Peripheral neuropathy (manifesting as paresthesia of the hands and feet) appears to be due to a relative pyridoxine deficiency. This can be avoided by supplementation of 25 to 50 mg per day of pyridoxine (vitamin B_6). Central nervous system (CNS) adverse effects can occur, including convulsions in patients prone to seizures. Hypersensitivity reactions with *isoniazid* include rashes and fever. Because *isoniazid* inhibits the metabolism of *carbamazepine* and *phenytoin* (Figure 41.6), *isoniazid* can potentiate the adverse effects of these drugs (for example, nystagmus and ataxia).

C. Rifamycins: rifampin, rifabutin, and rifapentine

Rifampin, *rifabutin*, and *rifapentine* are all considered rifamycins, a group of structurally similar macrocyclic antibiotics, which are first-line oral agents for tuberculosis.

1. **Rifampin:** *Rifampin* [ri-FAM-pin] has broader antimicrobial activity than *isoniazid* and can be used as part of treatment for several different bacterial infections. Because resistant strains rapidly emerge during monotherapy, it is never given as a single agent in the treatment of active tuberculosis.

    a. **Mechanism of action:** *Rifampin* blocks RNA transcription by interacting with the β subunit of mycobacterial DNA-dependent RNA polymerase.

    b. **Antimicrobial spectrum:** *Rifampin* is bactericidal for both intracellular and extracellular mycobacteria, including M. tuberculosis, and NTM, such as M. kansasii and Mycobacterium avium complex (MAC). It is effective against many gram-positive and gram-negative organisms and is used prophylactically for

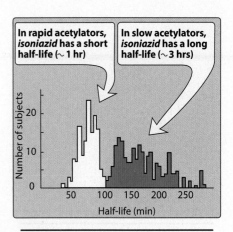

Figure 41.4
Bimodal distribution of *isoniazid* half-lives caused by rapid and slow acetylation of the drug.

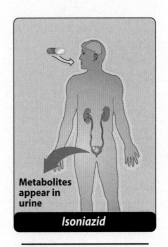

Figure 41.5
Administration and fate of *isoniazid*.

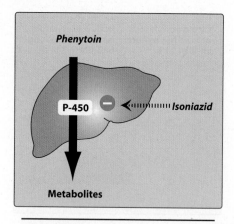

Figure 41.6
Isoniazid potentiates the adverse effects of *phenytoin*.

individuals exposed to meningitis caused by meningococci or Haemophilus influenzae. *Rifampin* also is highly active against M. leprae.

c. Resistance: Resistance to *rifampin* is caused by mutations in the affinity of the bacterial DNA-dependent RNA polymerase gene for the drug.

d. Pharmacokinetics: Absorption is adequate after oral administration. Distribution of *rifampin* occurs to all body fluids and organs. Concentrations attained in the CSF are variable, often 10% to 20% of blood concentrations. The drug is taken up by the liver and undergoes enterohepatic recycling. *Rifampin* can induce hepatic cytochrome P450 enzymes and transporters (see Chapter 1), leading to numerous drug interactions. Unrelated to its effects on cytochrome P450 enzymes, *rifampin* undergoes autoinduction, leading to a shortened elimination half-life over the first 1 to 2 weeks of dosing. Elimination of *rifampin* and its metabolites is primarily through the bile and into the feces; a small percentage is cleared in the urine (Figure 41.7). [Note: Urine, feces, and other secretions have an orange-red color, so patients should be forewarned. Tears may even stain soft contact lenses orange-red.]

e. Adverse effects: *Rifampin* is generally well tolerated. The most common adverse reactions include nausea, vomiting, and rash. Hepatitis and death due to liver failure are rare. However, the drug should be used judiciously in older patients, alcoholics, or those with chronic liver disease. There is a modest increase in the incidence of hepatic dysfunction when *rifampin* is coadministered with *isoniazid*. When *rifampin* is dosed intermittently, especially with doses of 1.2 g or greater, a flu-like syndrome can occur, with fever, chills, and myalgia, sometimes extending to acute renal failure, hemolytic anemia, and shock.

f. Drug interactions: Because *rifampin* induces a number of phase I cytochrome P450 enzymes and phase II enzymes (see Chapter 1), it can decrease the half-lives of coadministered drugs that are metabolized by these enzymes (Figure 41.8). This may necessitate higher dosages for coadministered drugs, a switch to drugs less affected by *rifampin*, or replacement of *rifampin* with *rifabutin*.

2. Rifabutin: *Rifabutin* [rif-a-BYOO-tin], a derivative of *rifampin*, is preferred for TB patients coinfected with the human immunodeficiency virus (HIV) who are receiving protease inhibitors (PIs) or several of the non-nucleoside reverse transcriptase inhibitors (NNRTIs). *Rifabutin* is a less potent inducer (approximately 40% less) of cytochrome P450 enzymes, thus lessening certain drug interactions. *Rifabutin* has adverse effects similar to those of *rifampin* but can also cause uveitis, skin hyperpigmentation, and neutropenia.

3. Rifapentine: *Rifapentine* [rih-fa-PEN-teen] has activity greater than that of *rifampin* in animal and in vitro studies, and it also has a longer half-life. In combination with *isoniazid*, *rifapentine* may be

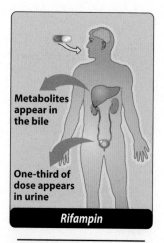

Figure 41.7
Administration and fate of *rifampin*. [Note: Patient should be warned that urine and tears may turn orange-red in color.]

used once weekly in patients with LTBI and in select HIV-negative patients with minimal pulmonary TB.

D. Pyrazinamide

Pyrazinamide [peer-a-ZIN-a-mide] is a synthetic, orally effective short-course agent used in combination with *isoniazid*, *rifampin*, and *ethambutol*. The precise mechanism of action is unclear. *Pyrazinamide* must be enzymatically hydrolyzed by pyrazinamidase to pyrazinoic acid, which is the active form of the drug. Some resistant strains lack the pyrazinamidase enzyme. *Pyrazinamide* is active against tuberculosis bacilli in acidic lesions and in macrophages. The drug distributes throughout the body, penetrating the CSF. *Pyrazinamide* may contribute to liver toxicity. Uric acid retention is common but rarely precipitates a gouty attack. Most of the clinical benefit from *pyrazinamide* occurs early in treatment. Therefore, this drug is usually discontinued after 2 months of a 6-month regimen.

E. Ethambutol

Ethambutol [e-THAM-byoo-tole] is bacteriostatic and specific for mycobacteria. *Ethambutol* inhibits arabinosyl transferase—an enzyme important for the synthesis of the mycobacterial cell wall. *Ethambutol* is used in combination with *pyrazinamide*, *isoniazid*, and *rifampin* pending culture and susceptibility data. [Note: *Ethambutol* may be discontinued if the isolate is determined to be susceptible to *isoniazid*, *rifampin*, and *pyrazinamide*.] *Ethambutol* is well distributed throughout the body. Penetration into the CNS is minimal, and it is questionably adequate for tuberculous meningitis. Both the parent drug and metabolites are primarily excreted in the urine. The most important adverse effect is optic neuritis, which results in diminished visual acuity and loss of ability to discriminate between red and green. The risk of optic neuritis increases with higher doses and in patients with renal impairment. Visual acuity and color discrimination should be tested prior to initiating therapy and periodically thereafter. Uric acid excretion is decreased by *ethambutol*, and caution should be exercised in patients with gout.

Figure 41.9 summarizes some of the characteristics of first-line drugs.

F. Alternate second-line drugs

Streptomycin [strep-toe-MY-sin], *para-aminosalicylic* [a-mee-noe-sal-i-SIL-ik] *acid*, *capreomycin* [kap-ree-oh-MYE-sin], *cycloserine* [sye-kloe-SER-een], *ethionamide* [e-thye-ON-am-ide], fluoroquinolones, and macrolides are second-line TB drugs. In general, these agents are less effective and more toxic than the first-line agents. Figure 41.10 summarizes some of the characteristics of second-line drugs.

1. **Streptomycin:** *Streptomycin*, an aminoglycoside antibiotic, was one of the first effective agents for TB (see Chapter 39). Its action appears to be greater against extracellular organisms. Infections due to *streptomycin*-resistant organisms may be treated with *kanamycin* or *amikacin*, to which these bacilli usually remain susceptible.

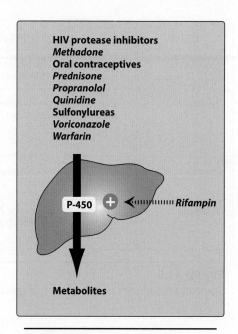

HIV protease inhibitors
Methadone
Oral contraceptives
Prednisone
Propranolol
Quinidine
Sulfonylureas
Voriconazole
Warfarin

P-450 + ⇐ *Rifampin*

Metabolites

Figure 41.8
Induces cytochrome P450, which can decrease the half-lives of coadministered drugs that are metabolized by this system.

DRUG	ADVERSE EFFECTS	COMMENTS
Ethambutol	Optic neuritis with blurred vision, red-green color blindness	Establish baseline visual acuity and color vision; test monthly.
Isoniazid	Hepatic enzyme elevation, hepatitis, peripheral neuropathy	Take baseline hepatic enzyme measurements; repeat if abnormal or patient is at risk or symptomatic. Clinically significant interaction with *phenytoin* and *carbamazepine*.
Pyrazinamide	Nausea, hepatitis, hyperuricemia, rash, joint ache, gout (rare)	Take baseline hepatic enzymes and uric acid measurements; repeat if abnormal or patient is at risk or symptomatic.
Rifampin	Hepatitis, GI upset, rash, flu-like syndrome, significant interaction with several drugs	Take baseline hepatic enzyme measurements and CBC; repeat if abnormal or patient is at risk or symptomatic. Warn patient that urine and tears may turn red-orange in color.

Figure 41.9
Some characteristics of first-line drugs used in treating tuberculosis. CBC = complete blood count. GI = gastrointestinal.

2. **Para-aminosalicylic acid:** *Para-aminosalicylic acid* (*PAS*) was another one of the original TB medications. From the early 1950s until well into the 1960s, *isoniazid*, *PAS*, plus *streptomycin* was the standard 18-month treatment regimen. While largely replaced by *ethambutol* for drug-susceptible TB, *PAS* remains an important component of many regimens for MDR-TB.

3. **Capreomycin:** This is a parenterally administered polypeptide that inhibits protein synthesis. *Capreomycin* is primarily reserved for the treatment of MDR-TB. Careful monitoring is necessary to minimize nephrotoxicity and ototoxicity.

DRUG	ADVERSE EFFECTS	COMMENTS
Fluoroquinolones	GI intolerance, tendonitis, CNS toxicity including caffeine-like effects	Monitor LFTs, serum creatinine / BUN, QT interval prolongation. Avoid concomitant ingestion with antacids, multivitamins or drugs containing di- or trivalent cations.
Aminoglycosides, Capreomycin	Nephrotoxicity, ototoxicity	Not available orally. Monitor for vestibular, auditory and renal toxicity.
Macrolides	GI intolerance, tinnitus	Monitor LFTs, serum creatinine / BUN, QT interval prolongation. Monitor for drug interactions due to CYP inhibition (except *azithromycin*).
Ethionamide	GI intolerance, hepatotoxicity, hypothyroidism	Monitor LFTs, TSH. A majority of patients experience GI intolerance. Cross-resistance with *isoniazid* is possible.
Para-aminosalicylic acid (PAS)	GI intolerance, hepatotoxicity, hypothyroidism	Monitor LFTs, TSH. Patients with glucose-6 phosphate dehydrogenase (G6PD) deficiency are at increased risk of hemolytic anemia.
Cycloserine	CNS toxicity	Close monitoring is needed for depression, anxiety, confusion, etc. Seizures may be exacerbated in patients with epilepsy. Monitor serum creatinine.

BUN = blood urea nitrogen; CNS = central nervous system; GI = gastrointestinal; LFTs = liver function tests; TSH = thyroid-stimulating hormone

Figure 41.10
Some characteristics of second-line drugs used in treating tuberculosis.

4. **Cycloserine:** This is an orally effective, tuberculostatic drug that disrupts D-alanine incorporation into the bacterial cell wall. It distributes well throughout body fluids, including the CSF. *Cycloserine* is primarily excreted unchanged in urine. Accumulation occurs with renal insufficiency. Adverse effects involve CNS disturbances (for example, lethargy, difficulty concentrating, anxiety, and suicidal tendency), and seizures may occur.

5. **Ethionamide:** This is a structural analog of *isoniazid* that also disrupts mycolic acid synthesis. The mechanism of action is not identical to *isoniazid*, but there is some overlap in the resistance patterns. *Ethionamide* is widely distributed throughout the body, including the CSF. Metabolism is extensive, most likely in the liver, to active and inactive metabolites. Adverse effects that limit its use include nausea, vomiting, and hepatotoxicity. Hypothyroidism, gynecomastia, alopecia, impotence, and CNS effects also have been reported.

6. **Fluoroquinolones:** The fluoroquinolones, specifically *moxifloxacin* and *levofloxacin*, have an important place in the treatment of multidrug-resistant tuberculosis. Some NTM also are susceptible. These drugs are discussed in detail in Chapter 40.

7. **Macrolides:** The macrolides *azithromycin* and *clarithromycin* are included in regimens for several NTM infections, including MAC. *Azithromycin* may be preferred for patients at greater risk for drug interactions (*clarithromycin* is a both a substrate and inhibitor of cytochrome P450 enzymes). Details about the pharmacology of macrolides are found in Chapter 39.

8. **Bedaquiline:** *Bedaquiline* [bed-AK-wi-leen], an ATP synthase inhibitor, is the first in a new class of drugs approved for the treatment of MDR-TB. *Bedaquiline* is administered orally, and it is active against many types of mycobacteria. *Bedaquiline* may cause QT prolongation, and monitoring of the electrocardiogram is recommended. This agent is a CYP3A4 substrate, and administration with strong CYP3A4 inducers (for example, *rifampin*) should be avoided.

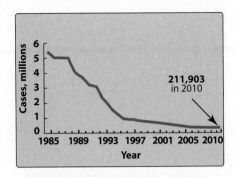

Figure 41.11
Reported prevalence of leprosy worldwide.

III. DRUGS FOR LEPROSY

Leprosy (or Hansen's disease) is uncommon in the United States; however, worldwide it is a much larger problem (Figure 41.11). Leprosy can be treated effectively with *dapsone* and *rifampin*, adding *clofazimine* in multibacillary cases (Figure 41.12).

A. Dapsone

Dapsone [DAP-sone] is structurally related to the sulfonamides and similarly inhibits dihydropteroate synthetase in the folate synthesis pathway. It is bacteriostatic for M. leprae, and resistant strains may be encountered. *Dapsone* also is used in the treatment of pneumonia caused by Pneumocystis jirovecii in immunosuppressed patients. The drug is well absorbed from the gastrointestinal tract and is distributed

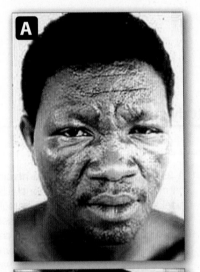

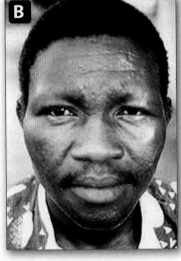

Figure 41.12
Leprosy patient. **A.** Before therapy. **B.** After 6 months of multidrug therapy.

throughout the body, with high concentrations in the skin. The parent drug undergoes hepatic acetylation. Both parent drug and metabolites are eliminated in the urine. Adverse reactions include hemolysis (especially in patients with glucose-6-phosphate dehydrogenase deficiency), methemoglobinemia, and peripheral neuropathy.

B. Clofazimine

Clofazimine [kloe-FAZ-i-meen] is a phenazine dye. Its mechanism of action may involve binding to DNA, although alternative mechanisms have been proposed. Its redox properties may lead to the generation of cytotoxic oxygen radicals that are toxic to the bacteria. *Clofazimine* is bactericidal to M. leprae, and it has potentially useful activity against M. tuberculosis and NTM. Following oral absorption, the drug accumulates in tissues, allowing intermittent therapy but does not enter the CNS. Patients typically develop a pink to brownish-black discoloration of the skin and should be informed of this in advance. Eosinophilic and other forms of enteritis, sometimes requiring surgery, have been reported. *Clofazimine* has some anti-inflammatory and anti-immune activities. Thus, erythema nodosum leprosum may not develop in patients treated with this drug.

Study Questions

Choose the ONE best answer.

41.1 A 35-year-old male, formerly a heroin abuser, has been on methadone maintenance for the last 13 months. Two weeks ago, he had a positive tuberculosis skin test (PPD test), and a chest radiograph showed evidence of right upper lobe infection. He was started on standard four-drug antimycobacterial therapy. He has come to the emergency department complaining of "withdrawal symptoms." Which of the following antimycobacterial drugs is likely to have caused this patient's acute withdrawal reaction?

A. Ethambutol.
B. Isoniazid.
C. Pyrazinamide.
D. Rifampin.
E. Streptomycin.

Correct answer = D. Rifampin is a potent inducer of cytochrome P450–dependent drug-metabolizing enzymes. The duration of action of methadone is dependent upon hepatic clearance, so enhanced drug metabolism will shorten the duration and increase the risk of withdrawal symptoms in individuals on methadone maintenance. None of the other drugs listed induce cytochrome P450 enzymes.

41.2 A 42-year-old male HIV patient was recently diagnosed with active tuberculosis. Currently, he is on a stable HIV regimen consisting of two protease inhibitors and two nucleoside reverse transcriptase inhibitors (NRTIs). What is the most appropriate regimen to use for treatment of his tuberculosis?

A. Rifampin + isoniazid + pyrazinamide + ethambutol.
B. Rifabutin + isoniazid + pyrazinamide + ethambutol.
C. Rifapentine + isoniazid + pyrazinamide + ethambutol.
D. Rifampin + moxifloxacin + pyrazinamide + ethambutol.
E. Amikacin + moxifloxacin + cycloserine + streptomycin.

Correct answer = B. Rifabutin is recommended in place of rifampin in patients coinfected with HIV, since it is a less potent inducer of CYP enzymes than rifampin. However, rifabutin is a CYP3A4 substrate and "bidirectional" interactions may result. Other medications, such as the protease inhibitors, may affect the concentration of rifabutin, requiring a dose adjustment. Answer E is incorrect as these are not first-line agents.

41.3 Which of the following is correct regarding clofazimine in the treatment of leprosy?

A. Clofazimine should not be used in patients with a deficiency in glucose-6-phosphate dehydrogenase (G6PD).

B. Peripheral neuropathy is one of the most common adverse effects seen with the drug.

C. Clofazimine may cause skin discoloration over time.

D. The risk of erythema nodosum leprosum is increased in patients given clofazimine.

Correct answer = C. Clofazimine is a phenazine dye and will cause bronzing (the skin pigment color will change color, from pink to brownish-black), especially in fair-skinned patients. This occurs in a majority of patients, and generally is not considered harmful but may take several months to years to fade after discontinuing the medication.

41.4 A 24-year-old male has returned to the clinic for his 1-month check-up after starting treatment for tuberculosis. He is receiving isoniazid, rifampin, pyrazinamide, and ethambutol. He states he feels fine, but now is having difficulty reading his morning newspaper and feels he may need to get glasses. Which of the following drugs may be causing his decline in vision?

A. Isoniazid.

B. Rifampin.

C. Pyrazinamide.

D. Ethambutol.

Correct answer = D. Optic neuritis, exhibited as a decrease in visual acuity or loss of color discrimination, is the most important side effect associated with ethambutol. Visual disturbances generally are dose related and more common in patients with reduced renal function. They are reversible (weeks to months) if ethambutol is discontinued promptly.

Antifungal Drugs

Jamie Kisgen

42

I. OVERVIEW

Infectious diseases caused by fungi are called mycoses, and they are often chronic in nature. Mycotic infections may be superficial and involve only the skin (cutaneous mycoses extending into the epidermis), while others may penetrate the skin, causing subcutaneous or systemic infections. The characteristics of fungi are so unique and diverse that they are classified in their own kingdom. Unlike bacteria, fungi are eukaryotic, with rigid cell walls composed largely of chitin rather than peptidoglycan (a characteristic component of most bacterial cell walls). In addition, the fungal cell membrane contains ergosterol rather than the cholesterol found in mammalian membranes. These structural characteristics are useful in targeting chemotherapeutic agents against fungal infections. Fungal infections are generally resistant to antibiotics, and, conversely, bacteria are resistant to antifungal agents. The incidence of fungal infections such as candidemia has been on the rise for the last few decades. This is attributed to an increased number of patients with chronic immune suppression due to organ transplantation, cancer chemotherapy, or infection with human immunodeficiency virus (HIV). During this same period, new therapeutic options have become available for the treatment of fungal infections. Figure 42.1 summarizes clinically useful agents for cutaneous and systemic mycoses. Figure 42.2 lists the common pathogenic organisms of the Kingdom Fungi, and Figure 42.3 provides an overview of the mechanism of action of the various antifungal agents.

II. DRUGS FOR SUBCUTANEOUS AND SYSTEMIC MYCOTIC INFECTIONS

A. Amphotericin B

Amphotericin [am-foe-TER-i-sin] *B* is a naturally occurring polyene antifungal produced by <u>Streptomyces</u> <u>nodosus</u>. In spite of its toxic potential, *amphotericin B* remains the drug of choice for the treatment of several life-threatening mycoses.

1. **Mechanism of action:** *Amphotericin B* binds to ergosterol in the plasma membranes of sensitive fungal cells. There, it forms pores (channels) that require hydrophobic interactions between

DRUGS FOR SUBCUTANEOUS AND SYSTEMIC MYCOSES
Amphotericin B VARIOUS
Anidulafungin ERAXIS
Caspofungin CANCIDAS
Fluconazole DIFLUCAN
Flucytosine ANCOBON
Itraconazole SPORANOX
Ketoconazole NIZORAL
Micafungin MYCAMINE
Posaconazole NOXAFIL
Voriconazole VFEND

DRUGS FOR CUTANEOUS MYCOSES
Butenafine LOTRIMIN ULTRA
Butoconazole GYNAZOLE
Clotrimazole LOTRIMIN AF
Ciclopirox PENLAC
Econazole ECOZA
Griseofulvin GRIFULVIN V, GRIS-PEG
Miconazole FUNGOID, MICATIN, MONISTAT
Naftifine NAFTIN
Nystatin MYCOSTATIN
Oxiconazole OXISTAT
Sertaconazole ERTACZO
Sulconazole EXELDERM
Terbinafine LAMISIL
Terconazole TERAZOL
Tioconazole VAGISTAT-1
Tolnaftate TINACTIN

Figure 42.1
Summary of antifungal drugs.

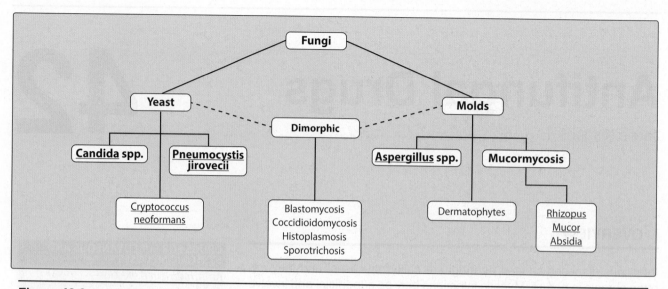

Figure 42.2
Common pathogenic organisms of Kingdom Fungi.

the lipophilic segment of the polyene antifungal and the sterol (Figure 42.4). The pores disrupt membrane function, allowing electrolytes (particularly potassium) and small molecules to leak from the cell, resulting in cell death.

2. **Antifungal spectrum:** *Amphotericin B* is either fungicidal or fungistatic, depending on the organism and the concentration of the drug. It is effective against a wide range of fungi, including <u>Candida albicans</u>, <u>Histoplasma capsulatum</u>, <u>Cryptococcus neoformans</u>,

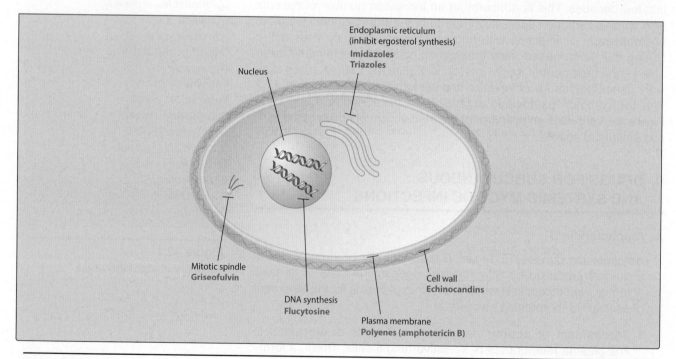

Figure 42.3
Cellular targets of antifungal drugs.

Coccidioides immitis, Blastomyces dermatitidis, and many strains of Aspergillus. [Note: *Amphotericin B* is also used in the treatment of the protozoal infection leishmaniasis.]

3. **Resistance:** Fungal resistance, although infrequent, is associated with decreased ergosterol content of the fungal membrane.

4. **Pharmacokinetics:** *Amphotericin B* is administered by slow, intravenous (IV) infusion (Figure 42.5). *Amphotericin B* is insoluble in water and must be coformulated with either sodium deoxycholate (conventional) or a variety of artificial lipids to form liposomes. The liposomal preparations have the primary advantage of reduced renal and infusion toxicity. However, due to high cost, liposomal preparations are reserved mainly as salvage therapy for patients who cannot tolerate conventional *amphotericin B*. *Amphotericin B* is extensively bound to plasma proteins and is distributed throughout the body. Inflammation favors penetration into various body fluids, but little of the drug is found in the CSF, vitreous humor, or amniotic fluid. However, *amphotericin B* does cross the placenta. Low levels of the drug and its metabolites appear in the urine over a long period of time, and some are also eliminated via the bile. Dosage adjustment is not required in patients with hepatic dysfunction, but when conventional *amphotericin B* causes renal dysfunction, the total daily dose is decreased by 50%.

5. **Adverse effects:** *Amphotericin B* has a low therapeutic index. The total adult daily dose of the conventional formulation should not exceed 1.5 mg/kg/d, whereas lipid formulations have been given safely in doses up to 10 mg/kg/d. Toxic manifestations are outlined below (Figure 42.6).

    a. **Fever and chills:** These occur most commonly 1 to 3 hours after starting the IV administration but usually subside with repeated administration of the drug. Premedication with a corticosteroid or an antipyretic helps to prevent this problem.

    b. **Renal impairment:** Despite the low levels of the drug excreted in the urine, patients may exhibit a decrease in glomerular filtration rate and renal tubular function. Serum creatinine may increase, creatinine clearance can decrease, and potassium and magnesium are lost. Renal function usually returns with discontinuation of the drug, but residual damage is likely at high doses. Azotemia is exacerbated by other nephrotoxic drugs, such as aminoglycosides, *cyclosporine, pentamidine,* and *vancomycin*, although adequate hydration can decrease its severity. To minimize nephrotoxicity, sodium loading with infusions of normal saline and the lipid-based *amphotericin B* products can be used.

    c. **Hypotension:** A shock-like fall in blood pressure accompanied by hypokalemia may occur, requiring potassium supplementation. Care must be exercised in patients taking *digoxin* and other drugs that can cause potassium fluctuations.

    d. **Thrombophlebitis:** Adding *heparin* to the infusion can alleviate this problem.

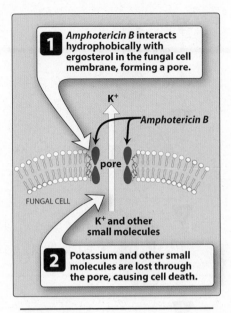

Figure 42.4
Model of a pore formed by *amphotericin B* in the lipid bilayer membrane.

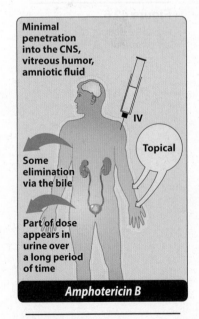

Figure 42.5
Administration and fate of *amphotericin B*. CNS = central nervous system.

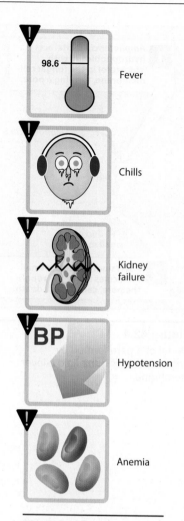

Figure 42.6
Adverse effects of
amphotericin B.

B. Antimetabolite antifungals

Flucytosine [floo-SYE-toe-seen] (*5-FC*) is a synthetic pyrimidine antimetabolite that is often used in combination with *amphotericin B*. This combination of drugs is administered for the treatment of systemic mycoses and for meningitis caused by C. neoformans and C. albicans.

1. **Mechanism of action:** *5-FC* enters the fungal cell via a cytosine-specific permease, an enzyme not found in mammalian cells. It is subsequently converted to a series of compounds, including *5-fluorouracil* and 5-fluorodeoxyuridine 5′-monophosphate, which disrupt nucleic acid and protein synthesis (Figure 42.7). [Note: *Amphotericin B* increases cell permeability, allowing more *5-FC* to penetrate the cell and leading to synergistic effects.]

2. **Antifungal spectrum:** *5-FC* is fungistatic. It is effective in combination with *itraconazole* for treating chromoblastomycosis (causes skin and subcutaneous infections) and in combination with *amphotericin B* for treating candidiasis and cryptococcosis. *Flucytosine* can also be used for Candida urinary tract infections when *fluconazole* is not appropriate; however, resistance can occur with repeated use.

3. **Resistance:** Resistance due to decreased levels of any of the enzymes in the conversion of *5-FC* to *5-fluorouracil* (*5-FU*) and beyond or from increased synthesis of cytosine can develop during therapy. This is the primary reason that *5-FC* is not used as a single antimycotic drug. The rate of emergence of resistant fungal cells is lower with a combination of *5-FC* plus a second antifungal agent than it is with *5-FC* alone.

4. **Pharmacokinetics:** *5-FC* is well absorbed by the oral route. It distributes throughout the body water and penetrates well into the CSF. *5-FU* is detectable in patients and is probably the result of metabolism of *5-FC* by intestinal bacteria. Excretion of both the parent drug and its minimal metabolites is by glomerular filtration, and the dose must be adjusted in patients with compromised renal function.

5. **Adverse effects:** *5-FC* causes reversible neutropenia, thrombocytopenia, and dose-related bone marrow depression. Caution must be exercised in patients undergoing radiation or chemotherapy with drugs that depress bone marrow. Reversible hepatic dysfunction with elevation of serum transaminases and alkaline phosphatase may occur. Gastrointestinal disturbances (nausea, vomiting, and diarrhea) are common, and severe enterocolitis may also occur.

C. Azole antifungals

Azole antifungals are made up of two different classes of drugs—imidazoles and triazoles. Although these drugs have similar mechanisms of action and spectra of activity, their pharmacokinetics and therapeutic uses vary significantly. In general, imidazoles are given topically for cutaneous infections, whereas triazoles are given systemically for the treatment or prophylaxis of cutaneous and systemic fungal infections. [Note: Imidazole antifungals are discussed in the section on agents for cutaneous mycotic infections.] The triazole antifungals include *fluconazole*, *itraconazole*, *posaconazole*, and *voriconazole*.

1. **Mechanism of action:** Azoles are predominantly fungistatic. They inhibit C-14 α-demethylase (a cytochrome P450 [CYP450] enzyme), thereby blocking the demethylation of lanosterol to ergosterol, the principal sterol of fungal membranes (Figure 42.8). The inhibition of ergosterol biosynthesis disrupts membrane structure and function, which, in turn, inhibits fungal cell growth.

2. **Resistance:** Resistance to azole antifungals is becoming a significant clinical problem, particularly with protracted therapy required in immunocompromised patients, such as those who have advanced HIV infection or bone marrow transplant. Mechanisms of resistance include mutations in the C-14 α-demethylase gene that lead to decreased azole binding. Additionally, some strains of fungi have developed efflux pumps that pump the azole out of the cell.

3. **Drug interactions:** All azoles inhibit the hepatic CYP450 3A4 isoenzyme to varying degrees. Patients on concomitant medications that are substrates for this isoenzyme may have increased concentrations and risk for toxicity. Several azoles, including *itraconazole* and *voriconazole*, are metabolized by CYP450 3A4 and other CYP450 isoenzymes. Therefore, concomitant use of potent CYP450 inhibitors (for example, *ritonavir*) and inducers (for example, *rifampin*) can lead to increased adverse effects or clinical failure of these azoles, respectively.

4. **Contraindications:** Azoles are considered teratogenic, and they should be avoided in pregnancy unless the potential benefit outweighs the risk to the fetus.

D. Fluconazole

Fluconazole [floo-KON-a-zole] was the first member of the triazole class of antifungal agents. It is the least active of all triazoles, with most of its spectrum limited to yeasts and some dimorphic fungi. It has no role in the treatment of aspergillosis or zygomycosis. It is highly active against <u>Cryptococcus neoformans</u> and certain species of <u>Candida</u>, including <u>C</u>. <u>albicans</u> and <u>C</u>. <u>parapsilosis</u>. Resistance is a concern, however, with other species, including <u>C</u>. <u>krusei</u> and <u>C</u>. <u>glabrata</u>. *Fluconazole* is used for prophylaxis against invasive fungal infections in recipients of bone marrow transplants. It also is the drug of choice for <u>Cryptococcus neoformans</u> after induction therapy with *amphotericin B* and *flucytosine* and is used for the treatment of candidemia and coccidioidomycosis. *Fluconazole* is effective against most forms of mucocutaneous candidiasis. It is commonly used as a single-dose oral treatment for vulvovaginal candidiasis. *Fluconazole* is available in oral or IV dosage formulations. It is well absorbed after oral administration and distributes widely to body fluids and tissues. The majority of the drug is excreted unchanged via the urine, and doses must be reduced in patients with renal dysfunction. The most common adverse effects with *fluconazole* are nausea, vomiting, headache, and skin rashes. Hepatotoxicity can also occur, and the drug should be used with caution in patients with liver dysfunction.

E. Itraconazole

Itraconazole [it-ra-KON-a-zole] is a synthetic triazole that has a broad antifungal spectrum compared to *fluconazole*. *Itraconazole* is the drug of choice for the treatment of blastomycosis, sporotrichosis,

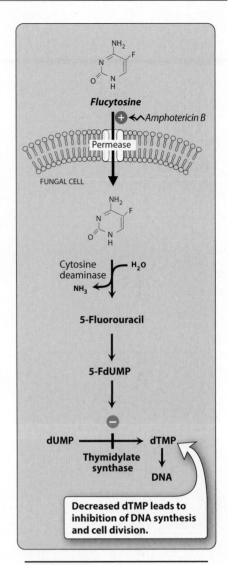

Figure 42.7
Mode of action of *flucytosine*. 5-FdUMP = 5-fluorodeoxyuridine 5′-monophosphate; dTMP = deoxythymidine 5′-monophosphate.

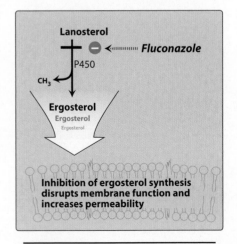

Figure 42.8
Mode of action of azole antifungals.

paracoccidioidomycosis, and histoplasmosis. It is rarely used for treatment of infections due to <u>Candida</u> and <u>Aspergillus</u> species because of the availability of newer and more effective agents. *Itraconazole* is available in two oral dosage forms, a capsule and an oral solution. The oral capsule should be taken with food, and ideally an acidic beverage, to increase absorption. In contrast, the solution should be taken on an empty stomach, as food decreases the absorption. The drug distributes well in most tissues, including bone and adipose tissues. *Itraconazole* is extensively metabolized by the liver, and the drug and inactive metabolites are excreted in the feces and urine. Adverse effects include nausea, vomiting, rash (especially in immunocompromised patients), hypokalemia, hypertension, edema, and headache. Hepatotoxicity can also occur, especially when given with other drugs that affect the liver. *Itraconazole* has a negative inotropic effect and should be avoided in patients with evidence of ventricular dysfunction, such as heart failure.

F. Posaconazole

Posaconazole [poe-sa-KONE-a-zole], a synthetic triazole, is a broad-spectrum antifungal structurally similar to *itraconazole*. It is available as an oral suspension, oral tablet, or IV formulation. *Posaconazole* is commonly used for the treatment and prophylaxis of invasive <u>Candida</u> and <u>Aspergillus</u> infections in severely immunocompromised patients. Due to its broad spectrum of activity, *posaconazole* is also used in the treatment of invasive fungal infections caused by <u>Scedosporium</u> and <u>Zygomycetes</u>. *Posaconazole* has a low oral bioavailability and should be given with food. Even though *posaconazole* has a long half-life, the suspension is usually given in divided doses throughout the day due to saturable absorption in the gut, whereas the tablet is given once daily. Unlike other azoles, *posaconazole* is not metabolized in the liver by CYP450 but is eliminated via glucuronidation. The most common adverse effects include gastrointestinal disturbances (nausea, vomiting, and diarrhea) and headaches. Like other azoles, *posaconazole* can cause an elevation in serum hepatic transaminases. Drugs that affect the gastric pH (for example, proton pump inhibitors) may decrease the absorption of oral *posaconazole* and should be avoided if possible. Due to its potent inhibition of CYP3A4, concomitant use of *posaconazole* with a number of agents (for example, ergot alkaloids, *atorvastatin*, *citalopram*, *risperidone*, *pimozide*, and *quinidine*) is contraindicated.

G. Voriconazole

Voriconazole [vor-i-KON-a-zole], a synthetic triazole related to *fluconazole*, has the advantage of being a broad-spectrum antifungal agent that is available in both IV and oral dosage forms. *Voriconazole* has replaced *amphotericin B* as the drug of choice for invasive aspergillosis. It is also approved for treatment of invasive candidiasis, as well as serious infections caused by <u>Scedosporium</u> and <u>Fusarium</u> species. *Voriconazole* has high oral bioavailability and penetrates into tissues well. Elimination is primarily by metabolism through the CYP450 enzymes. *Voriconazole* displays nonlinear kinetics, which can be affected by drug interactions and pharmacogenetic variability, particularly CYP450 2C19 polymorphisms. Adverse effects are similar to those of the other azoles; however, high trough concentrations are associated with visual and auditory hallucinations and an increased incidence of hepatotoxicity. *Voriconazole* is not only a substrate but also an inhibitor of CYP2C19, 2C9, and 3A4 isoenzymes. Inhibitors and inducers of these enzymes may impact levels of *voriconazole*, leading to toxicity or clinical failure, respectively. In addition, drugs that are substrates of these enzymes are impacted by *voriconazole* (Figure 42.9). Due to significant interactions, use of *voriconazole* is contraindicated with many drugs (for example, *rifampin, rifabutin, carbamazepine,* and the herb *St. John's wort*). Figures 42.10 and 42.11 summarize the azole antifungal agents.

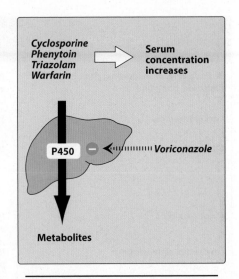

Figure 42.9
By inhibiting cytochrome P450, *voriconazole* can potentiate the toxicities of other drugs.

H. Echinocandins

Echinocandins interfere with the synthesis of the fungal cell wall by inhibiting the synthesis of $\beta(1,3)$-D-glucan, leading to lysis and cell death. *Caspofungin, micafungin,* and *anidulafungin* are available for IV administration once daily. *Micafungin* is the only echinocandin that does not require a loading dose. The echinocandins have potent activity against <u>Aspergillus</u> and most <u>Candida</u> species, including those species resistant to azoles. However, they have minimal activity against other fungi. All three agents are well tolerated, with the most common adverse effects being fever, rash, nausea, and phlebitis at the infusion site. They can also cause a histamine-like reaction (flushing) when infused too rapidly.

	FLUCONAZOLE	ITRACONAZOLE	VORICONAZOLE	POSACONAZOLE
SPECTRUM OF ACTIVITY	+	++	+++	++++
ROUTE(S) OF ADMINISTRATION	Oral, IV	Oral	Oral, IV	Oral, IV
ORAL BIOAVAILABILITY (%)	95	55 (solution)	96	Variable
DRUG LEVELS AFFECTED BY FOOD OR GASTRIC PH	No	Yes	No	Yes
PROTEIN BINDING (%)	10	99	58	99
PRIMARY ROUTE OF ELIMINATION	Renal	Hepatic CYP3A4	Hepatic CYP2C19, 2C9, 3A4	Hepatic Glucuronidation
CYTOCHROME P450 ENZYMES INHIBITED	CYP3A4, 2C9, 2C19	CYP3A4, 2C9	CYP2C19, 2C9, 3A4	CYP3A4
HALF-LIFE ($t_{1/2}$)	25 hours	30–40 hours	Dose Dependent	20–66 hours
CSF PENETRATION	Yes	No	Yes	Yes
RENAL EXCRETION OF ACTIVE DRUG (%)	> 90	< 2	< 2	< 2
TDM RECOMMENDED (RATIONALE)	No	Yes (Efficacy)	Yes (Efficacy and Safety)	Yes (Efficacy)

Figure 42.10
Summary of triazole antifungals. CSF = cerebrospinal fluid; TDM = therapeutic drug monitoring.

INTERACTING DRUG	DRUG	EFFECT ON DRUG EXPOSURE	MAIN CLINICAL CONSEQUENCE OF INTERACTION
Amiodarone, dronedarone, citalopram, pimozide, quinidine	*Itraconazole, fluconazole, voriconazole, posaconazole**	↑ exposure to interacting drugs	QT interval prolongation with risk of torsades de pointes
Carbamazepine	*Voriconazole*	↓ exposure to *voriconazole*	Treatment failure of *voriconazole*
Efavirenz	*Voriconazole*	↓ exposure to *voriconazole*	Treatment failure of *voriconazole*
		↑ exposure to *efavirenz*	Risk of *efavirenz* toxicity
Ergot alkaloids	*Itraconazole, fluconazole, voriconazole, posaconazole**	↑ exposure to ergot alkaloid	Ergotism
Lovastatin, simvastatin	*Itraconazole, voriconazole, posaconazole*	↑ exposure to HMG-CoA reductase inhibitor	Risk of rhabdomyolysis
Midazolam, triazolam	*Itraconazole, voriconazole, posaconazole*	↑ exposure to benzodiazepine	Sleepiness
Phenytoin	*Voriconazole, posaconazole*	↓ exposure to *voriconazole, posaconazole*	Treatment failure
		↑ exposure to *phenytoin*	Nystagmus, ataxia
Rifabutin	*Voriconazole, posaconazole*	↓ exposure to *voriconazole*	Treatment failure of *voriconazole*
		↑ exposure to *rifabutin*	Uveitis
Rifampicin (rifampin)	*Voriconazole, posaconazole*	↓ exposure to *voriconazole*	Treatment failure of *voriconazole*
High-dose *ritonavir* (400 mg twice daily)	*Voriconazole*	↓ exposure to *voriconazole*	Treatment failure of *voriconazole*
Vincristine, vinblastine	*Itraconazole, voriconazole, posaconazole*	↑ exposure to vinca alkaloids	Neurotoxicity
Sirolimus	*Voriconazole, posaconazole*	↑ exposure to *sirolimus*	Risk of *sirolimus* toxicity

Figure 42.11
Major or life-threatening drug interactions of azole drugs. ↑ indicates increased; ↓ indicates decreased. * Where an interaction has been reported for one triazole, the contraindication has been extended to all others.

1. **Caspofungin:** *Caspofungin* [kas-poh-FUN-jin] was the first member of the echinocandin class of antifungal drugs. *Caspofungin* is a first-line option for patients with invasive candidiasis, including candidemia, and a second-line option for invasive aspergillosis in patients who have failed or cannot tolerate *amphotericin B* or an azole. The dose of *caspofungin* does not need to be adjusted in renal impairment, but adjustment is warranted with moderate hepatic dysfunction. Concomitant administration of *caspofungin* with certain CYP450 enzyme inducers (for example, *rifampin*) may require an increase in the daily dose. *Caspofungin* should not be coadministered with *cyclosporine* due to a high incidence of elevated hepatic transaminases with concurrent use.

2. **Micafungin and anidulafungin:** *Micafungin* [mi-ka-FUN-jin] and *anidulafungin* [ay-nid-yoo-la-FUN-jin] are newer members of the echinocandin class of antifungal drugs. *Micafungin* and *anidulafungin* are first-line options for the treatment of invasive candidiasis, including candidemia. *Micafungin* is also indicated for the prophylaxis of invasive <u>Candida</u> infections in patients who are undergoing hematopoietic stem cell transplantation. *Micafungin* and *anidulafungin* do not need to be adjusted in renal impairment or mild to moderate hepatic dysfunction. *Anidulafungin* can be administered in severe hepatic dysfunction, but *micafungin* has not been studied in this condition. These agents are not substrates for CYP450 enzymes and do not have any associated drug interactions.

III. DRUGS FOR CUTANEOUS MYCOTIC INFECTIONS

Mold-like fungi that cause cutaneous infections are called dermatophytes or tinea. Tinea infections are classified by the affected site (for example, tinea pedis, which refers to an infection of the feet). Common dermatomycoses, such as tinea infections that appear as rings or round red patches with clear centers, are often referred to as "ringworm." This is a misnomer because fungi rather than worms cause the disease. The three different fungi that cause the majority of cutaneous infections are <u>Trichophyton</u>, <u>Microsporum</u>, and <u>Epidermophyton</u>. The drugs used in the treatment of cutaneous mycoses are listed in Figure 42.1.

A. Squalene epoxidase inhibitors

These agents act by inhibiting squalene epoxidase, thereby blocking the biosynthesis of ergosterol, an essential component of the fungal cell membrane (Figure 42.12). Accumulation of toxic amounts of squalene results in increased membrane permeability and death of the fungal cell.

1. **Terbinafine:** Oral *terbinafine* [TER-bin-a-feen] is the drug of choice for treating dermatophyte onychomycoses (fungal infections of nails). It is better tolerated, requires a shorter duration of therapy, and is more effective than either *itraconazole* or *griseofulvin*. Therapy is prolonged (usually about 3 months) but considerably shorter than that with *griseofulvin*. Oral *terbinafine* may also be used for tinea capitis (infection of the scalp). [Note: Oral antifungal therapy (*griseofulvin*, *terbinafine*, *itraconazole*) is needed for tinea capitis. Topical antifungals are ineffective.] Topical *terbinafine* (1% cream, gel or solution) is used to treat tinea pedis, tinea corporis (ringworm), and tinea cruris (infection of the groin). Duration of treatment is usually 1 week.

   a. **Antifungal spectrum:** *Terbinafine* is active against <u>Trichophyton</u>. It may also be effective against <u>Candida</u>, <u>Epidermophyton</u>, and <u>Scopulariopsis</u>, but the efficacy in treating clinical infections due to these pathogens has not been established.

   b. **Pharmacokinetics:** *Terbinafine* is available for oral and topical administration, although its bioavailability is only 40% due to first-pass metabolism. *Terbinafine* is highly protein bound and

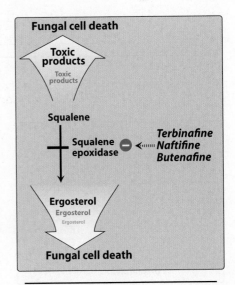

Figure 42.12
Mode of action of squalene epoxidase inhibitors.

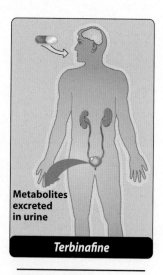

Figure 42.13
Administration and fate of *terbinafine*.

is deposited in the skin, nails, and adipose tissue. *Terbinafine* accumulates in breast milk and should not be given to nursing mothers. A prolonged terminal half-life of 200 to 400 hours may reflect the slow release from these tissues. Oral *terbinafine* is extensively metabolized by several CYP450 isoenzymes and is excreted mainly via the urine (Figure 42.13). The drug should be avoided in patients with moderate to severe renal impairment or hepatic dysfunction.

   c. Adverse effects: Common adverse effects of *terbinafine* include gastrointestinal disturbances (diarrhea, dyspepsia, and nausea), headache, and rash. Taste and visual disturbances have been reported, as well as transient elevations in serum hepatic transaminases. *Terbinafine* is an inhibitor of the CYP450 2D6 isoenzyme, and concomitant use with substrates of that isoenzyme may result in an increased risk of adverse effects with those agents.

2. Naftifine: *Naftifine* [NAF-ti-feen] is active against <u>Trichophyton</u>, <u>Microsporum</u>, and <u>Epidermophyton</u>. *Naftifine* 1% cream and gel are used for topical treatment of tinea corporis, tinea cruris, and tinea pedis. Duration of treatment is usually 2 weeks.

3. Butenafine: *Butenafine* [byoo-TEN-a-feen] is active against <u>Trichophyton</u> <u>rubrum</u>, <u>Epidermophyton</u>, and <u>Malassezia</u>. Like *naftifine*, *butenafine* 1% cream is used for topical treatment of tinea infections.

B. Griseofulvin

Griseofulvin [gris-ee-oh-FUL-vin] causes disruption of the mitotic spindle and inhibition of fungal mitosis (Figure 42.14). It has been largely replaced by oral *terbinafine* for the treatment of onychomycosis, although it is still used for dermatophytosis of the scalp and hair. *Griseofulvin* is fungistatic and requires a long duration of treatment (for example, 6 to 12 months for onychomycosis). Duration of therapy is dependent on the rate of replacement of healthy skin and nails. Ultrafine crystalline preparations are absorbed adequately from the gastrointestinal tract, and absorption is enhanced by high-fat meals. The drug concentrates in skin, hair, nails, and adipose tissue. *Griseofulvin* induces hepatic CYP450 activity, which increases the rate of metabolism of a number of drugs, including anticoagulants. The use of *griseofulvin* is contraindicated in pregnancy and patients with porphyria.

C. Nystatin

Nystatin [nye-STAT-in] is a polyene antifungal, and its structure, chemistry, mechanism of action, and resistance profile resemble those of *amphotericin B*. It is used for the treatment of cutaneous and oral <u>Candida</u> infections. The drug is negligibly absorbed from the gastrointestinal tract, and it is not used parenterally due to systemic toxicity (acute infusion-related adverse effects and nephrotoxicity). It is administered as an oral agent ("swish and swallow" or "swish and spit") for the treatment of oropharyngeal candidiasis (thrush), intravaginally for vulvovaginal candidiasis, or topically for cutaneous

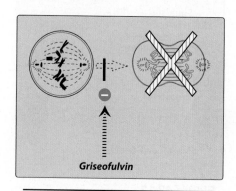

Figure 42.14
Inhibition of mitosis by *griseofulvin*.

candidiasis. Adverse effects are rare after oral administration, but nausea and vomiting occasionally occur. Topical and vaginal forms may cause skin irritation.

D. Imidazoles

Imidazoles are azole derivatives, which currently include *butoconazole* [byoo-toe-KON-a-zole], *clotrimazole* [kloe-TRIM-a-zole], *econazole* [e-KONE-a-zole], *ketoconazole* [kee-toe-KON-a-zole], *miconazole* [my-KON-a-zole], *oxiconazole* [oks-i-KON-a-zole], *sertaconazole* [ser-ta-KOE-na-zole], *sulconazole* [sul-KON-a-zole], *terconazole* [ter-KON-a-zole], and *tioconazole* [tye-oh-KONE-a-zole]. As a class of topical agents, they have a wide range of activity against Epidermophyton, Microsporum, Trichophyton, Candida, and Malassezia, depending on the agent. The topical imidazoles have a variety of uses, including tinea corporis, tinea cruris, tinea pedis, and oropharyngeal and vulvovaginal candidiasis. Topical use is associated with contact dermatitis, vulvar irritation, and edema. *Clotrimazole* is also available as a troche (lozenge), and *miconazole* is available as a buccal tablet for the treatment of thrush. Oral *ketoconazole* has historically been used for the treatment of systemic fungal infections but is rarely used today due to the risk for severe liver injury, adrenal insufficiency, and adverse drug interactions.

E. Ciclopirox

Ciclopirox [sye-kloe-PEER-oks] inhibits the transport of essential elements in the fungal cell, disrupting the synthesis of DNA, RNA, and proteins. *Ciclopirox* is active against Trichophyton, Epidermophyton, Microsporum, Candida, and Malassezia. It is available in a number of formulations. *Ciclopirox* 1% shampoo is used for treatment of seborrheic dermatitis. Tinea pedis, tinea corporis, tinea cruris, cutaneous candidiasis, and tinea versicolor may be treated with the 0.77% cream, gel, or suspension.

F. Tolnaftate

Tolnaftate [tole-NAF-tate] distorts the hyphae and stunts mycelial growth in susceptible fungi. *Tolnaftate* is active against Epidermophyton, Microsporum, and Malassezia furfur. [Note: *Tolnaftate* is not effective against Candida.] *Tolnaftate* is used to treat tinea pedis, tinea cruris, and tinea corporis. It is available as a 1% solution, cream, and powder.

Study Questions

Choose the ONE best answer.

42.1 Which of the following antifungal agents is MOST likely to cause renal insufficiency?

    A. Fluconazole.

    B. Amphotericin B.

    C. Itraconazole.

    D. Posaconazole.

Correct answer = B. Amphotericin B is the best choice since nephrotoxicity is commonly associated with this medication. Although the dose of fluconazole must be adjusted for renal insufficiency, it is not associated with causing nephrotoxicity. Itraconazole and posaconazole are metabolized by the liver and are not associated with nephrotoxicity.

42.2 A 55-year-old female presents to the hospital with shortness of breath, fever, and malaise. She has a history of breast cancer, which was diagnosed 3 months ago, and has been treated with chemotherapy. Her chest x-ray shows possible pneumonia, and respiratory cultures are positive for <u>Aspergillus fumigatus</u>. Which of the following is the MOST appropriate choice for treatment?

A. Voriconazole.

B. Fluconazole.

C. Flucytosine.

D. Ketoconazole.

> Correct answer = A. Voriconazole is the drug of choice for aspergillosis. Studies have found it to be superior to other regimens including amphotericin B. Fluconazole, flucytosine, and ketoconazole do not have reliable in vitro activity and are therefore not recommended.

42.3 Which of the following antifungal agents should be avoided in patients with evidence of ventricular dysfunction?

A. Micafungin.

B. Itraconazole.

C. Terbinafine.

D. Posaconazole.

> Correct answer = B. There is a black box warning that warns against the use of itraconazole in patients with evidence of ventricular dysfunction, including patients with heart failure.

42.4 A 56-year-old female with diabetes presents for routine foot evaluation with her podiatrist. The patient complains of thickening of the nail of the right big toe and a change in color (yellow). The podiatrist diagnoses the patient with onychomycosis of the toenails. Which of the following is the most appropriate choice for treating this infection?

A. Terbinafine.

B. Micafungin.

C. Itraconazole.

D. Griseofulvin.

> Correct answer = A. Terbinafine is better tolerated, requires a shorter duration of therapy, and is more effective than either itraconazole or griseofulvin. Micafungin is not active for this type of infection.

Antiprotozoal Drugs

Lisa Clayville Martin

43

I. OVERVIEW

Protozoal infections are common among people in underdeveloped tropical and subtropical countries, where sanitary conditions, hygienic practices, and control of the vectors of transmission are inadequate. However, with increased world travel, protozoal diseases are no longer confined to specific geographic locales. Because they are unicellular eukaryotes, the protozoal cells have metabolic processes closer to those of the human host than to prokaryotic bacterial pathogens. Therefore, protozoal diseases are less easily treated than bacterial infections, and many of the antiprotozoal drugs cause serious toxic effects in the host, particularly on cells showing high metabolic activity. Most antiprotozoal agents have not proven to be safe for pregnant patients. Drugs used to treat protozoal infections are summarized in Figure 43.1. [Note: Many of the drugs discussed below are not available in the United States; however, they are available in other world markets. In the United States, drugs for some protozoal infections may be obtained by contacting the Centers for Disease Control and Prevention.]

II. CHEMOTHERAPY FOR AMEBIASIS

Amebiasis (also called amebic dysentery) is an infection of the intestinal tract caused by <u>Entamoeba</u> <u>histolytica</u>. The disease can be acute or chronic, with varying degrees of illness, from no symptoms to mild diarrhea to fulminating dysentery. The diagnosis is established by isolating <u>E</u>. <u>histolytica</u> from feces. Therapy is indicated for acutely ill patients and asymptomatic carriers, since dormant <u>E</u>. <u>histolytica</u> may cause future infections in the carrier and be a potential source of infection for others. A summary of the life cycle of <u>E</u>. <u>histolytica</u> is presented in Figure 43.2. Therapeutic agents for amebiasis are classified as luminal, systemic, or mixed amebicides according to the site of action (Figure 43.2). For example, luminal amebicides act on the parasite in the lumen of the bowel, whereas systemic amebicides are effective against amebas in the intestinal wall and liver. Mixed amebicides are effective against both the luminal and systemic forms of the disease, although luminal concentrations are too low for single-drug treatment.

A. Mixed amebicides

   1. Metronidazole: *Metronidazole* [me-troe-NYE-da-zole], a nitroimidazole, is the mixed amebicide of choice for treating amebic infections. [Note: *Metronidazole* is also used in the treatment of

---

AMEBIASIS

Chloroquine ARALEN
Dehydroemetine DEHYDROEMETINE
Iodoquinol YODOXIN
Metronidazole FLAGYL
Paromomycin HUMATIN
Tinidazole TINDAMAX

MALARIA

Artemether/lumefantrine COARTEM
Atovaquone-proguanil MALARONE
Chloroquine ARALEN
Mefloquine LARIAM
Primaquine
Pyrimethamine DARAPRIM
Quinine/Quinidine QUALAQUIN,
QUINIDINE GLUCONATE

TRYPANOSOMIASIS

Benznidazole RADANIL
Eflornithine
Melarsoprol
Nifurtimox
Pentamidine NEBUPENT
Suramin GERMANIN

LEISHMANIASIS

Miltefosine IMPAVIDO
Sodium stibogluconate

TOXOPLASMOSIS

Pyrimethamine DARAPRIM

GIARDIASIS

Metronidazole FLAGYL
Nitazoxanide ALINIA
Tinidazole TINDAMAX

Figure 43.1
Summary of antiprotozoal agents.

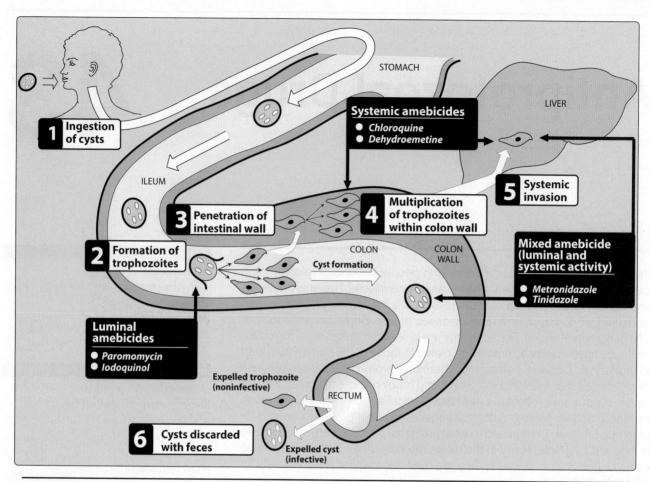

Figure 43.2
Life cycle of <u>Entamoeba</u> <u>histolytica</u>, showing the sites of action of amebicidal drugs.

infections caused by <u>Giardia</u> <u>lamblia</u>, <u>Trichomonas</u> <u>vaginalis</u>, anaerobic cocci, and anaerobic gram-negative bacilli (for example, <u>Bacteroides</u> species) and is the drug of choice for the treatment of pseudomembranous colitis caused by the anaerobic, gram-positive bacillus <u>Clostridium</u> <u>difficile</u>.]

a. **Mechanism of action:** Amebas possess ferredoxin-like, low-redox-potential, electron transport proteins that participate in metabolic electron removal reactions. The nitro group of *metronidazole* is able to serve as an electron acceptor, forming reduced cytotoxic compounds that bind to proteins and DNA, resulting in death of the <u>E</u>. <u>histolytica</u> trophozoites.

b. **Pharmacokinetics:** *Metronidazole* is completely and rapidly absorbed after oral administration. [Note: For the treatment of amebiasis, it is usually administered with a luminal amebicide, such as *iodoquinol* or *paromomycin*. This combination provides cure rates of greater than 90%.] *Metronidazole* distributes well throughout body tissues and fluids. Therapeutic levels can be found in vaginal and seminal fluids, saliva, breast milk, and cerebrospinal fluid (CSF). Metabolism of the drug depends on hepatic oxidation of the *metronidazole* side chain by mixed-function oxidase, followed by glucuronidation. Therefore, concomitant treatment with inducers of the cytochrome P450, such as *phenobarbital*, enhances the rate of metabolism, and inhibitors, such as *cimetidine*, prolong the plasma half-life of *metronidazole*. The drug accumulates in patients with severe hepatic disease. The parent drug and its metabolites are excreted in the urine.

c. **Adverse effects:** The most common adverse effects are nausea, vomiting, epigastric distress, and abdominal cramps (Figure 43.3). An unpleasant, metallic taste is commonly experienced. Other effects include oral moniliasis (yeast infection of the mouth) and, rarely, neurotoxicity (dizziness, vertigo, and numbness or paresthesia), which may necessitate discontinuation of the drug. If taken with alcohol, a *disulfiram*-like reaction may occur (see Chapter 15).

d. **Resistance:** Resistance to *metronidazole* is not a therapeutic problem for amebiasis, although strains of trichomonads resistant to the drug have been reported.

2. **Tinidazole:** *Tinidazole* [tye-NI-da-zole] is a second-generation nitroimidazole that is similar to *metronidazole* in spectrum of activity, absorption, adverse effects, and drug interactions. It is used for treatment of amebiasis, amebic liver abscess, giardiasis, and trichomoniasis. *Tinidazole* is as effective as *metronidazole*, with a shorter course of treatment, but it is more expensive. Alcohol consumption should be avoided during therapy.

B. Luminal amebicides

After treatment of invasive intestinal or extraintestinal amebic disease is complete, a luminal agent, such as *iodoquinol*, *diloxanide furoate*, or *paromomycin*, should be administered for treatment of the asymptomatic colonization state.

1. **Iodoquinol:** *Iodoquinol* [eye-oh-doe-QUIN-ole], a halogenated 8-hydroxyquinolone, is amebicidal against E. histolytica and is effective against the luminal trophozoite and cyst forms. Adverse effects of *iodoquinol* include rash, diarrhea, and dose-related peripheral neuropathy, including a rare optic neuritis. Long-term use of this drug should be avoided.

2. **Paromomycin:** *Paromomycin* [par-oh-moe-MYE-sin], an aminoglycoside antibiotic, is only effective against the intestinal (luminal) forms of E. histolytica, because it is not significantly absorbed from the gastrointestinal tract. *Paromomycin* is directly amebicidal and also exerts its antiamebic actions by reducing the population of intestinal flora. It is also an alternative agent for cryptosporidiosis and giardiasis. Gastrointestinal distress and diarrhea are the principal adverse effects.

C. Systemic amebicides

These drugs are useful for treating liver abscesses and intestinal wall infections caused by amebas.

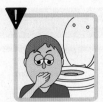
Nausea

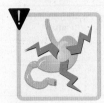
GI disturbance

Metallic taste

Figure 43.3
Adverse effects of *metronidazole*.

CLINICAL SYNDROME	DRUG
Asymptomatic cyst carriers	*Iodoquinol* or *paromomycin*
Diarrhea/dysentery Extraintestinal	*Metronidazole* plus *iodoquinol* or *paromomycin*
Amebic liver abscess	*Metronidazole* (or *tinidazole*) plus *iodoquinol* or *paromomycin*

Figure 43.4
Some commonly used therapeutic options for the treatment of amebiasis.

1. **Chloroquine:** *Chloroquine* [KLOR-oh-kwin] is used in combination with *metronidazole* (or as a substitute for one of the nitroimidazoles in the case of intolerance) to treat amebic liver abscesses. It eliminates trophozoites in liver abscesses, but it is not useful in treating luminal amebiasis. Therapy should be followed with a luminal amebicide. *Chloroquine* is also effective in the treatment of malaria.

2. **Dehydroemetine:** *Dehydroemetine* [de-hye-dro-EM-e-teen] is an alternative agent for the treatment of amebiasis. The drug inhibits protein synthesis by blocking chain elongation. Intramuscular injection is the preferred route, since it is an irritant when taken orally. The use of this ipecac alkaloid is limited by its toxicity, and it has largely been replaced by *metronidazole*. Adverse effects include pain at the site of injection, nausea, cardiotoxicity (arrhythmias and congestive heart failure), neuromuscular weakness, dizziness, and rash. A summary of the treatment of amebiasis is shown in Figure 43.4.

III. CHEMOTHERAPY FOR MALARIA

Malaria is an acute infectious disease caused by four species of the protozoal genus Plasmodium. It is transmitted to humans through the bite of a female Anopheles mosquito. Plasmodium falciparum is the most dangerous species, causing an acute, rapidly fulminating disease that is characterized by persistent high fever, orthostatic hypotension, and massive erythrocytosis (an abnormal elevation in the number of red blood cells accompanied by swollen, reddish limbs). P. falciparum infection can lead to capillary obstruction and death without prompt treatment. Plasmodium vivax causes a milder form of the disease. Plasmodium malariae is common to many tropical regions, but Plasmodium ovale is rarely encountered. Resistance acquired by the mosquito to insecticides, and by the parasite to drugs, has led to new therapeutic challenges, particularly in the treatment of P. falciparum. A summary of the life cycle of the parasite and the sites of action of the antimalarial drugs is presented in Figure 43.5.

A. Primaquine

Primaquine [PRIM-a-kwin], an 8-aminoquinoline, is an oral antimalarial drug that eradicates primary exoerythrocytic (tissue) forms of plasmodia and the secondary exoerythrocytic forms of recurring malarias (P. vivax and P. ovale). [Note: *Primaquine* is the only agent that prevents relapses of the P. vivax and P. ovale malarias, which may remain in the liver in the exoerythrocytic form after the erythrocytic form of the disease is eliminated.] The sexual (gametocytic) forms of all four plasmodia are destroyed in the plasma or are prevented from maturing later in the mosquito, thereby interrupting transmission of the disease. [Note: *Primaquine* is not effective against the erythrocytic stage of malaria and, therefore, is used in conjunction with agents to treat the erythrocytic form (for example, *chloroquine* and *mefloquine*).]

1. **Mechanism of action:** While not completely understood, metabolites of *primaquine* are believed to act as oxidants that are

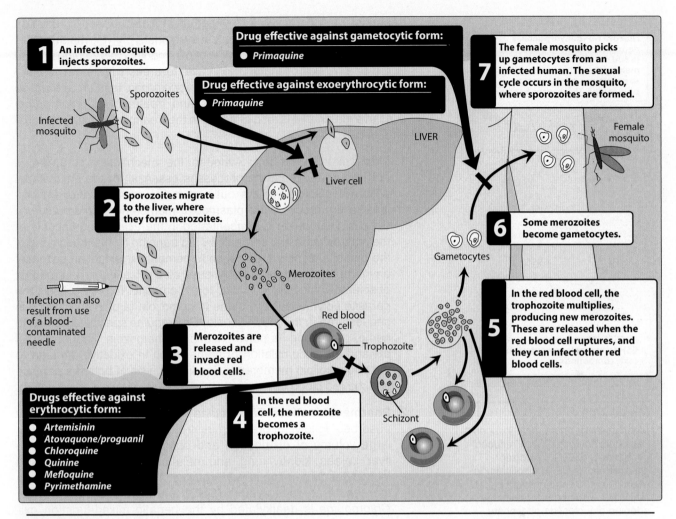

1 An infected mosquito injects sporozoites.

Drug effective against gametocytic form:
- *Primaquine*

Drug effective against exoerythrocytic form:
- *Primaquine*

7 The female mosquito picks up gametocytes from an infected human. The sexual cycle occurs in the mosquito, where sporozoites are formed.

Sporozoites

Infected mosquito

LIVER

Liver cell

Female mosquito

2 Sporozoites migrate to the liver, where they form merozoites.

Infection can also result from use of a blood-contaminated needle

Merozoites

6 Some merozoites become gametocytes.

Gametocytes

Red blood cell

Trophozoite

3 Merozoites are released and invade red blood cells.

5 In the red blood cell, the trophozoite multiplies, producing new merozoites. These are released when the red blood cell ruptures, and they can infect other red blood cells.

Drugs effective against erythrocytic form:
- *Artemisinin*
- *Atovaquone/proguanil*
- *Chloroquine*
- *Quinine*
- *Mefloquine*
- *Pyrimethamine*

4 In the red blood cell, the merozoite becomes a trophozoite.

Schizont

Figure 43.5
Life cycle of the malarial parasite, <u>Plasmodium</u> <u>falciparum</u>, showing the sites of action of antimalarial drugs.

responsible for the schizonticidal action as well as for the hemolysis and methemoglobinemia encountered as toxicities.

2. **Pharmacokinetics:** *Primaquine* is well absorbed after oral administration and is not concentrated in tissues. It is rapidly oxidized to many compounds, primarily the deaminated drug. Which compound possesses the schizonticidal activity has not been established. The drug is minimally excreted in the urine.

3. **Adverse effects:** *Primaquine* is associated with drug-induced hemolytic anemia in patients with glucose-6-phosphate dehydrogenase deficiency (Figure 43.6). Large doses of the drug may cause abdominal discomfort (especially when administered in combination with *chloroquine*) and occasional methemoglobinemia. *Primaquine* should not be used during pregnancy. All <u>Plasmodium</u> species may develop resistance to *primaquine*.

B. Chloroquine

Chloroquine is a synthetic 4-aminoquinoline that has been the mainstay of antimalarial therapy, and it is the drug of choice in the

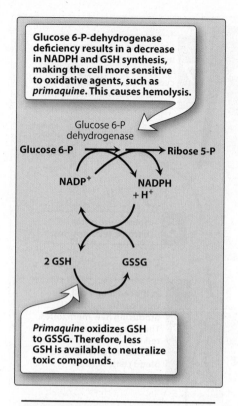

Figure 43.6

Mechanism of *primaquine-induced* hemolytic anemia. GSH = reduced glutathione; GSSG = oxidized glutathione; NADP$^+$ = nicotinamide adenine dinucleotide phosphate; NADPH = reduced nicotinamide adenine dinucleotide phosphate.

treatment of erythrocytic <u>P</u>. <u>falciparum</u> malaria, except in resistant strains. *Chloroquine* is less effective against <u>P</u>. <u>vivax</u> malaria. It is highly specific for the asexual form of plasmodia. *Chloroquine* is used in the prophylaxis of malaria for travel to areas with known *chloroquine*-sensitive malaria. [Note: *Hydroxychloroquine* is an alternative to *chloroquine* for the prophylaxis and treatment of *chloroquine*-sensitive malaria.] It is also effective in the treatment of extraintestinal amebiasis.

1. **Mechanism of action:** Although the mechanism of action is not fully understood, the processes essential for the antimalarial action of *chloroquine* are outlined in Figure 43.7. After traversing the erythrocytic and plasmodial membranes, *chloroquine* (a diprotic weak base) is concentrated in the acidic food vacuole of the malarial parasite, primarily by ion trapping. In the food vacuole, the parasite digests the host cell's hemoglobin to obtain essential amino acids. However, this process also releases large amounts of soluble heme, which is toxic to the parasite. To protect itself, the parasite polymerizes the heme to hemozoin (a pigment), which is sequestered in the food vacuole. *Chloroquine* specifically binds to heme, preventing its polymerization to hemozoin. The increased pH and the accumulation of heme result in oxidative damage to the phospholipid membranes, leading to lysis of both the parasite and the red blood cell.

2. **Pharmacokinetics:** *Chloroquine* is rapidly and completely absorbed following oral administration. The drug has a very large volume of distribution and concentrates in erythrocytes, liver, spleen, kidney, lung, and melanin-containing tissues, and leukocytes. It persists in erythrocytes. The drug also penetrates the central nervous system (CNS) and traverses the placenta. *Chloroquine* is dealkylated by the hepatic mixed-function oxidase system, and some metabolic products retain antimalarial activity. Both parent drug and metabolites are excreted predominantly in urine.

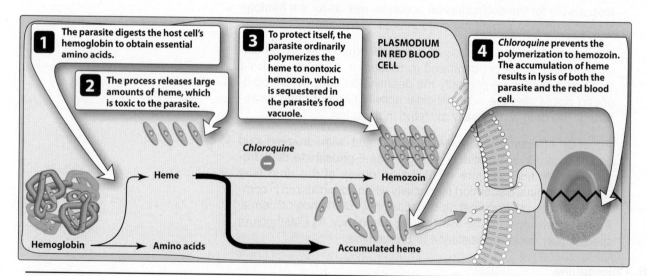

Figure 43.7

Action of *chloroquine* on the formation of hemozoin by <u>Plasmodium</u> species.

3. **Adverse effects:** Side effects are minimal at low prophylactic doses. At higher doses, gastrointestinal upset, pruritus, headaches, and blurred vision may occur (Figure 43.8). [Note: An ophthalmologic examination should be routinely performed.] Discoloration of the nail beds and mucous membranes may be seen on chronic administration. *Chloroquine* should be used cautiously in patients with hepatic dysfunction, severe gastrointestinal problems, or neurologic disorders. Patients with psoriasis or porphyria should not be treated with *chloroquine*, because an acute attack may be provoked. *Chloroquine* can prolong the QT interval, and use of other drugs that also cause QT prolongation should be avoided if possible.

4. **Resistance:** Resistance has become a serious medical problem throughout Africa, Asia, and most areas of Central and South America. *Chloroquine*-resistant P. falciparum exhibits multigenic alterations that confer a high level of resistance.

C. Atovaquone–proguanil

The combination of *atovaquone–proguanil* [a-TOE-va-kwone pro-GWA-nil] is effective for *chloroquine*-resistant strains of P. falciparum, and it is used in the prevention and treatment of malaria. *Atovaquone* inhibits mitochondrial processes such as electron transport, as well as ATP and pyrimidine biosynthesis. Cycloguanil, the active metabolite of *proguanil*, inhibits plasmodial dihydrofolate reductase, thereby preventing DNA synthesis. *Proguanil* is metabolized via CYP2C19, an isoenzyme that is known to exhibit a genetic polymorphism resulting in poor metabolism of the drug in some patients. The combination should be taken with food or milk to enhance absorption. Common adverse effects include nausea, vomiting, abdominal pain, headache, diarrhea, anorexia, and dizziness.

D. Mefloquine

Mefloquine [MEF-lo-kwin] is an effective single agent for prophylaxis and treatment of infections caused by multidrug-resistant forms of P. falciparum. Its exact mechanism of action remains undetermined. Resistant strains have been identified, particularly in Southeast Asia. *Mefloquine* is well absorbed after oral administration and is widely distributed to tissues. It has a long half-life (20 days) because of enterohepatic circulation and its concentration in various tissues. The drug undergoes extensive metabolism and is primarily excreted via the bile into the feces. Adverse reactions at high doses range from nausea, vomiting, and dizziness to disorientation, hallucinations, and depression. Because of the potential for neuropsychiatric reactions, *mefloquine* is usually reserved for treatment of malaria when other agents cannot be used. ECG abnormalities and cardiac arrest are possible if *mefloquine* is taken concurrently with *quinine* or *quinidine*.

E. Quinine

Quinine [KWYE-nine], originally isolated from the bark of the cinchona tree, interferes with heme polymerization, resulting in death of the erythrocytic form of the plasmodial parasite. It is reserved for severe infestations and for *chloroquine*-resistant malarial strains.

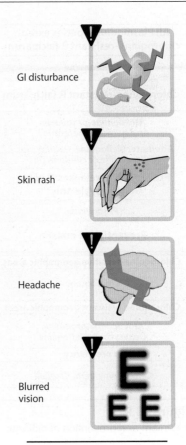

GI disturbance

Skin rash

Headache

Blurred vision

Figure 43.8
Some adverse effects commonly associated with *chloroquine*.

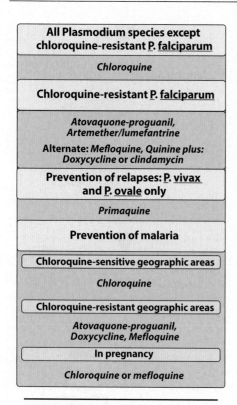

Figure 43.9
Treatment and prevention of malaria.

Quinine is usually administered in combination with *doxycycline*, *tetracycline*, or *clindamycin*. Taken orally, *quinine* is well distributed throughout the body. The major adverse effect of *quinine* is cinchonism, a syndrome causing nausea, vomiting, tinnitus, and vertigo. These effects are reversible and are not reasons for suspending therapy. However, *quinine* treatment should be suspended if hemolytic anemia occurs. Drug interactions include potentiation of neuromuscular-blocking agents and elevation of *digoxin* levels if taken concurrently. *Quinine* absorption is reduced by aluminum-containing antacids.

F. Artemisinin

Artemisinin [ar-te-MIS-in-in] is derived from the sweet wormwood plant, which has been used in traditional Chinese medicine for many centuries. *Artemisinin* and its derivatives are recommended first-line agents for the treatment of multidrug-resistant P. falciparum malaria. To prevent the development of resistance, these agents should not be used alone. For instance, *artemether* is coformulated with *lumefantrine* [AR-te-meth-er/loo-me-FAN-treen] and used for the treatment of uncomplicated malaria. [Note: *Lumefantrine* is an antimalarial drug similar in action to *quinine* or *mefloquine*.] *Artesunate* [ar-TEZ-oonate] may be combined with *sulfadoxine–pyrimethamine*, *mefloquine*, *clindamycin*, or others. The antimalarial action involves the production of free radicals resulting from cleavage of the drug's endoperoxide bridge by heme iron in the parasite food vacuole. These agents may also covalently bind to and damage specific malarial proteins. Oral, rectal, and intravenous (IV) preparations are available, but the short half-lives preclude the use of these drugs for prophylaxis. Adverse effects include nausea, vomiting, and diarrhea. High doses may cause prolongation of the QT interval. Hypersensitivity reactions and rash have occurred.

G. Pyrimethamine

Pyrimethamine [peer-i-METH-a-meen] inhibits plasmodial dihydrofolate reductase required for the synthesis of tetrahydrofolate (a cofactor needed for synthesis of nucleic acids). It acts as a blood schizonticide and a strong sporonticide when the mosquito ingests it with the blood of the human host. *Pyrimethamine* is not used alone for P. falciparum; it is available as a fixed-dose combination with *sulfadoxine*. Resistance to this combination has developed, so it is usually administered with other agents, such as *artemisinin* derivatives. *Pyrimethamine* in combination with *sulfadiazine* is also used against Toxoplasma gondii. If megaloblastic anemia occurs with *pyrimethamine* treatment, it may be reversed with *leucovorin*. Figure 43.9 shows some therapeutic options in the treatment of malaria.

IV. CHEMOTHERAPY FOR TRYPANOSOMIASIS

African trypanosomiasis (sleeping sickness) and American trypanosomiasis (also known as Chagas disease) are two chronic and, eventually, fatal diseases caused by species of Trypanosoma (Figure 43.10). In African sleeping sickness, T. brucei gambiense and T. brucei rhodesiense initially live and grow in the blood. The parasite later invades the CNS, causing inflammation of the brain and spinal cord that produces the characteristic lethargy and, eventually, continuous sleep. Chagas disease is caused by T. cruzi and is endemic in Central and South America. Antitrypanosomal drugs are outlined below.

A. Pentamidine

Pentamidine [pen-TAM-i-deen] is active against a variety of protozoal infections, including African trypanosomiasis due to T. brucei gambiense, for which it is used to treat the first stage (hemolymphatic stage without CNS involvement). *Pentamidine* is also an alternative for prophylaxis or treatment of infections caused by Pneumocystis jirovecii. [Note: P. jirovecii is an atypical fungus that causes pneumonia in immunocompromised patients, such as those with HIV infection. *Trimethoprim/sulfamethoxazole* is preferred in the treatment of P. jirovecii infections; however, *pentamidine* is an alternative in individuals who are allergic to sulfonamides.] *Pentamidine* is also an alternative drug for the treatment of leishmaniasis.

1. **Mechanism of action:** T. brucei concentrates *pentamidine* by an energy-dependent, high-affinity uptake system. [Note: Resistance is associated with inability to concentrate the drug.] Although its mechanism of action has not been defined, evidence exists that the drug interferes with parasite synthesis of RNA, DNA, phospholipids, and proteins.

2. **Pharmacokinetics:** *Pentamidine* is administered intramuscularly or intravenously for the treatment of trypanosomiasis and pneumonia caused by P. jirovecii. [Note: For prophylaxis of P. jirovecii pneumonia, *pentamidine* is administered via nebulizer.] The drug distributes widely and is concentrated in the liver, kidney, adrenals, spleen, and lungs. Because it does not enter the CSF, it is ineffective against the second stage (CNS involvement) of trypanosomiasis. The drug is not metabolized, and it is excreted very slowly in the urine.

3. **Adverse effects:** Serious renal dysfunction may occur, which is reversible on discontinuation. Other adverse reactions include hyperkalemia, hypotension, pancreatitis, hypoglycemia, hyperglycemia, and diabetes.

B. Suramin

Suramin [SOO-ra-min] is used primarily in the first stage (without CNS involvement) of African trypanosomiasis due to T. brucei rhodesiense. It is very reactive and inhibits many enzymes, especially those involved in energy metabolism, which appears to be the mechanism correlated with trypanocidal activity. *Suramin* must be injected intravenously. It binds to plasma proteins and does not penetrate the blood–brain barrier well. It has a long elimination half-life (more than 40 days) and is mainly excreted unchanged in the urine. Although infrequent, adverse reactions include nausea and vomiting, shock and loss of consciousness, acute urticaria, blepharitis, and neurologic problems, such as paresthesia, photophobia, and hyperesthesia of the hands and feet. Renal insufficiency may occur but tends

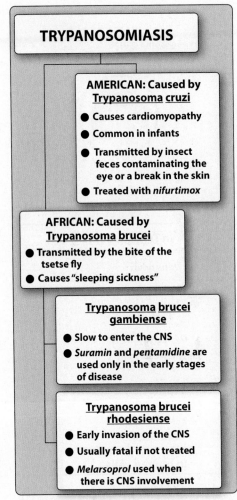

TRYPANOSOMIASIS

AMERICAN: Caused by Trypanosoma cruzi
- Causes cardiomyopathy
- Common in infants
- Transmitted by insect feces contaminating the eye or a break in the skin
- Treated with *nifurtimox*

AFRICAN: Caused by Trypanosoma brucei
- Transmitted by the bite of the tsetse fly
- Causes "sleeping sickness"

Trypanosoma brucei gambiense
- Slow to enter the CNS
- *Suramin* and *pentamidine* are used only in the early stages of disease

Trypanosoma brucei rhodesiense
- Early invasion of the CNS
- Usually fatal if not treated
- *Melarsoprol* used when there is CNS involvement

Figure 43.10
Summary of trypanosomiasis.
CNS = central nervous system.

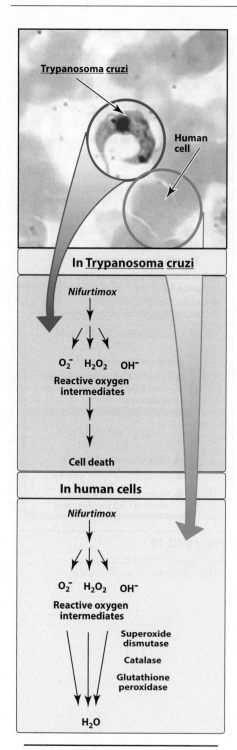

Figure 43.11
Generation of toxic intermediates by *nifurtimox*.

to resolve with discontinuation of treatment. Acute hypersensitivity reactions may occur, and a test dose should be given prior to drug administration.

C. Melarsoprol

Melarsoprol [mel-AR-so-prol], a trivalent arsenical compound, is used for the treatment of African trypanosomal infections in the second stage (CNS involvement). It is the only drug available for second-stage trypanosomiasis due to T. brucei rhodesiense. The drug reacts with sulfhydryl groups of various substances, including enzymes in both the organism and host. Some resistance has been noted, and it may be due to decreased transporter uptake of the drug. *Melarsoprol* is administered by slow IV injection and can be very irritating to the surrounding tissue. Adequate trypanocidal concentrations appear in the CSF, making *melarsoprol* the agent of choice in the treatment of T. brucei rhodesiense, which rapidly invades the CNS. The host readily oxidizes *melarsoprol* to a relatively nontoxic, pentavalent arsenic compound. The drug has a very short half-life and is rapidly excreted in urine. The use of *melarsoprol* is limited by CNS toxicity. Reactive encephalopathy may occur, which can be fatal in 10% of cases. Other adverse effects include peripheral neuropathy, hypertension, and albuminuria. Hypersensitivity reactions may also occur, and febrile reactions may follow injection. Hemolytic anemia has been seen in patients with glucose-6-phosphate dehydrogenase deficiency.

D. Eflornithine

Eflornithine [ee-FLOOR-nih-theen] is an irreversible inhibitor of ornithine decarboxylase. Inhibition of this enzyme halts the production of polyamines in the parasite, thereby leading to cessation of cell division. The IV formulation of *eflornithine* is a first-line treatment for second-stage African trypanosomiasis caused by T. brucei gambiense. [Note: Topical *eflornithine* is used as a treatment for unwanted facial hair in women.] The short half-life of *eflornithine* necessitates frequent IV administration, making the treatment regimen difficult to follow. *Eflornithine* is less toxic than *melarsoprol*, although the drug is associated with anemia, seizures, and temporary hearing loss.

E. Nifurtimox

Nifurtimox [nye-FER-tim-oks] is used in the treatment of T. cruzi infections (Chagas disease), although treatment of the chronic stage of such infections has led to variable results. It may also be useful for the treatment of second-stage T. brucei gambiense in combination with *eflornithine*. Being a nitroaromatic compound, *nifurtimox* undergoes reduction and eventually generates intracellular oxygen radicals, such as superoxide radicals and hydrogen peroxide (Figure 43.11). These highly reactive radicals are toxic to T. cruzi. *Nifurtimox* is administered orally. It is extensively metabolized, and the metabolites are excreted mainly in the urine. Adverse effects are common following chronic administration, particularly among the elderly. Major toxicities include hypersensitivity reactions (anaphylaxis, dermatitis) and gastrointestinal problems that may be severe enough to cause weight loss. Peripheral neuropathy is relatively common, and headache and dizziness may also occur.

F. Benznidazole

Benznidazole [benz-NI-da-zole] is a nitroimidazole derivative with a mechanism of action similar to *nifurtimox*. It tends to be better tolerated than *nifurtimox* and is an alternative for the treatment of Chagas disease. Adverse effects include dermatitis, peripheral neuropathy, insomnia, and anorexia.

V. CHEMOTHERAPY FOR LEISHMANIASIS

There are three types of leishmaniasis: cutaneous, mucocutaneous, and visceral. [Note: In the visceral type (liver and spleen), the parasite is in the bloodstream and can cause very serious problems.] Leishmaniasis is transmitted from animals to humans (and between humans) by the bite of infected sandflies. The diagnosis is established by demonstrating the parasite in biopsy material and skin lesions. For visceral leishmaniasis, parenteral treatments may include *amphotericin B* (see Chapter 42) and pentavalent antimonials, such as *sodium stibogluconate*, with *pentamidine* and *paromomycin* as alternative agents. *Miltefosine* is an orally active agent for visceral leishmaniasis. The choice of agent depends on the species of <u>Leishmania</u>, host factors, and resistance patterns noted in area of the world where the infection is acquired.

A. Sodium stibogluconate

The pentavalent antimonial *sodium stibogluconate* [stib-o-GLOO-koe-nate] is not effective in vitro. Therefore, it has been proposed that reduction to the trivalent antimonial compound is essential for activity. The exact mechanism of action has not been determined. Because it is not absorbed after oral administration, *sodium stibogluconate* must be administered parenterally, and it is distributed in the extravascular compartment. Metabolism is minimal, and the drug is excreted in urine. Adverse effects include injection site pain, pancreatitis, elevated liver enzymes, arthralgias, myalgias, gastrointestinal upset, and cardiac arrhythmias. Renal and hepatic function should be monitored periodically.

B. Miltefosine

Miltefosine [mil-te-FOE-zeen] is the first orally active drug for visceral leishmaniasis. It may also have some activity against cutaneous and mucocutaneous forms of the disease. The precise mechanism of action is not known, but *miltefosine* appears to interfere with phospholipids in the parasitic cell membrane to induce apoptosis. Nausea and vomiting are common adverse reactions. The drug is teratogenic and should be avoided in pregnancy.

VI. CHEMOTHERAPY FOR TOXOPLASMOSIS

One of the most common infections in humans is caused by the protozoan <u>T. gondii</u>, which is transmitted to humans when they consume raw or inadequately cooked infected meat. An infected pregnant woman can transmit the organism to her fetus. Cats are the only animals that shed oocysts, which can infect other animals as well as humans.

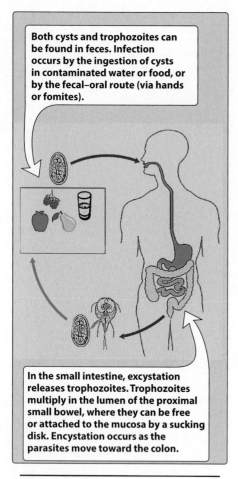

Both cysts and trophozoites can be found in feces. Infection occurs by the ingestion of cysts in contaminated water or food, or by the fecal–oral route (via hands or fomites).

In the small intestine, excystation releases trophozoites. Trophozoites multiply in the lumen of the proximal small bowel, where they can be free or attached to the mucosa by a sucking disk. Encystation occurs as the parasites move toward the colon.

Figure 43.12
Life cycle of Giardia lamblia.

The treatment of choice for this condition is a combination of *sulfadiazine* and *pyrimethamine*. *Leucovorin* is commonly administered to protect against folate deficiency. [Note: At the first appearance of a rash, *pyrimethamine* should be discontinued, because hypersensitivity to this drug can be severe.] *Pyrimethamine* with *clindamycin*, or the combination of *trimethoprim* and *sulfamethoxazole*, are alternative treatments. *Trimethoprim/sulfamethoxazole* is used for prophylaxis against toxoplasmosis (as well as P. jirovecii) in immunocompromised patients.

VII. CHEMOTHERAPY FOR GIARDIASIS

Giardia lamblia is the most commonly diagnosed intestinal parasite in the United States. It has two life cycle stages: the binucleate trophozoite with four flagella and the drug-resistant, four-nucleate cyst (Figure 43.12). Ingestion, usually from contaminated drinking water, leads to infection. The trophozoites exist in the small intestine and divide by binary fission. Occasionally, cysts are formed that pass out in stools. Although some infections are asymptomatic, severe diarrhea can occur, which can be very serious in immunocompromised patients. The treatment of choice is oral *metronidazole* for 5 days. An alternative is *tinidazole*, which is as effective as *metronidazole* in the treatment of giardiasis. This agent is administered orally as a single dose. *Nitazoxanide* [nye-ta-ZOX-a-nide], a nitrothiazole derivative, is also approved for the treatment of giardiasis. [Note: *Nitazoxanide* may also be used for cryptosporidiosis (a diarrheal illness most commonly seen in immunocompromised patients) caused by the parasite Cryptosporidium parvum.] For giardiasis, *nitazoxanide* is administered as a 3-day course of oral therapy. The anthelmintic drug *albendazole* may also be efficacious for giardiasis, and *paromomycin* is sometimes used for treatment of giardiasis in pregnant patients.

Study Questions

Choose the ONE best answer.

43.1 After the acute infection, which of the following medications is given to treat the asymptomatic colonization state of E. histolytica?

   A. Chloroquine.
   B. Iodoquinol.
   C. Metronidazole.
   D. Primaquine.

> Correct answer = B. Iodoquinol, diloxanide furoate, and paromomycin are luminal amebicides that are usually administered with mixed or systemic amebicides to treat the asymptomatic colonization state. Chloroquine is a systemic amebicide and an antimalarial. Metronidazole is a mixed amebicide. Primaquine is an antimalarial.

43.2 A group of college students are traveling to a chloroquine-resistant malaria area for a mission trip. Which of the following medications can be used for both prevention and treatment of malaria in these students?

   A. Pyrimethamine.
   B. Artemisinin.
   C. Atovaquone–proguanil.
   D. Melarsoprol.

> Correct answer = C. The combination of atovaquone–proguanil has been used for both prevention and treatment of malaria in chloroquine-resistant areas. Pyrimethamine is not recommended for prophylaxis of malaria. Artemisinin and its derivatives are not used for prophylaxis, only treatment of malaria. Melarsoprol is used for the treatment of African sleeping sickness.

43.3 Which of the following agents is available as an oral therapy for the treatment of visceral leishmaniasis?

A. Artemether/lumefantrine.
B. Miltefosine.
C. Nitazoxanide.
D. Tinidazole.

Correct answer = B. Miltefosine is the only oral agent available for the treatment of visceral leishmaniasis. All the other drugs are orally administered, but artemether/lumefantrine is used for the treatment of malaria, nitazoxanide is used for the treatment of giardiasis or cryptosporidiosis, and tinidazole is effective for amebiasis or giardiasis.

43.4 An 18-year-old male is diagnosed with Chagas disease. Which medication would be the best for this patient?

A. Nifurtimox.
B. Suramin.
C. Sodium stibogluconate.
D. Metronidazole.

Correct answer = A. Nifurtimox is indicated for the treatment of American trypanosomiasis (Chagas disease) caused by T. cruzi. Suramin is used for the treatment of first-stage African trypanosomiasis due to T. brucei rhodesiense. Sodium stibogluconate is used for the treatment of leishmaniasis. Metronidazole is used for the treatment of amebiasis and giardiasis.

Anthelmintic Drugs

44

Lisa Clayville Martin

I. OVERVIEW

Nematodes, trematodes, and cestodes are three major groups of helminths (worms) that infect humans. Anthelmintic drugs (Figure 44.1) are aimed at metabolic targets that are present in the parasite but either are absent from or have different characteristics than those of the host. Figure 44.2 illustrates the high incidence of helmintic infections worldwide. Most anthelmintics target eliminating the organisms from the host, as well as controlling spread of infections.

II. DRUGS FOR THE TREATMENT OF NEMATODES

Nematodes are elongated roundworms that possess a complete digestive system. They cause infections of the intestine as well as the blood and tissues.

A. Mebendazole

Mebendazole [me-BEN-da-zole], a synthetic benzimidazole compound, is a first-line agent for the treatment of infections caused by whipworms (<u>Trichuris</u> <u>trichiura</u>), pinworms (<u>Enterobius</u> <u>vermicularis</u>), hookworms (<u>Necator</u> <u>americanus</u> and <u>Ancylostoma</u> <u>duodenale</u>), and roundworms (<u>Ascaris</u> <u>lumbricoides</u>). *Mebendazole* acts by inhibiting the assembly of the microtubules in the parasite and also by irreversibly blocking glucose uptake. Affected parasites are expelled in the feces. Adverse effects include abdominal pain and diarrhea. *Mebendazole* should not be used in pregnant women. [Note: Many anthelmintics should be avoided in pregnancy (Figure 44.3); however, in mass prevention or treatment programs, certain agents (for example, *mebendazole* or *albendazole*) may be used in the second or third trimester.]

B. Pyrantel pamoate

Pyrantel pamoate [pi-RAN-tel PAM-oh-ate] is also effective in the treatment of infections caused by roundworms, pinworms, and hookworms (Figure 44.4). *Pyrantel pamoate* is poorly absorbed orally and exerts its effects in the intestinal tract. It acts as a depolarizing, neuromuscular-blocking agent, causing release of acetylcholine and inhibition of cholinesterase, leading to paralysis of the worm. The paralyzed

CHEMOTHERAPY OF HELMINTIC INFECTIONS: FOR NEMATODES
Diethylcarbamazine BANOCIDE
Ivermectin STROMECTOL
Mebendazole VERMOX
Pyrantel pamoate PIN-X
Thiabendazole MINTEZOL

CHEMOTHERAPY OF HELMINTIC INFECTIONS: FOR TREMATODES
Praziquantel BILTRICIDE

CHEMOTHERAPY OF HELMINTIC INFECTIONS: FOR CESTODES
Albendazole ALBENZA
Niclosamide

Figure 44.1
Summary of anthelmintic agents.

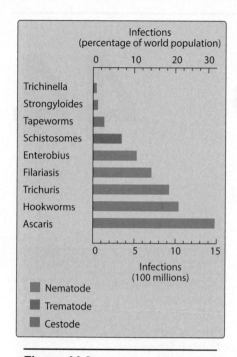

Figure 44.2
Relative incidence of helminth infections worldwide.

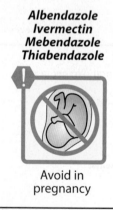

Avoid in
pregnancy

Figure 44.3
Albendazole, ivermectin, mebendazole, and *thiabendazole* should be avoided in pregnancy.

worm releases its hold on the intestinal tract and is expelled. Adverse effects are mild and include nausea, vomiting, and diarrhea.

C. Thiabendazole

Thiabendazole [thye-a-BEN-da-zole], a synthetic benzimidazole, is a potent broad-spectrum anthelmintic agent. Current use of *thiabendazole* is limited to the topical treatment of cutaneous larva migrans (creeping eruption). Because of its toxic effects, it has been largely replaced by other agents for many clinical applications.

D. Ivermectin

Ivermectin [eye-ver-MEK-tin] is the drug of choice for the treatment of cutaneous larva migrans, strongyloidiasis, and onchocerciasis (river blindness) caused by <u>Onchocerca</u> <u>volvulus</u> (kills microfilariae but has no activity against adult worms). [Note: *Ivermectin* is also useful in the treatment of pediculosis (lice) and scabies.] *Ivermectin* targets the glutamate-gated chloride channel receptors. Chloride influx is enhanced, and hyperpolarization occurs, resulting in paralysis and death of the worm. The drug is given orally and does not readily cross the blood–brain barrier. *Ivermectin* should not be used in pregnancy (Figure 44.3). The killing of the microfilaria in onchocerciasis can result in a dangerous Mazzotti reaction (fever, headache, dizziness, somnolence, and hypotension). The severity of this reaction is related to parasite load. Antihistamines or steroids may be given to ameliorate the symptoms.

E. Diethylcarbamazine

Diethylcarbamazine [dye-eth-il-kar-BAM-a-zeen] is the drug of choice for filariasis caused by infection with <u>Wuchereria</u> <u>bancrofti</u> and <u>Brugia</u> <u>malayi</u>. It kills the microfilariae and has activity against adult worms. [Note: In countries where filariasis is endemic, a combination of antifilarial drugs (either *diethylcarbamazine* and *albendazole* or *ivermectin* and *albendazole*) may be used as preventive chemotherapy.] *Diethylcarbamazine* is rapidly absorbed following oral administration with meals and is excreted mainly in the urine. Adverse effects may include fever, nausea, vomiting, arthralgia, and headache. [Note: *Diethylcarbamazine* can accelerate blindness and cause severe Mazzotti reactions in patients with onchocerciasis. It should be avoided in patients with this disorder.]

III. DRUGS FOR THE TREATMENT OF TREMATODES

The trematodes (flukes) are leaf-shaped flatworms that are generally characterized by the tissues they infect (for example, liver, lung, intestinal, or blood; Figure 44.5).

A. Praziquantel

Praziquantel [pray-zi-KWON-tel] is an agent of choice for the treatment of all forms of schistosomiasis, other trematode infections, and cestode infections such as taeniasis. *Praziquantel* is also used off-label in the treatment of cysticercosis (caused by

ONCHOCERCIASIS (RIVER BLINDNESS)

● Causative agent: <u>Onchocerca</u> <u>volvulus</u>.

● Common in areas of Mexico, South America, and tropical Africa.

● Characterized by subcutaneous nodules, a pruritic skin rash, and ocular lesions often resulting in blindness.

● Therapy: *Ivermectin*.

ENTEROBIASIS (PINWORM DISEASE)

● Causative agent: <u>Enterobius</u> <u>vermicularis</u>.

● Most common helminthic infection in the United States.

● Pruritus ani occurs, with white worms visible in stools or perianal region.

● Therapy: *Mebendazole* or *pyrantel pamoate*.

ASCARIASIS (ROUNDWORM DISEASE)

● Causative agent: <u>Ascaris</u> <u>lumbricoides</u>.

● Second only to pinworms as the most prevalent multicellular parasite in the United States; approximately one third of the world's population is infected with this worm.

● Ingested larvae grow in the intestine, causing abdominal symptoms, including intestinal obstruction; roundworms may pass to blood and infect the lungs.

● Therapy: *Pyrantel pamoate* or *mebendazole*.

FILARIASIS

● Causative agents: <u>Wuchereria</u> <u>bancrofti</u>, <u>Brugia</u> <u>malayi</u>.

● Worms cause blockage of lymph flow. Ultimately, local inflammation and fibrosis of the lymphatics occurs.

● After years of infestation, the arms, legs, and scrotum fill with fluid, causing elephantiasis.

● Therapy: A combination of *diethyl-carbamazine* and *albendazole*.

TRICHURIASIS (WHIPWORM DISEASE)

● Causative agent: <u>Trichuris</u> <u>trichiura</u>.

● Infection is usually asymptomatic; however, abdominal pain, diarrhea, and flatulence can occur.

● Therapy: *Mebendazole*.

HOOKWORM DISEASE

● Causative agents: <u>Ancylostoma</u> <u>duodenale</u> (Old World hookworm), <u>Necator</u> <u>americanus</u> (New World hookworm).

● Worm attaches to the intestinal mucosa, causing anorexia, ulcer-like symptoms, and chronic intestinal blood loss that leads to anemia.

● Treatment is unnecessary in asymptomatic individuals who are not anemic.

● Therapy: *Pyrantel pamoate* or *mebendazole*.

STRONGYLOIDIASIS (THREADWORM DISEASE)

● Causative agent: <u>Strongyloides</u> <u>stercoralis</u>.

● Relatively uncommon compared with other intestinal nematodes; a relatively benign disease in normal individuals that can progress to a fatal outcome in immuno-compromised patients.

● Therapy: *Ivermectin*.

TRICHINOSIS

● Causative agent: <u>Trichinella</u> <u>spiralis</u>.

● Usually caused by consumption of insufficiently cooked meat, especially pork.

● Therapy: *Albendazole* or *mebendazole*.

Figure 44.4
Characteristics of and therapy for commonly encountered nematode infections.

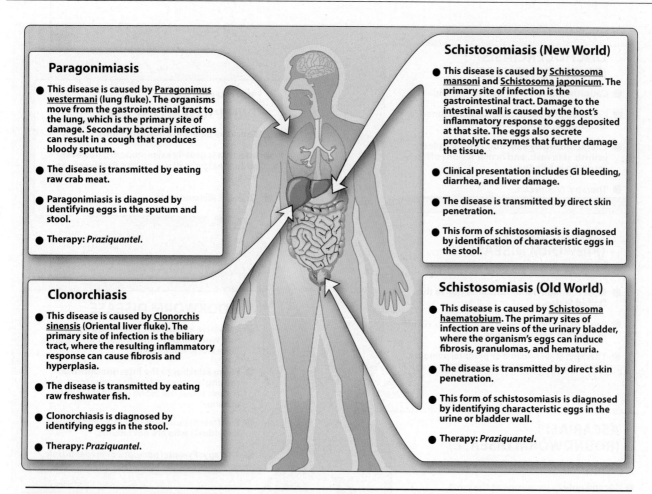

Figure 44.5
Characteristics of and therapy for commonly encountered trematode infections.

Taenia solium larvae; Figure 44.6). Permeability of the cell membrane to calcium is increased, causing contracture and paralysis of the parasite. *Praziquantel* should be taken with food and not chewed due to a bitter taste. It is rapidly absorbed after oral administration and distributes into the cerebrospinal fluid (CSF). The drug is extensively metabolized, and the inactive metabolites are excreted primarily in the urine. Common adverse effects include dizziness, malaise, and headache as well as gastrointestinal upset. *Dexamethasone*, *phenytoin*, *rifampin*, and *carbamazepine* may increase the metabolism of *praziquantel*. *Cimetidine* causes increased *praziquantel* levels. *Praziquantel* is contraindicated for the treatment of ocular cysticercosis, because destruction of the organism in the eye may cause irreversible damage.

IV. DRUGS FOR THE TREATMENT OF CESTODES

The cestodes, or "true tapeworms," typically have a flat, segmented body and attach to the host's intestine (Figure 44.6). Like the trematodes, the tapeworms lack a mouth and a digestive tract throughout their life cycle.

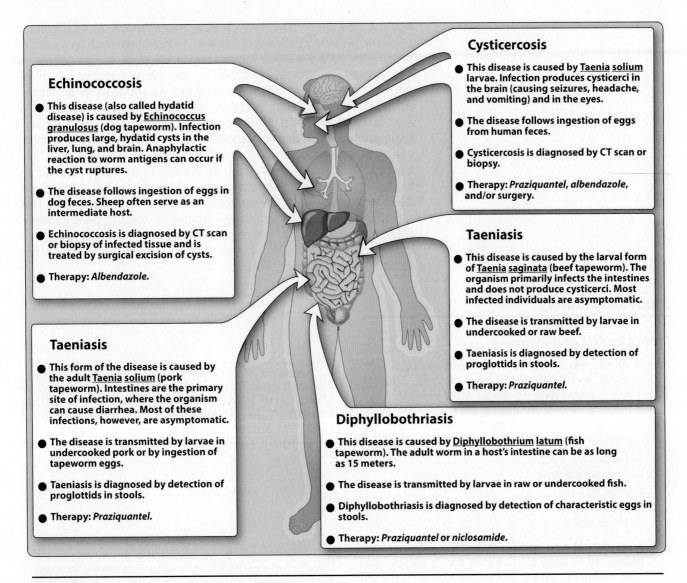

Echinococcosis

- This disease (also called hydatid disease) is caused by <u>Echinococcus granulosus</u> (dog tapeworm). Infection produces large, hydatid cysts in the liver, lung, and brain. Anaphylactic reaction to worm antigens can occur if the cyst ruptures.

- The disease follows ingestion of eggs in dog feces. Sheep often serve as an intermediate host.

- Echinococcosis is diagnosed by CT scan or biopsy of infected tissue and is treated by surgical excision of cysts.

- Therapy: *Albendazole.*

Taeniasis

- This form of the disease is caused by the adult <u>Taenia</u> <u>solium</u> (pork tapeworm). Intestines are the primary site of infection, where the organism can cause diarrhea. Most of these infections, however, are asymptomatic.

- The disease is transmitted by larvae in undercooked pork or by ingestion of tapeworm eggs.

- Taeniasis is diagnosed by detection of proglottids in stools.

- Therapy: *Praziquantel.*

Cysticercosis

- This disease is caused by <u>Taenia</u> <u>solium</u> larvae. Infection produces cysticerci in the brain (causing seizures, headache, and vomiting) and in the eyes.

- The disease follows ingestion of eggs from human feces.

- Cysticercosis is diagnosed by CT scan or biopsy.

- Therapy: *Praziquantel, albendazole,* and/or surgery.

Taeniasis

- This disease is caused by the larval form of <u>Taenia</u> <u>saginata</u> (beef tapeworm). The organism primarily infects the intestines and does not produce cysticerci. Most infected individuals are asymptomatic.

- The disease is transmitted by larvae in undercooked or raw beef.

- Taeniasis is diagnosed by detection of proglottids in stools.

- Therapy: *Praziquantel.*

Diphyllobothriasis

- This disease is caused by <u>Diphyllobothrium</u> <u>latum</u> (fish tapeworm). The adult worm in a host's intestine can be as long as 15 meters.

- The disease is transmitted by larvae in raw or undercooked fish.

- Diphyllobothriasis is diagnosed by detection of characteristic eggs in stools.

- Therapy: *Praziquantel* or *niclosamide.*

Figure 44.6
Characteristics of and therapy for commonly encountered cestode infections.

A. Niclosamide

Niclosamide [ni-KLOE-sa-mide] (no longer available in the United States) is an alternative to *praziquantel* for the treatment of taeniasis, diphyllobothriasis, and other cestode infections. It inhibits the mitochondrial phosphorylation of adenosine diphosphate (ADP) in the parasite, making it lethal for the cestode's scolex and segments but not for the ova. Anaerobic metabolism may also be inhibited. A laxative is administered prior to oral administration to purge the bowel of all dead segments and to enhance digestion and liberation of the ova. Alcohol should be avoided within 1 day of *niclosamide* use.

B. Albendazole

Albendazole [al-BEN-da-zole], another benzimidazole, inhibits microtubule synthesis and glucose uptake in nematodes and is effective against most nematodes known. Its primary therapeutic application, however, is in the treatment of cestodal infestations, such as cysticercosis and hydatid disease (caused by larval stage of <u>Echinococcus granulosus</u>). [Note: *Albendazole* is also very effective in treating microsporidiosis, a fungal infection.] *Albendazole* is erratically absorbed after oral administration, but absorption is enhanced by a high-fat meal. The drug distributes widely, including the CSF. It undergoes extensive first-pass metabolism, including formation of an active sulfoxide. *Albendazole* and its metabolites are primarily excreted in the bile. When used in short-course therapy (1 to 3 days) for nematodal infestations, adverse effects are mild and transient and include headache and nausea. Treatment of hydatid disease (3 months) has a risk of hepatotoxicity and, rarely, agranulocytosis or pancytopenia. Medical treatment of neurocysticercosis is associated with inflammatory responses to dying parasites in the CNS, including headache, vomiting, fever, and seizures.

Study Questions

Choose the ONE best answer.

44.1 A 48-year-old immigrant from Mexico presents with seizures and other neurologic symptoms. Eggs of T. solium are found upon examination of a stool specimen. A magnetic resonance image of the brain shows many cysts, some of which are calcified. Which one of the following drugs would be of benefit to this individual?

  A. Ivermectin.
  B. Pyrantel pamoate.
  C. Albendazole.
  D. Diethylcarbamazine.
  E. Niclosamide.

> Correct answer = C. The symptoms and other findings for this patient are consistent with neurocysticercosis. Albendazole is the drug of choice for the treatment of this infestation. The other drugs are not effective against the larval forms of tapeworms.

44.2 A 56-year-old man from South America is found to be parasitized by both schistosomes and T. solium—the pork tapeworm. Which of the following anthelmintic drugs would be effective for both infestations?

  A. Albendazole.
  B. Ivermectin.
  C. Mebendazole.
  D. Praziquantel.

> Correct answer = D. Praziquantel is a primary drug for the treatment of trematode and cestode infestations. Although albendazole is effective in cysticercosis, it is not active against flukes, and this patient has no evidence of cysticercosis. Ivermectin and mebendazole treat nematode infestations.

44.3 Which of the following medications inhibits the phosphorylation of adenosine diphosphate?

  A. Albendazole.
  B. Mebendazole.
  C. Niclosamide.
  D. Praziquantel.

> Correct answer = C. Niclosamide inhibits the parasite's mitochondrial phosphorylation of adenosine diphosphate (ADP), which produces usable energy in the form of adenosine triphosphate (ATP).

44.4 Which of the following medications used to treat river blindness targets chloride channels and can cause a Mazzotti reaction?

  A. Ivermectin.
  B. Praziquantel.
  C. Pyrantel pamoate.
  D. Albendazole.

> Correct answer = A. Ivermectin targets the parasite's glutamate-gated chloride channel receptors. Chloride influx and hyperpolarization occur, resulting in paralysis of the worm.

Antiviral Drugs

Elizabeth Sherman

45

I. OVERVIEW

Viruses are obligate intracellular parasites. They lack both a cell wall and a cell membrane, and they do not carry out metabolic processes. Viruses use much of the host's metabolic machinery, and few drugs are selective enough to prevent viral replication without injury to the infected host cells. Therapy for viral diseases is further complicated by the fact that the clinical symptoms appear late in the course of the disease, at a time when most of the virus particles have replicated. At this stage of viral infection, administration of drugs that block viral replication has limited effectiveness. However, some antiviral agents are useful as prophylactic agents. The few virus groups that respond to available antiviral drugs are discussed in this chapter. To assist in the review of these drugs, they are grouped according to the type of infection they target (Figure 45.1).

II. TREATMENT OF RESPIRATORY VIRAL INFECTIONS

Viral respiratory tract infections for which treatments exist include influenza A and B and respiratory syncytial virus (RSV). [Note: Immunization against influenza A is the preferred approach. However, antiviral agents are used when patients are allergic to the vaccine or outbreaks occur.]

A. Neuraminidase inhibitors

The neuraminidase inhibitors *oseltamivir* [os-el-TAM-i-veer] and *zanamivir* [za-NA-mi-veer] are effective against both type A and type B influenza viruses. They do not interfere with the immune response to influenza vaccine. Administered prior to exposure, neuraminidase inhibitors prevent infection and, when administered within 24 to 48 hours after the onset of symptoms, they modestly decrease the intensity and duration of symptoms.

1. **Mechanism of action:** Influenza viruses employ a specific neuraminidase that is inserted into the host cell membrane for the purpose of releasing newly formed virions. This enzyme is essential for the virus life cycle. *Oseltamivir* and *zanamivir* selectively inhibit neuraminidase, thereby preventing the release of new virions and their spread from cell to cell.

FOR RESPIRATORY VIRUS INFECTIONS
Amantadine SYMMETREL
Oseltamivir TAMIFLU
Ribavirin COPEGUS, REBETOL, RIBAPAK, RIBASPHERE, VIRAZOLE
Rimantadine FLUMADINE
Zanamivir RELENZA

FOR HEPATIC VIRAL INFECTIONS
Adefovir HEPSERA
Boceprevir VICTRELIS
Entecavir BARACLUDE
Interferon INTRON, AVONEX
Lamivudine EPIVIR-HBV
Pegylated interferon PEGASYS, PEG-INTRON
Telaprevir INCIVEK
Telbivudine TYZEKA
Tenofovir VIREAD

FOR HERPESVIRUS AND CYTOMEGALOVIRUS INFECTIONS
Acyclovir ZOVIRAX
Cidofovir VISTIDE
Famciclovir FAMVIR
Foscarnet FOSCAVIR
Ganciclovir CYTOVENE
Penciclovir DENAVIR
Trifluridine VIROPTIC
Valacyclovir VALTREX
Valganciclovir VALCYTE

FOR HIV: NUCLEOSIDE AND NUCLEOTIDE REVERSE TRANSCRIPTASE INHIBITORS
Abacavir ZIAGEN
Didanosine VIDEX
Emtricitabine EMTRIVA
Lamivudine EPIVIR
Stavudine ZERIT
Tenofovir VIREAD
Zidovudine RETROVIR

Figure 45.1
Summary of antiviral drugs.
HIV = human immunodeficiency virus.
(Continued on next page.)

FOR HIV: NONNUCLEOSIDE REVERSE TRANSCRIPTASE INHIBITORS
Delavirdine RESCRIPTOR
Efavirenz SUSTIVA
Etravirine INTELENCE
Nevirapine VIRAMUNE
Rilpivirine EDURANT
FOR HIV: PROTEASE INHIBITORS
Atazanavir REYATAZ
Darunavir PREZISTA
Fosamprenavir LEXIVA
Indinavir CRIXIVAN
Lopinavir/ritonavir KALETRA
Nelfinavir VIRACEPT
Ritonavir NORVIR
Saquinavir INVIRASE
Tipranavir APTIVUS
FOR HIV: ENTRY INHIBITORS
Enfuvirtide FUZEON
Maraviroc SELZENTRY
FOR HIV: INTEGRASE INHIBITORS
Dolutegravir TIVICAY
Elvitegravir
Raltegravir ISENTRESS
FOR HIV: FIXED DOSE COMBINATIONS
Lamivudine + abacavir EPZICOM
Emtricitabine + tenofovir TRUVADA
Zidovudine + lamivudine COMBIVIR
Efavirenz + emtricitabine + tenofovir ATRIPLA
Rilpivirine + tenofovir + emtricitabine COMPLERA
Zidovudine + lamivudine + abacavir TRIZIVIR
Elvitegravir + cobicistat + tenofovir + emtricitabine STRIBILD

Figure 45.1
Summary of antiviral drugs.
HIV = human immunodeficiency virus.

2. **Pharmacokinetics:** *Oseltamivir* is an orally active prodrug that is rapidly hydrolyzed by the liver to its active form. *Zanamivir* is not active orally and is administered via inhalation. Both drugs are eliminated unchanged in the urine (Figure 45.2).

3. **Adverse effects:** The most common adverse effects of *oseltamivir* are gastrointestinal (GI) discomfort and nausea, which can be alleviated by taking the drug with food. Irritation of the respiratory tract occurs with *zanamivir*. It should be used with caution in individuals with asthma or chronic obstructive pulmonary disease, because bronchospasm may occur.

4. **Resistance:** Mutations of the neuraminidase enzyme have been identified in adults treated with either of the neuraminidase inhibitors. These mutants, however, are often less infective and virulent than the wild type.

B. Adamantane antivirals

The therapeutic spectrum of the adamantane derivatives, *amantadine* [a-MAN-ta-deen] and *rimantadine* [ri-MAN-ta-deen], is limited to influenza A infections. Due to widespread resistance, the adamantanes are not recommended in the United States for the treatment or prophylaxis of influenza A.

1. **Mechanism of action:** *Amantadine* and *rimantadine* interfere with the function of the viral M2 protein, possibly blocking uncoating of the virus particle and preventing viral release within infected cells.

2. **Pharmacokinetics:** Both drugs are well absorbed after oral administration. *Amantadine* distributes throughout the body and readily penetrates into the central nervous system (CNS), whereas *rimantadine* does not cross the blood–brain barrier to the same extent. *Amantadine* is primarily excreted unchanged in the urine, and dosage reductions are needed in renal dysfunction. *Rimantadine* is extensively metabolized by the liver, and both the metabolites and the parent drug are eliminated by the kidney (Figure 45.3).

3. **Adverse effects:** *Amantadine* is mainly associated with CNS adverse effects, such as insomnia, dizziness, and ataxia. More serious adverse effects may include hallucinations and seizures. *Amantadine* should be employed cautiously in patients with psychiatric problems, cerebral atherosclerosis, renal impairment, or epilepsy. *Rimantadine* causes fewer CNS reactions. Both drugs cause GI intolerance. They should be used with caution in pregnant and nursing mothers.

4. **Resistance:** Resistance can develop rapidly, and resistant strains can be readily transmitted to close contacts. Resistance has been shown to result from a change in one amino acid of the M2 matrix protein. Cross-resistance occurs between the two drugs.

C. Ribavirin

Ribavirin [rye-ba-VYE-rin], a synthetic guanosine analog, is effective against a broad spectrum of RNA and DNA viruses. For example, *ribavirin* is used in treating immunosuppressed infants and young children with severe RSV infections. *Ribavirin* is also effective in chronic hepatitis C infections when used in combination with *interferon-α*.

1. **Mechanism of action:** *Ribavirin* inhibits replication of RNA and DNA viruses. The drug is first phosphorylated to the 5′-phosphate derivatives, the major product being the compound ribavirin triphosphate, which exerts its antiviral action by inhibiting guanosine triphosphate formation, preventing viral messenger RNA (mRNA) capping, and blocking RNA-dependent RNA polymerase.

2. **Pharmacokinetics:** *Ribavirin* is effective orally and by inhalation. An aerosol is used in the treatment of RSV infection. Absorption is increased if the drug is taken with a fatty meal. The drug and its metabolites are eliminated in urine (Figure 45.4).

3. **Adverse effects:** Side effects of *ribavirin* include dose-dependent transient anemia. Elevated bilirubin has also been reported. The aerosol may be safer, although respiratory function in infants can deteriorate quickly after initiation of aerosol treatment. Therefore, monitoring is essential. *Ribavirin* is contraindicated in pregnancy (Figure 45.5).

III. TREATMENT OF HEPATIC VIRAL INFECTIONS

The hepatitis viruses thus far identified (A, B, C, D, and E) each have a pathogenesis specifically involving replication in and destruction of hepatocytes. Of this group, hepatitis B (a DNA virus) and hepatitis C (an RNA virus) are the most common causes of chronic hepatitis, cirrhosis, and hepatocellular carcinoma (Figure 45.6) and are the only hepatic viral infections for which therapy is currently available. [Note: Hepatitis A is a commonly encountered infection caused by oral ingestion of the virus, but it is not a chronic disease.] Chronic hepatitis B may be treated with *peginterferon-α-2a*, which is injected subcutaneously once weekly. [Note: *Interferon-α-2b* injected intramuscularly or subcutaneously three times weekly is also useful in the treatment of hepatitis B, but *peginterferon-α-2a* has similar or slightly better efficacy with improved tolerability.] Oral therapy for chronic hepatitis B includes *lamivudine, adefovir, entecavir, tenofovir,* or *telbivudine*. The preferred treatment for chronic hepatitis C is the combination of *peginterferon-α-2a* or *peginterferon-α-2b* plus *ribavirin*, which is more effective than the combination of standard interferons and *ribavirin*. For genotype 1 chronic hepatitis C virus (HCV), an NS3/4A protease inhibitor (such as *boceprevir* or *telaprevir*) should be added to pegylated interferon and *ribavirin*.

A. Interferons

Interferons [in-ter-FEER-on] are a family of naturally occurring, inducible glycoproteins that interfere with the ability of viruses to infect cells. The interferons are synthesized by recombinant DNA technology. At least three types of interferons exist—α, β, and γ (Figure 45.7). One of the 15 interferon-α glycoproteins, *interferon-α-2b* has been approved for treatment of hepatitis B and C, condylomata acuminata, and cancers such as hairy cell leukemia and Kaposi sarcoma. In "pegylated" formulations, bis-monomethoxy polyethylene glycol has

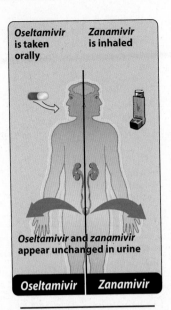

Figure 45.2
Administration and fate of *oseltamivir* and *zanamivir*.

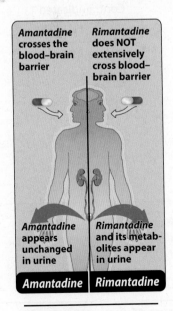

Figure 45.3
Administration and fate of *amantadine* and *rimantadine*.

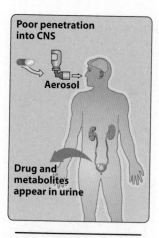

Figure 45.4
Administration and fate of *ribavirin*.

Ribavirin

Contraindicated
in pregnancy

Figure 45.5
Ribavirin
causes
teratogenic
effects.

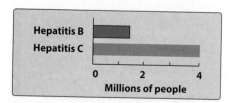

Figure 45.6
The prevalence of chronic hepatitis B and C in the United States.

been covalently attached to either *interferon-α-2a* or *-α-2b* to increase the size of the molecule. The larger molecular size delays absorption from the injection site, lengthens the duration of action of the drug, and also decreases its clearance.

1. **Mechanism of action:** The antiviral mechanism is incompletely understood. It appears to involve the induction of host cell enzymes that inhibit viral RNA translation, ultimately leading to the degradation of viral mRNA and tRNA.

2. **Pharmacokinetics:** *Interferon* is not active orally, but it may be administered intralesionally, subcutaneously, or intravenously. Very little active compound is found in the plasma, and its presence is not correlated with clinical responses. Cellular uptake and metabolism by the liver and kidney account for the disappearance of *interferon* from the plasma. Negligible renal elimination occurs.

3. **Adverse effects:** Adverse effects include flu-like symptoms, such as fever, chills, myalgias, arthralgias, and GI disturbances. Fatigue and mental depression are common. These symptoms subside with continued administration. The principal dose-limiting toxicities are bone marrow suppression, severe fatigue and weight loss, neurotoxicity characterized by somnolence and behavioral disturbances, autoimmune disorders such as thyroiditis and, rarely, cardiovascular problems such as heart failure. *Interferon* may also potentiate myelosuppression caused by other bone marrow–suppressive agents.

B. Lamivudine

This cytosine analog is an inhibitor of both hepatitis B virus (HBV) and human immunodeficiency virus (HIV) reverse transcriptases (RTs). *Lamivudine* [la-MI-vyoo-deen] must be phosphorylated by host cellular enzymes to the triphosphate (active) form. This compound competitively inhibits HBV RNA-dependent DNA polymerase. As with many nucleotide analogs, the intracellular half-life of the triphosphate is many hours longer than its plasma half-life. The rate of resistance is high following long-term therapy with *lamivudine*. *Lamivudine* is well absorbed orally and is widely distributed. It is mainly excreted unchanged in urine. Dose reductions are necessary when there is moderate renal insufficiency. *Lamivudine* is well tolerated, with rare occurrences of headache and dizziness.

C. Adefovir

Adefovir dipivoxil [ah-DEF-o-veer die-pih-VOCKS-ill] is a nucleotide analog that is phosphorylated by cellular kinases to adefovir diphosphate, which is then incorporated into viral DNA. This leads to termination of chain elongation and prevents replication of HBV. *Adefovir* is administered once a day and is renally excreted via glomerular filtration and tubular secretion. As with other agents, discontinuation of *adefovir* may result in severe exacerbation of hepatitis. Nephrotoxicity may occur with chronic use, and the drug should be used cautiously in patients with existing renal dysfunction. *Adefovir* may raise levels of *tenofovir* through competition for tubular secretion, and concurrent use should be avoided.

D. Entecavir

Entecavir [en-TECK-ah-veer] is a guanosine nucleoside analog for the treatment of HBV infections. Following intracellular phosphorylation to the triphosphate, it competes with the natural substrate, deoxyguanosine triphosphate, for viral RT. *Entecavir* is effective against *lamivudine*-resistant strains of HBV and is dosed once daily. The drug is primarily excreted unchanged in the urine and dosage adjustments are needed in renal dysfunction. Concomitant use of drugs with renal toxicity should be avoided.

E. Telbivudine

Telbivudine [tel-BIV-yoo-dine] is a thymidine analog that can be used in the treatment of HBV. *Telbivudine* is phosphorylated intracellularly to the triphosphate, which can either compete with endogenous thymidine triphosphate for incorporation into DNA or be incorporated into viral DNA, where it serves to terminate further elongation of the DNA chain. The drug is administered orally, once a day. *Telbivudine* is eliminated by glomerular filtration as the unchanged drug. The dose must be adjusted in renal failure. Adverse reactions include fatigue, headache, diarrhea, and elevations in liver enzymes and creatine kinase.

F. Tenofovir (see tenofovir under Section VI - NRTIs)

G. Boceprevir and telaprevir

Boceprevir [boe-SE-pre-vir] and *telaprevir* [tel-A-pre-vir] are the first oral direct-acting antiviral agents for the adjunctive treatment of chronic HCV genotype 1. These HCV NS3/4A serine protease inhibitors covalently and reversibly bind to the NS3 protease active site, thus inhibiting viral replication in host cells. Both drugs are potent inhibitors of viral replication; however, they have a low barrier to resistance and, when used as monotherapy, resistance quickly develops. Therefore, *boceprevir* or *telaprevir* should be used in combination with *peginterferon alfa* and *ribavirin* in order to improve response rates and reduce the emergence of viral resistance. *Boceprevir* is administered with food to improve absorption. The absorption of *telaprevir* is enhanced when it is administered with non–low-fat food. The metabolism of *boceprevir* and *telaprevir* occurs via CYP450 isoenzymes. Because both drugs are strong inhibitors of CYP3A4/5 and are also partially metabolized by CYP3A4/5, they have the potential for complex drug interactions. Common adverse events with *boceprevir* include anemia and dysgeusia. *Telaprevir* is associated with rash, anemia, and anorectal discomfort.

IV. TREATMENT OF HERPESVIRUS INFECTIONS

Herpes viruses are associated with a broad spectrum of diseases, for example, cold sores, viral encephalitis, and genital infections. The drugs that are effective against these viruses exert their actions during the acute phase of viral infections and are without effect during the latent phase.

Interferon-α	*Interferon-β*	*Interferon-γ*
Chronic hepatitis B and C	**Relapsing-remitting multiple sclerosis**	**Chronic granulomatous disease**
Genital warts caused by papillomavirus		
Leukemia, hairy-cell		
Leukemia, chronic myelogenous		
Kaposi sarcoma		

Figure 45.7
Some approved indications for *interferon*.

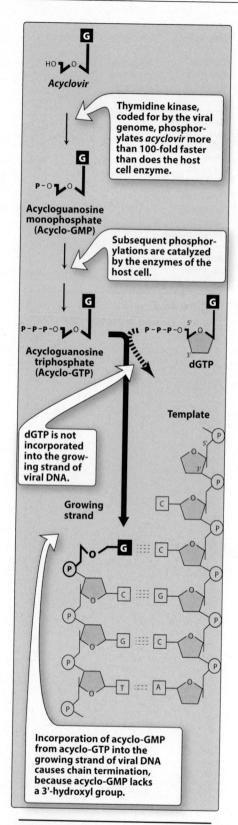

Figure 45.8

Incorporation of *acyclovir* into replicating viral DNA, causing chain termination. dGTP = deoxyguanosine triphosphate.

A. Acyclovir

Acyclovir [ay-SYE-kloe-veer] (*acycloguanosine*) is the prototypic antiherpetic therapeutic agent. Herpes simplex virus (HSV) types 1 and 2, varicella-zoster virus (VZV), and some Epstein-Barr virus–mediated infections are sensitive to *acyclovir*. It is the treatment of choice in HSV encephalitis. The most common use of *acyclovir* is in therapy for genital herpes infections. It is also given prophylactically to seropositive patients before bone marrow transplant and post–heart transplant to protect such individuals from herpetic infections.

1. **Mechanism of action:** *Acyclovir*, a guanosine analog, is monophosphorylated in the cell by the herpesvirus-encoded enzyme thymidine kinase (Figure 45.8). Therefore, virus-infected cells are most susceptible. The monophosphate analog is converted to the di- and triphosphate forms by the host cell kinases. Acyclovir triphosphate competes with deoxyguanosine triphosphate as a substrate for viral DNA polymerase and is itself incorporated into the viral DNA, causing premature DNA chain termination.

2. **Pharmacokinetics:** *Acyclovir* is administered by intravenous (IV), oral, or topical routes. [Note: The efficacy of topical applications is questionable.] The drug distributes well throughout the body, including the cerebrospinal fluid (CSF). *Acyclovir* is partially metabolized to an inactive product. Excretion into the urine occurs both by glomerular filtration and tubular secretion (Figure 45.9). *Acyclovir* accumulates in patients with renal failure. The valyl ester, *valacyclovir* [val-a-SYE-kloe-veer], has greater oral bioavailability than *acyclovir*. This ester is rapidly hydrolyzed to *acyclovir* and achieves levels of the latter comparable to those of *acyclovir* following IV administration.

3. **Adverse effects:** Side effects of *acyclovir* treatment depend on the route of administration. For example, local irritation may occur from topical application; headache, diarrhea, nausea, and vomiting may result after oral administration. Transient renal dysfunction may occur at high doses or in a dehydrated patient receiving the drug intravenously.

4. **Resistance:** Altered or deficient thymidine kinase and DNA polymerases have been found in some resistant viral strains and are most commonly isolated from immunocompromised patients. Cross-resistance to the other agents in this family occurs.

B. Cidofovir

Cidofovir [si-DOE-foe-veer] is approved for the treatment of cytomegalovirus (CMV) retinitis in patients with AIDS. [Note: CMV is a member of the herpesvirus family.] *Cidofovir* is a nucleotide analog of cytosine, the phosphorylation of which is not dependent on viral or cellular enzymes. It inhibits viral DNA synthesis. Slow elimination of the active intracellular metabolite permits prolonged dosage intervals and eliminates the permanent venous access needed for *ganciclovir* therapy. *Cidofovir* is administered intravenously. Intravitreal injection (injection into the vitreous humor between the lens and the retina) of *cidofovir* is associated with risk of hypotony and uveitis and is reserved for extraordinary cases. *Cidofovir* produces significant renal toxicity

(Figure 45.10), and it is contraindicated in patients with preexisting renal impairment and in those taking nephrotoxic drugs. Neutropenia and metabolic acidosis also occur. Oral *probenecid* and IV normal saline are coadministered with *cidofovir* to reduce the risk of nephrotoxicity. Since the introduction of highly active antiretroviral therapy (HAART), the prevalence of CMV infections in immunocompromised hosts has markedly declined, as has the importance of *cidofovir* in the treatment of these patients.

C. Foscarnet

Unlike most antiviral agents, *foscarnet* [fos-KAR-net] is not a purine or pyrimidine analog. Instead, it is a phosphonoformate (a pyrophosphate derivative) and does not require activation by viral (or cellular) kinases. *Foscarnet* is approved for CMV retinitis in immunocompromised hosts and for *acyclovir*-resistant HSV infections. *Foscarnet* works by reversibly inhibiting viral DNA and RNA polymerases, thereby interfering with viral DNA and RNA synthesis. Mutation of the polymerase structure is responsible for resistant viruses. *Foscarnet* is poorly absorbed orally and must be injected intravenously. It must also be given frequently to avoid relapse when plasma levels fall. It is dispersed throughout the body, and greater than 10% enters the bone matrix, from which it slowly leaves. The parent drug is eliminated by glomerular filtration and tubular secretion (Figure 45.11). Adverse effects include nephrotoxicity, anemia, nausea, and fever. Due to chelation with divalent cations, hypocalcemia and hypomagnesemia are also seen. In addition, hypokalemia, hypo- and hyperphosphatemia, seizures, and arrhythmias have been reported.

D. Ganciclovir

Ganciclovir [gan-SYE-kloe-veer] is an analog of *acyclovir* that has greater activity against CMV. It is used for the treatment of CMV retinitis in immunocompromised patients and for CMV prophylaxis in transplant patients.

1. **Mechanism of action:** Like *acyclovir*, *ganciclovir* is activated through conversion to the nucleoside triphosphate by viral and cellular enzymes. The nucleotide inhibits viral DNA polymerase and can be incorporated into the DNA resulting in chain termination.

2. **Pharmacokinetics:** *Ganciclovir* is administered IV and distributes throughout the body, including the CSF. Excretion into the urine occurs through glomerular filtration and tubular secretion (Figure 45.12). Like *acyclovir*, *ganciclovir* accumulates in patients with renal failure. *Valganciclovir* [val-gan-SYE-kloe-veer], an oral drug, is the valyl ester of *ganciclovir*. Like *valacyclovir*, *valganciclovir* has high oral bioavailability, because rapid hydrolysis in the intestine and liver after oral administration leads to high levels of *ganciclovir*.

3. **Adverse effects:** Adverse effects include severe, dose-dependent neutropenia. *Ganciclovir* is carcinogenic as well as embryotoxic and teratogenic in experimental animals.

4. **Resistance:** Resistant CMV strains have been detected that have lower levels of ganciclovir triphosphate.

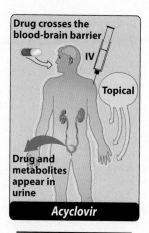

Figure 45.9
Administration and fate of *acyclovir*. IV = intravenous.

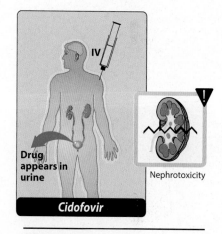

Figure 45.10
Administration, fate, and toxicity of *cidofovir*. IV = intravenous.

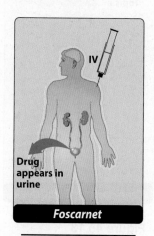

Figure 45.11
Administration and fate of *foscarnet*.

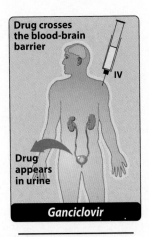

Figure 45.12
Administration and
fate of *ganciclovir*.

E. Penciclovir and famciclovir

Penciclovir [pen-SYE-kloe-veer] is an acyclic guanosine nucleoside derivative that is active against HSV-1, HSV-2, and VZV. *Penciclovir* is only administered topically (Figure 45.13). It is monophosphorylated by viral thymidine kinase, and cellular enzymes form the nucleoside triphosphate, which inhibits HSV DNA polymerase. *Penciclovir* triphosphate has an intracellular half-life much longer than acyclovir triphosphate. *Penciclovir* is negligibly absorbed upon topical application and is well tolerated. *Famciclovir* [fam-SYE-kloe-veer], another acyclic analog of 2′-deoxyguanosine, is a prodrug that is metabolized to the active *penciclovir*. The antiviral spectrum is similar to that of *ganciclovir*, and it is approved for treatment of acute herpes zoster, genital HSV infection, and recurrent herpes labialis. The drug is effective orally (Figure 45.13). Adverse effects include headache and nausea.

F. Trifluridine

Trifluridine [trye-FLURE-i-deen] is a fluorinated pyrimidine nucleoside analog that is structurally similar to thymidine. Once converted to the triphosphate, the agent is believed to inhibit the incorporation of thymidine triphosphate into viral DNA and, to a lesser extent, lead to the synthesis of defective DNA that renders the virus unable to replicate. *Trifluridine* is active against HSV-1, HSV-2, and vaccinia virus. It is indicated for treatment of HSV keratoconjunctivitis and recurrent epithelial keratitis. Because the triphosphate form of *trifluridine* can also incorporate to some degree into cellular DNA, the drug is considered to be too toxic for systemic use. Therefore, the use of *trifluridine* is restricted to a topical ophthalmic preparation. A short half-life necessitates that the drug be applied frequently. Adverse effects include a transient irritation of the eye and palpebral (eyelid) edema.

Figure 45.14 summarizes selected antiviral agents.

V. OVERVIEW OF THE TREATMENT FOR HIV INFECTION

Prior to approval of *zidovudine* in 1987, treatment of HIV infections focused on decreasing the occurrence of opportunistic infections that caused a high degree of morbidity and mortality in AIDS patients. Today, the viral life cycle is understood (Figure 45.15), and a combination of drugs is used to suppress replication of HIV and restore the number of CD4 cells and immunocompetence to the host. This multidrug regimen is commonly referred to as "highly active antiretroviral therapy," or HAART (Figure 45.16). There are five classes of antiretroviral drugs, each of which targets one of the four viral processes. These classes of drugs are nucleoside and nucleotide reverse transcriptase inhibitors (NRTIs), nonnucleoside reverse transcriptase inhibitors (NNRTIs), protease inhibitors (PIs), entry inhibitors, and the integrase inhibitors. The preferred initial therapy is a combination of two NRTIs with a PI, an NNRTI, or an integrase inhibitor. Selection of the appropriate combination is based on 1) avoiding the use of two agents of the same nucleoside analog; 2) avoiding overlapping toxicities and genotypic and phenotypic characteristics of the virus; 3) patient factors, such as disease symptoms and concurrent

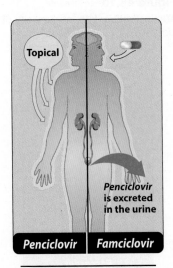

Figure 45.13
Administration and
fate of *penciclovir* and
famciclovir.

Antiviral drug	Mechanism of action	Viruses or diseases affected
Acyclovir	Metabolized to acyclovir triphosphate, which inhibits viral DNA polymerase	Herpes simplex, varicella-zoster, cytomegalovirus
Amantadine	Blockage of the M2 protein ion channel and its ability to modulate intracellular pH	Influenza A
Cidofovir	Inhibition of viral DNA polymerase	Cytomegalovirus; indicated only for virus-induced retinitis
Famciclovir	Same as *penciclovir*	Herpes simplex, varicella-zoster
Foscarnet	Inhibition of viral DNA polymerase and reverse transcriptase at the pyrophosphate-binding site	Cytomegalovirus, *acyclovir*-resistant herpes simplex, *acyclovir*-resistant varicella-zoster
Ganciclovir	Inhibits viral DNA polymerase	Cytomegalovirus
Interferon-α	Induction of cellular enzymes that interfere with viral protein synthesis	Hepatitis B and C, human herpesvirus 8, papilloma virus, Kaposi sarcoma, hairy cell leukemia, chronic myelogenous leukemia
Lamivudine	Inhibition of viral DNA polymerase and reverse transcriptase	Hepatitis B (chronic cases), human immunodeficiency virus type 1
Oseltamivir	Inhibition of viral neuraminidase	Influenza A
Penciclovir	Metabolized to penciclovir triphosphate, which inhibits viral DNA polymerase	Herpes simplex
Ribavirin	Interference with viral messenger RNA	Lassa fever, hantavirus (hemorrhagic fever renal syndrome), hepatitis C (in chronic cases in combination with *interferon-α* and in combination both with *interferon-α* and HCV protease inhibitor for HCV genotype I), RSV in children and infants
Rimantadine	Blockage of the M2 protein ion channel and its ability to modulate intracellular pH	Influenza A
Valacyclovir	Same as *acyclovir*	Herpes simplex, varicella-zoster, cytomegalovirus
Zanamivir	Inhibition of viral neuraminidase	Influenza A

Figure 45.14
Summary of selected antiviral agents. RSV = respiratory syncytial virus.

illnesses; 4) impact of drug interactions; and 5) ease of adherence to the regimen. The goals of therapy are to maximally and durably suppress HIV RNA replication, to restore and preserve immunologic function, to reduce HIV-related morbidity and mortality, and to improve quality of life.

VI. NRTIS USED TO TREAT HIV INFECTION

A. Overview of NRTIs

1. **Mechanism of action:** NRTIs are analogs of native ribosides (nucleosides or nucleotides containing ribose), which all lack a 3′-hydroxyl group. Once they enter cells, they are phosphorylated by cellular enzymes to the corresponding triphosphate analog, which is preferentially incorporated into the viral DNA by RT. Because the 3′-hydroxyl group is not present, a 3′,5′-phosphodiester bond between an incoming nucleoside triphosphate and the growing DNA

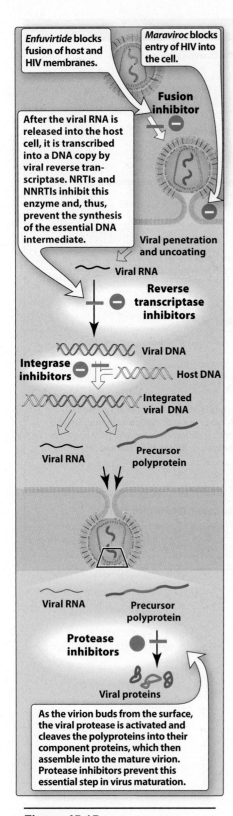

Enfuvirtide blocks fusion of host and HIV membranes.

Maraviroc blocks entry of HIV into the cell.

After the viral RNA is released into the host cell, it is transcribed into a DNA copy by viral reverse transcriptase. NRTIs and NNRTIs inhibit this enzyme and, thus, prevent the synthesis of the essential DNA intermediate.

Fusion inhibitor

Viral penetration and uncoating

Viral RNA

Reverse transcriptase inhibitors

Viral DNA

Integrase inhibitors

Host DNA

Integrated viral DNA

Viral RNA

Precursor polyprotein

Viral RNA

Precursor polyprotein

Protease inhibitors

Viral proteins

As the virion buds from the surface, the viral protease is activated and cleaves the polyproteins into their component proteins, which then assemble into the mature virion. Protease inhibitors prevent this essential step in virus maturation.

Figure 45.15
Drugs used to prevent HIV from replicating. NRTI = nucleoside and nucleotide reverse transcriptase inhibitor; NNRTI = nonnucleoside reverse transcriptase inhibitor.

chain cannot be formed, and DNA chain elongation is terminated. Affinities of the drugs for many host cell DNA polymerases are lower than they are for HIV RT, although mitochondrial DNA polymerase γ appears to be susceptible at therapeutic concentrations.

2. **Pharmacokinetics:** The NRTIs are primarily renally excreted, and all require dosage adjustment in renal insufficiency except *abacavir*, which is metabolized by alcohol dehydrogenase and glucuronyl transferase.

3. **Adverse effects:** Many of the toxicities of the NRTIs are believed to be due to inhibition of the mitochondrial DNA polymerase in certain tissues. As a general rule, the dideoxynucleosides, such as *didanosine* and *stavudine*, have a greater affinity for the mitochondrial DNA polymerase, leading to toxicities such as peripheral neuropathy, pancreatitis, and lipoatrophy. When more than one NRTI is given, care is taken to avoid overlapping toxicities. All of the NRTIs have been associated with a potentially fatal liver toxicity characterized by lactic acidosis and hepatomegaly with steatosis.

4. **Drug interactions:** Due to the renal excretion of the NRTIs, there are not many drug interactions encountered with these agents except for *zidovudine* and *tenofovir*.

5. **Resistance:** NRTI resistance is well characterized, and the most common resistance pattern is a mutation at viral RT codon 184, which confers a high degree of resistance to *lamivudine* and *emtricitabine* but, more importantly, restores sensitivity to *zidovudine* and *tenofovir*. Because cross-resistance and antagonism occur between agents of the same analog class (thymidine, cytosine, guanosine, and adenosine), concomitant use of agents with the same analog target is contraindicated (for example, *zidovudine* and *stavudine* are both analogs of thymidine and should not be used together).

B. Zidovudine (AZT)

Zidovudine [zye-DOE-vyoo-deen], the pyrimidine analog, *3′-azido-3′-deoxythymidine* (*AZT*), was the first agent available for the treatment of HIV infection. *AZT* is approved for the treatment of HIV in children and adults and to prevent perinatal transmission of HIV. It is also used for prophylaxis in individuals exposed to HIV infection. *AZT* is well absorbed after oral administration. Penetration across the blood–brain barrier is excellent, and the drug has a half-life of 1 hour with an intracellular half-life of approximately 3 hours. Most of the drug is glucuronidated by the liver and then excreted in the urine (Figure 45.17). *AZT* is toxic to bone marrow and can cause anemia and neutropenia. Headaches are also common. Both *stavudine* and *ribavirin* are activated by the same intracellular pathways and should not be given with *AZT*.

C. Stavudine (d4T)

Stavudine [STAV-yoo-deen] is an analog of thymidine approved for the treatment of HIV. The drug is well absorbed after oral administration, and it penetrates the blood–brain barrier. The majority of the drug is excreted unchanged in the urine. Renal impairment interferes with clearance. *Stavudine* is a strong inhibitor of cellular enzymes such as the DNA polymerases, thus reducing mitochondrial DNA synthesis and resulting in toxicity. The major and most common clinical toxicity is peripheral neuropathy, along with headache, rash, diarrhea, and lipoatrophy.

D. Didanosine (ddI)

Upon entry of *didanosine* [dye-DAN-oh-seen] (*dideoxyinosine, ddI*) into the host cell, *ddI* is biotransformed into dideoxyadenosine triphosphate (ddATP) through a series of reactions that involve phosphorylations and aminations. Like *AZT*, the resulting ddATP is incorporated into the DNA chain, causing termination of chain elongation. Due to its acid lability, absorption is best if *ddI* is taken in the fasting state. The drug penetrates into the CSF but to a lesser extent than does *AZT*. Most of the parent drug appears in the urine (Figure 45.18). Pancreatitis, which may be fatal, is a major toxicity with *ddI* and requires monitoring of serum amylase. The dose-limiting toxicity of *ddI* is peripheral neuropathy. Because of its similar adverse effect profile, concurrent use of *stavudine* is not recommended.

E. Tenofovir (TDF)

Tenofovir [te-NOE-fo-veer] is a nucleotide analog, namely, an acyclic nucleoside phosphonate analog of adenosine 5′-monophosphate. It is converted by cellular enzymes to the diphosphate, which is the inhibitor of HIV RT. Cross-resistance with other NRTIs may occur. *Tenofovir* has a long half-life, allowing once-daily dosing. Most of the drug is recovered unchanged in the urine. Serum creatinine must be monitored and doses adjusted in renal insufficiency. GI complaints are frequent and include nausea and bloating (Figure 45.19). The drug should not be used with *ddI* due to drug interactions. *Tenofovir* decreases the concentrations of the PI *atazanavir* such that *atazanavir* must be boosted with *ritonavir* if these agents are given concurrently.

F. Lamivudine (3TC)

Lamivudine [la-MI-vyoo-deen] (*2′-deoxy-3′-thiacytidine, 3TC*) inhibits the RT of both HIV and HBV. However, it does not affect mitochondrial DNA synthesis or bone marrow precursor cells, resulting in less toxicity. It has good bioavailability on oral administration, depends on the kidney for excretion, and is well tolerated.

G. Emtricitabine (FTC)

Emtricitabine [em-tri-SIGH-ta-been], a fluoro derivative of *lamivudine*, inhibits both HIV and HBV RT. *Emtricitabine* is well absorbed after oral administration. Plasma half-life is about 10 hours, whereas it has a long intracellular half-life of 39 hours. *Emtricitabine* is eliminated essentially unchanged in urine. It has no significant interactions with other drugs. Headache, diarrhea, nausea, and rash are the most common adverse effects. *Emtricitabine* may also cause hyperpigmentation of the soles and palms. Withdrawal of *emtricitabine* in HBV-infected patients may result in worsening hepatitis.

H. Abacavir (ABC)

Abacavir [a-BA-ka-veer] is a guanosine analog. *Abacavir* is well absorbed orally. It is metabolized to inactive metabolites via alcohol

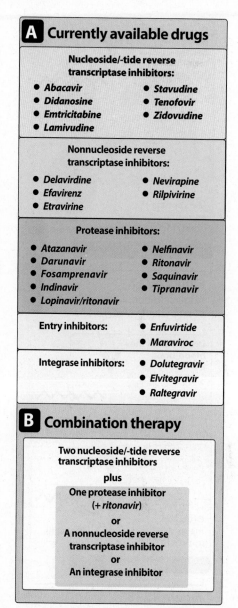

A **Currently available drugs**

Nucleoside/-tide reverse transcriptase inhibitors:
- *Abacavir*
- *Didanosine*
- *Emtricitabine*
- *Lamivudine*
- *Stavudine*
- *Tenofovir*
- *Zidovudine*

Nonnucleoside reverse transcriptase inhibitors:
- *Delavirdine*
- *Efavirenz*
- *Etravirine*
- *Nevirapine*
- *Rilpivirine*

Protease inhibitors:
- *Atazanavir*
- *Darunavir*
- *Fosamprenavir*
- *Indinavir*
- *Lopinavir/ritonavir*
- *Nelfinavir*
- *Ritonavir*
- *Saquinavir*
- *Tipranavir*

Entry inhibitors:
- *Enfuvirtide*
- *Maraviroc*

Integrase inhibitors:
- *Dolutegravir*
- *Elvitegravir*
- *Raltegravir*

B **Combination therapy**

Two nucleoside/-tide reverse transcriptase inhibitors

plus

One protease inhibitor (+ *ritonavir*)

or

A nonnucleoside reverse transcriptase inhibitor

or

An integrase inhibitor

Figure 45.16
Highly active antiretroviral therapy (HAART).

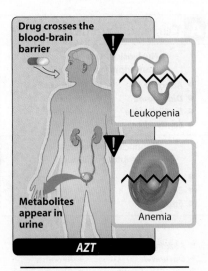

Figure 45.17
Administration, fate, and toxicity
of *zidovudine* (*AZT*).

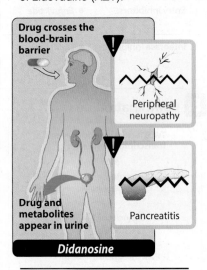

Figure 45.18
Administration, fate, and toxicity
of *didanosine*.

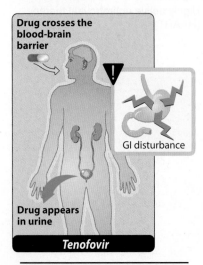

Figure 45.19
Administration, fate, and toxicity
of *tenofovir*.

dehydrogenase and glucuronyl transferase, and metabolites appear in the urine (Figure 45.20). Common adverse effects include GI disturbances, headache, and dizziness. Approximately 5% of patients exhibit the "hypersensitivity reaction," which is usually characterized by drug fever, plus a rash, GI symptoms, malaise, or respiratory distress (Figure 45.21). Sensitized individuals should *never* be rechallenged because of rapidly appearing, severe reactions that may lead to death. A genetic test (HLA-B*5701) is available to screen patients for the potential of this reaction. Figure 45.22 shows some adverse reactions commonly seen with nucleoside analogs.

VII. NNRTIS USED TO TREAT HIV INFECTION

NNRTIs are highly selective, noncompetitive inhibitors of HIV-1 RT. They bind to HIV RT at an allosteric hydrophobic site adjacent to the active site, inducing a conformational change that results in enzyme inhibition. They do not require activation by cellular enzymes. These drugs have common characteristics that include cross-resistance with other NNRTIs, drug interactions, and a high incidence of hypersensitivity reactions, including rash.

A. Nevirapine (NVP)

Nevirapine [ne-VYE-ra-peen] is used in combination with other antiretroviral drugs for the treatment of HIV infections in adults and children. Due to the potential for severe hepatotoxicity, *nevirapine* should not be initiated in women with CD4 cell counts greater than 250 cells/mm^3 or in men with CD4 cell counts greater than 400 cells/mm^3. *Nevirapine* is well absorbed orally. The lipophilic nature of *nevirapine* accounts for its wide tissue distribution, including the CNS, placenta (transfers to the fetus), and breast milk. *Nevirapine* is metabolized via hydroxylation and subsequent glucuronide conjugation. The metabolites are excreted in urine (Figure 45.23). *Nevirapine* is an inducer of the CYP3A4 isoenzymes, and it increases the metabolism of a number of drugs, such as oral contraceptives, *ketoconazole, methadone, quinidine,* and *warfarin*. The most frequently observed adverse effects are rash, fever, headache, and elevated serum transaminases and fatal hepatotoxicity. Severe dermatologic effects have been encountered, including Stevens-Johnson syndrome and toxic epidermal necrolysis. A 14-day titration period at half the dose is mandatory to reduce the risk of serious epidermal reactions and hepatotoxicity.

B. Delavirdine (DLV)

Delavirdine [de-LA-vir-deen] is not recommended as a preferred or alternate NNRTI in the current HIV guidelines due to its inferior antiviral efficacy and inconvenient (three times daily) dosing.

C. Efavirenz (EFV)

Efavirenz [e-FA-veer-enz] is the preferred NNRTI. Following oral administration, *efavirenz* is well distributed, including to the CNS (Figure 45.24). It should be administered on an empty stomach to reduce adverse CNS effects. Most of the drug is bound to plasma albumin at therapeutic doses. A half-life of more than 40 hours accounts for its recommended once-a-day dosing. *Efavirenz* is extensively metabolized to inactive products. The drug is a potent inducer of CYP450 enzymes and, therefore, may reduce the concentrations of drugs that are substrates of the CYP450. Most adverse effects are tolerable and are associated with the CNS, including dizziness, headache, vivid dreams, and loss of concentration (Figure 45.25). Nearly half of patients experience these complaints, which usually resolve within a few weeks. Rash is another common adverse effect. *Efavirenz* should be avoided in pregnant women.

D. Etravirine (ETR)

Etravirine [et-ra-VYE-rine] is a second-generation NNRTI active against many HIV strains that are resistant to the first-generation NNRTIs. HIV strains with the common K103N mutation that are resistant to the first-generation NNRTIs are fully susceptible to *etravirine*. *Etravirine* is indicated for HIV treatment–experienced, multidrug-resistant patients who have evidence of ongoing viral replication. The bioavailability of *etravirine* is enhanced when taken with a high-fat meal. Although it has a half-life of approximately 40 hours, it is indicated for twice-daily dosing. *Etravirine* is extensively metabolized to inactive products and excreted mainly in the feces. Because *etravirine* is a potent inducer of CYP450, the doses of CYP450 substrates may need to be increased when given with *etravirine*. Rash is the most common adverse effect.

E. Rilpivirine (RPV)

Rilpivirine [ril-pi-VIR-een] is approved for HIV treatment-naïve patients in combination with other antiretroviral agents. It is administered orally once daily with meals and has pH-dependent absorption. Therefore, it should not be coadministered with proton pump inhibitors and requires dose separation from H_2-receptor antagonists and antacids. *Rilpivirine* is highly bound to plasma proteins, primarily albumin. *Rilpivirine* is a substrate of CYP3A4, and coadministration with other medications that are inducers or inhibitors of this isoenzyme may affect levels of the drug. *Rilpivirine* is mainly excreted in the feces. Cross-resistance to other NNRTIs is likely after virologic failure and development of *rilpivirine* resistance. The most common adverse reactions are depressive disorders, headache, insomnia, and rash.

VIII. PROTEASE INHIBITORS USED TO TREAT HIV INFECTION

Inhibitors of HIV protease have significantly altered the course of this devastating viral disease. Within a year of their introduction in 1995, the number of deaths in the United States due to AIDS declined, although the trend appears to be leveling off (Figure 45.26).

A. Overview

These potent agents have several common features that characterize their pharmacology.

1. **Mechanism of action:** All of the drugs in this group are reversible inhibitors of the HIV aspartyl protease (retropepsin), which is the viral enzyme responsible for cleavage of the viral polyprotein

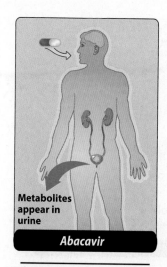

Figure 45.20
Administration and fate of *abacavir*.

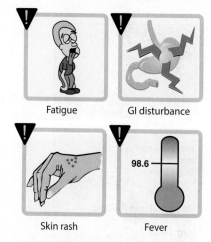

Fatigue   GI disturbance

Skin rash   Fever

Figure 45.21
Hypersensitivity reactions to *abacavir*.

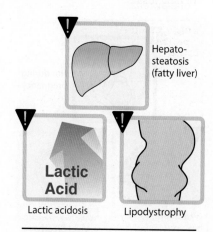

Hepato-steatosis (fatty liver)

Lactic Acid

Lactic acidosis   Lipodystrophy

Figure 45.22
Some adverse reactions of nucleoside analogs.

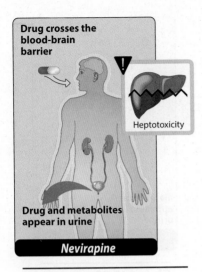

Figure 45.23
Administration, fate, and toxicity of *nevirapine*.

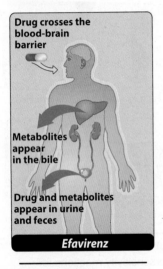

Figure 45.24
Administration and fate of *efavirenz*.

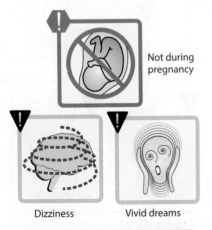

Figure 45.25
Adverse reactions of *efavirenz*.

into a number of essential enzymes (RT, protease, and integrase) and several structural proteins. The inhibition prevents maturation of the viral particles and results in the production of noninfectious virions.

2. **Pharmacokinetics:** High-fat meals substantially increase the bioavailability of some PIs, such as *nelfinavir* and *saquinavir*, whereas the bioavailability of *indinavir* is decreased, and others are essentially unaffected. The HIV PIs are all substantially bound to plasma proteins. All are substrates for the CYP3A4 isoenzyme, and individual PIs are also metabolized by other CYP450 isoenzymes. Metabolism is extensive, and very little of the PIs are excreted unchanged in urine. Dosage adjustments are unnecessary in renal impairment.

3. **Adverse effects:** PIs commonly cause nausea, vomiting, and diarrhea (Figure 45.27). Disturbances in glucose and lipid metabolism also occur, including diabetes, hypertriglyceridemia, and hypercholesterolemia. Chronic administration results in fat redistribution, including loss of fat from the extremities, fat accumulation in the abdomen and the base of the neck ("buffalo hump"; Figure 45.28), and breast enlargement. These physical changes may indicate to others that an individual is HIV infected.

4. **Drug interactions:** Drug interactions are a common problem for all PIs, because they are not only substrates but also potent inhibitors of CYP450 isoenzymes. Drug interactions are, therefore, quite common. Drugs that rely on metabolism for their termination of action may accumulate to toxic levels. Examples of potentially dangerous interactions from drugs that are contraindicated with PIs include rhabdomyolysis from *simvastatin* or *lovastatin*, excessive sedation from *midazolam* or *triazolam*, and respiratory depression from *fentanyl* (Figure 45.29). Other drug interactions that require dosage modification and cautious use include *warfarin, sildenafil,* and *phenytoin* (Figure 45.30). In addition, inducers of CYP450 isoenzymes may decrease PI plasma concentrations to suboptimal levels, contributing to treatment failures. Thus, drugs such as *rifampin* and *St. John's wort* are also contraindicated with PIs.

5. **Resistance:** Resistance occurs as an accumulation of stepwise mutations of the protease gene. Initial mutations result in decreased ability of the virus to replicate, but as the mutations accumulate, virions with high levels of resistance to the protease inhibitors emerge. Suboptimal concentrations of PI result in the more rapid appearance of resistant strains.

B. Ritonavir (RTV)

Ritonavir [ri-TOE-na-veer] is no longer used as a single PI but, instead, is used as a pharmacokinetic enhancer or "booster" of other PIs. *Ritonavir* is a potent inhibitor of CYP3A, and concomitant *ritonavir* administration at low doses increases the bioavailability of the second PI, often allowing for longer dosing intervals. The resulting higher C_{min} levels of the "boosted" PI also help to prevent the development of resistance. Therefore, "boosted" PIs are preferred agents in the HIV treatment guidelines. Metabolism and biliary excretion are the primary methods of elimination. *Ritonavir* has a half-life of 3 to 5 hours. Because it is primarily an inhibitor of CYP450 isoenzymes, numerous drug interactions have been identified. Nausea, vomiting, diarrhea, headache, and circumoral paresthesias are among the more common adverse effects.

C. Saquinavir (SQV)

To maximize bioavailability, *saquinavir* [sa-KWIH-na-veer] is always given along with a low dose of *ritonavir.* High-fat meals also enhance absorption. Elimination of *saquinavir* is primarily by hepatic metabolism, followed by biliary excretion. Its half-life is 7 to 12 hours, requiring twice-daily dosing. The most common adverse effects of *saquinavir* include headache, fatigue, diarrhea, nausea, and other GI disturbances. Increased levels of hepatic aminotransferases have been noted, particularly in patients with concurrent hepatitis B or C infections.

D. Indinavir (IDV)

Indinavir [in-DIH-na-veer] is well absorbed orally and, of all the PIs, is the least protein bound. Acidic gastric conditions are necessary for absorption. Absorption is decreased when administered with meals, although a light, low-fat snack is permissible. *Indinavir* has the shortest half-life of the PIs, at 1.8 hours. Boosting with *ritonavir* overcomes this problem and also permits twice-daily dosing. *Indinavir* is extensively metabolized, and the metabolites are excreted in the feces and urine. The dosage should, therefore, be reduced in the presence of hepatic insufficiency. GI symptoms and headache are the predominant adverse effects. *Indinavir* characteristically causes nephrolithiasis and hyperbilirubinemia. Adequate hydration is important to reduce the incidence of kidney stone formation, and patients should drink at least 1.5 L of water per day. Fat redistribution is particularly troublesome with this drug.

E. Nelfinavir (NFV)

Nelfinavir [nel-FIN-a-veer] is well absorbed and does not require strict food or fluid conditions, although it is usually given with food. *Nelfinavir* undergoes metabolism by several CYP450 isoenzymes. It is the only PI that cannot be boosted by *ritonavir,* because it is not extensively metabolized by CYP3A. The half-life of *nelfinavir* is 5 hours. Diarrhea is the most common adverse effect and can be controlled with *loperamide.*

F. Fosamprenavir (FPV)

Fosamprenavir [fos-am-PREN-a-veer] is a prodrug that is metabolized to *amprenavir* following oral absorption. Its long plasma half-life permits twice-daily dosing. Coadministration of *ritonavir* increases the plasma levels of *amprenavir* and lowers the total daily dose. *Fosamprenavir* boosted with *ritonavir* is one of the alternative PIs according to the current HIV treatment guidelines. Nausea, vomiting, diarrhea, fatigue, paresthesias, and headache are common adverse effects.

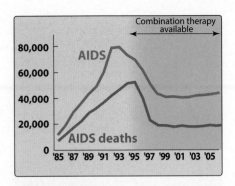

Figure 45.26
Estimated number of AIDS cases and deaths due to AIDS in the United States. *Green* background indicates years in which combination antiretroviral therapy came into common usage.

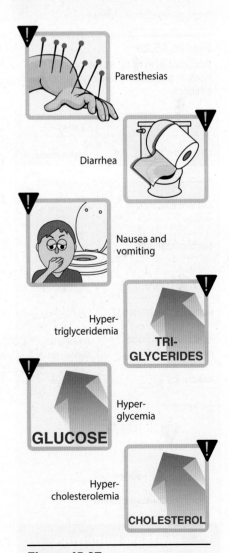

Figure 45.27
Some adverse effects of the HIV protease inhibitors.

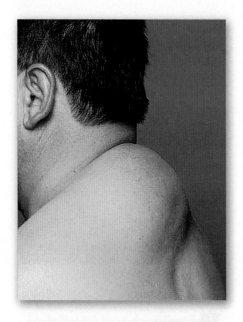

Figure 45.28
Accumulation of fat at the base of the neck in a patient receiving a protease inhibitor.

DRUG CLASS	EXAMPLE
ANTIARRHYTHMICS	*Amiodarone*
ERGOT DERIVATIVES	*Ergotamine*
ANTIMYCOBACTERIAL DRUGS	*Rifampin*
BENZODIAZEPINES	*Triazolam*
INHALED STEROIDS	*Fluticasone*
HERBAL SUPPLEMENTS	*St. John's wort*
HMG CoA REDUCTASE INHIBITORS	*Lovastatin Simvastatin*
NARCOTICS	*Fentanyl*
β-2 AGONIST	*Salmeterol*

Contraindicated

PROTEASE INHIBITORS

Figure 45.29
Drugs that should not be coadministered with any protease inhibitor.

G. Lopinavir (LPV/r)

Lopinavir [loe-PIN-a-veer] is an alternative PI, according to the HIV treatment guidelines. *Lopinavir* has very poor bioavailability, which is substantially enhanced by including a low-dose *ritonavir* booster in the formulation. GI adverse effects and hypertriglyceridemia are the most common adverse effects of *lopinavir*. Enzyme inducers as well as *St. John's wort* should be avoided, because they lower the plasma concentrations of *lopinavir*. Because the oral solution contains alcohol, *disulfiram* or *metronidazole* administration can cause unpleasant reactions.

H. Atazanavir (ATV)

Atazanavir [ah-ta-ZA-na-veer] is a preferred PI. *Atazanavir* is well absorbed orally. It must be taken with food, because food increases absorption and bioavailability. The drug is highly protein bound and undergoes extensive metabolism by CYP3A4 isoenzymes. It is excreted primarily in bile. It has a half-life of about 7 hours, but it may be administered once daily. *Atazanavir* is a competitive inhibitor of glucuronyl transferase, and benign hyperbilirubinemia and jaundice are known adverse effects. In the heart, *atazanavir* prolongs the PR interval. *Atazanavir* exhibits a decreased risk of hyperlipidemia compared with other PIs. Unboosted *atazanavir* is contraindicated with concurrent use of proton pump inhibitors, and administration must be spaced apart from H_2-blockers and antacids.

I. Tipranavir (TPV)

Tipranavir [ti-PRA-na-veer] is a nonpeptide PI that inhibits HIV protease in viruses that are resistant to the other PIs. *Tipranavir* is well absorbed when taken with food. The half-life is 6 hours, and it must be administered twice daily in combination with *ritonavir*. Adverse effects are similar to those of the other PIs, with the exception of severe and fatal hepatitis and rare cases of intracranial hemorrhage. Most patients experiencing these severe adverse effects have underlying comorbidities. *Tipranavir* is useful in "salvage" regimens in patients with multidrug resistance.

J. Darunavir (DRV)

Darunavir [da-RU-na-veer] is a preferred PI and is always given along with a low dose of *ritonavir*. *Darunavir* is approved for initial therapy in treatment-naïve HIV-infected patients, as well as for treatment-experienced patients with HIV that is resistant to other PIs. *Darunavir* must be taken with food to increase absorption. The elimination half-life is 15 hours when combined with *ritonavir*. *Darunavir* is extensively metabolized by the CYP3A enzymes and is also an inhibitor of the CYP3A4 isoenzyme. Adverse effects are similar to those of the other PIs. In addition, *darunavir* therapy has been associated with a rash.

A summary of PIs is presented in Figure 45.31.

IX. ENTRY INHIBITORS USED TO TREAT HIV INFECTION

A. Enfuvirtide

Enfuvirtide [en-FU-veer-tide] is a fusion inhibitor. For HIV to gain entry into the host cell, it must fuse its membrane with that of the host cell. This is accomplished by changes in the conformation of the viral transmembrane glycoprotein gp41, which occurs when HIV binds to the host cell surface. *Enfuvirtide* is a polypeptide that binds to gp41, preventing the conformational change. *Enfuvirtide*, in combination with other antiretroviral agents, is approved for therapy of treatment-experienced patients with evidence of viral replication despite ongoing antiretroviral drug therapy. As a peptide, it must be given subcutaneously. Most of the adverse effects are related to the injection, including pain, erythema, induration, and nodules, which occur in almost all patients. *Enfuvirtide* must be reconstituted prior to administration.

B. Maraviroc

Maraviroc [ma-RAV-i-rok] is another entry inhibitor. Because it is well absorbed orally, it is formulated as an oral tablet. *Maraviroc* blocks the CCR5 coreceptor that works together with gp41 to facilitate HIV entry through the membrane into the cell. HIV may express preference for either the CCR5 coreceptor or the CXCR4 coreceptor, or both (dual-tropic). Prior to use of *maraviroc*, a test to determine viral tropism is required to distinguish whether the strain of HIV virus uses the CCR5 coreceptor, the CXCR4 coreceptor, or is dual-tropic. Only strains of HIV that use CCR5 to gain access to the cell can be successfully treated with *maraviroc*. *Maraviroc* is metabolized by CYP450 liver enzymes, and the dose must be reduced when given with most PIs or strong CYP450 inhibitors. Conversely, it should be increased in patients receiving *efavirenz*, *etravirine*, or strong CYP450 inducers. *Maraviroc* is generally well tolerated.

X. INTEGRASE INHIBITORS USED TO TREAT HIV INFECTION

The integrase strand transfer inhibitors (INSTIs), often called integrase inhibitors, work by inhibiting the insertion of proviral DNA into the host cell genome. The active site of the integrase enzyme binds to the host cell DNA and includes two divalent metal cations that serve as chelation targets for the INSTIs. As a result, when an INSTI is present, the active site of the enzyme is occupied and the integration process is halted. The INSTIs are generally well tolerated, with nausea and diarrhea being the most commonly reported adverse effects. Importantly, INSTIs are subject to chelation interactions with antacids resulting in significant reductions in bioavailability. It is therefore recommended that INSTI doses are separated from antacids and other polyvalent cations by several hours. Resistance to INSTIs occurs with single-point mutations within the integrase gene. Cross-resistance between *raltegravir* and *elvitegravir* can occur, although *dolutegravir* has limited cross-resistance to other INSTIs.

DRUG CLASS	EXAMPLE
ANTICOAGULANTS	*Warfarin*
ANTICONVULSANTS	*Phenytoin*
ANTIFUNGALS	*Voriconazole*
ANTIMYCOBACTERIALS	*Rifabutin*
ERECTILE DYSFUNCTION AGENTS	*Sildenafil* *Tadalafil* *Vardenafil*
LIPID-LOWERING AGENTS	*Atorvastatin*
NARCOTICS	*Methadone*

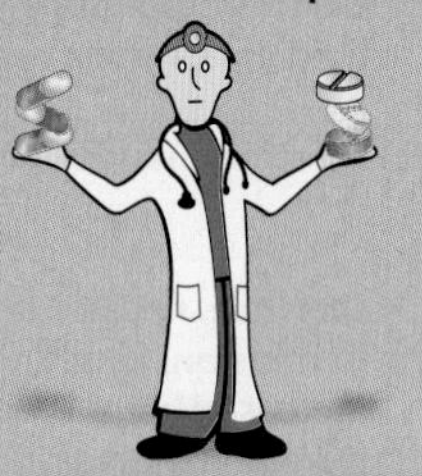

PROTEASE INHIBITORS

Figure 45.30
Drugs that require dose modifications or cautious use with any protease inhibitor.

DRUGS	MAJOR TOXICITIES AND CONCERNS
Atazanavir	Nausea, abdominal discomfort, skin rash, hyperbilirubinemia
Darunavir	Nausea, abdominal discomfort, headache, skin rash
Fosamprenavir	Nausea, diarrhea, vomiting, oral and perioral paresthesia, and rash
Indinavir	Benign hyperbilirubinemia, nephrolithiasis; take 1 hour before or 2 hours after food; may take with skim milk or a low-fat meal; drink >1.5 L of liquid daily
Lopinavir	Gastrointestinal, hyperlipidemia, insulin resistance
Nelfinavir	Diarrhea, nausea, flatulence, rash
Ritonavir	Diarrhea, nausea, taste perversion, vomiting, anemia, increased hepatic enzymes, increased triglycerides. Capsules require refrigeration, tablets do not. Take with meals; chocolate milk improves the taste
Saquinavir	Diarrhea, nausea, abdominal discomfort, elevated transaminase levels. Take with high-fat meal or within 2 hours of a full meal
Tipranavir	Nausea, vomiting, diarrhea, rash, severe hepatotoxicity, intracranial hemorrhage

Figure 45.31

Summary of protease inhibitors. [Note: *Lopinavir* is coformulated with *ritonavir*. *Ritonavir* inhibits the metabolism of *lopinavir*, thereby increasing its level in the plasma.]

A. Raltegravir

In combination with other antiretroviral agents, *raltegravir* [ral-TEG-ra-veer] is approved for both initial therapy of treatment-naïve patients and treatment-experienced patients with evidence of viral replication despite ongoing antiretroviral drug therapy. *Raltegravir* has a half-life of approximately 9 hours and is dosed twice daily. The route of metabolism is UDP-glucuronosyltransferase (UGT)1A1-mediated glucuronidation and, therefore, drug interactions with CYP450 inducers, inhibitors, or substrates do not occur. *Raltegravir* is well tolerated, although serious adverse effects, such as elevated creatine kinase with muscle pain and rhabdomyolysis and possible depression with suicidal ideation, have been reported.

B. Elvitegravir

Elvitegravir [el-vi-TEG-ra-vir] is currently only available in a fixed-dose combination single tablet containing *tenofovir*, *emtricitabine*, *elvitegravir*, and *cobicistat*. [Note: *Cobicistat* is a pharmacokinetic enhancer or booster drug used in combination treatments of HIV since it inhibits CYP3A enzymes.] The half-life of *elvitegravir* is 3 hours when administered alone, but increases to approximately 9 hours when boosted by *cobicistat*. Pharmacokinetic boosting of *elvitegravir* allows it to be dosed orally once daily with food. However, it can also lead to clinically significant drug interactions. *Elvitegravir* is highly bound to plasma proteins and is primarily metabolized in the liver via CYP3A, and to a lesser extent via UGT1A1/3 glucuronidation. It is mainly excreted in the feces. The most common adverse effect of *elvitegravir* is nausea, although *cobicistat* may also cause elevations in serum creatinine due to inhibition of tubular creatinine secretion. Cross-resistance between *raltegravir* and *elvitegravir* is high.

C. Dolutegravir

Dolutegravir [doe-loo-TEG-ra-vir] is rapidly absorbed following oral administration. *Dolutegravir* is highly protein bound and undergoes extensive hepatic metabolism. Metabolism primarily occurs through UGT1A1 with minor contributions from CYP3A4. Potent inducers and/or inhibitors of UGT1A1 and CYP3A4 can significantly alter *dolutegravir* concentrations. More than half the dose is eliminated unchanged in the feces; nearly a third is eliminated as metabolites in the urine. It is an inhibitor of the renal transport protein OCT2 and can result in mild, benign, and reversible elevation in serum creatinine. *Dolutegravir* can be given once daily without the use of a pharmacokinetic booster in patients without preexisting INSTI resistance. Twice-daily dosing is recommended for INSTI treatment-experienced patients or when strong UGT1A1 or CYP3A inducers are present. Depending on the specific genetic profile, some patients with *raltegravir* and *elvitegravir* resistance mutations maintain susceptibility to *dolutegravir*.

Study Questions

Choose the ONE best answer.

45.1 A 30-year-old male patient with human immuno-deficiency virus infection is being treated with a HAART (highly active antiretroviral therapy) regimen. Four weeks after initiating therapy, he presents to the emergency department complaining of fever, rash, and gastrointestinal upset. Which one of the following drugs is most likely the cause of his symptoms?

A. Zidovudine.

B. Nelfinavir.

C. Abacavir.

D. Efavirenz.

E. Darunavir.

Correct answer = C. The abacavir hypersensitivity reaction is characterized by fever, rash, and gastrointestinal upset. The patient must stop therapy and not be rechallenged.

45.2 A 75-year-old man with chronic obstructive pulmonary disease is diagnosed with suspected influenza based on his complaints of flu-like symptoms that began 24 hours ago. Which of the following agents is most appropriate to initiate for the treatment of influenza?

A. Ribavirin.

B. Oseltamivir.

C. Zanamivir.

D. Rimantadine.

E. Amantadine.

Correct answer = B. Oseltamivir is the best choice since it is administered orally and not associated with resistance. Zanamivir is administered via inhalation and is not recommended for patients with underlying COPD. High rates of resistance have developed to adamantanes (amantadine, rimantadine), and these drugs are infrequently indicated. Ribavirin is not indicated for treatment of influenza.

45.3 A 24-year-old female is diagnosed with genital herpes simplex virus infection. Which of the following agents is indicated for use in this diagnosis?

A. Valacyclovir.

B. Cidofovir.

C. Ganciclovir.

D. Zanamivir.

E. Lamivudine.

Correct answer = A. Valacyclovir, famciclovir, penciclovir, and acyclovir are all indicated for herpes simplex virus infection. Cidofovir and ganciclovir are used for CMV retinitis. Zanamivir is indicated for influenza. Lamivudine is indicated for HIV and hepatitis B.

45.4 A female patient who is being treated for chronic hepatitis B develops nephrotoxicity while on treatment. Which is the most likely medication she is taking for HBV treatment?

A. Entecavir.

B. Telbivudine.

C. Lamivudine.

D. Adefovir.

Correct answer = D. Nephrotoxicity is the most commonly seen with adefovir.

Anticancer Drugs

46

Kourtney LaPlant and Paige Louzon

I. OVERVIEW

It is estimated that over 25% of the population of the United States will face a diagnosis of cancer during their lifetime, with more than 1.6 million new cancer patients diagnosed each year. Less than a quarter of these patients will be cured solely by surgery and/or local radiation. Most of the remainder will receive systemic chemotherapy at some time during their illness. In a small fraction (approximately 10%) of patients with cancer representing selected neoplasms, the chemotherapy will result in a cure or a prolonged remission. However, in most cases, the drug therapy will produce only a regression of the disease, and complications and/or relapse may eventually lead to death. Thus, the overall 5-year survival rate for cancer patients is about 68%, ranking cancer second only to cardiovascular disease as a cause of mortality. Figure 46.1 provides a list of the anticancer agents discussed in this chapter.

II. PRINCIPLES OF CANCER CHEMOTHERAPY

Cancer chemotherapy strives to cause a lethal cytotoxic event or apoptosis in the cancer cells that can arrest a tumor's progression. The attack is generally directed toward DNA or against metabolic sites essential to cell replication, for example, the availability of purines and pyrimidines, which are the building blocks for DNA or RNA synthesis (Figure 46.2). Ideally, these anticancer drugs should interfere only with cellular processes that are unique to malignant cells. Unfortunately, most currently available anticancer drugs do not specifically recognize neoplastic cells but, rather, affect all kinds of proliferating cells, both normal and abnormal. Therefore, almost all antitumor agents have a steep dose–response curve for both therapeutic and toxic effects.

A. Treatment strategies

1. **Goals of treatment:** The ultimate goal of chemotherapy is a cure (that is, long-term, disease-free survival). A true cure requires the eradication of every neoplastic cell. If a cure is not attainable, then the goal becomes control of the disease (stop the cancer from enlarging and spreading) to extend survival and maintain the best quality of life. Thus, the individual maintains a "near-normal" existence, with the cancer being treated as a chronic disease. In either case, the neoplastic cell burden is initially reduced (debulked),

ANTIMETABOLITES
Azacitidine VIDAZA
Capecitabine XELODA
Cladribine LEUSTATIN
Cytarabine CYTOSINE ARABINOSIDE (ARA-C)
Fludarabine FLUDARA
5-Fluorouracil ADRUCIL
Gemcitabine GEMZAR
6-Mercaptopurine PURINETHOL
Methotrexate (MTX) TREXALL
Pemetrexed ALIMTA
Pralatrexate FOLOTYN

ANTIBIOTICS
Bleomycin BLENOXANE
Daunorubicin CERUBIDINE
Doxorubicin ADRIAMYCIN
Epirubicin ELLENCE
Idarubicin IDAMYCIN
Mitoxantrone

ALKYLATING AGENTS
Busulfan MYLERAN
Carmustine BICNU
Chlorambucil LEUKERAN
Cyclophosphamide CYTOXAN
Dacarbazine DTIC-DOME
Ifosfamide IFEX
Lomustine CEENU
Melphalan ALKERAN
Temozolomide TEMODAR

MICROTUBULE INHIBITORS
Docetaxel TAXOTERE
Paclitaxel TAXOL
Vinblastine
Vincristine VINCASAR PFS
Vinorelbine NAVELBINE

Figure 46.1
Summary of chemotherapeutic agents.
(Figure continues on next page.)

STEROID HORMONES AND THEIR ANTAGONISTS

Anastrozole ARIMIDEX
Bicalutamide CASODEX
Estrogens VARIOUS
Exemestane AROMASIN
Flutamide
Fulvestrant FASLODEX
Goserelin ZOLADEX
Letrozole FEMARA
Leuprolide LUPRON
Megestrol acetate MEGACE
Nilutamide NILANDRON
Prednisone
Raloxifene EVISTA
Tamoxifen
Triptorelin TRELSTAR

MONOCLONAL ANTIBODIES

Bevacizumab AVASTIN
Cetuximab ERBITUX
Rituximab RITUXAN
Trastuzumab HERCEPTIN

TYROSINE KINASE INHIBITORS

Dasatinib SPRYCEL
Erlotinib TARCEVA
Imatinib GLEEVEC
Nilotinib TASIGNA
Sorafenib NEXAVAR
Sunitinib SUTENT

OTHERS

Abiraterone ZYTIGA
Asparaginase ERWINAZE
Carboplatin
Cisplatin PLATINOL
Enzalutamide XTANDI
Etoposide TOPOSAR, VEPESID
Interferons PEG-INTRON
Irinotecan CAMPTOSAR
Oxaliplatin ELOXATIN
Procarbazine MATULANE
Topotecan HYCAMTIN

Figure 46.1 (Continued)
Summary of chemotherapeutic agents.

either by surgery and/or by radiation, followed by chemotherapy, immunotherapy, therapy using biological modifiers, or a combination of these treatment modalities (Figure 46.3). In advanced stages of cancer, the likelihood of controlling the cancer is far from reality and the goal is palliation (alleviation of symptoms and avoidance of life-threatening toxicity). This means that chemotherapeutic drugs may be used to relieve symptoms caused by the cancer and improve the quality of life, even though the drugs may not extend survival. The goal of treatment should always be kept in mind, as it often influences treatment decisions. Figure 46.4 illustrates how treatment goals can be dynamic.

2. **Indications for treatment:** Chemotherapy is sometimes used when neoplasms are disseminated and are not amenable to surgery. Chemotherapy may also be used as a supplemental treatment to attack micrometastases following surgery and radiation treatment, in which case it is called adjuvant chemotherapy. Chemotherapy given prior to the surgical procedure in an attempt to shrink the cancer is referred to as neoadjuvant chemotherapy, and chemotherapy given in lower doses to assist in prolonging a remission is known as maintenance chemotherapy.

3. **Tumor susceptibility and the growth cycle:** The fraction of tumor cells that are in the replicative cycle ("growth fraction") influences their susceptibility to most cancer chemotherapeutic agents. Rapidly dividing cells are generally more sensitive to chemotherapy, whereas slowly proliferating cells are less sensitive to chemotherapy. In general, nondividing cells (those in the G_0 phase; Figure 46.5) usually survive the toxic effects of many of these agents.

   a. **Cell cycle specificity of drugs:** Both normal cells and tumor cells go through growth cycles (Figure 46.5). However, the number of cells that are in various stages of the cycle may differ in normal and neoplastic tissues. Chemotherapeutic agents that are effective only against replicating cells (that is, those cells that are dividing) are said to be cell cycle specific (Figure 46.5), whereas other agents are said to be cell cycle nonspecific. The nonspecific drugs, although having generally more toxicity in cycling cells, are also useful against tumors that have a low percentage of replicating cells.

   b. **Tumor growth rate:** The growth rate of most solid tumors in vivo is initially rapid, but growth rate usually decreases as the tumor size increases (Figure 46.3). This is due to the unavailability of nutrients and oxygen caused by inadequate vascularization and lack of blood circulation. Tumor burden can be reduced through surgery, radiation, or by using cell cycle–nonspecific drugs to promote the remaining cells into active proliferation, thus increasing their susceptibility to cell cycle–specific chemotherapeutic agents.

B. Treatment regimens and scheduling

Drug dosages are usually calculated on the basis of body surface area, in an effort to tailor the medications to each patient.

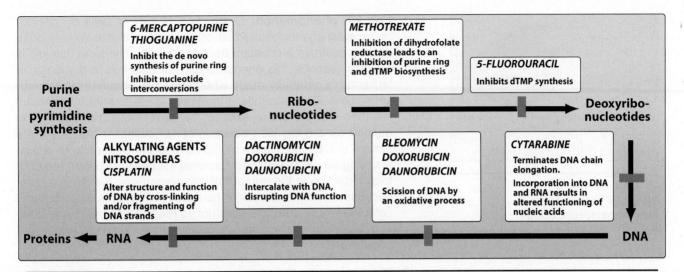

Figure 46.2
Examples of chemotherapeutic agents affecting RNA and DNA. dTMP = deoxythymidine monophosphate.

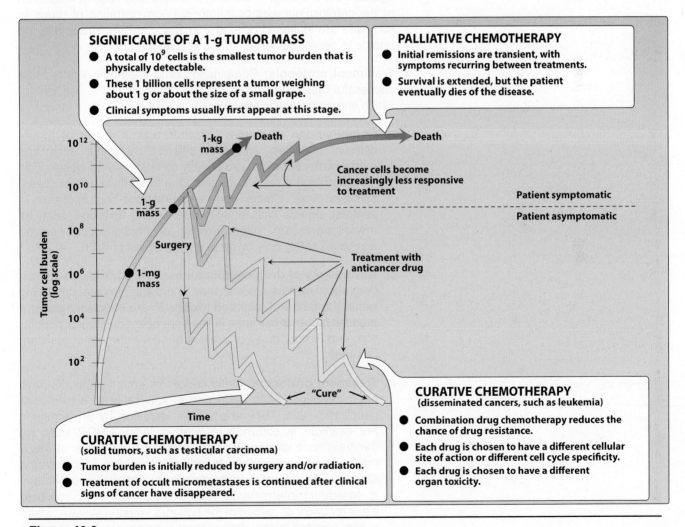

Figure 46.3
Effects of various treatments on the cancer cell burden in a hypothetical patient.

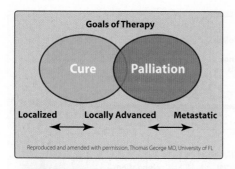

Figure 46.4
Goals of treatment with chemotherapeutic agents.

1. **Log kill phenomenon:** Destruction of cancer cells by chemotherapeutic agents follows first-order kinetics (that is, a given dose of drug destroys a constant fraction of cells). The term "log kill" is used to describe this phenomenon. For example, a diagnosis of leukemia is generally made when there are about 10^9 (total) leukemic cells. Consequently, if treatment leads to a 99.999-percent kill, then 0.001% of 10^9 cells (or 10^4 cells) would remain. This is defined as a 5-log kill (reduction of 10^5 cells). At this point, the patient will become asymptomatic, and the patient is in remission (Figure 46.3). For most bacterial infections, a 5-log (100,000-fold) reduction in the number of microorganisms results in a cure, because the immune system can destroy the remaining bacterial cells. However, tumor cells are not as readily eliminated, and additional treatment is required to totally eradicate the leukemic cell population.

2. **Pharmacologic sanctuaries:** Leukemic or other tumor cells find sanctuary in tissues such as the central nervous system (CNS), where transport constraints prevent certain chemotherapeutic agents from entering. Therefore, a patient may require irradiation of the craniospinal axis or intrathecal administration of drugs to eliminate the leukemic cells at that site. Similarly, drugs may be unable to penetrate certain areas of solid tumors.

3. **Treatment protocols:** Combination drug chemotherapy is more successful than single-drug treatment in most of the cancers for which chemotherapy is effective.

   a. **Combinations of drugs:** Cytotoxic agents with qualitatively different toxicities, and with different molecular sites and mechanisms of action, are usually combined at full doses. This results in higher response rates, due to additive and/or potentiated cytotoxic effects, and nonoverlapping host toxicities. In contrast, agents with similar dose-limiting toxicities, such as myelosuppression, nephrotoxicity, or cardiotoxicity, can be combined safely only by reducing the doses of each.

   b. **Advantages of drug combinations:** The advantages of such drug combinations are that they 1) provide maximal cell killing within the range of tolerated toxicity, 2) are effective against a broader range of cell lines in the heterogeneous tumor population, and 3) may delay or prevent the development of resistant cell lines.

   c. **Treatment protocols:** Many cancer treatment protocols have been developed, and each one is applicable to a particular neoplastic state. They are usually identified by an acronym. For example, a common regimen called R-CHOP, used for the treatment of non-Hodgkin lymphoma, consists of *rituximab*, **c**yclophosphamide, **h**ydroxydaunorubicin (doxorubicin), **O**ncovin (vincristine), and **p**rednisone or prednisolone. Therapy is scheduled intermittently (approximately 21 days apart) to allow recovery or rescue of the patient's immune system, which is also affected by the chemotherapeutic agents, thus reducing the risk of serious infection.

C. Problems associated with chemotherapy

Cancer drugs are toxins that present a lethal threat to the cells. It is, therefore, not surprising that cells have evolved elaborate defense mechanisms to protect themselves from chemical toxins, including chemotherapeutic agents.

1. **Resistance:** Some neoplastic cells (for example, melanoma) are inherently resistant to most anticancer drugs. Other tumor types may acquire resistance to the cytotoxic effects of a medication by mutating, particularly after prolonged administration of suboptimal drug doses. The development of drug resistance is minimized by short-term, intensive, intermittent therapy with combinations of drugs. Drug combinations are also effective against a broader range of resistant cells in the tumor population.

2. **Multidrug resistance:** Stepwise selection of an amplified gene that codes for a transmembrane protein (P-glycoprotein for "permeability" glycoprotein; Figure 46.6) is responsible for multidrug resistance. This resistance is due to adenosine triphosphate–dependent pumping of drugs out of the cell in the presence of P-glycoprotein. Cross-resistance following the use of structurally unrelated agents also occurs. For example, cells that are resistant to the cytotoxic effects of the Vinca alkaloids are also resistant to *dactinomycin* and to the anthracycline antibiotics, as well as to *colchicine*, and vice versa. These drugs are all naturally occurring substances, each of which has a hydrophobic aromatic ring and a positive charge at neutral pH. [Note: P-glycoprotein is normally expressed at low levels in most cell types, but higher levels are found in the kidney, liver, pancreas, small intestine, colon, and adrenal gland. It has been suggested that the presence of P-glycoprotein may account for the intrinsic resistance to chemotherapy observed with adenocarcinomas.] Certain drugs at high concentrations (for example, *verapamil*) can inhibit the pump and, thus, interfere with the efflux of the anticancer agent. However, these drugs are undesirable because of adverse pharmacologic actions of their own. Pharmacologically inert pump blockers are being sought.

3. **Toxicity:** Therapy aimed at killing rapidly dividing cancer cells also affects normal cells undergoing rapid proliferation (for example, cells of the buccal mucosa, bone marrow, gastrointestinal [GI] mucosa, and hair follicles), contributing to the toxic manifestations of chemotherapy.

   a. **Common adverse effects:** Most chemotherapeutic agents have a narrow therapeutic index. Severe vomiting, stomatitis, bone marrow suppression, and alopecia occur to a lesser or greater extent during therapy with all antineoplastic agents. Vomiting is often controlled by administration of antiemetic drugs. Some toxicities, such as myelosuppression that predisposes to infection, are common to many chemotherapeutic agents (Figure 46.7), whereas other adverse reactions are confined to specific agents, such as bladder toxicity with *cyclophosphamide,* cardiotoxicity with *doxorubicin,* and pulmonary fibrosis with *bleomycin*. The duration of the side effects varies

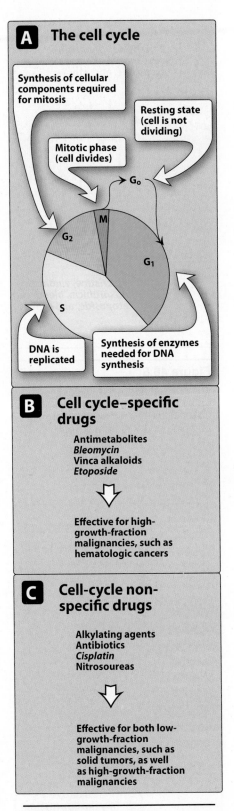

A The cell cycle

Synthesis of cellular components required for mitosis

Resting state (cell is not dividing)

Mitotic phase (cell divides)

G_0

M

G_2

G_1

S

DNA is replicated

Synthesis of enzymes needed for DNA synthesis

B Cell cycle–specific drugs

Antimetabolites
Bleomycin
Vinca alkaloids
Etoposide

Effective for high-growth-fraction malignancies, such as hematologic cancers

C Cell-cycle non-specific drugs

Alkylating agents
Antibiotics
Cisplatin
Nitrosoureas

Effective for both low-growth-fraction malignancies, such as solid tumors, as well as high-growth-fraction malignancies

Figure 46.5
Effects of chemotherapeutic agents on the growth cycle of mammalian cells.

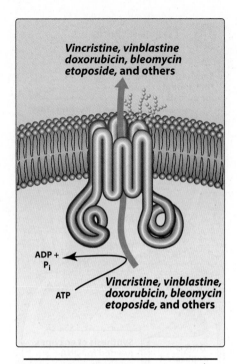

Figure 46.6
The six membrane-spanning loops of the P-glycoprotein form a central channel for the ATP-dependent pumping of drugs from the cell.

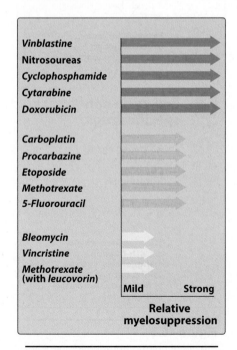

Figure 46.7
Comparison of myelosuppressive potential of chemotherapeutic drugs.

widely. For example, alopecia is transient, but the cardiac, pulmonary, and bladder toxicities can be irreversible.

b. Minimizing adverse effects: Some toxic reactions may be ameliorated by interventions, such as the use of cytoprotectant drugs, perfusing the tumor locally (for example, a sarcoma of the arm), removing some of the patient's marrow prior to intensive treatment and then reimplanting it, or promoting intensive diuresis to prevent bladder toxicities. The megaloblastic anemia that occurs with *methotrexate* can be effectively counteracted by administering *folinic acid* (*leucovorin*). With the availability of human granulocyte colony–stimulating factor (*filgrastim*), the neutropenia associated with treatment of cancer by many drugs can be partially reversed.

4. Treatment-induced tumors: Because most antineoplastic agents are mutagens, neoplasms (for example, acute nonlymphocytic leukemia) may arise 10 or more years after the original cancer was cured. [Note: Treatment-induced neoplasms are especially a problem after therapy with alkylating agents.] Most tumors that develop from cancer chemotherapeutic agents respond well to treatment strategies.

III. ANTIMETABOLITES

Antimetabolites are structurally related to normal compounds that exist within the cell (Figure 46.8). They generally interfere with the availability of normal purine or pyrimidine nucleotide precursors, either by inhibiting their synthesis or by competing with them in DNA or RNA synthesis. Their maximal cytotoxic effects are in S-phase and are, therefore, cell cycle specific.

A. Methotrexate, pemetrexed, and pralatrexate

The vitamin folic acid plays a central role in a variety of metabolic reactions involving the transfer of one-carbon units and is essential for cell replication. Folic acid is obtained mainly from dietary sources and from that produced by intestinal flora. *Methotrexate* [meth-oh-TREK-sate] (*MTX*), *pemetrexed* [pem-e-TREX-ed], and *pralatrexate* [pral-a-TREX-ate] are antifolate agents.

1. Mechanism of action: *MTX* is structurally related to folic acid and acts as an antagonist of the vitamin by inhibiting mammalian dihydrofolate reductase (DHFR), the enzyme that converts folic acid to its active, coenzyme form, tetrahydrofolic acid (FH_4) (Figure 46.9). The inhibition of DHFR can only be reversed by a 1000-fold excess of the natural substrate, dihydrofolate (FH_2), or by administration of *leucovorin,* which bypasses the blocked enzyme and replenishes the folate pool (Figure 46.9). [Note: *Leucovorin,* or *folinic acid,* is the N^5-formyl group–carrying form of FH_4.] *MTX* is specific for the S-phase of the cell cycle. *Pemetrexed* is an antimetabolite similar in mechanism to *methotrexate*. However, in addition to inhibiting DHFR, it also inhibits thymidylate synthase and other enzymes involved in folate metabolism and DNA synthesis. *Pralatrexate* is a newer antimetabolite that also inhibits DHFR.

DRUG	ROUTE	ADVERSE EFFECTS	NOTABLE DRUG INTERACTIONS	MONITORING PARAMETERS	NOTES
Methotrexate	IV/PO/ IM/IT	N/V/D, stomatitis, rash, alopecia, myelosuppression, high-dose: renal damage IT: neurologic toxicities	*Omeprazole, folic acid, warfarin,* NSAIDs, penicillins, cephalosporins	CBC; renal, hepatic function; *methotrexate* levels (after high-dose infusion)	Some adverse effects can be prevented or reversed by administering *leucovorin.* Dose adjust in renal impairment
6-Mercaptopurine (6-MP)	PO	N/V/D, myelosuppression, anorexia, hepatotoxicity (jaundice)	*Warfarin, allopurinol,* SMZ/TMP	CBC; renal, hepatic function	Reduce dose of *6-MP* by 50%–75% when used with *allopurinol* to prevent toxicity
Fludarabine	IV	N/V/D, myelosuppression, rash, immunosuppression, fever, edema, neurologic toxicity	*Cytarabine, cyclophosphamide, cisplatin, mitoxantrone, pentostatin*	CBC; renal, hepatic function; tumor lysis syndrome	Immunosuppression increases risk of opportunistic infections. Dose adjust in renal impairment
Cladribine	IV/SC	Neutropenia, immunosuppression, fever, N/V, teratogenic, peripheral neuropathy		CBC; renal function; tumor lysis syndrome	Immunosuppression increases risk of opportunistic infections.
5-Fluorouracil (5-FU)	IV	Diarrhea, alopecia, severe mucositis, myelosuppression (bolus), "hand-foot syndrome" (continuous infusion), coronary vasospasm	*Methotrexate* (antifolate analogs)	CBC; renal, hepatic function; diarrhea	"Hand-foot syndrome"/palmar-plantar erythrodysesthesia (PPE) is an erythematous desquamation of the palms and soles
Capecitabine	PO	Diarrhea, mucositis, myelosuppression, "hand-foot syndrome", chest pain	*Warfarin, phenytoin*	CBC; renal, hepatic function; diarrhea	Should be taken within 30 min of a meal; keep skin well moisturized
Cytarabine	IV/IT	N/V/D, myelosuppression, hepatotoxicity; neurologic toxicity, conjunctivitis (high dose)	*Digoxin,* alkylating agents, *methotrexate*	CBC; renal, hepatic function; CNS toxicity	Administer steroid eye drops with high dose to prevent conjunctivitis
Azacitidine	IV/SC	Myelosuppression (neutropenia, thrombocytopenia), N/V, constipation, hypokalemia, renal toxicity		CBC; renal, hepatic function	Stability of prepared drug (IV) is only 60 min
Gemcitabine	IV	Myelosuppression, (thrombocytopenia), N/V, alopecia, rash, flu-like syndrome	Potent radiosensitizer	CBC; hepatic function, rash	

IV= intravenous; PO= oral; SC=subcutaneous; IM=intramuscular; IT=intrathecal; N=nausea; V=vomiting; D=diarrhea; SMZ/TMP=sulfamethoxazole/trimethoprim; CBC=complete blood count.

Figure 46.8
Summary of antimetabolites.

2. **Therapeutic uses:** *MTX,* usually in combination with other drugs, is effective against acute lymphocytic leukemia, Burkitt lymphoma in children, breast cancer, bladder cancer, and head and neck carcinomas. In addition, low-dose *MTX* is effective as a single agent against certain inflammatory diseases, such as severe psoriasis and rheumatoid arthritis, as well as Crohn disease. All patients receiving *MTX* require close monitoring for possible toxic effects. *Pemetrexed* is primarily used in non–small cell lung cancer. *Pralatrexate* is used in relapsed or refractory T-cell lymphoma.

3. **Resistance:** Nonproliferating cells are resistant to *MTX,* probably because of a relative lack of DHFR, thymidylate synthase, and/ or the glutamylating enzyme. Decreased levels of the *MTX* polyglutamate have been reported in resistant cells and may be due to its decreased formation or increased breakdown. Resistance in neoplastic cells can be due to amplification (production of additional copies) of the gene that codes for DHFR, resulting in increased levels of this enzyme. The enzyme affinity for *MTX* may also be diminished. Resistance can also occur from a reduced influx of

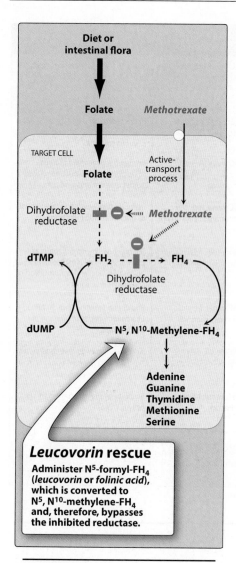

Figure 46.9
Mechanism of action of *methotrexate* and the effect of administration of *leucovorin*. FH_2 = dihydrofolate; FH_4 = tetrahydrofolate; dTMP = deoxythymidine monophosphate; dUMP = deoxyuridine monophosphate.

MTX, apparently caused by a change in the carrier-mediated transport responsible for pumping the drug into the cell.

4. **Pharmacokinetics:** *MTX* is variably absorbed at low doses from the GI tract, but it can also be administered by intramuscular, intravenous (IV), and intrathecal routes (Figure 46.10). Because *MTX* does not easily penetrate the blood–brain barrier, it can be administered intrathecally to destroy neoplastic cells that are thriving in the sanctuary of the CNS. High concentrations of the drug are found in the intestinal epithelium, liver, and kidney, as well as in ascites and pleural effusions. *MTX is* also distributed to the skin. High doses of *MTX* undergo hydroxylation at the 7 position and become 7-hydroxymethotrexate. This derivative is much less active as an antimetabolite. It is less water soluble than *MTX* and may lead to crystalluria. Therefore, it is important to keep the urine alkaline and the patient well hydrated to avoid renal toxicity. Excretion of the parent drug and the 7-OH metabolite occurs primarily via urine, although some of the drug and its metabolite appear in feces due to enterohepatic excretion.

5. **Adverse effects:** Adverse effects of MTX are outlined in Figure 46.8. *Pemetrexed* should be given with folic acid and vitamin B_{12} supplements to reduce hematologic and GI toxicities. It is also recommended to pretreat with corticosteroids to prevent cutaneous reactions. One of the more common side effects of *pralatrexate* is mucositis. Doses must be adjusted or withheld based on the severity of mucositis. *Pralatrexate* also requires supplementation with folic acid and vitamin B_{12}.

B. 6-Mercaptopurine

6-Mercaptopurine [mer-kap-toe-PYOOR-een] (*6-MP*) is the thiol analog of hypoxanthine. *6-MP* and *6-thioguanine* were the first purine analogs to prove beneficial for treating neoplastic disease. [Note: *Azathioprine,* an immunosuppressant, exerts its cytotoxic effects after conversion to *6-MP.*] *6-MP* is used principally in the maintenance of remission in acute lymphoblastic leukemia. *6-MP* and its analog, *azathioprine,* are also beneficial in the treatment of Crohn disease.

1. **Mechanism of action:**

a. **Nucleotide formation:** To exert its antileukemic effect, *6-MP* must penetrate target cells and be converted to the nucleotide analog, 6-MP-ribose phosphate (better known as 6-thioinosinic acid or TIMP; Figure 46.11). The addition of the ribose phosphate is catalyzed by the salvage pathway enzyme, hypoxanthine–guanine phosphoribosyltransferase (HGPRT).

b. **Inhibition of purine synthesis:** A number of metabolic processes involving purine biosynthesis and interconversions are affected by the nucleotide analog, TIMP. Similar to nucleotide monophosphates, TIMP can inhibit the first step of de novo purine ring biosynthesis (catalyzed by glutamine phosphoribosyl pyrophosphate amidotransferase). TIMP also blocks the formation of adenosine monophosphate and xanthinuric acid from inosinic acid.

c. **Incorporation into nucleic acids:** TIMP is converted to thioguanine monophosphate, which after phosphorylation to di- and triphosphates can be incorporated into RNA. The deoxyribonucleotide analogs that are also formed are incorporated into DNA. This results in nonfunctional RNA and DNA.

2. **Resistance:** Resistance is associated with 1) an inability to biotransform *6-MP* to the corresponding nucleotide because of decreased levels of HGPRT, 2) increased dephosphorylation, or 3) increased metabolism of the drug to thiouric acid or other metabolites.

3. **Pharmacokinetics:** Oral absorption is erratic and incomplete. Once it enters the blood circulation, the drug is widely distributed throughout the body, except for the cerebrospinal fluid (CSF). The bioavailability of *6-MP* can be reduced by first-pass metabolism in the liver. *6-MP* is converted in the liver to the 6-methylmercaptopurine derivative or to thiouric acid (an inactive metabolite). [Note: The latter reaction is catalyzed by xanthine oxidase.] The parent drug and its metabolites are excreted by the kidney.

C. Fludarabine

Fludarabine [floo-DARE-a-been] is the 5′-phosphate of 2-fluoroadenine arabinoside, a purine nucleotide analog. It is useful in the treatment of chronic lymphocytic leukemia, hairy cell leukemia, and indolent non-Hodgkin lymphoma. *Fludarabine* is a prodrug, the phosphate being removed in the plasma to form 2-F-araA, which is taken up into cells and again phosphorylated (initially by deoxycytidine kinase). Although the exact cytotoxic mechanism is uncertain, the triphosphate is incorporated into both DNA and RNA. This decreases their synthesis in the S-phase and affects their function. Resistance is associated with reduced uptake into cells, lack of deoxycytidine kinase, and decreased affinity for DNA polymerase, as well as other mechanisms. *Fludarabine* is administered IV rather than orally, because intestinal bacteria split off the sugar to yield the very toxic metabolite, fluoroadenine. Urinary excretion accounts for partial elimination.

D. Cladribine

Another purine analog, *2-chlorodeoxyadenosine* or *cladribine* [KLA-dri-been], undergoes reactions similar to those of *fludarabine,* and it must be phosphorylated to a nucleotide to be cytotoxic. It becomes incorporated at the 3′-terminus of DNA and, thus, hinders elongation. It also affects DNA repair and is a potent inhibitor of ribonucleotide reductase. Resistance may be due to mechanisms analogous to those that affect *fludarabine,* although cross-resistance is not observed. *Cladribine* is effective against hairy cell leukemia, chronic lymphocytic leukemia, and non-Hodgkin lymphoma. The drug is given as a single, continuous infusion. *Cladribine* distributes throughout the body, including into the CSF.

E. 5-Fluorouracil

5-Fluorouracil [flure-oh-YOOR-ah-sil] (*5-FU*), a pyrimidine analog, has a stable fluorine atom in place of a hydrogen atom at position 5 of the

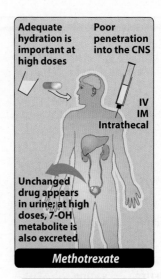

Figure 46.10
Administration and fate of *methotrexate*. CNS = central nervous system; IV = intravenous; IM = intramuscular.

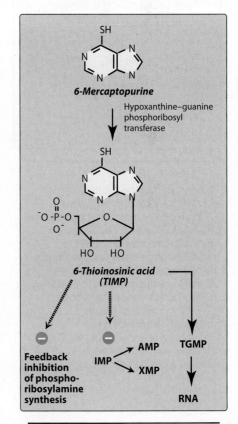

Figure 46.11
Actions of *6-mercaptopurine*. GMP = guanosine monophosphate; AMP = adenosine monophosphate; XMP = xanthosine monophosphate.

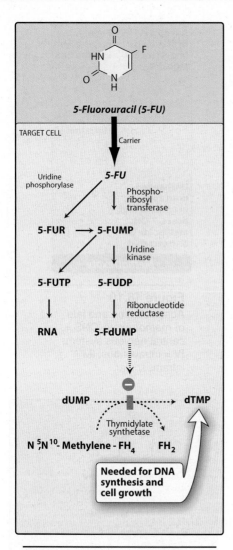

Figure 46.12
Mechanism of the cytotoxic action of *5-FU*. *5-FU* is converted to 5-fluorodeoxyuridine monophosphate (5-FdUMP), which competes with deoxyuridine monophosphate (dUMP) for the enzyme thymidylate synthetase. 5-FU = *5-fluorouracil*; 5-FUR = 5-fluorouridine; 5-FUMP = 5-fluorouridine monophosphate; 5-FUDP = 5-fluorouridine diphosphate; 5-FUTP = 5-fluorouridine triphosphate; dUMP = deoxyuridine monophosphate; dTMP = deoxythymidine monophosphate.

uracil ring. The fluorine interferes with the conversion of deoxyuridylic acid to thymidylic acid, thus depriving the cell of thymidine, one of the essential precursors for DNA synthesis. *5-FU* is employed primarily in the treatment of slowly growing solid tumors (for example, colorectal, breast, ovarian, pancreatic, and gastric carcinomas). When applied topically, *5-FU* is also effective for the treatment of superficial basal cell carcinomas.

1. **Mechanism of action:** *5-FU* itself is devoid of antineoplastic activity. It enters the cell through a carrier-mediated transport system and is converted to the corresponding deoxynucleotide (5-fluorodeoxyuridine monophosphate [5-FdUMP]; Figure 46.12), which competes with deoxyuridine monophosphate for thymidylate synthase, thus inhibiting its action. DNA synthesis decreases due to lack of thymidine, leading to imbalanced cell growth and "thymidine-less death" of rapidly dividing cells. [Note: *Leucovorin* is administered with *5-FU,* because the reduced folate coenzyme is required in the thymidylate synthase inhibition. For example, a standard regimen for advanced colorectal cancer is *irinotecan* plus *5-FU/leucovorin*.] *5-FU* is also incorporated into RNA, and low levels have been detected in DNA. In the latter case, a glycosylase excises the *5-FU,* damaging the DNA. *5-FU* produces the anticancer effect in the S-phase of the cell cycle.

2. **Resistance:** Resistance is encountered when the cells have lost their ability to convert *5-FU* into its active form (5-FdUMP) or when they have altered or increased thymidylate synthase levels.

3. **Pharmacokinetics:** Because of its severe toxicity to the GI tract, *5-FU* is given IV or, in the case of skin cancer, topically. The drug penetrates well into all tissues, including the CNS. *5-FU* is rapidly metabolized in the liver, lung, and kidney. It is eventually converted to fluoro-β-alanine, which is removed in the urine. The dose of *5-FU* must be adjusted in impaired hepatic function. Elevated levels of dihydropyrimidine dehydrogenase (DPD) can increase the rate of *5-FU* catabolism and decrease its bioavailability. The DPD level varies from individual to individual and may differ by as much as sixfold in the general population. Patients with DPD deficiency may experience severe toxicity manifested by pancytopenia, mucositis, and life-threatening diarrhea. Knowledge of an individual's DPD activity should allow more appropriate dosing of 5-FU.

F. Capecitabine

Capecitabine [cape-SITE-a-been] is a novel, oral fluoropyrimidine carbamate. It is used in the treatment of colorectal and metastatic breast cancer. After being absorbed, *capecitabine,* which is itself nontoxic, undergoes a series of enzymatic reactions, the last of which is hydrolysis to *5-FU*. This step is catalyzed by thymidine phosphorylase, an enzyme that is concentrated primarily in tumors (Figure 46.13). Thus, the cytotoxic activity of *capecitabine* is the same as that of *5-FU* and is tumor specific. The most important enzyme inhibited by *5-FU* (and, thus, *capecitabine*) is thymidylate synthase. *Capecitabine* is well absorbed following oral administration. It is extensively metabolized to *5-FU* and is eventually biotransformed into fluoro-β-alanine. Metabolites are primarily eliminated in the urine.

G. Cytarabine

Cytarabine [sye-TARE-ah-been] (*cytosine arabinoside* or *ara-C*) is an analog of 2′-deoxycytidine in which the natural ribose residue is replaced by D-arabinose. *Cytarabine* acts as a pyrimidine antagonist. The major clinical use of *cytarabine* is in acute nonlymphocytic (myelogenous) leukemia (AML). *Cytarabine* enters the cell by a carrier-mediated process and, like the other purine and pyrimidine antagonists, must be sequentially phosphorylated by deoxycytidine kinase and other nucleotide kinases to the nucleotide form (cytosine arabinoside triphosphate or ara-CTP) to be cytotoxic. Ara-CTP is an effective inhibitor of DNA polymerase. The nucleotide is also incorporated into nuclear DNA and can terminate chain elongation. It is, therefore, S-phase (and, hence, cell cycle) specific.

1. **Resistance:** Resistance to *cytarabine* may result from a defect in the transport process, a change in activity of phosphorylating enzymes (especially deoxycytidine kinase), or an increased pool of the natural dCTP nucleotide. Increased deamination of the drug to uracil arabinoside (ara-U) can also cause resistance.

2. **Pharmacokinetics:** *Cytarabine* is not effective when given orally, because of its deamination to the noncytotoxic ara-U by cytidine deaminase in the intestinal mucosa and liver. Given IV, it distributes throughout the body but does not penetrate the CNS in sufficient amounts. Therefore, it may also be injected intrathecally. A liposomal preparation that provides slow release into the CSF is also available. *Cytarabine* undergoes extensive oxidative deamination in the body to ara-U, a pharmacologically inactive metabolite. Both *cytarabine* and ara-U are excreted in urine.

H. Azacitidine

Azacitidine [A-zuh-SITE-i-dine] is a pyrimidine nucleoside analog of cytidine. It is used for the treatment of myelodysplastic syndromes and AML. *Azacitidine* undergoes activation to the nucleotide metabolite azacitidine triphosphate and gets incorporated into RNA to inhibit RNA processing and function. It is S-phase cell cycle specific. The mechanism of resistance is not well described.

I. Gemcitabine

Gemcitabine [jem-SITE-ah-been] is an analog of the nucleoside deoxycytidine. It is used most commonly for pancreatic cancer and non–small cell lung cancer. *Gemcitabine* is a substrate for deoxycytidine kinase, which phosphorylates the drug to 2′,2′-difluorodeoxycytidine triphosphate (Figure 46.14). Resistance to the drug is probably due to its inability to be converted to a nucleotide, caused by an alteration in deoxycytidine kinase. In addition, the tumor cell can produce increased levels of endogenous deoxycytidine that compete for the kinase, thus overcoming the inhibition. *Gemcitabine* is infused IV. It is deaminated to difluorodeoxyuridine, which is not cytotoxic, and is excreted in urine.

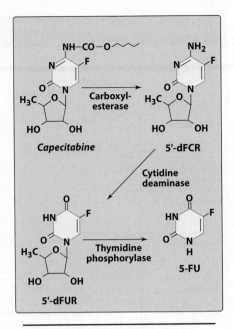

Figure 46.13
Metabolic pathway of *capecitabine* to *5-fluorouracil (5-FU)*. 5′-dFCR = 5′-deoxy-5-fluorocytidine; 5′-dFUR = 5′-deoxy-5-fluorouridine.

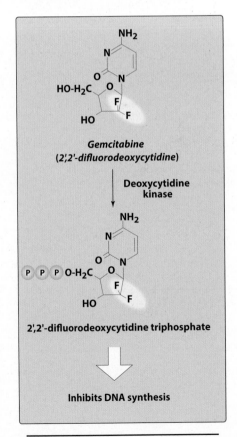

Figure 46.14
Mechanism of action of *gemcitabine*.

DRUG	ROUTE	ADVERSE EFFECTS	NOTABLE DRUG INTERACTIONS	MONITORING PARAMETERS	NOTES
Doxorubicin	IV	Myelosuppression, N/V/D, mucositis, cardiac toxicity, alopecia, red coloration of urine. Strong vesicants	*Phenytoin, trastuzumab* (cardiotoxicity), *digoxin*	CBC; Renal, hepatic function; cardiac function (ECHO or MUGA); adjust in hepatic dysfunction	Cumulative doses >450mg/m^2 increase risk of cardiotoxicity. Vesicant!
Daunorubicin	IV				Cumulative doses >550mg/m^2 increase risk of cardiotoxicity. Vesicant!
Liposomal Doxorubicin	IV				Not a substitute for *doxorubicin*, less cardiotoxicity
Epirubicin	IV		*Cimetidine*		Cumulative doses >900 mg/m^2 increase risk of cardiotoxicity. Vesicant! Less N/V
Idarubicin	IV			As with other anthracyclines plus tumor lysis syndrome	Cumulative doses >150 mg/m^2 increase risk of cardiotoxicity. Vesicant!
Bleomycin	IV/SC/IM	Pulmonary fibrosis, alopecia, skin reactions, hyperpigmentation of hands, fever, chills, anaphylaxis	Phenothiazines, *cisplatin* (renal), radiation (pulmonary)	Pulmonary function tests (PFTs); adjust in renal dysfunction; anaphylaxis	"Bleomycin lung" pulmonary fibrosis can be fatal . Discontinue if any signs of lung dysfunction

IV= intravenous; SC=subcutaneous; IM=intramuscular; N=nausea; V=vomiting; D=diarrhea; CBC=complete blood count.

Figure 46.15
Summary of antitumor antibiotics.

IV. ANTIBIOTICS

The antitumor antibiotics (Figure 46.15) owe their cytotoxic action primarily to their interactions with DNA, leading to disruption of DNA function. In addition to intercalation, their abilities to inhibit topoisomerases (I and II) and produce free radicals also play a major role in their cytotoxic effect. They are cell cycle nonspecific with *bleomycin* as an exception.

A. Anthracyclines: Doxorubicin, daunorubicin, idarubicin, epirubicin, and mitoxantrone

Doxorubicin [dox-oh-ROO-bi-sin] and *daunorubicin* [daw-noe-ROO-bi-sin] are classified as anthracycline antibiotics. *Doxorubicin* is the hydroxylated analog of *daunorubicin*. *Idarubicin* [eye-da-ROO-bi-sin], the 4-demethoxy analog of *daunorubicin*, *epirubicin* [eh-pee-ROO-bih-sin], and *mitoxantrone* [mye-toe-ZAN-trone] are also available. Applications for these agents differ despite their structural similarity and their apparently similar mechanisms of action. *Doxorubicin* is one of the most important and widely used anticancer drugs. It is used in combination with other agents for treatment of sarcomas and a variety of carcinomas, including breast and lung, as well as for treatment of acute lymphocytic leukemia and lymphomas. *Daunorubicin* and *idarubicin* are used in the treatment of acute leukemias, and *mitoxantrone* is used in prostate cancer.

1. **Mechanism of action:** *Doxorubicin* and other anthracyclines induce cytotoxicity through several different mechanisms. For example, *doxorubicin*-derived free radicals can induce membrane

lipid peroxidation, DNA strand scission, and direct oxidation of purine or pyrimidine bases, thiols, and amines (Figure 46.16).

2. **Pharmacokinetics:** All these drugs must be administered IV, because they are inactivated in the GI tract. Extravasation is a serious problem that can lead to tissue necrosis. The anthracycline antibiotics bind to plasma proteins as well as to other tissue components, where they are widely distributed. They do not penetrate the blood–brain barrier or the testes. These agents undergo extensive hepatic metabolism, and dosage adjustments are needed in patients with impaired hepatic function. Biliary excretion is the major route of elimination. Some renal excretion also occurs, but dosage adjustments are generally not needed in renal dysfunction. Because of the dark red color of the anthracycline drugs, the veins may become visible surrounding the site of infusion, and red discoloration of urine may occur.

3. **Adverse effects:** Irreversible, dose-dependent cardiotoxicity, apparently a result of the generation of free radicals and lipid peroxidation, is the most serious adverse reaction and is more common with *daunorubicin* and *doxorubicin* than with *idarubicin* and *epirubicin*. Addition of *trastuzumab* to protocols with *doxorubicin* or *epirubicin* increases congestive heart failure. There has been some success with the iron chelator *dexrazoxane* in protecting against the cardiotoxicity of *doxorubicin*. The liposomal-encapsulated *doxorubicin* is reported to be less cardiotoxic than the usual formulation.

B. Bleomycin

Bleomycin [blee-oh-MYE-sin] is a mixture of different copper-chelating glycopeptides that, like the anthracycline antibiotics, cause scission of DNA by an oxidative process. *Bleomycin* is cell cycle specific and causes cells to accumulate in the G_2 phase. It is primarily used in the treatment of testicular cancers and Hodgkin lymphoma.

1. **Mechanism of action:** A DNA–*bleomycin*–Fe^{2+} complex appears to undergo oxidation to *bleomycin*–Fe^{3+}. The liberated electrons react with oxygen to form superoxide or hydroxyl radicals, which, in turn, attack the phosphodiester bonds of DNA, resulting in strand breakage and chromosomal aberrations (Figure 46.17).

2. **Resistance:** Although the mechanisms of resistance have not been elucidated, increased levels of bleomycin hydrolase (or deaminase), glutathione *S*-transferase, and possibly, increased efflux of the drug have been implicated. DNA repair also may contribute.

3. **Pharmacokinetics:** *Bleomycin* is administered by a number of routes. The *bleomycin*-inactivating enzyme (a hydrolase) is high in a number of tissues (for example, liver and spleen) but is low in the lung and is absent in skin (accounting for the drug's toxicity in those tissues). Most of the parent drug is excreted unchanged in the urine, necessitating dose adjustment in patients with renal failure.

4. **Adverse effects:** Mucocutaneous reactions and alopecia are common. Hypertrophic skin changes and hyperpigmentation of

Figure 46.16
Doxorubicin interacts with molecular oxygen, producing superoxide ions and hydrogen peroxide, which cause single-strand breaks in DNA.

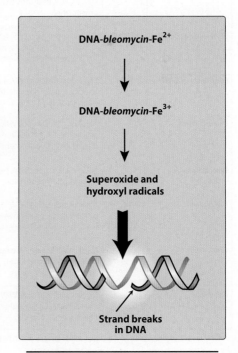

Figure 46.17
Bleomycin causes breaks in DNA by an oxidative process.

the hands are prevalent. There is a high incidence of fever and chills and a low incidence of serious anaphylactoid reactions. Pulmonary toxicity is the most serious adverse effect, progressing from rales, cough, and infiltrate to potentially fatal fibrosis. The pulmonary fibrosis that is caused by *bleomycin* is often referred as "bleomycin lung." *Bleomycin* is unusual in that myelosuppression is rare.

V. ALKYLATING AGENTS

Alkylating agents (Figure 46.18) exert their cytotoxic effects by covalently binding to nucleophilic groups on various cell constituents. Alkylation of DNA is probably the crucial cytotoxic reaction that is lethal to the tumor cells. Alkylating agents do not discriminate between cycling and resting cells, even though they are most toxic for rapidly dividing cells. They are used in combination with other agents to treat a wide variety of lymphatic and solid cancers. In addition to being cytotoxic, all are mutagenic and carcinogenic and can lead to secondary malignancies such as acute leukemia.

DRUG	ROUTE	ADVERSE EFFECTS	NOTABLE DRUG INTERACTIONS	MONITORING PARAMETERS	NOTES
Cyclophosphamide	IV/PO	Myelosuppression, hemorrhagic cystitis, N/V/D, alopecia, amenorrhea, secondary malignancies	*Phenobarbital, phenytoin* (P450); *digoxin*, anticoagulants	Urinalysis; CBC; renal, hepatic function	Good hydration to prevent bladder toxicity (mesna with high doses)
Ifosfamide	IV	Myelosuppression, hemorrhagic cystitis, N/V, neurotoxicity, alopecia, amenorrhea	*Phenobarbital, phenytoin* (P450); *cimetidine, allopurinol, warfarin*	Urinalysis; neurotoxicity	Use mesna and hydration to prevent bladder toxicity
Carmustine (BCNU)	IV	Myelosuppression, N/V, facial flushing, hepatotoxicity, pulmonary toxicity, impotence, infertility	*Cimetidine, amphotericin B, digoxin, phenytoin*	CBC; PFTs; renal, hepatic function	Also available as an implantable wafer (brain)
Lomustine (CCNU)	PO	Myelosuppression, N/V, pulmonary toxicity, impotence, infertility, neurotoxicity	*Cimetidine*, alcohol	CBC; PFTs; renal function	Administer on an empty stomach
Dacarbazine	IV	Myelosuppression, N/V, flu-like syndrome, CNS toxicity, hepatotoxicity, photosensitivity	*Phenytoin, phenobarbital* (P450)	CBC; renal, hepatic function	Vesicant
Temozolomide	PO	N/V, myelosuppression, headache, fatigue, photosensitivity		CBC; renal, hepatic function	Requires PCP prophylaxis
Melphalan	IV/PO	Myelosuppression, N/V/D, mucositis, hypersensitivity (IV)	*Cimetidine*, steroids, *cyclosporine*	CBC; renal, hepatic function; Adjust in renal dysfunction	Take on an empty stomach
Chlorambucil	PO	Myelosuppression, skin rash, pulmonary fibrosis (rare), hyperuricemia, seizures	*Phenobarbital, phenytoin* (P450)	CBC; renal, hepatic function; uric acid	Take with food
Busulfan	IV	Myelosuppression, N/V/D, mucositis, skin rash, pulmonary fibrosis, hepatotoxicity	*Acetaminophen, itraconazole, phenytoin*	CBC; pulmonary symptoms; renal, hepatic function	"Busulfan lung"

IV= intravenous; PO= oral; N=nausea; V=vomiting; D=diarrhea; CBC=complete blood count; PFTs=pulmonary function tests.

Figure 46.18
Summary of alkylating agents.

A. Cyclophosphamide and ifosfamide

These drugs are very closely related mustard agents that share most of the same primary mechanisms and toxicities. They are cytotoxic only after generation of their alkylating species, which are produced through hydroxylation by cytochrome P450 (CYP450). These agents have a broad clinical spectrum, being used either singly or as part of a regimen in the treatment of a wide variety of neoplastic diseases, such as non-Hodgkin lymphoma, sarcoma, and breast cancer.

1. **Mechanism of action:** *Cyclophosphamide* [sye-kloe-FOSS-fah-mide] is the most commonly used alkylating agent. Both *cyclophosphamide* and *ifosfamide* [eye-FOSS-fah-mide] are first biotransformed to hydroxylated intermediates primarily in the liver by the CYP450 system (Figure 46.19).The hydroxylated intermediates then undergo breakdown to form the active compounds, phosphoramide mustard and acrolein. Reaction of the phosphoramide mustard with DNA is considered to be the cytotoxic step. The parent drug and its metabolites are primarily excreted in urine.

2. **Pharmacokinetics:** *Cyclophosphamide* is available in oral or IV preparations, whereas *ifosfamide* is IV only. *Cyclophosphamide* is metabolized in the liver to active and inactive metabolites, and minimal amounts are excreted in the urine as unchanged drug. *Ifosfamide* is metabolized primarily by CYP450 3A4 and 2B6 isoenzymes. It is mainly renally excreted.

3. **Resistance:** Resistance results from increased DNA repair, decreased drug permeability, and reaction of the drug with thiols (for example, glutathione). Cross-resistance does not always occur.

4. **Adverse effects:** A unique toxicity of both drugs is hemorrhagic cystitis, which can lead to fibrosis of the bladder. Bladder toxicity has been attributed to acrolein in the urine in the case of *cyclophosphamide* and to toxic metabolites of *ifosfamide*. Adequate hydration as well as IV injection of mesna (sodium 2-mercaptoethane sulfonate), which neutralizes the toxic metabolites, can minimize this problem. A fairly high incidence of neurotoxicity has been reported in patients on high-dose *ifosfamide,* probably due to the metabolite, chloroacetaldehyde.

B. Nitrosoureas

Carmustine [KAR-mus-teen, BCNU] and *lomustine* [LOE-mus-teen, CCNU] are closely related nitrosoureas. Because of their ability to penetrate the CNS, the nitrosoureas are primarily employed in the treatment of brain tumors.

1. **Mechanism of action:** The nitrosoureas exert cytotoxic effects by an alkylation that inhibits replication and, eventually, RNA and protein synthesis. Although they alkylate DNA in resting cells, cytotoxicity is expressed primarily on cells that are actively dividing. Therefore, nondividing cells can escape death if DNA repair occurs. Nitrosoureas also inhibit several key enzymatic processes by carbamoylation of amino acids in proteins in the targeted cells.

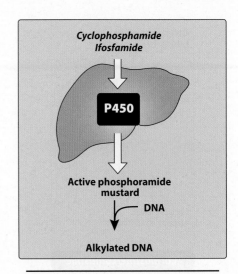

Figure 46.19
Activation of *cyclophosphamide* and *ifosfamide* by hepatic cytochrome P450.

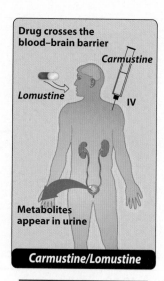

Figure 46.20
Administration and fate
of *carmustine/lomustine*.
IV = intravenous.

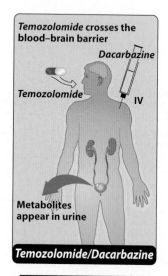

Figure 46.21
Administration and
fate of *temozolomide*
and *dacarbazine*. IV =
intravenous.

2. Pharmacokinetics: In spite of the similarities in their structures, *carmustine* is administered IV and as chemotherapy wafer implants, whereas *lomustine* is given orally. Because of their lipophilicity, they distribute widely in the body, but their most striking property is their ability to readily penetrate the CNS. The drugs undergo extensive metabolism. *Lomustine* is metabolized to active products. The kidney is the major excretory route for the nitrosoureas (Figure 46.20).

C. Dacarbazine

Dacarbazine [dah-KAR-bah-zeen] is an alkylating agent that must undergo biotransformation to an active metabolite, methyltriazeno-imidazole carboxamide (MTIC). This metabolite is responsible for the drug's activity as an alkylating agent by forming methylcarbonium ions that can attack the nucleophilic groups in the DNA molecule. Thus, similar to other alkylating agents, the cytotoxic action of dacarbazine has been attributed to the ability of its metabolite to methylate DNA on the O^6 position of guanine. *Dacarbazine* has found use in the treatment of melanoma and Hodgkin lymphoma.

D. Temozolomide

The treatment of tumors in the brain is particularly difficult. *Temozolomide* [te-moe-ZOE-loe-mide], a triazene agent, has been approved for use against glioblastomas and anaplastic astrocytomas. It is also used in metastatic melanoma. *Temozolomide* is related to *dacarbazine,* because both must undergo biotransformation to an active metabolite, MTIC, which probably is responsible for the methylation of DNA on the 6 position of guanine. Unlike *dacarbazine, temozolomide* does not require the CYP450 system for metabolic transformation, and it undergoes chemical transformation at normal physiological pH. *Temozolomide* also has the property of inhibiting the repair enzyme, O^6-guanine-DNA alkyltransferase. *Temozolomide* differs from *dacarbazine* in that it crosses the blood–brain barrier. *Temozolomide* is administered intravenously or orally and has excellent bioavailability after oral administration. The parent drug and metabolites are excreted in urine (Figure 46.21).

E. Other alkylating agents

Mechlorethamine [mek-lor-ETH-ah-meen] was developed as a vesicant (nitrogen mustard) during World War I. Its ability to cause lymphocytopenia led to its use in lymphatic cancers. *Melphalan* [MEL-fah-lan], a phenylalanine derivative of nitrogen mustard, is used in the treatment of multiple myeloma. This is a bifunctional alkylating agent that can be given orally. Although *melphalan* can be given orally, the plasma concentration differs from patient to patient due to variation in intestinal absorption and metabolism. The dose of *melphalan* is carefully adjusted by monitoring the platelet and white blood cell counts. *Chlorambucil* [clor-AM-byoo-sil] is another bifunctional alkylating agent that is used in the treatment of chronic lymphocytic leukemia. Both *melphalan* and *chlorambucil* have moderate hematologic toxicities and upset the GI tract. *Busulfan* [byoo-SUL-fan] is another oral agent that is effective against chronic granulocytic leukemia. In aged patients, *busulfan* can cause pulmonary fibrosis ("busulfan lung"). Like other alkylating agents, all of these agents are leukemogenic.

VI. MICROTUBULE INHIBITORS

The mitotic spindle is part of a larger, intracellular skeleton (cytoskeleton) that is essential for the movements of structures occurring in the cytoplasm of all eukaryotic cells. The mitotic spindle consists of chromatin plus a system of microtubules composed of the protein tubulin. The mitotic spindle is essential for the equal partitioning of DNA into the two daughter cells that are formed when a eukaryotic cell divides. Several plant-derived substances used as anticancer drugs disrupt this process by affecting the equilibrium between the polymerized and depolymerized forms of the microtubules, thereby causing cytotoxicity. The microtubule inhibitors are summarized in Figure 46.22.

A. Vincristine and vinblastine

Vincristine [vin-KRIS-teen] (*VX*) and *vinblastine* [vin-BLAS-teen] (*VBL*) are structurally related compounds derived from the periwinkle plant, <u>Vinca</u> <u>rosea</u>. They are, therefore, referred to as the Vinca alkaloids. A less neurotoxic agent is *vinorelbine* [vye-NOR-el-been] (*VRB*). Although the Vinca alkaloids are structurally similar to one another, their therapeutic indications are different. They are generally administered in combination with other drugs. *VX* is used in the treatment of acute lymphoblastic leukemia in children, Wilms tumor, Ewing soft tissue sarcoma, and Hodgkin and non-Hodgkin lymphomas, as well as some other rapidly proliferating neoplasms. [Note: *VX* (former trade name, Oncovin) is the "O" in the R-CHOP regimen for lymphoma. Due to relatively mild myelosuppressive activity, *VX* is used in a number of other protocols.] *VBL* is administered with *bleomycin* and *cisplatin* for the treatment of metastatic testicular carcinoma. It is also used in the treatment of systemic Hodgkin and non-Hodgkin lymphomas. *VRB* is beneficial in the treatment of advanced non–small cell lung cancer, either as a single agent or with *cisplatin*.

DRUG	ROUTE	ADVERSE EFFECTS	NOTABLE DRUG INTERACTIONS	MONITORING PARAMETERS	NOTES
Vincristine	IV	Neurotoxicity, constipation	*Phenytoin, phenobarbital, carbamazepine,* azole antifungal drugs	CBC, hepatic function, peripheral neuropathy	Vesicants, IT administration may result in death.
Vinblastine	IV	Myelosuppression, neurotoxicity		CBC, hepatic function	
Vinorelbine	IV	Granulocytopenia			
Paclitaxel	IV	Neutropenia, neurotoxicity, alopecia, N, V	*Repaglinide, gemfibrozil, rifampin* (CYP2C8)	CBC, hepatic function, peripheral neuropathy	Hypersensitivity reactions (dyspnea, urticaria, hypotension), require premedications
Docetaxel	IV	Neutropenia, neurotoxicity, fluid retention, alopecia, N, V, D	*Ketoconazole, ritonavir* (CYP3A4)		

IV= intravenous; IT=intrathecal; N=nausea; V=vomiting; D=diarrhea; CBC=complete blood count.

Figure 46.22
Summary of microtubule inhibitors.

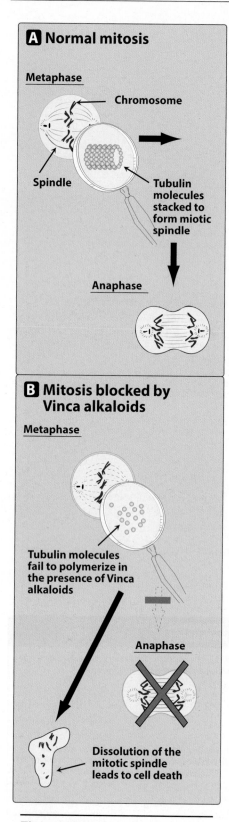

A **Normal mitosis**

Metaphase

Chromosome

Spindle

Tubulin molecules stacked to form miotic spindle

Anaphase

B **Mitosis blocked by Vinca alkaloids**

Metaphase

Tubulin molecules fail to polymerize in the presence of Vinca alkaloids

Anaphase

Dissolution of the mitotic spindle leads to cell death

Figure 46.23
Mechanism of action of the microtubule inhibitors.

1. **Mechanism of action:** *VX, VRB,* and *VBL* are all cell cycle specific and phase specific, because they block mitosis in metaphase (M-phase). Their binding to the microtubular protein, tubulin, blocks the ability of tubulin to polymerize to form microtubules. Instead, paracrystalline aggregates consisting of tubulin dimers and the alkaloid drug are formed. The resulting dysfunctional spindle apparatus, frozen in metaphase, prevents chromosomal segregation and cell proliferation (Figure 46.23).

2. **Pharmacokinetics:** IV injection of these agents leads to rapid cytotoxic effects and cell destruction. This, in turn, can cause hyperuricemia due to the oxidation of purines that are released from fragmenting DNA molecules. The Vinca alkaloids are concentrated and metabolized in the liver by the CYP450 pathway and eliminated in bile and feces. Doses must be modified in patients with impaired hepatic function or biliary obstruction.

3. **Adverse effects:** *VX* and *VBL* have certain toxicities in common. These include phlebitis or cellulitis, if the drugs extravasate during injection, as well as nausea, vomiting, diarrhea, and alopecia. However, the adverse effects of *VX* and *VBL* are not identical. *VBL* is a more potent myelosuppressant than *VX*, whereas peripheral neuropathy (paresthesias, loss of reflexes, foot drop, and ataxia) is associated with *VX*. Constipation is more frequently encountered with *VX*. These agents should not be administered intrathecally. This potential drug error can result in death, and special precautions should be in place for administration.

B. Paclitaxel and docetaxel

Paclitaxel [PAK-li-tax-el] was the first member of the taxane family to be used in cancer chemotherapy. A semisynthetic *paclitaxel* is now available through chemical modification of a precursor found in the needles of Pacific yew species. An albumin-bound form is also available. Substitution of a side chain has resulted in *docetaxel* [doe-see-TAX-el], which is the more potent of the two drugs. *Paclitaxel* has shown good activity against advanced ovarian cancer and metastatic breast cancer. Favorable results have been obtained in non–small cell lung cancer when administered with *cisplatin*. *Docetaxel* is commonly used in prostate, breast, GI, and non–small cell lung cancers.

1. **Mechanism of action:** Both drugs are active in the G_2/M-phase of the cell cycle, but unlike the Vinca alkaloids, they promote polymerization and stabilization of the polymer rather than disassembly, leading to the accumulation of microtubules (Figure 46.24). The overly stable microtubules formed are nonfunctional, and chromosome desegregation does not occur. This results in death of the cell.

2. **Pharmacokinetics:** These agents undergo hepatic metabolism by the CYP450 system and are excreted via the biliary system. Dose modification is not required in patients with renal impairment, but doses should be reduced in patients with hepatic dysfunction.

3. **Adverse effects:** The dose-limiting toxicities of *paclitaxel* and *docetaxel* are neutropenia and leukopenia. Alopecia occurs, but

vomiting and diarrhea are uncommon. [Note: Because of serious hypersensitivity reactions (including dyspnea, urticaria, and hypotension), patients who are treated with *paclitaxel* should be premedicated with *dexamethasone* and *diphenhydramine*, as well as with an H$_2$ blocker.]

VII. STEROID HORMONES AND THEIR ANTAGONISTS

Tumors that are steroid hormone sensitive may be either 1) hormone responsive, in which the tumor regresses following treatment with a specific hormone; or 2) hormone dependent, in which removal of a hormonal stimulus causes tumor regression; or 3) both. Removal of hormonal stimuli from hormone-dependent tumors can be accomplished by surgery (for example, in the case of orchiectomy—surgical removal of one or both testes—for patients with advanced prostate cancer) or by drugs (for example, in breast cancer, for which treatment with the antiestrogen *tamoxifen* is used to prevent estrogen stimulation of breast cancer cells; Figure 46.25). For a steroid hormone to influence a cell, that cell must have intracellular (cytosolic) receptors that are specific for that hormone (Figure 46.26A).

A. Prednisone

Prednisone [PRED-ni-sone] is a potent, synthetic, anti-inflammatory corticosteroid with less mineralocorticoid activity than *cortisol* (see Chapter 27). [Note: At high doses, *cortisol* is lymphocytolytic and leads to hyperuricemia due to the breakdown of lymphocytes.] *Prednisone* is primarily employed to induce remission in patients with acute lymphocytic leukemia and in the treatment of both Hodgkin and non-Hodgkin lymphomas. *Prednisone* is readily absorbed orally. Like other glucocorticoids, it is bound to plasma albumin and transcortin. *Prednisone* itself is inactive and must first undergo 11-β-hydroxylation to *prednisolone* in the liver. *Prednisolone* is the active drug. This steroid then binds to a receptor that triggers the production of specific proteins (Figure 46.26A). The latter is glucuronidated and excreted in urine along with the parent compound.

B. Tamoxifen

Tamoxifen [tah-MOX-ih-fen] is an estrogen antagonist with some estrogenic activity, and it is classified as a selective estrogen receptor modulator (SERM). It is used for first-line therapy in the treatment of estrogen receptor–positive breast cancer. It also finds use prophylactically in reducing breast cancer occurrence in women who are at high risk. However, because of possible stimulation of premalignant lesions due to its estrogenic properties, patients should be closely monitored during therapy.

1. **Mechanism of action:** *Tamoxifen* binds to estrogen receptors in the breast tissue, but the complex is unable to translocate into the nucleus for its action of initiating transcriptions. That is, the complex fails to induce estrogen-responsive genes, and RNA synthesis does not ensue (Figure 46.26B). The result is a depletion (down-regulation) of estrogen receptors, and the growth-promoting

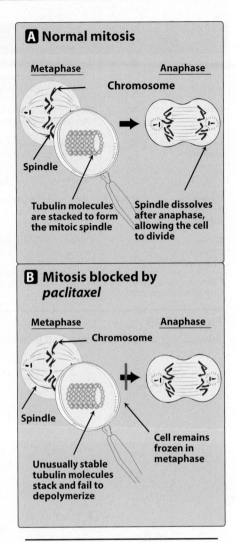

A Normal mitosis

Metaphase — Anaphase
Chromosome
Spindle

Tubulin molecules are stacked to form the mitoic spindle

Spindle dissolves after anaphase, allowing the cell to divide

B Mitosis blocked by *paclitaxel*

Metaphase — Anaphase
Chromosome
Spindle

Unusually stable tubulin molecules stack and fail to depolymerize

Cell remains frozen in metaphase

Figure 46.24
Paclitaxel stabilizes microtubules, rendering them nonfunctional.

DRUG	ROUTE	ADVERSE EFFECTS	NOTABLE DRUG INTERACTIONS	MONITORING PARAMETERS	NOTES
Prednisone	PO	Hyperglycemia, infection, ulcers, pancreatitis, mood changes, cataract formation, osteoporosis		Glucose, CBC	Administer with food
Tamoxifen	PO	Hot flashes, N,V, vaginal bleeding, hypercalcemia, thromboembolism	*Warfarin, rifampin*	Vaginal bleeding, new breast lumps	May cause endometrial cancer
Anastrozole and *Letrozole*	PO	Hot flashes, N, joint pain, ischemic cardiovascular events, osteoporosis	Estrogen-containing products	Hepatic function, bone mineral density monitoring, cholesterol monitoring	Contraindicated in premenopausal or pregnant women
Leuprolide, Goserelin, Triptorelin	Depot, Sub-Q, IM	Tumor flare, hot flashes, asthenia, gynecomastia		Bone mineral density monitoring, serum testosterone, PSA	
Flutamide, Nilutamide, Bicalutamide	PO	Hot flashes, N, gynecomastia, pain, constipation	*Warfarin*	Hepatic function, PSA	Combined with LHRH agonists or surgical castration

PO=oral administration; N=nausea; V=vomiting; CBC=complete blood count; Sub-Q=subcutaneous; IM=intramuscular; PSA=prostate-specific antigen; LHRH=luteinizing hormone–releasing hormone.

Figure 46.25
Summary of steroid hormones and their antagonists.

effects of the natural hormone and other growth factors are suppressed. [Note: Estrogen competes with *tamoxifen*. Therefore, in premenopausal women, the drug is used with a gonadotropin-releasing hormone (GnRH) analog such as *leuprolide,* which lowers estrogen levels.]

2. **Pharmacokinetics:** *Tamoxifen* is effective after oral administration. It is partially metabolized by the liver. Some metabolites possess antagonist activity, whereas others have agonist activity. Unchanged drug and metabolites are excreted predominantly through the bile into the feces. *Tamoxifen* is an inhibitor of CYP3A4 and P-glycoprotein.

3. **Adverse effects:** Side effects caused by *tamoxifen* include hot flashes, nausea, vomiting, skin rash, and vaginal bleeding and discharge (due to estrogenic activity of the drug and some of its metabolites). Hypercalcemia may occur, requiring cessation of the drug. *Tamoxifen* can also lead to increased pain if the tumor has metastasized to bone. *Tamoxifen* has the potential to cause endometrial cancer. Other toxicities include thromboembolism and effects on vision. [Note: Because of a more favorable adverse effect profile, aromatase inhibitors are making an impact in the treatment of breast cancer.]

C. **Fulvestrant and raloxifene**

Fulvestrant [fool-VES-trant] and *raloxifene* [ral-OKS-i-feen] are two agents that interact with the estrogen receptor to prevent some of the downstream effects. *Fulvestrant* is an estrogen receptor antagonist that is given via intramuscular injection to patients with hormone receptor–positive metastatic breast cancer. This agent binds to and causes estrogen receptor down-regulation on tumors and other targets. *Raloxifene* is a SERM given orally that acts to block estrogen effects in the uterine and breast tissues, while promoting effects in the bone to inhibit resorption. This agent has been shown to reduce the risk of estrogen receptor–positive invasive breast cancer in postmenopausal women. These agents are known to cause hot flashes, arthralgias, and myalgias.

D. Aromatase inhibitors

The aromatase reaction is responsible for the extra-adrenal synthesis of estrogen from androstenedione, which takes place in liver, fat, muscle, skin, and breast tissues, including breast malignancies. Peripheral aromatization is an important source of estrogen in postmenopausal women. Aromatase inhibitors decrease the production of estrogen in these women.

1. **Anastrozole and letrozole:** The imidazole aromatase inhibitors, such as *anastrozole* [an-AS-troe-zole] and *letrozole* [LE-troe-zole], are nonsteroidal aromatase inhibitors. They do not predispose patients to endometrial cancer and are devoid of the androgenic side effects that occur with the steroidal aromatase inhibitors such as *aminoglutethimide*. Although *anastrozole* and *letrozole* are considered second-line therapy after *tamoxifen* for hormone-dependent breast cancer in the United States, they have become first-line drugs in other countries for the treatment of breast cancer in postmenopausal women. They are orally active and cause almost a total suppression of estrogen synthesis. Both drugs are extensively metabolized in the liver, and metabolites and parent drug are excreted primarily in the urine.

2. **Exemestane:** A steroidal, irreversible inhibitor of aromatase, *exemestane* [ex-uh-MES-tane], is orally well absorbed and widely distributed. Hepatic metabolism is by the CYP3A4 isoenzyme. Because the metabolites are excreted in urine, doses of the drug must be adjusted in patients with renal failure. Its major toxicities are nausea, fatigue, and hot flashes. Alopecia and dermatitis have also been noted.

E. Progestins

Megestrol [me-JESS-trole] *acetate* is a progestin that was widely used in treating metastatic hormone-responsive breast and endometrial neoplasms. It is orally effective. Other agents are usually compared to it in clinical trials; however, the aromatase inhibitors are replacing it in therapy.

F. Leuprolide, goserelin, and triptorelin

GnRH is normally secreted by the hypothalamus and stimulates the anterior pituitary to secrete the gonadotropic hormones: 1) luteinizing hormone (LH), the primary stimulus for the secretion of testosterone by the testes, and 2) follicle-stimulating hormone (FSH), which stimulates the secretion of estrogen. *Leuprolide* [loo-PROE-lide], *goserelin* [GOE-se-rel-in], and *triptorelin* [TRIP-to-rel-in] are synthetic analogs of GnRH. As GnRH analogs, they occupy the GnRH receptor in the pituitary, which leads to its desensitization and, consequently, inhibition of release of FSH and LH. Thus, both androgen and estrogen syntheses are reduced (Figure 46.27). Response to *leuprolide* in prostatic cancer is equivalent to that of orchiectomy with regression of tumor and relief of bone pain. These drugs have some benefit in premenopausal

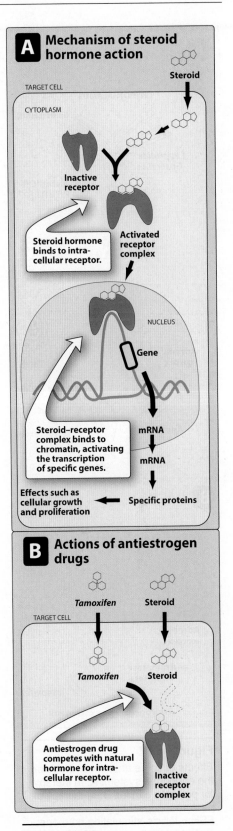

Figure 46.26
Action of steroid hormones and antiestrogen agents. mRNA = messenger RNA.

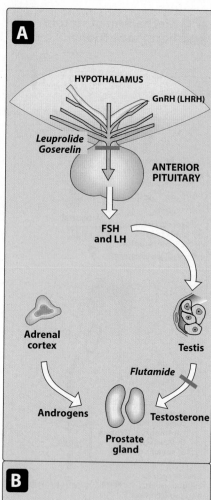

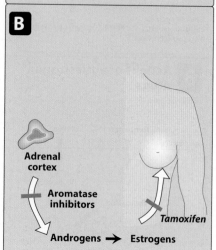

Figure 46.27
Effects of some anticancer drugs on the endocrine system. **A.** In therapy for prostatic cancer. **B.** In therapy of postmenopausal breast cancer. FSH = follicle-stimulating hormone; GnRH (LHRH) = gonadotropin-releasing hormone (luteinizing hormone–releasing hormone); LH = luteinizing hormone.

women with advanced breast cancer and have largely replaced estrogens in therapy for prostate cancer. *Leuprolide* is available as 1) a sustained-release intradermal implant, 2) a subcutaneous depot injection, or 3) an intramuscular depot injection to treat metastatic carcinoma of the prostate. *Goserelin acetate* is a subcutaneous implant, and *triptorelin pamoate* is injected intramuscularly. Levels of androgen may initially rise but then fall to castration levels. The adverse effects of these drugs, including impotence, hot flashes, and tumor flare, are minimal compared to those experienced with estrogen treatment.

G. Estrogens

Estrogens, such as *ethinyl estradiol,* had been used in the treatment of prostatic cancer. However, they have been largely replaced by the GnRH analogs because of fewer adverse effects. Estrogens inhibit the growth of prostatic tissue by blocking the production of LH, thereby decreasing the synthesis of androgens in the testis. Thus, tumors that are dependent on androgens are affected. Estrogen treatment can cause serious complications, such as thromboemboli, myocardial infarction, strokes, and hypercalcemia. Men who are taking estrogens may experience gynecomastia and impotence.

H. Flutamide, nilutamide, and bicalutamide

Flutamide [FLOO-tah-mide], *nilutamide* [nye-LOO-ta-mide], and *bicalutamide* [bye-ka-LOO-ta-mide] are synthetic, nonsteroidal antiandrogens used in the treatment of prostate cancer. They compete with the natural hormone for binding to the androgen receptor and prevent its translocation into the nucleus (Figure 46.27). These antiandrogens are taken orally and are cleared through the kidney. [Note: *Flutamide* requires dosing three times a day and the others once a day.] Side effects include gynecomastia and GI distress. Rarely, liver failure has occurred with *flutamide. Nilutamide* can cause visual problems.

VIII. MONOCLONAL ANTIBODIES

Monoclonal antibodies (Figure 46.28) have become an active area of drug development for anticancer therapy and other nonneoplastic diseases, because they are directed at specific targets and often have fewer adverse effects. They are created from B lymphocytes (from immunized mice or hamsters) fused with "immortal" B-lymphocyte tumor cells. The resulting hybrid cells can be individually cloned, and each clone will produce antibodies directed against a single antigen type. Recombinant technology has led to the creation of "humanized" antibodies that overcome the immunologic problems previously observed following administration of mouse (murine) antibodies. The use of the monoclonal antibodies *trastuzumab, rituximab, bevacizumab,* and *cetuximab* in the treatment of cancer is described below. Many other monoclonal antibody treatments are available, examples of which include *alemtuzumab,* which is used in the treatment of refractory B-cell chronic lymphocytic leukemia, *panitumumab,* which is effective in metastatic colorectal tumors, and *I*[131]-*tositumomab,* which is used in relapsed non-Hodgkin lymphoma. [Note: Monoclonal antibodies also find application in a number of other disorders, such as inflammatory bowel disease, psoriasis, and rheumatoid arthritis.]

DRUG	ROUTE	ADVERSE EFFECTS	NOTABLE DRUG INTERACTIONS	MONITORING PARAMETERS	NOTES
Trastuzumab	IV	Cardiomyopathy, infusion-related fever and chills, pulmonary toxicity, headache, N, V, neutropenia in combination with chemotherapy		LVEF, CBC, pulmonary toxicity due to infusion reaction	Embryo-fetal toxicity
Rituximab	IV	Fatal infusion reaction, TLS, mucocutaneous reactions, PML	*Cisplatin*	Vital signs during infusion, TLS labs	Fatal reactivation of hepatitis B, premedication required prior to infusion to prevent reaction
Bevacizumab	IV	Hypertension, GI perforation, proteinuria, wound-healing problems, bleeding		BP, urine protein, signs and symptoms of bleeding	Hold for recent or upcoming surgical procedures
Cetuximab	IV	Skin rash, electrolyte wasting, infusion reaction, D		Electrolytes, vital signs during infusion	Premedication required prior to infusion, rash equated with increased response

IV=intravenous; N=nausea; V=vomiting; LVEF=left ventricular ejection fraction; CBC=complete blood count; GI=gastrointestinal; BP=blood pressure; D=diarrhea; TLS=tumor lysis syndrome; PML=progressive multifocal leukoencephalopathy.

Figure 46.28
Summary of monoclonal antibodies.

A. Trastuzumab

In patients with metastatic breast cancer, overexpression of transmembrane human epidermal growth factor receptor protein 2 (HER2) is seen in 25% to 30% of patients. HER2 overexpression is also noted in gastric and gastroesophageal cancers. *Trastuzumab* [tra-STEW-zoo-mab], a humanized monoclonal antibody, specifically targets the extracellular domain of the HER2 growth receptor that has intrinsic tyrosine kinase activity. [Note: At least 50 tyrosine kinases mediate cell growth or division by phosphorylating signaling proteins. They have been implicated in the development of many neoplasms by an unknown mechanism.]

1. **Mechanism of action:** *Trastuzumab* binds to HER2 sites in breast cancer, gastric cancer, and gastroesophageal tissues and inhibits the proliferation of cells that overexpress the HER2 protein, thereby decreasing the number of cells in the S-phase. By binding to HER2, it blocks downstream signaling pathways, induces antibody-dependent cytotoxicity, and prevents the release of HER2.

2. **Adverse effects:** The most serious toxicity associated with the use of *trastuzumab* is congestive heart failure. The toxicity is worsened if given in combination with anthracyclines. Extreme caution should be exercised when giving the drug to patients with preexisting cardiac dysfunction.

B. Rituximab

Rituximab [ri-TUCKS-ih-mab] was the first monoclonal antibody to be approved for the treatment of cancer. It is a genetically engineered, chimeric monoclonal antibody directed against the CD20 antigen that is found on the surfaces of normal and malignant B lymphocytes. CD20 plays a role in the activation process for cell cycle initiation and differentiation. The CD20 antigen is expressed on nearly all B-cell non-Hodgkin lymphomas but not in other bone marrow cells.

Rituximab is effective in the treatment of lymphomas, chronic lympho-cytic leukemia, and rheumatoid arthritis.

1. **Mechanism of action:** The Fab domain of *rituximab* binds to the CD20 antigen on the B lymphocytes, and its Fc domain recruits immune effector functions, inducing complement and antibody-dependent, cell-mediated cytotoxicity of the B cells. The antibody is commonly used with other combinations of anticancer agents, such as *cyclophosphamide, doxorubicin, vincristine* (Oncovin), and *prednisone* (CHOP).

2. **Adverse effects:** Severe adverse reactions have been fatal. It is important to infuse *rituximab* slowly. Hypotension, bronchospasm, and angioedema may occur. Chills and fever commonly accom-pany the first infusion (especially in patients with high circulating levels of neoplastic cells), because of rapid activation of comple-ment which results in the release of tumor necrosis factor-α and interleukins. Pretreatment with *diphenhydramine, acetaminophen,* and corticosteroids can ameliorate these problems. Tumor lysis syndrome has been reported within 24 hours of the first dose of *rituximab.* This syndrome consists of hyperkalemia, hypocalcemia, hyperuricemia, hyperphosphatasemia (an abnormally high content of alkaline phosphatase in the blood), and acute renal failure that may require dialysis.

C. Bevacizumab

The monoclonal antibody *bevacizumab* [be-vah-SEE-zoo-mab] is an IV antiangiogenesis agent. *Bevacizumab* is approved for use as a first-line drug against metastatic colorectal cancer and is given with *5-FU*–based chemotherapy. It attaches to and stops vascular endo-thelial growth factor from stimulating the formation of new blood ves-sels (neovascularization). Without new blood vessels, tumors do not receive the oxygen and essential nutrients necessary for growth and proliferation.

D. Cetuximab and panitumumab

Cetuximab [see-TUX-i-mab] is another chimeric monoclonal antibody infused intravenously and approved to treat KRAS wild-type metastatic colorectal cancer and head and neck cancers. [Note: KRAS is a form of RAS proteins, which are mediators of proliferation and differentia-tion.] It exerts its antineoplastic effect by targeting the epidermal growth factor receptor (EGFR) on the surface of cancer cells and interfering with their growth. *Cetuximab, panitumumab* [pan-i-TUE-moo-mab], and other agents that target this receptor cause a distinct acneiform-type rash. The appearance of this rash has been associated with a positive response to therapy.

IX. PLATINUM COORDINATION COMPLEXES

A. Cisplatin, carboplatin, and oxaliplatin

Cisplatin [SIS-pla-tin] was the first member of the platinum coordi-nation complex class of anticancer drugs, but because of its severe toxicity, *carboplatin* [KAR-boe-pla-tin] was developed. The mechanisms of action of the two drugs are similar, but their potency, pharmacokinetics, patterns of distribution, and dose-limiting toxicities differ significantly (Figure 46.29). *Cisplatin* has synergistic cytotoxicity with radiation and other chemotherapeutic agents. It has found wide application in the treatment of solid tumors, such as metastatic testicular carcinoma in combination with *VBL* and *bleomycin,* ovarian carcinoma in combination with *cyclophosphamide,* or alone for bladder carcinoma. *Carboplatin* is used when patients cannot be vigorously hydrated, as is required for *cisplatin* treatment, or if they suffer from kidney dysfunction or are prone to neuro- or ototoxicity. *Oxaliplatin* [ox-AL-ih-pla-tin] is a closely related analog of *carboplatin* used in the setting of colorectal cancer.

1. **Mechanism of action:** The mechanism of action for this class of drugs is similar to that of the alkylating agents. In the high-chloride milieu of the plasma, *cisplatin* persists as the neutral species, which enters the cell and loses its chlorides in the low-chloride milieu. It then binds to guanine in DNA, forming inter- and intrastrand crosslinks. The resulting cytotoxic lesion inhibits both polymerases for DNA replication and RNA synthesis. Cytotoxicity can occur at any stage of the cell cycle, but cells are most vulnerable to the actions of these drugs in the G_1 and S-phases.

2. **Pharmacokinetics:** These agents are administered via IV infusion. *Cisplatin and carboplatin* can also be given intraperitoneally for ovarian cancer and intra-arterially to perfuse other organs. The highest concentrations of the drugs are found in the liver, kidney, and intestinal, testicular, and ovarian cells, but little penetrates into the CSF. The renal route is the main avenue for excretion.

3. **Adverse effects:** Severe, persistent vomiting occurs for at least 1 hour after administration of *cisplatin* and may continue for as long as 5 days. Premedication with antiemetic agents is required. The major limiting toxicity is dose-related nephrotoxicity, involving the distal convoluted tubule and collecting ducts. This can be prevented by aggressive hydration. Other toxicities include ototoxicity with high-frequency hearing loss and tinnitus. Unlike *cisplatin,* *carboplatin* causes only mild nausea and vomiting, and it is rarely

DRUG	ROUTE	ADVERSE EFFECTS	NOTABLE DRUG INTERACTIONS	MONITORING PARAMETERS	NOTES
Cisplatin	IV, IP, IA	Neurotoxicity, myelosuppression, ototoxicity, N, V, electrolyte wasting, infusion reaction, nephrotoxicity	Anticonvulsants	CBC, CMP, electrolytes, hearing	Aggressive pre- and posthydration required, high incidence of nausea and vomiting
Carboplatin	IV, IP, IA	Myelosuppression, N, V, infusion reaction	Aminoglycosides	CBC	Dose calculated using AUC
Oxaliplatin	IV	Neurotoxicity, N, V, infusion reaction, hepatotoxicity, myelosuppression	*Warfarin*	CBC, neurologic function, hepatic function	Cold-related and cumulative peripheral neuropathy

IV=intravenous; IP=intraperitoneally; IA=intraarterially; AUC=area under the curve; N=nausea; V=vomiting; CBC=complete blood count; CMP=complete metabolic panel.

Figure 46.29
Summary of platinum coordination complexes.

nephro-, neuro-, or ototoxic. Its dose-limiting toxicity is myelosuppression. *Oxaliplatin* has a distinct side effect of cold-induced peripheral neuropathy that usually resolves within 72 hours of administration. It also causes myelosuppression and cumulative peripheral neuropathy. Hepatotoxicity has also been reported. These agents may cause hypersensitivity reactions ranging from skin rashes to anaphylaxis.

X. TOPOISOMERASE INHIBITORS

These agents exert their mechanism of action via inhibition of topoisomerase enzymes, a class of enzymes that reduce supercoiling of DNA (Figure 46.30).

A. Camptothecins

Camptothecins are plant alkaloids originally isolated from the Chinese tree Camptotheca. *Irinotecan* [eye-rin-oh-TEE-kan] and *topotecan* [toe-poe-TEE-kan] are semisynthetic derivatives of *camptothecin* [camp-toe-THEE-sin]. *Topotecan* is used in metastatic ovarian cancer when primary therapy has failed and also in the treatment of small cell lung cancer. *Irinotecan* is used with *5-FU* and *leucovorin* for the treatment of colorectal carcinoma.

1. **Mechanism of action:** These drugs are S-phase specific and inhibit topoisomerase I, which is essential for the replication of DNA in human cells (Figure 46.31). SN-38 (the active metabolite of *irinotecan*) is approximately 1000 times as potent as *irinotecan* as an inhibitor of topoisomerase I. The topoisomerases relieve torsional strain in DNA by causing reversible, single-strand breaks.

2. **Adverse effects:** Bone marrow suppression, particularly neutropenia, is the dose-limiting toxicity for *topotecan*. Frequent blood counts should be performed on patients taking this drug. Myelosuppression is also seen with *irinotecan*. Acute and delayed diarrhea may be severe and require treatment with *atropine* during the infusion or high doses of *loperamide* in the days following the infusion.

B. Etoposide

Etoposide [e-toe-POE-side] is a semisynthetic derivative of the plant alkaloid, podophyllotoxin. It blocks cells in the late S- to G_2 phase

DRUG	ROUTE	ADVERSE EFFECTS	NOTABLE DRUG INTERACTIONS	MONITORING PARAMETERS	NOTES
Irinotecan	IV	Diarrhea, myelosuppression, N, V	CYP3A4 substrates	CBC, electrolytes	Acute and delayed (life-threatening) diarrhea
Topotecan	IV, PO	Myelosuppression, N, V	P-glycoprotein inhibitors (PO)	CBC	Diarrhea common with PO
Etoposide	IV, PO	Myelosuppression, hypotension, alopecia, N, V		CBC	May cause secondary malignancies (leukemias)

IV=intravenous; PO=oral administration; N=nausea; V=vomiting; CBC=complete blood count.

Figure 46.30
Summary of topoisomerase inhibitors.

of the cell cycle. Its major target is topoisomerase II. Binding of the drug to the enzyme–DNA complex results in persistence of the transient, cleavable form of the complex and, thus, renders it susceptible to irreversible double-strand breaks (Figure 46.32). *Etoposide* finds its major clinical use in the treatment of lung cancer and in combination with *bleomycin* and *cisplatin* for testicular carcinoma. *Etoposide* may be administered either IV or orally. Dose-limiting myelosuppression (primarily leukopenia) is the major toxicity.

XI. TYROSINE KINASE INHIBITORS

The tyrosine kinases are a family of enzymes that are involved in several important processes within a cell, including signal transduction and cell division. Many tyrosine kinase inhibitors are available, and these agents have a wide variety of applications in the treatment of cancer (Figure 46.33). Some of the more common agents are discussed below.

A. Imatinib, dasatinib, and nilotinib

Imatinib [i-MAT-in-ib] *mesylate* is used for the treatment of chronic myelogenous leukemia (CML) as well as GI stromal tumors. It acts as a signal transduction inhibitor, used specifically to inhibit tumor tyrosine kinase activity. A deregulated BCR-ABL kinase is present in the leukemia cells of almost every patient with CML. In the case of GI stromal tumors, an unregulated expression of tyrosine kinase is associated with a growth factor. The ability of *imatinib* to occupy the "kinase pocket" prevents the phosphorylation of tyrosine on the substrate molecule and, hence, inhibits subsequent steps that lead to cell proliferation. *Nilotinib* [ni-LOT-in-ib] and *dasatinib* [da-SAT-in-ib] are also first-line options for CML. These agents are all available in oral formulations, and they are associated with notable toxicities, such as fluid retention and QT prolongation (Figure 46.33).

B. Erlotinib

Erlotinib [er-LOT-tih-nib] is an inhibitor of the epidermal growth factor receptor tyrosine kinase. It is an oral agent approved for the treatment of non–small cell lung cancer and pancreatic cancer. *Erlotinib* is absorbed after oral administration and undergoes extensive metabolism in the liver by the CYP3A4 isoenzyme. The most common adverse effects are diarrhea, nausea, acne-like skin rashes, and ocular disorders. A rare but potentially fatal adverse effect is interstitial lung disease, which presents as acute dyspnea with cough.

C. Sorafenib and sunitinib

Sorafenib [SOR-af-i-nib] and *sunitinib* [su-NIT-ti-nib] are oral serine/threonine and tyrosine kinase inhibitors used mainly in renal cell carcinoma. *Sorafenib* is also part of the treatment strategy for hepatocellular carcinoma, and *sunitinib* is used in GI stromal tumors and pancreatic neuroendocrine tumors. These agents target cell surface kinases that are involved in tumor signaling, angiogenesis, and apoptosis, thus slowing tumor growth. Adverse effects include diarrhea, fatigue, hand and foot syndrome, and hypertension.

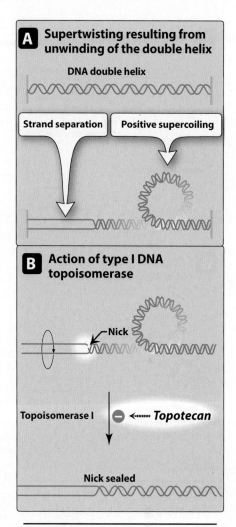

A Supertwisting resulting from unwinding of the double helix

DNA double helix

Strand separation

Positive supercoiling

B Action of type I DNA topoisomerase

Nick

Topoisomerase I ⊖ ←---- *Topotecan*

Nick sealed

Figure 46.31
Action of type I DNA topoisomerases.

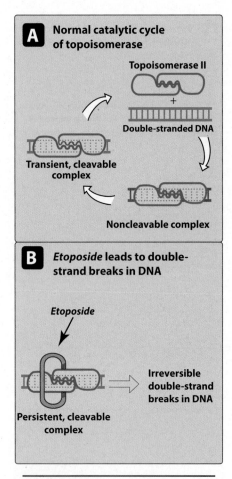

A Normal catalytic cycle of topoisomerase

Topoisomerase II

+

Double-stranded DNA

Transient, cleavable complex

Noncleavable complex

B *Etoposide* leads to double-strand breaks in DNA

Etoposide

Irreversible double-strand breaks in DNA

Persistent, cleavable complex

Figure 46.32
Mechanism of action of *etoposide*.

XII. MISCELLANEOUS AGENTS

A. Procarbazine

Procarbazine [proe-KAR-ba-zeen] is used in the treatment of Hodgkin disease and other cancers. *Procarbazine* rapidly equilibrates between the plasma and the CSF after oral administration. It must undergo a series of oxidative reactions to exert its cytotoxic action that causes inhibition of DNA, RNA, and protein synthesis. Metabolites and the parent drug are excreted via the kidney. Bone marrow depression is the major toxicity, and nausea, vomiting, and diarrhea are common. The drug is also neurotoxic, causing symptoms ranging from drowsiness to hallucinations to paresthesias. Because it inhibits monoamine oxidase, patients should be warned against ingesting foods that contain high levels of tyramine (for example, aged cheeses, beer, and wine) as this could cause a hypertensive crisis. Ingestion of alcohol leads to a disulfiram-like reaction. *Procarbazine* is both mutagenic and teratogenic. Nonlymphocytic leukemia has developed in patients treated with the drug.

B. Asparaginase and pegaspargase

Some neoplastic cells require an external source of asparagine because of limited capacity to synthesize sufficient amounts of the amino acid to support growth and function. L-*Asparaginase* [ah-SPAR-a-gi-nase] and the pegylated formulation *pegaspargase* [peg-ah-SPAR-jase] catalyze the deamination of asparagine to aspartic acid and ammonia, thus depriving the tumor cells of this amino acid, which is needed for protein synthesis. The form of the enzyme used chemotherapeutically is derived from bacteria. L-*Asparaginase* is used to treat childhood acute lymphocytic leukemia in combination with *VX* and *prednisone*. The enzyme must be administered either IV or intramuscularly, because it is destroyed by gastric enzymes.

DRUG	ROUTE	ADVERSE EFFECTS	NOTABLE DRUG INTERACTIONS	MONITORING PARAMETERS	NOTES
Imatinib	PO	Myelosuppression, fluid retention, CHF	CYP3A4 substrates, *warfarin*	CBC, BCR-ABL	Monitor for development of heart failure
Dasatinib	PO	Myelosuppression, fluid retention, diarrhea	CYP3A4 substrates, acid-reducing agents	CBC, BCR-ABL, electrolytes	QT prolongation
Nilotinib	PO	Myelosuppression, QT prolongation, hepatotoxicity	CYP3A4 substrates, acid-reducing agents	CBC, BCR-ABL, electrolytes	QT prolongation, administer on empty stomach
Erlotinib	PO	Rash, ILD, hepatotoxicity	CYP3A4 substrates, acid-reducing agents, *warfarin*	CMP	Rash equated with increased response
Sorafenib	PO	Hypertension, hand-foot syndrome, rash, diarrhea, fatigue	CYP3A4 inducers, *warfarin*	BP, CMP	Wound-healing complications, cardiac events
Sunitinib	PO	Hypertension, hand-foot syndrome, rash, diarrhea, fatigue, hepatotoxicity, hypothyroidism	CYP3A4 substrates	BP, CMP, TSH	Monitor for development of heart failure

PO=oral administration; ILD=interstitial lung disease; CMP=complete metabolic panel; CBC=complete blood count; TSH=thyroid stimulating hormone; BP=blood pressure.

Figure 46.33
Summary of tyrosine kinase inhibitors.

Toxicities include a range of hypersensitivity reactions (because it is a foreign protein), a decrease in clotting factors, liver abnormalities, pancreatitis, seizures, and coma due to ammonia toxicity.

C. Interferons

Human interferons are biological response modifiers and have been classified into the three types α, β, and γ on the basis of their antigenicity. The α interferons are primarily leukocytic, whereas the β and γ interferons are produced by connective tissue fibroblasts and T lymphocytes, respectively. Recombinant DNA techniques in bacteria have made it possible to produce large quantities of pure interferons, including two species designated *interferon-α-2a* and *2b* that are employed in treating neoplastic diseases. *Interferon-α-2a* is currently approved for the management of hairy cell leukemia, CML, and acquired immunodeficiency syndrome (AIDS)-related Kaposi sarcoma. *Interferon-α-2b* is approved for the treatment of hairy cell leukemia, melanoma, AIDS-related Kaposi sarcoma, and follicular lymphoma. Interferons interact with surface receptors on other cells, at which site they exert their effects. Bound interferons are neither internalized nor degraded. As a consequence of the binding of interferon, a series of complex intracellular reactions take place. These include synthesis of enzymes, suppression of cell proliferation, activation of macrophages, and increased cytotoxicity of lymphocytes. However, the exact mechanism by which the interferons are cytotoxic is unknown. Interferons are well absorbed after intramuscular or subcutaneous injections. An IV form of *interferon-α-2b* is also available. Interferons undergo glomerular filtration and are degraded during reabsorption, but liver metabolism is minimal. Flu-like symptoms and GI upset are common with these agents. Suicidal ideation and seizures have been reported.

D. Abiraterone acetate

Abiraterone [ab-er-AT-er-own] *acetate* is an oral agent used in the treatment of metastatic castration–resistant prostate cancer (Figure 46.34). *Abiraterone acetate* is used in conjunction with *prednisone* to inhibit the CYP17 enzyme (an enzyme required for androgen synthesis), resulting in reduced testosterone production. Coadministration with *prednisone* is required to help lessen the effects of mineralocorticoid excess resulting from CYP17 inhibition. Hepatotoxicity may occur, and patients should be closely monitored for hypertension, hypokalemia,

DRUG	ROUTE	ADVERSE EFFECTS	NOTABLE DRUG INTERACTIONS	MONITORING PARAMETERS	NOTES
Abiraterone acetate	PO	Hypertension, fluid retention, diarrhea, hot flushes, hepatotoxicity	CYP2D6 substrates	PSA, BP, LFTs	Administer with *prednisone*, administer on empty stomach twice daily
Enzalutamide	PO	Asthenia/fatigue, fluid retention, hot flushes, joint/muscle pain	*Gemfibrozil*, CYP3A4, CYP2C9, CYP2C19 substrate	PSA	Seizure precaution, administer once daily

PO=oral administration; PSA=prostate-specific antigen; BP=blood pressure; LFTs=liver function tests.

Figure 46.34
Summary of miscellaneous chemotherapeutic agents.

and fluid retention. Joint and muscle discomfort, hot flushes, and diarrhea are common side effects with this agent.

E. Enzalutamide

Enzalutamide [enz-a-LOOT-a-mide] is an oral agent that works at the level of the androgen-signaling pathway in the treatment of metastatic castrate-resistant prostate cancer in patients that have previously received *docetaxel* chemotherapy. *Enzalutamide* inhibits the binding of androgen to receptors and inhibits androgen receptor nuclear translocation and interaction with DNA. Notable adverse effects include asthenia, back pain, fluid retention, and risk of seizure. Multiple drug interactions potentially exist, as this drug is a strong inducer of CYP3A4 and a moderate inducer of CYP2C9 and CYP2C19.

Anticancer therapy strives to cure disease, prolong life, and ameliorate symptoms caused by tumor invasion. These agents may have severe, life-threatening side effects, but with careful consideration and monitoring, these agents can be very useful in the treatment of cancer. "Chemo Man" is a useful tool to help remember the most common toxicities of these drugs (Figure 46.35).

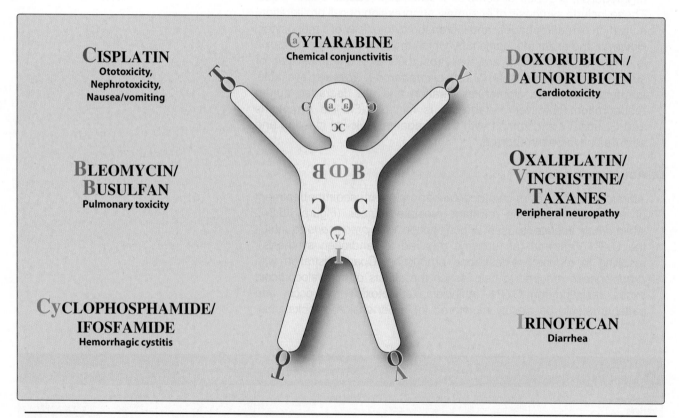

Figure 46.35
Chemo Man—a summary of toxicity of chemotherapeutic agents.

Study Questions

Choose the ONE best answer.

46.1 A patient is about to undergo three cycles of chemotherapy prior to surgery for bladder cancer. Which of the following best describes chemotherapy in this setting?

A. Adjuvant.
B. Neoadjuvant.
C. Palliative.
D. Maintenance.

Correct answer = B. Since the chemotherapy is being given *before* the surgery, it is considered neoadjuvant. Chemotherapy is indicated when neoplasms are disseminated and are not amenable to surgery (palliative). Chemotherapy is also used as a supplemental treatment to attack micrometastases following surgery and radiation treatment, in which case it is called adjuvant chemotherapy. Chemotherapy given prior to the surgical procedure in an attempt to shrink the cancer is referred to as neoadjuvant chemotherapy, and chemotherapy given in lower doses to assist in prolonging a remission is known as maintenance chemotherapy.

46.2 A 45-year-old male patient is being treated with ABVD chemotherapy for Hodgkin lymphoma. He presents for cycle 4 of a planned 6 cycles with a new-onset cough. He states it started a week ago and he also feels like he has a little trouble catching his breath. Which drug in the ABVD regimen is the most likely cause of his pulmonary toxicity?

A. Doxorubicin (**A**driamycin).
B. Bleomycin.
C. Vinblastine.
D. Dacarbazine.

Correct answer = B. Pulmonary toxicity is the most serious adverse effect of bleomycin, progressing from rales, cough, and infiltrate to potentially fatal fibrosis. The pulmonary fibrosis that is caused by bleomycin is often referred as "bleomycin lung."

46.3 FL is a 64-year-old male about to undergo therapy for rhabdomyosarcoma. His chemotherapy includes ifosfamide. Which of the following is most appropriate to include in chemotherapy orders for this patient?

A. IV hydration, mesna, and frequent urinalyses.
B. Leucovorin and frequent urinalyses.
C. Allopurinol and frequent urinalyses.
D. IV hydration, prophylactic antibiotics, and frequent urinalyses.

Correct answer = A. A unique toxicity of ifosfamide is hemorrhagic cystitis. This bladder toxicity has been attributed to toxic metabolites of *ifosfamide*. Adequate hydration as well as IV injection of mesna (sodium 2-mercaptoethane sulfonate), which neutralizes the toxic metabolites, can minimize this problem. Frequent urinalyses to monitor for red blood cells should be ordered. Leucovorin is used with methotrexate or 5-FU (not ifosfamide). Allopurinol has a drug interaction with ifosfamide and is not an agent that prevents hemorrhagic cystitis. Prophylactic antibiotics are not needed.

46.4 The appearance of a facial rash with cetuximab is associated with which of the following?

A. A negative response to therapy.
B. A positive response to therapy.
C. A drug allergy.
D. An infusion reaction.

Correct answer = B. Patients undergoing therapy with an EGFR inhibitor such as cetuximab often develop an acne-like rash on the face, chest, upper back, and arms. The appearance of such a rash has been correlated with an increased response as compared to patients who do not experience a rash during therapy.

Immunosuppressants 47

Sony Tuteja

I. OVERVIEW

The importance of the immune system in protecting the body against harmful foreign molecules is well recognized. However, in the case of organ transplantation, the immune system can elicit a damaging immune response, causing rejection of the transplanted tissue. Transplantation of organs and tissues (for example, kidney, heart, or bone marrow) has become routine due to improved surgical techniques and better tissue typing. Also, drugs are now available that more selectively inhibit rejection of transplanted tissues while preventing the patient from becoming immunologically compromised (Figure 47.1). Earlier drugs were nonselective, and patients frequently succumbed to infection due to suppression of both the antibody-mediated (humoral) and cell-mediated arms of the immune system. Today, the principal approach to immunosuppressive therapy is to alter lymphocyte function using drugs or antibodies against immune proteins. Because of their severe toxicities when used as monotherapy, a combination of immunosuppressive agents, usually at lower doses, is generally employed. Immunosuppressive drug regimens usually consist of anywhere from two to four agents with different mechanisms of action that disrupt various levels of T-cell activation. [Note: Although this chapter focuses on immunosuppressive agents in the context of organ transplantation, these agents may be used in the treatment of other disorders. For example, cyclosporine may be useful in the treatment of psoriasis, and various monoclonal antibodies have applications in a number of disorders, including rheumatoid arthritis, multiple sclerosis, Crohn disease, and ulcerative colitis.]

The immune activation cascade can be described as a three-signal model. Signal 1 constitutes T-cell triggering at the CD3 receptor complex by an antigen on the surface of an antigen-presenting cell (APC). Signal 1 alone is insufficient for T-cell activation and requires signal 2. Signal 2, also referred to as costimulation, occurs when CD80 and CD86 on the surface of APCs engage CD28 on T cells. Both signals 1 and 2 activate several intracellular signal transduction pathways, one of which is the calcium–calcineurin pathway. These pathways trigger the production of cytokines such as interleukin (IL)-2 and T-cell dependent activation of B lymphocytes. IL-2 then binds to the IL-2 receptor (also known as CD25) on the surface of other T cells to activate mammalian target of rapamycin (mTOR), providing signal 3, the stimulus for T-cell proliferation. Immunosuppressive drugs can be categorized by their mechanism of action: 1) interference with cytokine production or action; 2) disruption of

SELECTIVE INHIBITORS OF CYTOKINE PRODUCTION AND FUNCTION
Belatacept NULOJIX
Cyclosporine NEORAL, SANDIMMUNE
Everolimus AFINITOR, ZORTRESS
Sirolimus RAPAMUNE
Tacrolimus PROGRAF

IMMUNOSUPPRESSIVE ANTIMETABOLITES
Azathioprine IMURAN
Mycophenolate mofetil CELLCEPT
Mycophenolate sodium MYFORTIC

ANTIBODIES
Antithymocyte globulins ATGAM, THYMOGLOBULIN
Basiliximab SIMULECT

ADRENOCORTICOIDS
Methylprednisolone MEDROL
Prednisolone ORAPRED, PRELONE
Prednisone

Figure 47.1
Immunosuppressant drugs.

Cytokine	Actions
IL-1	• Enhances activity of NK cells • Attracts neutrophils and macrophages
IL-2	• Induces proliferation of antigen-primed T cells • Enhances activity of NK cells
IFN-γ	• Enhances activity of macrophages and NK cells • Increases expression of MHC molecules • Enhances production of IgG$_{2a}$
TNF-α	• Cytotoxic effect on tumor cells • Induces cytokine secretion in the inflammatory response

Figure 47.2

Summary of selected cytokines. IL = interleukin; IFN = interferon; TNF = tumor necrosis factor; NK = natural killer; MHC = major histocompatibility complex; IgG = immunoglobulin G.

cell metabolism, preventing lymphocyte proliferation; and 3) mono- and polyclonal antibodies that block T-cell surface molecules.

II. SELECTIVE INHIBITORS OF CYTOKINE PRODUCTION AND FUNCTION

Cytokines are soluble, antigen-nonspecific signaling proteins that bind to cell surface receptors on a variety of cells. The term cytokine includes interleukins (ILs), interferons (IFNs), tumor necrosis factors (TNFs), transforming growth factors, and colony-stimulating factors. Of particular interest is IL-2, a growth factor that stimulates the proliferation of antigen-primed (helper) T cells, which subsequently produce more IL-2, IFN-γ, and TNF-α (Figure 47.2). These cytokines collectively activate natural killer cells, macrophages, and cytotoxic T lymphocytes. Drugs that interfere with the production or activity of IL-2 significantly dampen the immune response and, thereby, decrease graft rejection. These drugs can be further divided into three main classes: 1) calcineurin inhibitors (*cyclosporine* and *tacrolimus*), 2) costimulation blockers (*belatacept*), and 3) mTOR inhibitors (*sirolimus* and *everolimus*).

A. Cyclosporine

Cyclosporine [sye-kloe-SPOR-een], a calcineurin inhibitor, is a lipophilic cyclic polypeptide extracted from the soil fungus <u>Beauveria nivea</u>.

1. **Mechanism of action:** *Cyclosporine* preferentially suppresses cell-mediated immune reactions, whereas humoral immunity is affected to a far lesser extent. After diffusing into the T cell, *cyclosporine* binds to a cyclophilin (more generally called an immunophilin) to form a complex that binds to calcineurin (Figure 47.3). Calcineurin is responsible for dephosphorylating NFATc (**c**ytosolic **N**uclear **F**actor of **A**ctivated **T** cells). Because the cyclosporine–calcineurin complex cannot perform this reaction, NFATc cannot enter the nucleus to promote reactions that are required for the synthesis of cytokines, including IL-2. The end result is a decrease in IL-2, which is the primary chemical stimulus for increasing the number of T lymphocytes.

2. **Therapeutic uses:** *Cyclosporine* is used to prevent rejection of kidney, liver, and cardiac allogeneic transplants and is typically combined in a double-drug or triple-drug regimen with corticosteroids and an antimetabolite such as *mycophenolate mofetil. Cyclosporine* may also be used for recalcitrant psoriasis.

3. **Pharmacokinetics:** *Cyclosporine* may be given either orally or by intravenous (IV) infusion. Oral absorption is variable due to metabolism by a cytochrome P450 (CYP3A4) isoenzyme in the gastrointestinal (GI) tract and efflux by P-glycoprotein (P-gp), which limits *cyclosporine* absorption by pumping the drug back into the gut lumen. About 50% of the drug is bound to erythrocytes. *Cyclosporine* is extensively metabolized, primarily by hepatic CYP3A4. [Note: When other drug substrates for this enzyme are given concomitantly, many drug interactions have been reported.]

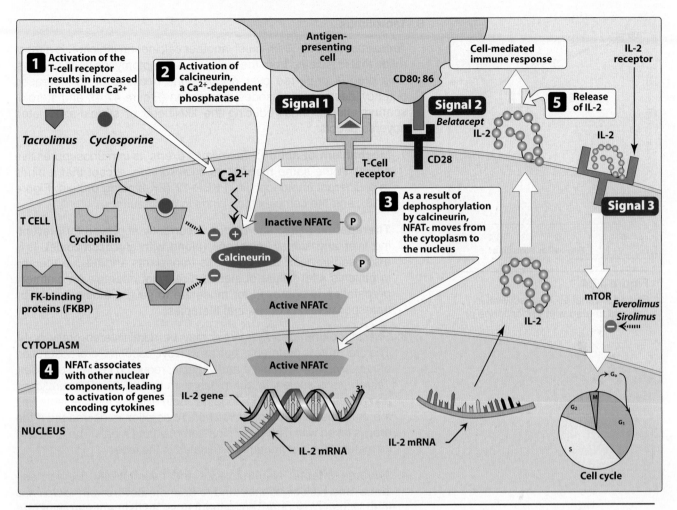

Figure 47.3
Mechanism of action of immunosuppressive *agents*. IL-2 = interleukin-2; mTOR = mammalian target of rapamycin; NFATc = cytosolic nuclear factor of activated T cells; mRNA = messenger RNA.

Excretion of the metabolites is primarily through the biliary route into the feces.

4. **Adverse effects:** Many of the adverse effects caused by *cyclosporine* are dose dependent. Therefore, it is important to monitor blood levels of the drug. Nephrotoxicity is the most common and important adverse effect of *cyclosporine*, and it is critical to monitor kidney function. Reduction of the *cyclosporine* dosage can result in reversal of nephrotoxicity in most cases. [Note: Coadministration of drugs that also can cause kidney dysfunction, such as aminoglycosides and nonsteroidal anti-inflammatory drugs, can potentiate the nephrotoxicity of *cyclosporine*.] Because hepatotoxicity can also occur, liver function should be periodically assessed. In patients taking *cyclosporine*, infections are common and may be life threatening. Viral infections due to the herpes group and cytomegalovirus (CMV) are prevalent. Lymphoma may occur in transplanted patients due to the net level of immunosuppression. Other toxicities include hypertension, hyperlipidemia, hyperkalemia (K⁺-sparing diuretics should be avoided in these patients), tremor, hirsutism, glucose intolerance, and gum hyperplasia.

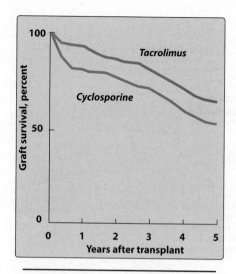

Figure 47.4
Five-year renal allograft survival in patients treated with *cyclosporine* or *tacrolimus*.

B. Tacrolimus

Tacrolimus [ta-CRAW-lih-mus], another calcineurin inhibitor, is a macrolide that is isolated from the soil fungus <u>Streptomyces</u> <u>tsukubaensis</u>. This drug is preferred over *cyclosporine* because of its increased potency, decreased episodes of rejection (Figure 47.4), and steroid-sparing effects, thus reducing the likelihood of steroid-associated adverse effects.

1. **Mechanism of action:** *Tacrolimus* exerts its immunosuppressive effects in the same manner as *cyclosporine*, except that it binds to a different immunophilin, FKBP-12 (FK-**b**inding **p**rotein; Figure 47.3), and the complex then binds to calcineurin.

2. **Therapeutic uses:** *Tacrolimus* is currently approved for preventing liver and kidney rejections (along with glucocorticoids). It is also used in heart and pancreas transplants and rescue therapy in patients after failure of standard rejection therapy. An ointment preparation is approved for moderate to severe atopic dermatitis unresponsive to conventional therapies.

3. **Pharmacokinetics:** *Tacrolimus* may be administered orally or IV. The oral route is preferable, but, as with *cyclosporine*, oral absorption of *tacrolimus* is incomplete and variable, requiring tailoring of doses. *Tacrolimus* is subject to gut metabolism by CYP3A4/5 isoenzymes and is a substrate for P-gp. Together, both of these mechanisms limit the oral bioavailability of *tacrolimus*. Absorption is decreased if the drug is taken with high-fat or high-carbohydrate meals. The drug and its metabolites are primarily eliminated in the feces.

4. **Adverse effects:** Nephrotoxicity and neurotoxicity (tremor, seizures, and hallucinations) tend to be more severe with *tacrolimus* than with *cyclosporine,* but careful dose adjustment can minimize this problem. Development of posttransplant insulin-dependent diabetes mellitus is a problem, especially in black and Hispanic patients. Other toxicities are similar to *cyclosporine*, except that *tacrolimus* does not cause hirsutism or gingival hyperplasia, but it can cause alopecia. Compared with *cyclosporine, tacrolimus* has a lower incidence of cardiovascular toxicities, such as hypertension and hyperlipidemia, both of which are common comorbidities in kidney transplant recipients. Drug interactions are similar to *cyclosporine.*

C. Costimulation blocker

Belatacept [bel-AT-a-sept], a second-generation costimulation blocker, is a recombinant fusion protein that targets signal 2 in the immune activation cascade. It is used for long-term maintenance immunosuppressive therapy.

1. **Mechanism of action:** *Belatacept* blocks CD28-mediated costimulation of T lymphocytes (signal 2) by binding to CD80 and CD86 on APCs. This prevents the downstream stimulatory signals promoting T-cell survival, proliferation, and IL-2 production.

2. **Therapeutic uses:** *Belatacept* is used in kidney transplantation in combination with *basiliximab, mycophenolate mofetil,* and

corticosteroids. This drug can take the place of the calcineurin inhibitors in an effort to avoid the detrimental long-term cardiovascular, metabolic, and renal complications seen with *cyclosporine* and *tacrolimus*. [Note: The first-generation costimulation blocker a*batacept* is approved for rheumatoid arthritis.]

3. **Pharmacokinetics:** *Belatacept* is the first IV maintenance immunosuppressant and is dosed in two phases. The initial high-dose phase is administered on a more frequent interval. In the maintenance phase, the dose is decreased and administered once a month. Monthly dosing may be beneficial in patients for whom medication compliance is an issue. *Belatacept* clearance is not affected by age, sex, race, renal, or hepatic function.

4. **Adverse effects:** *Belatacept* increases the risk of posttransplant lymphoproliferative disorder (PTLD), particularly of the central nervous system. Therefore, it is contraindicated in those patients who have never been exposed to the Epstein-Barr virus (EBV), a common cause of PTLD. Serological titers to EBV are typically obtained to confirm exposure. Common adverse events include anemia, diarrhea, urinary tract infection, and edema.

D. Sirolimus

Sirolimus [sih-ROW-lih-mus] (also known as *rapamycin*) is a macrolide obtained from fermentations of the soil mold <u>Streptomyces hygroscopicus</u>.

1. **Mechanism of action:** *Sirolimus* binds to the same cytoplasmic FK-binding protein as *tacrolimus*, but instead of forming a complex with calcineurin, *sirolimus* binds to mTOR (a serine/threonine kinase), interfering with signal 3. [Note: TOR proteins are essential for many cellular functions, such as cell cycle progression, DNA repair, and as regulators involved in protein translation.] Binding of *sirolimus* to mTOR blocks the progression of activated T cells from the G_1 to the S phase of the cell cycle and, consequently, the proliferation of these cells (Figure 47.5). Unlike *cyclosporine* and *tacrolimus*, *sirolimus* does not lower IL-2 production but, rather, inhibits the cellular response to IL-2.

2. **Therapeutic uses:** *Sirolimus* is approved for use in renal transplantation, in combination with *cyclosporine* and corticosteroids, thereby allowing lower doses of those medications to be used and lowering their toxic potential. The combination of *sirolimus* and *cyclosporine* is synergistic because *sirolimus* works later in the immune activation cascade. To limit the long-term adverse effects of *cyclosporine*, *sirolimus* is often used in calcineurin inhibitor withdrawal protocols in patients who remain rejection free during the first 3 months posttransplant. The antiproliferative action of *sirolimus* is also valuable in cardiology where *sirolimus*-coated stents are used to inhibit restenosis of the blood vessels by reducing proliferation of the endothelial cells.

3. **Pharmacokinetics:** The drug is available as an oral solution or tablet. Although it is readily absorbed, high-fat meals can decrease the absorption. *Sirolimus* has a long half-life (57 to 62 hours), allowing

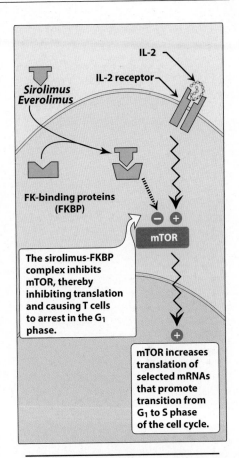

Figure 47.5

Mechanism of action of *sirolimus* and *everolimus*. mTOR = molecular target of *rapamycin* (*sirolimus*); IL = interleukin; mRNA = messenger RNA.

for once-daily dosing. A loading dose is recommended at the time of initiation of therapy. Like both *cyclosporine* and *tacrolimus*, *sirolimus* is metabolized by the CYP3A4 isoenzyme, is a substrate for P-gp, and has similar drug interactions. *Sirolimus* also increases the concentrations of *cyclosporine*, and careful blood level monitoring of both agents must be done to avoid harmful drug toxicities.

4. **Adverse effects:** A common adverse effect of *sirolimus* is hyperlipidemia (elevated cholesterol and triglycerides), which may require treatment. The combination of *cyclosporine* and *sirolimus* is more nephrotoxic than *cyclosporine* alone due to the drug interaction between the two, necessitating lower doses. Other untoward problems are headache, nausea and diarrhea, leukopenia, and thrombocytopenia. Impaired wound healing has been noted with *sirolimus* in obese patients and those with diabetes, which can be especially problematic immediately following the transplant surgery and in patients receiving corticosteroids.

E. Everolimus

Everolimus [e-ve-RO-li-mus], another mTOR inhibitor, is approved for use in renal transplantation. It is also indicated for second-line treatment in patients with advanced renal cell carcinoma.

1. **Mechanism of action:** *Everolimus* has the same mechanism of action as *sirolimus*. It inhibits activation of T cells by forming a complex with FKBP-12 and subsequently blocking mTOR.

2. **Therapeutic uses:** *Everolimus* is used to prevent rejection in kidney transplant recipients in combination with *basiliximab, cyclosporine,* and corticosteroids.

3. **Pharmacokinetics:** *Everolimus* is rapidly absorbed, but absorption is decreased with high-fat meals. *Everolimus* is a substrate of CYP3A4 and P-gp and, thus, is subject to the same drug interactions as previously mentioned. *Everolimus* avidly binds erythrocytes, and monitoring of whole blood trough concentrations is recommended. It has a much shorter half-life than *sirolimus* and requires twice-daily dosing. *Everolimus* increases drug concentrations of *cyclosporine*, thereby enhancing the nephrotoxic effects of *cyclosporine*, and is, therefore, recommended to be used with reduced doses of *cyclosporine*.

4. **Adverse effects:** *Everolimus* has adverse effects similar to *sirolimus*. An additional adverse effect noted with *everolimus* is angioedema, which may increase with concomitant use of angiotensin-converting enzyme inhibitors. There is also an increased risk of kidney arterial and venous thrombosis, resulting in graft loss, usually in the first 30 days posttransplantation.

III. IMMUNOSUPPRESSIVE ANTIMETABOLITES

Immunosuppressive antimetabolite agents are generally used in combination with corticosteroids and the calcineurin inhibitors, *cyclosporine* and *tacrolimus*.

A. Azathioprine

Azathioprine [ay-za-THYE-oh-preen] was the first agent to achieve widespread use in organ transplantation. It is a prodrug that is converted first to *6-mercaptopurine* (*6-MP*) and then to the corresponding nucleotide, thioinosinic acid. The immunosuppressive effects of *azathioprine* are due to this nucleotide analog. Because of their rapid proliferation in the immune response and their dependence on the de novo synthesis of purines required for cell division, lymphocytes are predominantly affected by the cytotoxic effects of *azathioprine*. Its major nonimmune toxicity is bone marrow suppression. Concomitant use with angiotensin-converting enzyme inhibitors or *cotrimoxazole* in renal transplant patients can lead to an exaggerated leukopenic response. *Allopurinol,* an agent used to treat gout, significantly inhibits the metabolism of *azathioprine.* Therefore, the dose of *azathioprine* must be reduced. Nausea and vomiting are also encountered. (See Chapter 46 for a thorough discussion of *6-MP.*)

B. Mycophenolate mofetil

Mycophenolate mofetil [mye-koe-FEN-oh-late MAW-feh-til] has, for the most part, replaced *azathioprine* because of its safety and efficacy in prolonging graft survival. It has been successfully used in heart, kidney, and liver transplants. As an ester, it is rapidly hydrolyzed in the GI tract to mycophenolic acid. This is a potent, reversible, noncompetitive inhibitor of inosine monophosphate dehydrogenase, which blocks the de novo formation of guanosine phosphate. Thus, like *6-MP*, it deprives the rapidly proliferating T and B cells of a key component of nucleic acids (Figure 47.6). [Note: Lymphocytes lack the salvage pathway for purine synthesis and, therefore, are dependent on de novo purine production.] Mycophenolic acid is quickly and almost completely absorbed after oral administration. The glucuronide metabolite is excreted predominantly in urine. The most common adverse effects of *mycophenolate mofetil* are GI, including diarrhea, nausea, vomiting, and abdominal pain. High doses of *mycophenolate mofetil* are associated with a higher risk of CMV infection. Concomitant administration with antacids containing magnesium or aluminum, or with *cholestyramine,* can decrease absorption of the drug.

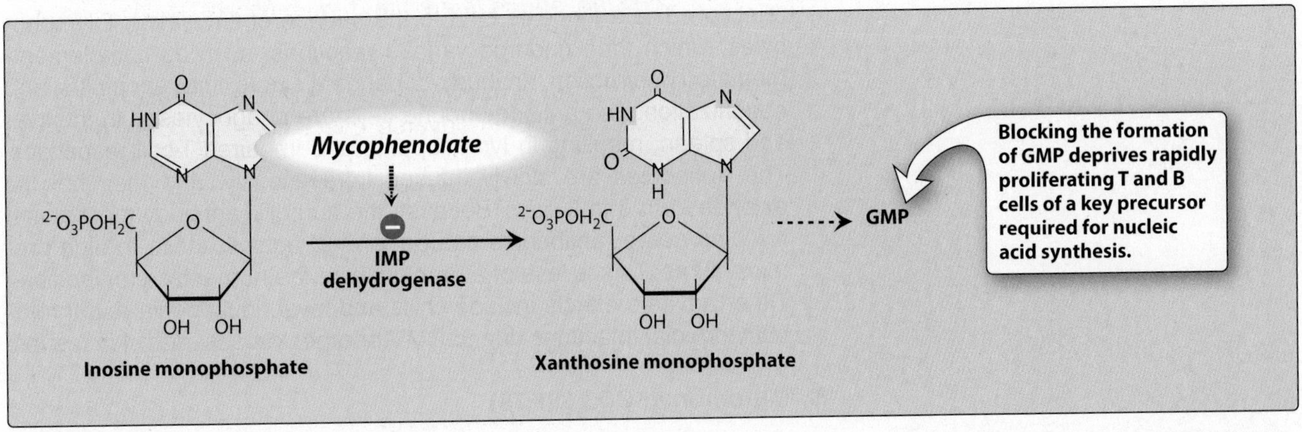

Figure 47.6
Mechanism of action of *mycophenolate.* GMP = guanosine monophosphate.

C. Enteric-coated mycophenolate sodium

In an effort to minimize the GI effects associated with *mycophenolate mofetil*, enteric-coated *mycophenolate sodium* is contained within a delayed-release formulation designed to release in the neutral pH of the small intestine. This formulation is equivalent to *mycophenolate mofetil* in the prevention of acute rejection episodes in kidney transplant recipients. However, the rate of GI adverse events is similar to that with *mycophenolate mofetil*.

IV. ANTIBODIES

The use of antibodies plays a central role in prolonging allograft survival. [Note: An allograft is transplant of an organ or tissue from one person to another who is not genetically identical.] They are prepared by immunization of either rabbits or horses with human lymphoid cells (producing a mixture of polyclonal antibodies or monoclonal antibodies) or by hybridoma technology (producing antigen-specific monoclonal antibodies). Hybridomas are produced by fusing mouse antibody-producing cells with tumor cells. Hybrid cells are selected and cloned, and the antibody specificity of the clones is determined. Clones of interest can be cultured in large quantities to produce clinically useful amounts of the desired antibody. Recombinant DNA technology can also be used to replace part of the mouse gene sequence with human genetic material, thus "humanizing" the antibodies and making them less antigenic. The names of monoclonal antibodies conventionally contain "xi" or "zu" if they are chimerized or humanized, respectively. The suffix "-mab" (monoclonal antibody) identifies the category of drug. The polyclonal antibodies, although relatively inexpensive to produce, are variable and less specific, which is in contrast to monoclonal antibodies, which are homogeneous and specific.

A. Antithymocyte globulins

Antithymocyte globulins are polyclonal antibodies that are primarily used at the time of transplantation to prevent early allograft rejection along with other immunosuppressive agents. They may also be used to treat severe rejection episodes or corticosteroid-resistant acute rejection. The antibodies bind to the surface of circulating T lymphocytes, which then undergo various reactions, such as complement-mediated destruction, antibody-dependent cytotoxicity, apoptosis, and opsonization. The antibody-bound cells are phagocytosed in the liver and spleen, resulting in lymphopenia and impaired T-cell responses. The antibodies are slowly infused intravenously, and their half-life extends from 3 to 9 days. Because the humoral antibody mechanism remains active, antibodies can be formed against these foreign proteins. [Note: This is less of a problem with the humanized antibodies.] Other adverse effects include chills and fever, leukopenia and thrombocytopenia, infections due to CMV or other viruses, and skin rashes.

B. Muromonab-CD3 (OKT3)

Muromonab-CD3 [myoo-roe-MOE-nab] is a murine (mouse) monoclonal antibody that is directed against the glycoprotein CD3 antigen of human T cells. *Muromonab-CD3* was the first monoclonal antibody approved for clinical use in 1986, indicated for the treatment of corticosteroid-resistant acute rejection of kidney, heart, and liver allografts. The drug has been discontinued from the market due to the availability of newer biologic drugs with similar efficacy and fewer side effects.

C. Basiliximab

The antigenicity and short serum half-life of the murine monoclonal antibody have been averted by replacing most of the murine amino acid sequences with human ones by genetic engineering. *Basiliximab* [bah-si-LIK-si-mab] is said to be "chimerized" because it consists of 25% murine and 75% human protein. [Note: "Humanized" monoclonal antibodies (for example, *trastuzumab* used for breast cancer; see Chapter 46) have a smaller stretch of nonhuman protein.] *Basiliximab* is approved for prophylaxis of acute rejection in renal transplantation in combination with *cyclosporine* and corticosteroids. It is not used for the treatment of ongoing rejection. *Basiliximab* is an anti-CD25 antibody that binds to the α chain of the IL-2 receptor on activated T cells and, thus, interferes with the proliferation of these cells. Blockade of this receptor foils the ability of any antigenic stimulus to activate the T-cell response system. *Basiliximab* is given as an IV infusion. The serum half-life of *basiliximab* is about 7 days. Usually, two doses of this drug are administered—the first at 2 hours prior to transplantation and the second at 4 days after the surgery. The drug is generally well tolerated, with GI toxicity as the main adverse effect.

A summary of the major immunosuppressive drugs is presented in Figure 47.7.

V. CORTICOSTEROIDS

The corticosteroids were the first pharmacologic agents to be used as immunosuppressives, both in transplantation and in various autoimmune disorders. They are still one of the mainstays for attenuating rejection episodes. For transplantation, the most common agents are *prednisone* and *methylprednisolone,* whereas *prednisone* and *prednisolone* are used for autoimmune conditions. [Note: In transplantation, they are used in combination with agents described previously in this chapter.] The steroids are used to suppress acute rejection of solid organ allografts and in chronic graft-versus-host disease. In addition, they are effective against a wide variety of autoimmune conditions, including refractory rheumatoid arthritis, systemic lupus erythematosus, temporal arthritis, and asthma. The exact mechanism responsible for the immunosuppressive action of the corticosteroids is unclear. The T lymphocytes are affected most. The steroids are able to rapidly reduce lymphocyte populations by lysis or redistribution. On entering cells, they bind to the glucocorticoid receptor. The complex passes into the nucleus and regulates the transcription of DNA. Among the genes affected are those involved in inflammatory responses. The use of these agents is associated with numerous adverse effects. For example, they are diabetogenic and can cause hypercholesterolemia, cataracts, osteoporosis, and hypertension with prolonged use. Consequently, efforts are being directed toward reducing or eliminating the use of steroids in the maintenance of allografts.

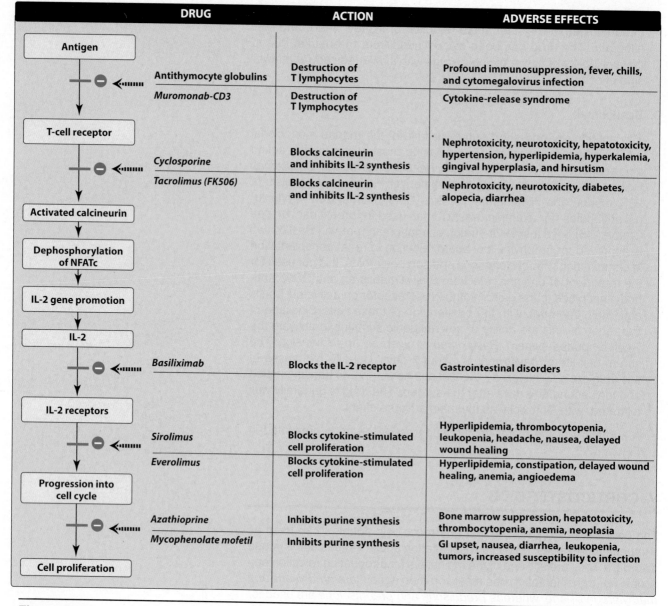

Figure 47.7

Sites of action of immunosuppressants. IL-2 = interleukin-2; NFATc = cytosolic nuclear factor of activated T cells; GI = gastrointestinal.

Study Questions

Choose the ONE best answer.

47.1 A 45-year-old male who received a renal transplant 3 months previously and is being maintained on prednisone, cyclosporine, and mycophenolate mofetil is found to have increased creatinine levels and a kidney biopsy indicating severe rejection. Which of the following courses of therapy would be appropriate?

A. Increased dose of prednisone.
B. Hemodialysis.
C. Treatment with rabbit antithymocyte globulin.
D. Treatment with sirolimus.
E. Treatment with azathioprine.

Correct answer = C. This patient is apparently undergoing an acute rejection of the kidney. The most effective treatment would be administration of an antibody. Increasing the dose of prednisone may have some effect but would not be enough to treat the rejection. Sirolimus is used prophylactically with cyclosporine to prevent renal rejection but is less effective when an episode is occurring. Furthermore, the combination of cyclosporine and sirolimus is more nephrotoxic than cyclosporine alone. Azathioprine has no benefit over mycophenolate.

47.2 All of the following are reasonable combinations of immunosuppressive drugs except:

A. Basiliximab, belatacept, mycophenolate mofetil, and prednisone.
B. Thymoglobulin, cyclosporine, azathioprine, and prednisone.
C. Tacrolimus, mycophenolate mofetil, and prednisone.
D. Tacrolimus, cyclosporine, and prednisone.
E. Tacrolimus, sirolimus, and prednisone.

Correct answer = D. Tacrolimus and cyclosporine are both calcineurin inhibitors and have the same mechanism of action. Immunosuppressive drug regimens should work synergistically at different places in the T-cell activation cascade. Additionally, cyclosporine and tacrolimus are both extremely nephrotoxic and when used together would cause harm to the patients.

47.3 Which of the following drugs used to prevent allograft rejection can cause hyperlipidemia?

A. Azathioprine.
B. Basiliximab.
C. Belatacept.
D. Mycophenolate mofetil.
E. Sirolimus.

Correct answer = E. Patients who are receiving sirolimus can develop elevated cholesterol and triglyceride levels, which can be controlled by statin therapy. None of the other agents has this adverse effect.

47.4 Which of the following drugs specifically inhibits calcineurin in the activated T lymphocytes?

A. Basiliximab.
B. Tacrolimus.
C. Prednisone.
D. Sirolimus.
E. Mycophenolate mofetil.

Correct answer = B. Tacrolimus binds to FKBP-12, which, in turn, inhibits calcineurin and interferes in the cascade of reactions that synthesize interleukin-2 (IL-2) and lead to T-lymphocyte proliferation. Although basiliximab also interferes with T-lymphocyte proliferation, it does so by binding to the CD25 site on the IL-2 receptor. Prednisone can affect not only T-cell proliferation but also that of B cells and is, therefore, nonspecific. Sirolimus, while also binding to FKBP-12, does not inhibit calcineurin. Mycophenolate mofetil exerts its immunosuppressive action by inhibiting inosine monophosphate dehydrogenase, thus depriving the cells of guanosine, a key component of nucleic acids.

Clinical Toxicology

48

Dawn Sollee

I. OVERVIEW

For thousands of years, poisons and the study of them (toxicology) have been woven into the rich fabric of the human experience. Homer and Aristotle described the poison arrow; Socrates was executed with poison hemlock; Cleopatra used an African Cobra to commit suicide; lead poisoning may have helped bring down the Roman Empire; Marilyn Monroe, Elvis Presley, and actor Heath Ledger all fatally overdosed on prescription medication. Toxins can be inhaled, insufflated (snorted), orally ingested, injected, and absorbed dermally (Figure 48.1). Once in the body, some of the common targets of toxicity include the central nervous system, the lungs, the kidney, the heart, the liver, the blood, and even the intricate acid/base and electrolyte balance of the body. An understanding of the varied mechanisms of toxicity helps to provide an explanation for the clinical manifestations and a basis for the approach to treatment. This chapter provides an overview of the emergent management of the poisoned patient. In addition, a brief review of some of the more common and interesting toxins, their mechanisms, clinical presentations, and clinical management is presented.

II. EMERGENCY TREATMENT OF THE POISONED PATIENT

The first principle in the management of the poisoned patient is to treat the patient, not the poison. Airway, breathing, and circulation are assessed and addressed initially, along with any other immediately life-threatening toxic effect (for example, profound increases or decreases in blood pressure, heart rate, breathing, or body temperature, or any dangerous dysrhythmias). Acid/base and electrolyte disturbances, along with an *acetaminophen* and salicylate blood level, can be further assessed as laboratory results are obtained. After administering oxygen, obtaining intravenous access, and placing the patient on a cardiac monitor, the poisoned patient with altered mental status should be considered

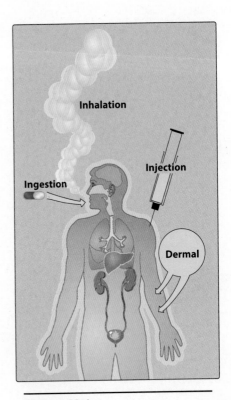

Figure 48.1
Routes of exposure for toxins.

for administration of the "coma cocktail" as possibly diagnostic and therapeutic. The "coma cocktail" consists of intravenous dextrose to treat hypoglycemia, a possible toxicological cause of altered mental status, along with *naloxone* to treat possible opioid or *clonidine* toxicity, and *thiamine* for ethanol-induced Wernicke encephalopathy. [Note: Hypoglycemia may be caused by oral hypoglycemics, *insulin*, ackee plant, and ethanol.]

A. Decontamination

Once the patient is stabilized, the assessment for decontamination can occur. This may include flushing of the eyes with saline or tepid water to a neutral pH for ocular exposures, rinsing of the skin for dermal exposures, as well as administration of gastrointestinal (GI) decontamination with gastric lavage, activated charcoal, or whole bowel irrigation (utilizing a polyethylene glycol electrolyte balanced solution) for selected ingestions. Several substances do not adsorb to activated charcoal (for example, lead and other heavy metals, *iron, lithium, potassium*, and alcohols), limiting the use of activated charcoal unless there are coingested products.

B. Elimination enhancement

1. **Hemodialysis:** The elimination of some medications/toxins may be enhanced by hemodialysis if certain properties are met: low protein binding, small volume of distribution, small molecular weight, and water solubility of the toxin. Some examples of medications or substances that can be removed with hemodialysis include methanol, ethylene glycol, salicylates, *theophylline, phenobarbital*, and *lithium*.

2. **Urinary alkalinization:** Alkalinization of the urine enhances the elimination of salicylates or *phenobarbital*. Increasing the urine pH with intravenous *sodium bicarbonate* transforms the drug into an ionized form that prevents reabsorption, thereby trapping it in the urine to be eliminated by the kidney. The goal urine pH is within the range of 7.5 to 8, while ensuring that the serum pH does not exceed 7.55.

3. **Multiple-dose activated charcoal:** Multiple-dose activated charcoal therapy enhances the elimination of certain drugs (for example, *theophylline, phenobarbital, digoxin, carbamazepine, valproic acid*) by creating a gradient across the lumen of the gut. Medications traverse from areas of high concentration to low concentration, promoting medication already absorbed to cross back into the gut to be adsorbed by the activated charcoal present. In addition, activated charcoal blocks the reabsorption of medications that undergo enterohepatic recirculation (such as *phenytoin*), by adsorbing the substance to the activated charcoal. Bowel sounds must be present prior to each activated charcoal dose to ensure movement of the GI tract and prevent obstruction.

III. SELECT PHARMACEUTICAL AND OCCUPATIONAL TOXICITIES

A. Acetaminophen

Acetaminophen produces toxicity when its usual metabolic pathways become saturated. Usually, *acetaminophen* undergoes metabolism by sulfation, glucuronidation, and *N*-hydroxylation by the cytochrome

P450 system. When a toxic amount of *acetaminophen* is ingested, the first two processes are overwhelmed and more *acetaminophen* is metabolized by the cytochrome P450 system to a hepatotoxic metabolite (*N*-acetyl-*p*-benzoquinoneimine, NAPQI). In therapeutic *acetaminophen* ingestions, the liver generates glutathione, which detoxifies NAPQI. However, in overdose, the glutathione is depleted, leaving the metabolite to produce toxicity. There are four phases typically describing *acetaminophen* toxicity (Figure 48.2). The antidote for *acetaminophen* toxicity, *N*-acetylcysteine (*NAC*), initially works as a glutathione precursor and glutathione substitute and assists with sulfation. Later on, *NAC* may function as an antioxidant to aid in recovery. *NAC* is the most effective when initiated 8 to 10 hours postingestion. The Rumack-Matthew nomogram (Figure 48.3), which is based on the time of ingestion and the serum *acetaminophen* level, is utilized after an acute ingestion to determine if *NAC* therapy is needed. The

Phase 1 (0 to 24 hours): loss of appetite, nausea, vomiting, general malaise

Phase 2 (24 to 72 hours): abdominal pain, increased liver enzymes

Phase 3 (72 to 96 hours): liver necrosis, jaundice, encephalopathy, renal failure, death

Phase 4 (>4 days to 2 weeks): complete resolution of symptoms and organ failure

Figure 48.2
Phases of *acetaminophen* toxicity.

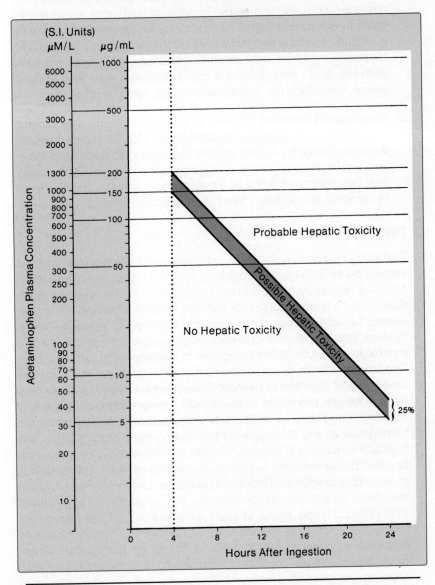

Figure 48.3
Rumack-Matthew nomogram for *acetaminophen* poisoning. *Acetaminophen* concentration plotted vs. time after exposure to predict potential toxicity and antidote use.

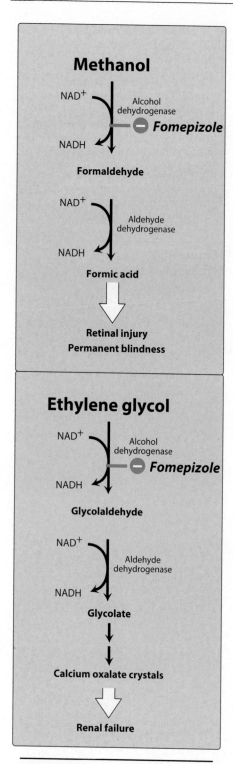

Figure 48.4
Metabolism of methanol and ethylene glycol.

nomogram is helpful for acute *acetaminophen* ingestions when levels can be obtained between 4 and 24 hours postingestion.

B. Alcohols

1. **Methanol (wood alcohol) and ethylene glycol:** Methanol is found in such products as windshield washer fluid and model airplane fuel. Ethylene glycol is most commonly found in radiator antifreeze. These primary alcohols are themselves relatively nontoxic and cause mainly CNS sedation. However, methanol and ethylene glycol are oxidized to toxic products: formic acid in the case of methanol and glycolic, glyoxylic, and oxalic acids in the case of ethylene glycol. *Fomepizole* inhibits this oxidative pathway by blocking alcohol dehydrogenase. It prevents the formation of toxic metabolites and allows the parent alcohols to be excreted by the kidney (Figure 48.4). Hemodialysis is often utilized to remove the already-produced toxic acids. In addition, cofactors are administered to encourage metabolism to nontoxic metabolites (*folate* for methanol, *thiamine* and *pyridoxine* for ethylene glycol). If untreated, methanol ingestion may produce blindness, metabolic acidosis, seizures, and coma. Ethylene glycol ingestion may lead to renal failure, hypocalcemia, metabolic acidosis, and heart failure.

2. **Isopropanol (rubbing alcohol, isopropyl alcohol):** This secondary alcohol is metabolized to acetone via alcohol dehydrogenase. Acetone cannot be further oxidized to carboxylic acids, and therefore, acidemia does not occur. Isopropanol is a known CNS depressant (approximately twice as intoxicating as ethanol) and GI irritant. No antidote is necessary to treat an isopropyl alcohol ingestion.

C. Carbon monoxide

Carbon monoxide is a colorless, odorless, and tasteless gas, which is impossible for individuals to detect without a carbon monoxide detector. It is a natural by-product of the combustion of carbonaceous materials, and common sources of this gas include automobiles, poorly vented furnaces, fireplaces, wood-burning stoves, kerosene space heaters, house fires, and charcoal grills. Following inhalation, carbon monoxide rapidly binds to hemoglobin to produce carboxyhemoglobin. The binding affinity of carbon monoxide to hemoglobin is 230 to 270 times greater than that of oxygen. Consequently, even low concentrations of carbon monoxide in the air can produce significant levels of carboxyhemoglobin. In addition, bound carbon monoxide increases hemoglobin affinity for oxygen at the other oxygen-binding sites. This high-affinity binding of oxygen prevents the unloading of oxygen at the tissues, further reducing oxygen delivery (Figure 48.5). The presence of this highly oxygenated blood may produce "cherry red" skin. Carbon monoxide toxicity can occur following the inhalation or ingestion of methylene chloride found in paint strippers also. Once absorbed, methylene chloride is metabolized by the liver to carbon monoxide through the cytochrome P450 pathway. The symptoms of carbon monoxide intoxication are consistent with hypoxia, with the brain and heart showing the greatest sensitivity. Symptoms include headache, dyspnea, lethargy, confusion, and drowsiness, whereas higher exposure levels can lead to seizures, coma, and death. The management of a carbon monoxide–poisoned patient includes prompt removal from the source of carbon monoxide and institution of 100% oxygen by non-rebreathing face mask or endotracheal tube. In patients with severe intoxication, oxygenation in a hyperbaric chamber is recommended.

D. Cyanide

Cyanide is just one of the toxic products of combustion produced during house fires. Additionally, cyanide salts are used in electroplating, and hydrogen cyanide may be produced during photographic developing and petroleum refining. Once absorbed into the body, cyanide quickly binds to many metalloenzymes, thereby rendering them inactive. Its principal toxicity occurs as a result of the inactivation of the enzyme cytochrome oxidase (cytochrome a_3), leading to the inhibition of cellular respiration. Therefore, even in the presence of oxygen, tissues such as the brain and heart, which require a high oxygen demand, are adversely affected. Death can occur quickly due to respiratory arrest of oxidative phosphorylation and production of adenosine triphosphate. The most recently developed antidote, *hydroxocobalamin* (vitamin B_{12a}), is administered intravenously to bind the cyanide and produce *cyanocobalamin* (vitamin B_{12}) without the worry of hypotension or methemoglobin production. The older cyanide antidote kit comprises *sodium nitrite* to form cyanomethemoglobin and *sodium thiosulfate* to accelerate the production of thiocyanate, which is much less toxic than cyanide and is also quickly excreted in urine. In patients with smoke inhalation and cyanide toxicity, the induction of methemoglobin with *sodium nitrite* should be avoided unless the carboxyhemoglobin concentration is less than 10%. Otherwise, the oxygen-carrying capacity of blood becomes too low.

E. Iron

Previously, ingestion of iron was the leading cause of poisoning death in children. However, the incidence of pediatric iron toxicity has greatly diminished during the past two decades due to education and changes in packaging. Iron is radiopaque and may show up on an abdominal radiograph if the product contains a sufficient concentration of elemental iron. Toxic effects can be expected with as little as 20 mg/kg of elemental iron ingested, and doses of 60 mg/kg may be lethal. Each iron salt contains a different concentration of elemental iron (Figure 48.6). Based on the quantity ingested, the patient's weight, and the elemental iron concentration, an assessment of potential toxicity can be made. A serum iron level should be obtained, since levels between 500 and 1000 µg/dL have been associated with shock and levels higher than 1000 µg/dL with morbidity and mortality. If a significant amount of iron has been ingested, the patient usually presents with nausea, vomiting, and abdominal pain. Depending on the amount of elemental iron ingested, the patient may experience a latent period or may progress quickly to hypovolemia, metabolic acidosis, hypotension, and coagulopathy. Ultimately, hepatic failure and multisystem failure, coma, and death may occur. *Deferoxamine,* an iron-specific chelator, binds free iron, creating ferrioxamine to be excreted in the urine. The intravenous route for *deferoxamine* is preferred, but hypotension may occur if rapid boluses are administered instead of a continuous infusion.

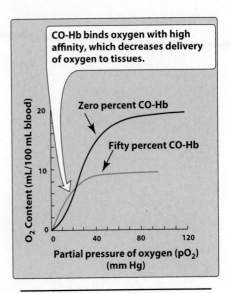

Figure 48.5
Effect of carbon monoxide on the oxygen affinity of hemoglobin.
CO-Hb = carbon monoxyhemoglobin.

Content	Elemental iron (%)
Ferrous fumarate	33
Ferrous gluconate	12
Ferrous sulfate	20

Figure 48.6
Elemental iron contained in various iron preparations.

F. Lead

Lead is ubiquitous in the environment, with sources of exposure including old paint, drinking water, industrial pollution, food, and contaminated dust. However, with the elimination of tetraethyl lead in gasoline during the mid-1980s in the United States, environmental exposure to organic lead has been reduced, and most chronic exposure to lead occurs with inorganic lead salts, such as those in paint used in housing constructed prior to 1978. Age-dependent differences in the absorption of ingested lead are known to occur. Adults absorb about 10% of an ingested dose, whereas children absorb about 40%. Inorganic forms of lead are initially distributed to the soft tissues and more slowly redistribute to bone, teeth, and hair. When lead makes its way to the bone, it impairs new bone formation and causes increased calcium deposition in long bones visible on x-ray. Ingested lead is radiopaque and may appear on an abdominal radiograph if present in the GI tract. Lead has an apparent blood half-life of about 1 to 2 months, whereas its half-life in the bone is 20 to 30 years. Chronic exposure to lead can have serious effects on several tissues (Figure 48.7).

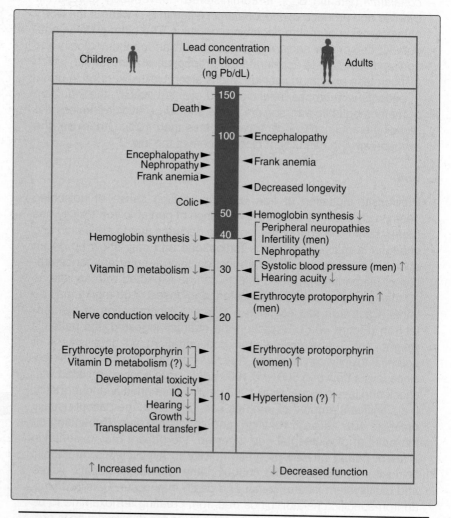

Figure 48.7

Comparison of effects of lead on children and adults.

1. **Central nervous system:** The CNS effects of lead have often been termed lead encephalopathy. Symptoms include headaches, confusion, clumsiness, insomnia, fatigue, and impaired concentration. As the disease progresses, clonic convulsions and coma can occur. Death is rare, given the ability to treat lead intoxication with chelation therapy. Children are more susceptible than adults to the CNS effects of lead. Furthermore, blood levels of 5 to 20 µg/dL in children have been shown to lower IQ in the absence of other symptoms. It has been estimated that as many as 9% of the children in the United States may have blood lead levels greater than 10 µg/dL.

2. **Gastrointestinal system:** Early symptoms can include discomfort and constipation (and, occasionally, diarrhea), whereas higher exposures can produce painful intestinal spasms.

3. **Blood:** Lead has complex effects on the constituents of blood, leading to hypochromic, microcytic anemia as a result of a shortened erythrocyte life span and disruption of heme synthesis. Elevated blood lead levels can be used diagnostically for determining lead intoxication, provided that blood lead levels are greater than about 25 µg/dL.

Multiple chelators can be utilized in the treatment of lead toxicity. When levels are greater than 45 µg/dL, but less than 70 µg/dL in children, *succimer (dimercaptosuccinic acid, DMSA),* an oral chelator, is the treatment of choice. With lead levels greater than 70 µg/dL or if encephalopathy is present, dual parenteral therapy is required with *dimercaprol* given intramuscularly and *calcium disodium edetate* given intravenously. *Dimercaprol* is suspended in peanut oil and should not be given to those with a peanut allergy.

G. Organophosphate and carbamate insecticides

These insecticides exert their toxicity through inhibition of acetylcholinesterase, with subsequent accumulation of excess acetylcholine producing nicotinic (mydriasis, fasciculations, muscle weakness, hypertension) and muscarinic (diarrhea, urination, miosis, bradycardia, bronchorrhea, emesis, lacrimation, salivation) effects. Carbamates reversibly bind to acetylcholinesterase, whereas organophosphates undergo an aging process to ultimately irreversibly inactivate the enzyme. Organophosphate nerve agents, such as sarin, soman, and tabun, have the same mechanism of action, but the aging process is much more rapid compared to insecticides. *Atropine*, a muscarinic receptor antagonist, and *pralidoxime*, an oxime to reactivate cholinesterase, should be administered intravenously or intramuscularly to treat the muscarinic and nicotinic effects, respectively.

IV. ANTIDOTES

Specific chemical antidotes for poisoning have been developed for a number of chemicals or classes of toxicants (Figure 48.8). This is not an all-inclusive list.

POISON	ANTIDOTE(S)
Acetaminophen	*N-Acetylcysteine*
Anticholinergic agents (antihistamines, etc.)	*Physostigmine*
Arsenic	*Succimer (dimercaptosuccinic acid, DMSA), dimercaprol*
Benzodiazepine	*Flumazenil*
Carbon monoxide	*Oxygen (± hyperbaric chamber)*
Cyanide	*Hydroxocobalamin Sodium nitrite and sodium thiosulfate*
Digitalis	*Digoxin-immune Fab*
Hydrofluoric acid	*Calcium*
Iron	*Deferoxamine*
Isoniazid and gyromitra mushrooms	*Pyridoxine*
Methanol and ethylene glycol	*Fomepizole*
Heparin	*Protamine sulfate*
Lead	*Succimer (dimercaptosuccinic acid, DMSA), dimercaprol, calcium disodium edetate*
Methemoglobinemia	*Methylene blue*
Opiates, clonidine	*Naloxone*
Organophosphates, nerve gases	*Atropine, pralidoxime*
Warfarin	*Vitamin K1 (phytonadione)*

Figure 48.8
Common antidotes.

Study Questions

Choose the ONE best answer.

48.1 A 3-year-old boy is brought to the emergency department by his mother, who reports that he has been crying continuously and "does not want to play or eat" for the last few days. She also states that he has not had regular bowel movements, with mostly constipation and occasional diarrhea, and frequently complains of abdominal pain. The child now has an altered level of consciousness, is difficult to arouse, and begins to seize. The clinician rules out infection and other medical causes. Upon questioning, the mother states that the house is in an older neighborhood, that her house has not been remodeled or repainted since the 1940s, and that the paint is chipping around the windows and doors. The child is otherwise breathing on his own and urinating normally. Which toxin would you expect to be producing such severe effects in this child?

A. Iron.

B. Lead.

C. Carbon monoxide.

D. Cyanide.

E. Ethylene glycol.

Correct answer = B. Lead poisoning is common among children in older homes painted before lead was removed from paint. Paint chips with lead are easily ingested by toddlers, and excessively high lead levels can lead to the signs and symptoms described plus clumsiness, confusion, headaches, coma, constipation, intestinal spasms, and anemia. Death is rare when chelation therapy is instituted. Iron can produce abdominal pain, but more often would cause diarrhea, vomiting, and volume loss. If he had cyanide poisoning, death would have occurred quickly following respiratory arrest of oxidative phosphorylation and production of adenosine triphosphate, but this child has been exhibiting symptoms over several days. Carbon monoxide would affect the entire household, depending on the source. Clinical effects from carbon monoxide would include headache, nausea, and CNS depression. Ethylene glycol is sweet and may be ingested by a toddler. The presentation of ethylene glycol toxicity would include initial appearance of intoxication, which was not mentioned.

48.2 A 41-year-old male pocket watch maker presents to the emergency department after he was found unconscious on the floor of the shop by a coworker. The coworker states that the patient complained of being cold this morning around 8 AM (the central heat was broken, and the outdoor temperature was 34°F) and that since noon, he had been complaining of headache, drowsiness, confusion, and nausea. The clinician notices that he has cherry red skin. What is the most likely toxin causing his signs and symptoms?

A. Ethylene glycol.

B. Cyanide.

C. Acetaminophen.

D. Carbon monoxide.

E. Methanol.

Correct answer = D. Although watch makers and other professionals who use electroplating may be at higher risk for cyanide exposure because many plating baths use cyanide-containing ingredients (for example, potassium cyanide), this patient shows signs of carbon monoxide poisoning, such as cherry red skin, headache, confusion, nausea, and drowsiness leading to unconsciousness. The history also leads us to believe that this person may have been using a space heater to stay warm, which would be consistent with the description. A carboxyhemoglobin level should be obtained to confirm the exposure. Cyanide in low doses from such an occupational exposure can present with loss of consciousness, flushing, headache, and confusion. Chronically, workers may develop a rash after handling cyanide solutions. Also, an odor of bitter almonds may be present. An arterial blood gas and a venous blood gas could be obtained and compared to determine if cyanide is present (a lack of oxygen extraction would be present on the venous side). Ethylene glycol and methanol toxicity may cause alterations in mental status, but the history did not include anything suggesting a toxic alcohol ingestion. Acetaminophen toxicity is not consistent with this presentation.

48.3 A 50-year-old migrant worker comes to the emergency department from the field he was working in and complains of diarrhea, tearing, nausea and vomiting, and sweating. The clinician notices that he looks generally anxious and has fine fasciculations in the muscles of the upper chest as well as pinpoint pupils. Which antidote should he receive first?

A. *N*-acetylcysteine.
B. Sodium nitrite.
C. Deferoxamine.
D. Atropine.
E. Fomepizole.

Correct answer = D. Atropine is appropriate for this patient, who has symptoms consistent with organophosphate (insecticide) poisoning. The mnemonic DUMBBELS (diarrhea, urination, miosis, bronchorrhea/bradycardia, emesis, lacrimation, salivation) can be used to remember the signs and symptoms of cholinergic toxicity. An anticholinergic antidote, atropine, controls these muscarinic symptoms, whereas the antidote pralidoxime treats the nicotinic symptoms like fasciculations (involuntary muscle quivering or twitching). *N*-acetylcysteine is the antidote for acetaminophen overdose and acts as a sulfhydryl donor. Sodium nitrite is one of the antidotes included in the old cyanide antidote kit (sodium nitrite and sodium thiosulfate). Deferoxamine is the chelating agent for iron. Fomepizole is the antidote for methanol and ethylene glycol.

48.4 A 45-year-old male presented to the emergency department 18 hours after ingesting an unknown product. On presentation, he is tachycardic, hypertensive, tachypneic, and complaining of flank pain. A metabolic panel is obtained, and the patient has a large anion gap acidosis, an increased creatinine, and hypocalcemia. Which substance was most likely ingested?

A. Methanol.
B. Acetaminophen.
C. Ethylene glycol.
D. Iron.
E. Opioids.

Correct answer = C. Ethylene glycol produces a metabolic acidosis from the toxic metabolites. The formation of calcium oxalate crystals, which can be found on urinalysis, leads to hypocalcemia and renal failure. The treatment regimen for this patient would include intravenous fomepizole, if some of the parent compound was still present, and hemodialysis. Thiamine and pyridoxine are the cofactors involved in the metabolism of ethylene glycol. Methanol may produce a metabolic acidosis as well, but its target organ of toxicity is the eyes instead of the kidneys as with ethylene glycol. Acetaminophen toxicity may produce upper quadrant pain within the first 24 hours, but vital sign abnormalities are not usually found during this time frame. Iron toxicity may also produce a metabolic acidosis and tachycardia. However, hypocalcemia does not occur. Opioid toxicity, as mentioned in Chapter 14, usually presents with CNS and respiratory depression, not tachycardia and hypertension.

48.5 A 27-year-old female presents to the emergency department 6 hours after reportedly ingesting 20 tablets of acetaminophen 500 mg. An acetaminophen level is drawn, but it has to be sent out to another lab and will not return for another 6 hours. What is the most appropriate next step in management of this patient?

A. Administer a dose (50 g) of activated charcoal.
B. Empirically start *N*-acetylcysteine therapy.
C. Administer a dose of intravenous naloxone.
D. Wait for the level to return and then decide what to do.
E. Draw a NAPQI level.

Correct answer = B. *N*-acetylcysteine should be started empirically on the basis of the history, and then, once the level returns and is plotted on the Rumack-Matthew nomogram, a final decision on whether to continue therapy can be made. Activated charcoal would not be of any benefit 6 hours post–acetaminophen ingestion. Naloxone is utilized for opioid toxicity, not acetaminophen toxicity. The optimal time frame to give *N*-acetylcysteine is within 8 to 10 hours postingestion. So, waiting on the level to return would put the patient more than 12 hours postingestion. Therefore, initiation of *N*-acetylcysteine therapy should happen, if possible during the optimal time frame. Clinicians are unable to draw a NAPQI level and therefore cannot utilize this to guide therapy.

48.6 A 4-year-old female presents to the emergency department with CNS depression. Her vital signs indicate that she is slightly bradycardic and slightly hypotensive for her age. Upon further questioning, the mother admits that there are two clonidine 0.2 mg tablets missing from the home. Which of the following antidotes might be beneficial for this patient?

A. Flumazenil.
B. Atropine.
C. Deferoxamine.
D. Naloxone.
E. Succimer.

Correct answer = D. Naloxone has a reversal rate of the CNS effects of approximately 50% in clonidine ingestions. Flumazenil reverses benzodiazepines and has no effect on clonidine. Atropine is an anticholinergic agent and would not improve the CNS depression. Deferoxamine is the chelator for iron, and succimer is a lead chelator.

48.7 A 40-year-old male presents to the emergency department with a complaint of abdominal pain. The patient appears intoxicated, but an ethanol level returns as negative and his basic metabolic panel is unremarkable. Which of these substances did he probably ingest?

 A. Isopropyl alcohol.
 B. Methanol.
 C. Ethylene glycol.
 D. Ethanol.
 E. Organophosphates.

Correct answer = A. Isopropyl alcohol produces twice as much CNS depression as ethanol and is known to cause GI distress. Isopropyl alcohol is metabolized to acetone, so a metabolic acidosis does not result (which is in contrast to the acidosis generated by methanol and ethylene glycol). The ethanol level was negative, eliminating ethanol as an ingestion. Organophosphate toxicity yields nicotinic and muscarinic effects, which are not described in the history.

48.8 A 5-year-old male is brought in to the health care facility for being irritable and failure to thrive. He is alert, and his vital signs are normal. The doctor diagnoses him with lead toxicity when the blood lead level returns as 50 μg/dL. Which chelator regimen should be started?

 A. Dimercaprol.
 B. Calcium disodium edetate.
 C. Both dimercaprol and calcium disodium edetate.
 D. Succimer.
 E. Deferoxamine.

Correct answer = D. Succimer (dimercaptosuccinic acid, DMSA) is utilized when the lead level is greater than 45 μg/dL, without encephalopathy. If encephalopathy is present, or the lead level is greater than 70 μg/dL in a child, then dual parenteral therapy with dimercaprol and calcium disodium edetate is indicated. Dimercaprol intramuscular therapy is initiated 4 hours prior to the intravenous administration of calcium disodium edetate when both medications are required. Deferoxamine is not indicated since it is the chelator for iron.

48.9 A 3-year-old healthy female ingested one of her mother's 1 mg alprazolam tablets 45 minutes ago. The child presented to the emergency department with CNS depression but a normal heart rate and blood pressure. Her bedside glucose check is also normal. Which of the following antidotes might be helpful?

 A. Flumazenil.
 B. Naloxone.
 C. Physostigmine.
 D. Atropine.
 E. Fomepizole.

Correct answer = A. Flumazenil is a competitive benzodiazepine antagonist that reverses the CNS depression from benzodiazepines such as alprazolam. After flumazenil administration, resedation usually occurs, since the duration of the benzodiazepine is longer than that of the flumazenil. Naloxone reverses the effects from opioids and clonidine, not benzodiazepines. Physostigmine is the antidote for anticholinergic toxicity, and atropine is an anticholinergic agent. Fomepizole is the antidote for methanol or ethylene glycol toxicity.

48.10 A 34-year-old male with a history of a seizure disorder, maintained on phenytoin and phenobarbital, presented to the emergency department for CNS depression. The phenobarbital level was 70 mg/L (15 to 40 mg/L therapeutic range) and the phenytoin level was 15 mg/L (10 to 20 mg/L therapeutic range). He denies any acute ingestion. What therapy can be considered to enhance the elimination of phenobarbital without impacting the phenytoin?

 A. Multiple doses of activated charcoal.
 B. Gastric lavage.
 C. Urinary alkalinization.
 D. Whole bowel irrigation.
 E. Urinary acidification.

Correct answer = C. Urinary alkalinization enhances the elimination of the phenobarbital but does not affect the therapeutic phenytoin level. Sodium bicarbonate, 1 mEq/kg, is administered intravenously initially and then a sodium bicarbonate continuous infusion is titrated to maintain a urine pH of 7.5 to 8, without exceeding a serum pH of 7.55. Multiple doses of activated charcoal would lower the concentration of both medications, rendering the phenytoin subtherapeutic. Gastric lavage is a GI decontamination technique employed usually within the first hour after an acute ingestion of a life-threatening amount, to remove approximately 30% of the product in the stomach. Whole bowel irrigation is another GI decontamination modality involving administration of large quantities (up to 2 L/hour in adults) of a polyethylene glycol–balanced electrolyte solution via a nasogastric tube until the patient generates clear rectal effluent. Urinary acidification is no longer performed for substances such as amphetamines and quinidine.

Index

Figure Sources

Figure 1.21. Modified from H. P. Range, and M. M. Dale, Pharmacology, Churchill Livingstone (1987).

Figure 1.27. Modified from Figure 6-3, Libby: Braunwald's Heart Disease: A Textbook of Cardiovascular Medicine, 8th ed., Philadelphia, PA, Saunders (2007).

Figures 6.9, 6.11. Modified from M. J. Allwood, A. F. Cobbold, and J. Ginsburg. Peripheral vascular effects of noradrenaline, isopropylnoradrenaline and dopamine. Br. Med. Bull. 19: 132 (1963).

Figure 8.13. Modified from R. Young. Update on Parkinson's disease. Am. Fam. Physician 59: 2155 (1999).

Figure 9.5. Modified from A. Kales, Excertpa Medical Congress Series 899: 149 (1989).

Figure 9.6. From data of E. C. Dimitrion, A. J. Parashos, and J. S. Giouzepas, Drug Invest. 4: 316 (1992).

Figure 12.10. Science Source, New York, NY.

Figure 14.11. Modified from T. R. Kosten, and P. G. O'Connor. N. Engl. J. Med. 348: 1786 (2003).

Figure 16.4. Modified from N. L. Benowitz, Science 319: 1318 (1988).

Figure 16.5. Modified from B. J. Materson, Drug Therapy 157 (1985).

Figure 19.6. Data from Results of the Cooperative North Scandinavian Enalapril Survival Study, N. Engl. J. Med. 316: 80 (1988).

Figure 19.7. Modified from the Effect of metoprolol CR/XL in chronic heart failure: metoprolol CR/XL Randomised Intervention Trial in Congestive Heart Failure (MERIT-HF). Lancet 353: 2001 (1999).

Figure 19.10. Modified from M Jessup, and S Brozena, N. Engl. J. Med. 348: 2007 (2003).

Figure 19.11. Modified from T. B. Young, M. Gheorghiade, and B. F. Uretsky. Superiority of "triple" drug therapy in heart failure: insights from the PROVED and RADIANCE trials Prospective Randomized Study of Ventricular Function and Efficacy of Digoxin. Randomized Assessment of Digoxin and Inhibitors of Angiotensin-Converting Enzyme. J. Am. Coll. Cardiol. 32: 686 (1998).

Figure 20.3. Modified from J. A. Beven, and J. H. Thompson, Essentials of Pharmacology, Philadelphia, PA, Harper and Row (1983).

Figure 23.7. Modified from D. J. Schneider, P. B. Tracy, and B. E. Sobel, Hosp. Pract. 107 (1998).

Figure 23.6. Modified from M. K. S. Leow, C. L. Addy, and C. S. Mantzoros. Clinical review 159: human immunodeficiency virus/ highly active antiretroviral therapy-associated metabolic syndrome: clinical presentation, pathophysiology, and therapeutic strategies. J. Clin. Endocrinol. Metab. 88: 1961 (2003).

Figures 24.2. Modified from B. G. Katzung, Basic and Clinical Pharmacology, Appleton and Lange, (1987).

Figure 24.9. Modified from K. Okamura, H. Ikenoue, and A. Shiroozu. Reevaluation of the effects of methylmercaptoimidazole and propylthiouracil in patients with Graves' hyperthyroidism. J. Clin. Endocrinol. Metab. 65: 719 (1987).

Figure 25.5. Modified from M. C. Riddle, Postgrad. Med. 92: 89 (1992).

Figure 25.7. Modified from I. R. Hirsch. Insulin analogues. N. Engl. J. Med. 352: 174 (2005).

Figure 25.9. Modified from O. B. Crofford. Diabetes control and complications. Annu. Rev. Med. 46: 267 (1995).

Figures 26.6 and 26.7. Modified from D. R. Mishell, Jr.. Medical progress: contraception. N. Engl. J. Med. 320: 777 (1989).

Figure 26.9. Modified from A. S. Dobs, A. W. Meikle, S. Arver, et al. Pharmacokinetics, efficacy, and safety of a permeation-enhanced testosterone transdermal system in comparison with bi-weekly injections of testosterone enanthate for the treatment of hypogonadal men. J. Clin. Endocrinol. Metab. 84: 3469 (1999).

Figure 26.10. Modified from J. D. McConnell, C. G. Roehrborn, and O. M. Bautista. The long-term effect of doxazosin, finasteride, and combination therapy on the clinical progression of benign prostatic hyperplasia. N. Engl. J. Med. 349: 2387 (2003).

Figure 27.7. Modified from K. G. Saag, R. Koehnke, and J. R. Caldwell, et al. Low dose long-term corticosteroid therapy in rheumatoid arthritis: an analysis of serious adverse events. Am. J. Med. 96: 115 (1994).

Figure 31.2. Modified from D. Cave, Hosp. Pract. (1992).

Figure 31.5. Modified from F. E. Silverstein, D. Y. Graham, and J. R. Senior. Misoprostol reduces serious gastrointestinal complications in patients with rheumatoid arthritis receiving nonsteroidal anti-inflammatory drugs. A randomized, double-blind, placebo-controlled trial. Ann. Intern. Med. 123: 241 (1995).

Figure 31.6. Modified from S. M. Grunberg, and P. J. Hesketh. Control of chemotherapy-induced emesis. N. Engl. J. Med. 329: 1790 (1993).

Figures 31.8, 31.9. From data of S. Bilgrami, and B. G. Fallon. Chemotherapy-induced nausea and vomiting. Easing patients' fear and discomfort with effective antiemetic regimens. Postgrad. Med. 94: 55 (1993).

Figure 36.14. Adapted from T. D. Warner, F. Giuliano, I. Vojnovic, et al. Nonsteroid drug selectivities for cyclo-oxygenase-1 rather than cyclo-oxygenase-2 are associated with human gastrointestinal toxicity: a full in vitro analysis. Proc. Natl. Acad. Sci. U. S. A. 96: 7563 (1999).

Figure 36.22. Modified from D. D. Dubose, A. C. Cutlip, and W. D. Cutlip. Migraines and other headaches: an approach to diagnosis and classification. Am. Fam. Physician 51: 1498 (1995).

Figure 41.4. Modified from data of D. A. Evans, K. A. Maley, and V. A. McRusick. Genetic control of isoniazid metabolism in man. Br. Med. J. 2: 485 (1960).

Figure 41.5. Modified from data of P. J. Neuvonen, K. T. Kivisto, and P. Lehto, Clin. Pharm. Therapy 50: 499 (1991).

Figure 41.12. Modified from Y. Nivoix, D. Leveque, and R. Herbrecht, et al. The enzymatic basis of drug-drug interactions with systemic triazole antifungals. Clin. Pharmacokinet. 47: 779 (2008).

Figure 45.14. Modified from H. H. Balfour. Antiviral drugs. N. Engl. J. Med. 340: 1255 (1999).

Figure 46.4. Reprinted with permission from Dr. Thomas George, MD.

Figure 46.6. Modified from N. Kartner, and V. Ling, Sci. Am. (1989).

Figure 48.3. Reprinted with permission from B. H. Rumack. Acetaminophen overdose in children and adolescents. Pediatr. Clin. Noth Am. 33: 691 (1986).

Figure 48.7. Reprinted with permission from the Centers for Disease Control and Prevention. http://wonder.cdc.gov/